Health Informatics

More information about this series at http://www.springer.com/series/1114

Morris F. Collen • Marion J. Ball
Editors

The History of Medical Informatics in the United States

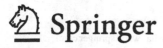
Springer

Editors
Morris F. Collen (deceased)

Marion J. Ball
IBM Research
Baltimore, MD, USA

Johns Hopkins University
Baltimore, MD, USA

ISSN 1431-1917   ISSN 2197-3741 (electronic)
Health Informatics
ISBN 978-1-4471-7112-6   ISBN 978-1-4471-6732-7 (eBook)
DOI 10.1007/978-1-4471-6732-7

Springer London Heidelberg New York Dordrecht

Printed on acid-free paper

Springer-Verlag London Ltd. is part of Springer Science+Business Media (www.springer.com)

To the future of informatics and its evolving branches

Foreword I

How often does a person envision a new medical discipline and then live to see this vision come into reality? He not only practiced his discipline, he established professional associations to promote it, and he mentored generations of practitioners. As a result of his pioneering efforts, we now have a field of clinical informatics. Information and communication technology is now used to improve health and healthcare in our hospitals, our clinicians' offices, our places of work, our schools, and our homes. Physicians and nurses now train in clinical informatics, and physicians can be board certified in what has become a new subspecialty.

One year ago, we celebrated Dr. Collen's 100th birthday near his home in San Francisco. Luminaries from the field of clinical informatics and health service research came to reflect on their interactions with this great man and to celebrate the field he grandfathered. After a day of celebrations, Dr. Collen delivered a 20-minute talk that was insightful, modest, and caring.

The story of his life and work has been well told, by Howard Bleich at the time of his 80th birthday, by Jochen Moehr on his 90th, and by Donald Lindberg and Marion Ball on his 100th birthday. Published in *MD Computing* (1994;11(3):136–139), the *Journal of the American Medical Informatics Association* (2003;10(6):613–615), and *Methods of Information in Medicine* (2013;52(5):371–373), these accounts stand as tributes to the man identified as "pioneer in computerized medicine" in his obituary in *The New York Times* of October 5, 2014.

This book, the second edition of *A History of Medical Informatics in the United States*, is not only a labor of Dr. Collen's love for our field but is also a comprehensive updating of his original work, first published in 1995. The same luminaries who gathered to celebrate his life came forward to help to update, edit, and revise the manuscript he left behind. Like the original, it serves as an invaluable resource documenting the infrastructure that is transforming care delivery in the twenty-first century. Dr. Collen's book will serve as a reminder to future generations of the important contributions of this wonderful clinician, mentor, and gentleman.

2014 Recipient of the Morris F. Collen Award   Charles Safran
Professor of Medicine, Harvard Medical School
Boston, MA, USA

Foreword II

Director of the Division of Research,

Morris F. Collen, MD, developed his groundbreaking contributions to medical informatics amid the fertile environment of Kaiser Permanente, one of the nation's first and most renowned integrated healthcare systems. As one of the founding partners of The Permanente Medical Group, now the largest medical group in the United States, Morrie championed the principle that physicians should manage healthcare for both individual patients and large populations. He and the organization's other founders weathered controversy during the 1940s and 1950s for their beliefs. Today, the concepts of prepayment for services, comprehensive electronic medical records, and an emphasis on preventive care have been widely embraced throughout the country.

Morrie's approach to medical informatics was informed by his work as a physician providing medical care to a socioeconomically diverse group of patients. During World War II, he treated thousands of workers in the Richmond shipyards, and he later served as the physician-in-chief of Kaiser Permanente's San Francisco medical center. He related that in the late 1950s, the leader of The Permanente Medical Group, Sidney R. Garfield, MD, thought that the time had come for computers to be useful in the practice of medicine and dispatched him to figure out how.

Inspired by a major conference on medical electronics in New York in 1960, Morrie founded the group that became the Division of Research in Kaiser Permanente's Northern California region. He began to collect medical information on patients via new multiphasic preventive examinations and entered the data into a mainframe computer – using punch cards. This work and the information obtained led to major improvements in medical practice decades ahead of the rest of healthcare. Since that era, the Division of Research has grown into an internationally respected group of researchers who continue to use informatics in hundreds of ongoing studies to identify the drivers of health and disease and to find innovative ways to enhance healthcare.

This book reflects Morrie's visionary leadership as well as the dedication of his many colleagues, especially his beloved editor, Marion Ball, EdD. At a time when the most advanced computers had less power than a watch today, he saw what was possible and the ultimate potential for big data to revolutionize medical care. In sharing ways we can harness information to take better care of patients in real-world settings, this work stands as a beacon on the path to better healthcare for modern society.

Director of the Division of Research   Tracy Lieu
Kaiser Permanente Northern California
Oakland, CA, USA

Executive Director and CEO, The Permanente Medical Group   Robert Pearl
Kaiser Permanente, Oakland, CA, USA

Preface

This volume is the legacy of Morris F. Collen, a vital force in medical informatics in the United States since its birth. In the last years of his life, up until his death at age 100 in September 2014, Dr. Collen – Morrie to many of us – worked every day to update his *History of Medical Informatics in the United States*, published in 1995. In the original edition, Morrie compiled a meticulously detailed chronological record of significant events in the history of medical informatics and their impact on direct patient care and clinical research. His intent was to offer a representative sampling of published contributions to the field; his vision was that this would serve as a useful bridge between medical informatics of the past and of the future.

As he revised his *History*, Morrie restructured the book, replacing the original seven chapters with eighteen to reflect the transformation medical informatics had undergone in the years since 1990. The systems that were once exclusively institutionally driven – hospital, multihospital, and outpatient information systems – are today joined by systems that are driven by clinical subspecialties, nursing, pathology, clinical laboratory, pharmacy, imaging, and more. At the core is the person – not the clinician, not the institution – whose health all these systems are designed to serve, a foundational belief that guided Morrie throughout his career, from his early work with multiphasic health testing, with the computer-based patient record at the height of his career, and finally to the completion of this new *History*.

Of course he knew that time was not on his side and enlisted me to help. He worked on the manuscript each day, and we spoke every evening by telephone. The review was exacting, adding new material was time-consuming, and in the summer before Morrie died, he asked me to assume control of the project and do what needed to be done to see the *History* into print when he was no longer here. I realized this was a daunting task with an ambitious goal, and, upon his death, I asked his colleagues, the medical informatics community, for help.

Nineteen informaticians, whose names appear on the chapters in the finished book, agreed to help. Most of them had known him for years. Several had been leaders, along with Morrie, when the field was in its infancy, not yet named; others met him and worked with him as the field grew and matured; and a lucky few claimed him as their mentor. Recognized leaders in medical informatics today (and many of them recipients of the Morris F. Collen Award in Medical Informatics), they carefully reviewed the draft chapters, editing and updating the material Morrie left behind. They gave of their time and expertise to bring Morrie's work to completion – a task that proved more difficult than I and my colleagues had initially imagined.

The chapters in the manuscript Morrie left behind were in different states of completion and posed different challenges. Some colleagues edited chapters that Morrie had spent considerable time revising; their task, as they saw it, was to do a final edit on his behalf, smoothing or restructuring for clarity and, in some instances, adding to and commenting on Morrie's text. Other colleagues took on chapters that Morrie was in the midst of revising; for them, the challenge was to add their insights to Morrie's while maintaining his vision. And three colleagues contributed the chapter on imaging that Morrie had planned but not yet developed. All their efforts honor Morrie and serve the field. To them I owe heartfelt thanks.

Like the field of medical informatics it describes, this new *History* reflects the changes made possible by information technology. Like the earlier version that sits on bookshelves around the country, it is available as a hardcover book. Comprehensive in its coverage, it preserves much of the history recounted in the first edition – history now growing ever more distant and difficult to trace. This new *History* provides an unrivaled repository of the literature – much of it in hard-to-locate proceedings and reports from professional and industry groups – that guided informatics as it matured. Yet it is much more than a repository. It sets forth Morrie's last assessments of the field he pioneered and cultivated, and it is enriched by the contributions of his colleagues who reviewed his chapters and helped bring this volume to completion. Always collegial, Morrie himself would welcome these new perspectives on the work that engaged him so completely up to the end of his life.

Mirroring the advances in healthcare computing it describes, this new *History* is available as an e-book in its entirety or as individual chapters. Morrie prepared each chapter to be complete unto itself, including all the information the reader needed to understand the area covered. A quick chapter-by-chapter guide to the concepts and topics discussed in this richly detailed book appears below. For readers, Morrie's approach and the guide mean quick and easy access to specific material when they first seek it. Once downloaded, it can remain readily available, retrievable by a mouse click or finger swipe. To all those who look to the evolving field of informatics for tools and approaches to providing healthcare that is efficient, effective, evidence-based, and of the highest quality possible, this is Morrie's gift.

Marion J. Ball

A Brief Overview of Concepts and Topics

The short summaries below provide an overview of the material covered in this lengthy and comprehensive volume:

Chapter 1 The Development of Digital Computers

A multi-decade perspective on the evolution of computers, operating systems, and programming languages; workstations and other interface devices; communication technologies, networks, and databases in society and specifically in healthcare.

Chapter 2 The Creation of a New Discipline

Medical informatics as a distinct field, the origin of the term itself, and the various nuances of the discipline as it has taken shape over the past six decades, with attention to roles played by publications, professional organizations, industry, academia, and government.

Chapter 3 Development of Medical Information Systems (MISs)

Medical information systems, their scope, different architectural and developmental approaches, the role of textual and non-textual data, the databases they require, the role of standards, and the use of natural language processing for textual data.

Chapter 4 Medical Databases and Patient Record Systems

Data for medical information systems; electronic patient records and the expanded electronic health record; the evolution from separate databases to more integrated models; and their role in capturing information for care, making it available in a timely fashion and affecting the care process.

Chapter 5 Outpatient Information Systems (OISs) for Ambulatory Care

Information system capabilities for patients outside of the hospital; priorities, requirements, and design implications, with emphasis on patient identification and record linkage, on capturing patient history and physician examination data; also telemedicine and mobile healthcare.

Chapter 6 The Early History of Hospital Information Systems

Early hospital information systems and the external factors influencing their development, with descriptions of early systems; admission, discharge, and transfer systems and the evolution of concept sharing during development; and functional requirements and technical designs.

Chapter 7 Nursing Informatics: Past, Present, and Future

Evolution from terminals and workstations at nursing stations to point of care devices; order entry, staffing, and scheduling functions; systems for patient classification, quality assurance, care planning, decision support, nursing education and research; nursing informatics as a specialty.

Chapter 8 Specialized High-Intensity Clinical Settings: A Brief Review

Early development of specialized systems for intensive care units and emergency departments; current status and interoperability challenges arising from incompatible equipment for intensive care and the exchange of patient information between emergency department and other settings.

Chapter 9 Information Systems for Clinical Subspecialties

Functional and technical requirements for various medical subspecialties and the development of systems to support their differing needs, focusing primarily on internal medicine, surgery, obstetrics/gynecology, pediatrics, and mental health subspecialties.

Chapter 10 Multi-Hospital Information Systems (MHISs)

Added requirements as healthcare organizations formed alliances and acquired hospitals and practices; the need for translation among databases; evolution of multi-hospital information systems in the Federal sector (Veterans Administration, Department of Defense), mental health, and commercial sector.

Chapter 11 Clinical Support Information Systems (CSISs)

Development of systems to address internal scheduling, workflow processing, and material handling of the clinical laboratory, pathology department, pharmacy, and imaging; their function to produce results available to the physician and integrated into the electronic medical record.

Chapter 12 Clinical Laboratory (LAB) Information Systems

Requirements for specimen processing and analysis, their early evolution and evaluation; special characteristics of lab subsystems for chemistry, hematology, microbiology, and other specialized analyses; developments in result and interpretive analysis reporting.

Chapter 13 Anatomic Pathology Information Laboratory Information Systems and Natural Language Processing: Early History

Development of systems for specimen management and interpretation in anatomic pathology and its subareas, of coding systems and systematized nomenclature, and of natural language processing (NLP) for extraction of findings from narrative reports; later work on image processing and telepathology.

Chapter 14 Pharmacy Information (PHARM) Systems

Requirements for pharmacy information management; the development of systems to support it, including identification and surveillance of adverse drug events and polypharmacy; and the development of systems for pharmacotherapy.

Chapter 15 Imaging Information Systems

Early emphasis on scheduling, workflow, etc.; advances in digital imaging, including Picture Archiving and Communication Systems (PACS), and digital image interpretation workstations; coding, structured input methods, the incorporation of voice dictation, and distribution of image-enhanced reports.

Chapter 16 Public and Personal Health Testing Systems

Systems for public and personal health testing; public health monitoring; multiphasic health testing and systems to automate it and the integration of those functions into the electronic patient record; development of advanced biosurveillance systems and public health informatics.

Chapter 17 Decision Support Systems

Evolution of tools and knowledge bases for decision support, administrative and quality management, and clinical decision making; the National Library of Medicine as a major resource provider; development of methods for data mining, data analytics, and knowledge discovery.

Chapter 18 Medical Informatics: Past and Future

Analysis of the past six decades; projections for the next decade, including transforming trends: an aging population with multiple diseases and polypharmacy; mHealth and personal biosensors; patient genotyping; cloud computing and big data; patient data security; public health in disaster scenarios.

Robert A. Greenes
Judith V. Douglas
Marion J. Ball

Acknowledgments

Let me open by thanking the most important person of all, Morris F. Collen, who would first thank his late wife Bobbie, who persuaded him to enter the field of medicine. This was and is his book, even after so many others have helped to complete it. Honored for his pioneering work in medical informatics, Morrie is remembered as well for his generosity of spirit and would join with me in thanking all those I mention below for help in bringing this volume to publication.

Kaiser Permanente, Morrie's professional home throughout his career and his long and productive retirement, continued their support for his work even after his death. Their unwavering commitment to seeing his new *History* into print never wavered and kept me on course. My heartfelt thanks go to Lincoln Cushing, Archivist, Kaiser Permanente Heritage Resources; Bryan Culp, Archivist Emeritus; Tracy Lieu, Director, and Joe Selby, Gary Friedman, and Ted Van Brunt, former Directors of the Kaiser Permanente Division of Research; Joe Terdiman and Jamila Gul, who worked with Morrie in Research; Brenda Cooke and Marlene Rozofsky Rogers, the Research librarians upon whom Morrie relied; and Morrie's many colleagues and friends in the Division of Research. I am also deeply grateful to Robert Pearl, Executive Director and CEO; Francis J. Crosson, Sharon Levine, Phil Madvig, and Holly Ruehlin, of The Permanente Medical Group, for their unflagging support of Morrie's work; and to the Board of Directors and Executive Staff of The Permanente Medical Group for their consistent and ongoing support of the Morris F. Collen Research Award since 2003.

I owe a tremendous debt to all my colleagues from the world of informatics whose names appear elsewhere in this volume, alongside the chapters they completed. Several among them did still more. Bob Greenes served as my adviser throughout, looking at the overall structure of the book; preparing the short descriptions of each chapter that appear elsewhere in the front matter; recruiting two eminent colleagues, Brad Erickson and Ron Arenson, to join with him in authoring the one completely new chapter on imaging that Morrie had envisioned; and taking Morrie's vision forward in the final chapter of the book. John Silva helped recruit Mike Becich, who in turn enlisted Alexis Carter; and Harold Lehmann helped bring on Bob Miller and involve Anne Seymour in the project.

At the Johns Hopkins University, Anne Seymour, Director of the Welch Medical Library, and Associate Director Stella Seal committed valuable staff time to complete the reference work for this volume. Associate Director and Senior Reference Specialist Ivy Linwood Garner served as lead, together with Reference Specialists Christopher Henry and Vivian McCall.

Charles Ball, Debbie Ball, Alex Ball, and Ryan Ball located materials for Morrie and brought them to him to use in his research. Evelyn Graetz and Rabbi Robert Graetz of Temple Isaiah helped Morrie every day, and Vicki Shambaugh of the Pacific Health Research and Education Institute urged him on. Randall Collen, Morrie's son, and John Ball, my husband, offered continued belief in this project, and Matthew Douglas, Judy Douglas's son, helped check citations and prepare the materials that appear at the back of the book.

I would like to thank Grant Weston at Springer, who unstintingly supported Morrie over the last few years, encouraging him to complete *Computer Medical Databases* in 2012 and agreeing to see this new *History of Medical Informatics* through the publication process after Morrie's death.

Finally, I want to acknowledge Judy Douglas, who has spent the last six months almost full time working with all of the contributing editors and coauthors as well as with the Johns Hopkins Welch Medical Library staff to bring this work to fruition. Years ago, Judy helped Morrie and me bring *Aspects of the Computer-Based Patient Record* (Springer, 1992) to publication. That experience and Judy's memory of reading the first edition of *The History of Medical Informatics in the United States* when it was still in manuscript form made her determined to make this new edition measure up to the first – and to the standards of excellence that characterized Morrie professionally and personally.

                                                                                    Marion J. Ball

Contents

Contributors

Ronald L. Arenson, M.D. Department of Radiology and Biomedical Imaging, University of California, San Francisco, CA, USA

Marion J. Ball, Ed.D. IBM Research, Baltimore, MD, USA

Johns Hopkins University, Baltimore, MD, USA

Howard L. Bleich, M.D. Harvard Medical School, Division of Clinical Informatics, Department of Medicine, Beth Israel Deaconess Medical Center, Brookline, MA, USA

Michael J. Becich, M.D., Ph.D. Department of Biomedical Informatics, University of Pittsburgh School of Medicine, Pittsburgh, PA, USA

Alexis B. Carter, M.D., F.C.A.P., F.A.S.C.P. Department of Pathology and Laboratory Medicine, Emory University, Atlanta, GA, USA

Morris F. Collen, B.E.E., M.D., D.Sc. (Hon) Author was deceased at the time of publication

Don Eugene Detmer, M.D., M.A. Department of Public Health Sciences, University of Virginia, Charlottesville, VA, USA

Bradley James Erickson, M.D., Ph.D. Department of Radiology, Mayo Clinic, Rochester, MN, USA

Robert A. Greenes, M.D., Ph.D. Arizona State University, Tempe, AZ, USA

Department of Biomedical Informatics, Mayo Clinic, Rochester, MN, USA

W. Ed Hammond Duke Center for Health Informatics, Duke University, Durham, NC, USA

Casimir A. Kulikowski, Ph.D. Department of Computer Science Hill Center, Rutgers University, Piscataway, NJ, USA

Harold P. Lehmann, M.D., Ph.D. Division of Health Sciences Informatics, Johns Hopkins School of Medicine, Baltimore, MD, USA

Nancy M. Lorenzi, Ph.D., M.A., M.S. School of Medicine, Department of Biomedical Informatics, School of Nursing, Vanderbilt University, Medical Center, Nashville, TN, USA

Alexa T. McCray Center for Biomedical Informatics, Harvard Medical School, Boston, MA, USA

Randolph A. Miller, M.D. Department of Biomedical Informatics, School of Medicine, Vanderbilt University Medical Center, Nashville, TN, USA

Robert E. Miller, M.D. Departments of Pathology and Biomedical Engineering, Division of Health Sciences Informatics, Johns Hopkins University School of Medicine, Baltimore, MD, USA

Department of Health Policy and Management, Bloomberg School of Public Health, Johns Hopkins University, Baltimore, MD, USA

Stuart J. Nelson, M.D., F.A.C.P., F.A.C.M.I. Health Sciences Library and Informatics Center, University of New Mexico, Albuquerque, AZ, USA

John S. Silva, M.D., F.A.C.M.I. Silva Consulting Services, LLC, Eldersburg, MD, USA

Edward H. Shortliffe, M.D., Ph.D. Arizona State University, Phoenix, AZ, USA

Columbia University, New York, NY, USA

Weill Cornell Medical College, New York, NY, USA

New York Academy of Medicine, New York, NY, USA

Warner V. Slack, M.D. Harvard Medical School, Division of Clinical Informatics, Department of Medicine, Beth Israel Deaconess Medical Center, Brookline, MA, USA

Patricia Hinton Walker, Ph.D., RN, FAAN, DNAP, PCC Strategic Initiatives and Graduate School of Nursing, Uniformed Services University of the Health Sciences, Bethesda, MD, USA

Part I
Prologue

Chapter 1
The Development of Digital Computers

Morris F. Collen and Casimir A. Kulikowski

Abstract In the 1950s, the transistor replaced the vacuum tubes that had empowered Eniac, Colossus, and other early computers in the 1940s. In the 1960s and 1970s, computing moved from slow, expensive mainframes to faster mini- and microcomputers and multiprocessors, empowered by chip technology and integrated circuits, and leveraged by increasingly sophisticated operating systems and programming languages. By the 1980s, commercially available programs were able to perform commonly needed computational functions. With the growth of computer capabilities and computer storage capacities, database technology and database management systems gave rise to the development of distributed database systems. Efficient computer-stored databases proved essential to many medical computing applications, making vast amounts of data available to users. Over time computer applications became more numerous and complex, with software claiming a larger fraction of computing costs. Display terminals and clinical workstations offered graphic displays and supported structured data entry and reporting. Devices, such as the mouse, light pens, touch screens, and input technologies, such as speech and handwriting recognition, were developed to ease the user's tasks and foster physician acceptance. Over the same span of time, computer communications evolved as well, moving from copper wire to fiber optic cable and, most recently, to wireless systems. The Internet and the World Wide Web became the main modes used for local and global communications. By the 2010s laptops replaced desktop computers, and tablets and smart phones were commonplace in health care.

Keywords Early computers • Computer languages • Computer communication networks • Computer terminals • Data storage • Clinical records and systems • User computer interfaces • Networking and the World Wide Web

---

Author was deceased at the time of publication.

M.F. Collen (deceased)

C.A. Kulikowski, Ph.D. (✉)
Department of Computer Science Hill Center, Rutgers University,
Busch Campus, Piscataway, NJ, USA
e-mail: kulikow@rutgers.edu

© Springer-Verlag London 2015
M.F. Collen, M.J. Ball (eds.), *The History of Medical Informatics in the United States*, Health Informatics, DOI 10.1007/978-1-4471-6732-7_1

In the latter part of the nineteenth century, John Shaw Billings, a physician and the director of the Army Surgeon General's Library (later to become the National Library of Medicine) initiated a series of events that led to the development of the modern digital computer in the United States [114]. Asked to assist the Census Bureau with the 1880 and with the 1890 census, Billings suggested to Hollerith, an engineer, that there should be a machine for doing the purely mechanical work of tabulating population and similar statistics. Hollerith used paper cards the size of a dollar bill, allowing him to store the cards using Treasury Department equipment and eliminate the need for new storage devices. Descriptions were printed on the edge of the cards for individual data items punched into corresponding specific locations on the card [6]. In 1882 Hollerith invented the paper punch card with 288 locations for holes, punched out by a hand-operated device, until he built a machine for electrically punching the holes; and next he built machines for reading and sorting the punched cards. The 1890 census data on 62 million people were processed in 1 month using 56 of Hollerith's machines. In 1896 Hollerith established the Tabulating Machines Company which became the Computing-Tabulating-Recording (CTR) Corporation in 1911, but soon after lost most of its business to a rival more up-to-date firm. However, when Thomas J. Watson Sr. joined the CTR Corporation and became its executive in 1918, CTR recovered, and in 1924 changed its name to the International Business Machines (IBM) Corporation. Thus, a physician, Billings, laid the foundation for the development of digital computing in the United States.

1.1 Electro-Mechanical Digital Computers

The earliest digital data computers were mechanical calculators Pascal invented in France in the mid-1600s. In the 1830s Babbage, a British mathematician, built an automated mechanical computing machine with gears and linkages that he called a Difference Engine. Babbage then conceived a more advanced Analytical Engine that would have become the first mechanical digital computer. During the 1840s, Ada Byron, the Countess of Lovelace and daughter of Lord Byron, collaborated with Babbage to develop programs for his Analytical Engine, which he never actually completed; she is credited by some as the first programmer of a digital computer [264].

In 1940 Stibitz and his colleagues at Bell Laboratories developed a partially automated digital computer that used electrically controlled, mechanical magnetic switches as relay switches. The "on" and "off" positions of the relay switches represented the numbers 0 and 1 as the binary-bits in the base-2 system [47]. Stibitz exploited the relative simplicity of using the binary system for a digital computer since every number, letter, symbol, and punctuation could be represented by a unique combination of bits. Previous calculators and computers had processed numbers using the base-10 decimal system, which required multiples of ten-gear teeth to turn switches on and off in order to count. Later the American Standard Code for Information Exchange (ASCII) assigned an eight-digit binary code to each letter, so

that 01000001 was the letter A, 01000010 was letter B, 01000011 was letter C, and
so forth in the ASCII code.

In 1941 Zuse built the world's first fully functional, program-controlled, general-
purpose, electro-mechanical digital computer in Germany. This machine used relay
switches and was based on the binary system; thus, when a switch was turned "on"
it represented the number "1", and when turned "off" it represented "0". Due to
World War II, Zuse's invention received little recognition in the United States.

In 1943 the Mark I computer was designed by Aiken at the Harvard Computation
Laboratory. Built by the International Business Machine (IBM) Company as the
Automatic Sequence Controlled Calculator (ASCC), in 1944 it was installed at
Harvard University, where it was called Mark I. Run by an electric motor, it was a
program-controlled computer based on the decimal system; all machine operations
were performed electro-mechanically by its wheel counters and relay switches [6, 80].

1.2   Early Electronic Digital Computers

With the advent of modern electronics, the flow of electric current replaced mechanical moving parts of earlier computers, and vacuum tubes replaced electromechani-
cal switches. First generation computers were "hardwired", and their circuits were
their programs. As computer processors advanced, new computer system architectures were developed.

Colossus is generally credited to have been the first all-electronic digital computer in the world. Guided by the mathematicians Turing, Newman, and their colleagues at the Bletchley Park Research Establishment in England [173], the Colossus
was installed and working in December 1944. Used by the British during World War
II to carry out the many logical steps needed to break German coded messages, it
showed that computers could be used for purposes other than just processing numbers [133]. Atanasoff's computer is considered by some to be the very first, fully
electronic, digital computer built in the United States. Invented by Atanasoff, a
physicist at Iowa State University and operational in 1942, it was a single-purpose
computer that used the binary system [52, 173].

However, ENIAC (Electronic Numerical Integrator and Calculator) is more generally credited to be the first electronic digital computer built in the United States.
Invented in 1946 by Mauchly, Eckert, and their coworkers at the Moore School of
the University of Pennsylvania [221], ENIAC occupied a space 30×50 ft, weighed
30 tons, used 18,000 vacuum tubes for its active arithmetic and logic elements, and
was based on a decimal numeral system. Secretly built under contract with the
U.S. Army Ballistics Research Laboratory to calculate the trajectories for gunnery
in World War II, ENIAC was capable of solving a wide variety of problems in science, engineering, and statistics. The computations were electronic, but the problems had to be entered manually by setting switches and plugging in cables [53].
EDVAC (Electronic Discrete Variable Automatic Computer) was also designed by
Mauchly and Eckert in 1944, even before the ENIAC was completed. Delivered in

1949, EDVAC was a binary-based computer that had 6,000 vacuum tubes and covered 490 ft^2 of floor space. UNIVAC (Universal Automatic Computer) was developed in the late 1940s; it used von Neumann's computer-stored program technology. The first computer to process both numeric and alphabetic data, UNIVAC had 5,000 vacuum tubes and was still based on the decimal system.

SEAC (Standard Eastern Automatic Computer) was used by Ledley, a pioneer in the use of digital computers for medical purposes in the United States, when in 1950 he conducted research in computer applications to dental projects at the National Bureau of Standards. Since at that date the UNIVAC was not yet operational, Ledley [157] claimed that SEAC was the world's first high-speed electronic digital computer in which the programs were stored digitally in the computer's memory. Demonstrated in 1951, the first real-time computer, the Whirlwind, was the source of several significant technological innovations. In addition to having the first magnetic core, random-access memory, it was the first 16-bit computer and paved the way for the development of the minicomputer in the mid-1960s [6].

When Eckert and Mauchly recognized the potential usefulness of computers in science and industry, and obtained patents for their inventions, they left the University of Pennsylvania and set up the first commercial computer company in the United States, the Eckert and Mauchly Electronic Control Company of Philadelphia. In 1950 Remington Rand, founded in 1911 to make typewriters and tabulating equipment, took control of the Eckert and Mauchly Company; a year later, in 1951, Remington Rand completed the first UNIVAC for the Census Bureau to be used in analyzing the 1950 census data.

International Business Machines (IBM) Company, which in 1939 had financed the construction of Aiken's Mark I at the Harvard Computation Laboratory, initiated work in 1945 on its first internally developed computer, the IBM 604. Marketed in 1948, the 604 was an electronic multiplier with 1,400 vacuum tubes and a plug board for wiring simple instructions. In 1952 Watson Jr. became the president of IBM; there he directed the manufacturing of the IBM 701 Defense Calculator. A binary-based computer with 4,000 vacuum tubes that was faster than the UNIVAC, the IBM 701 computer supported the U.S. Army's needs during the Korean War [30]. In 1950 IBM released its 704 scientific computer; with magnetic core memory, a cathode-ray tube (CRT) display monitor, FORTRAN programming and some graphics capability, it was among the earliest computers used for medical research [217].

Transistor-based, second generation digital computers were introduced in the late 1950s. Instead of using vacuum tubes these computers employed transistors, invented in 1947 by Shockley, Bardeen, and Brattain at AT&T's Bell Laboratories. In their work, for which they won the 1956 Nobel prize for physics, the three scientists had observed an electric signal was produced when two contacts were applied to a crystal. Their initial point-contact transistor served as an electric switch with four components: a source where the electric current entered, a drain where the current left, a channel linking the two, and a device that acted as a gate to the channel. By opening and closing the channel, the gate governed whether an electric current could flow along a thin metal film of a semiconductor, and thus defined the on-or-off state that provided a computer's binary function. In 1951 Shockley and his team also developed a junction transistor which used the internal properties of semiconductors rather than the surface effects on which point-contact devices depended. Shockley "doped" a silicon semiconductor with impurities (such as arsenic or boron) that created free electrons to produce a negative charge, or stole electrons from the semiconductor's lattice to create positively charged "holes". When joined together, the negatively charged electrons and the positively charged holes flowed toward the junction where they joined and others took their place, creating a current that flowed in one direction [105].

Computer transistor chips were invented in 1959 when Kilby at Texas Instruments and Noyce at Fairchild Semiconductor were independently able to make the crystal in a transistor serve as its own circuit board [38]. Kilby's device required putting the circuit components together by hand. Noyce's group fabricated the components of a circuit (the resistors, capacitors, transistors, and the interconnecting wireless conductive pathways) all on one surface of a flat wafer of silicon. They thereby created the first miniature integrated circuit on a chip [200]. Transistor-based computers are wired much the same way as vacuum tube-based computers; but they are much smaller, require less power, and are more reliable. In 1959 IBM began marketing its first transistorized computer, the IBM 7090, which contained 32,768 words of memory, with each word being 36-bits in length instead of the prior 16-bit word length; it employed magnetic tape for secondary storage [34]. By the end of the 1950s, IBM had three-fourths of the computer market in the United States [50]. Friedel [105] noted that within a decade transistors were used in hundreds of devices, including telephones, radios, hearing aids, pocket calculators, and digital computers. In 1961 Fairchild and Texas Instruments introduced logic chips that, in addition to the arithmetic *AND* function, performed the Boolean operations *OR* and *NOR* (not OR). By stringing logic chips as gates together in different ways, the engineers could endow computers with the power to support decision making processes [6]. The invention of the computer chip with its integrated circuits produced dramatic changes in computers, and was probably the most important event that ushered in the information age.

Third generation computers appeared in 1963 in the form of solid state integrated circuits that consisted of hundreds of transistors, diodes, and resistors embedded on one or more tiny silicon chips, in a process called large scale integration (LSI) [32]. Once again computers became smaller and more reliable, and required less power. The manufacture of computer circuits became more like a printing process and less like a traditional assembly process, since the chip makers worked like photoengravers with masks and light-sensitive chemicals etching the silicon layers [83]. In 1964 IBM introduced its system/360 series of computers, a family of the earliest third generation computers all using the same operating system (OS/360) that allowed data processing operations to expand from the smallest machine in the series to the largest without the need to rewrite essential programs. The IBM series/360 computer with its Systems Network Architecture (SNA) led the industry into modern commercial computing, and was the basis for IBM's spectacular growth [271].

In the early 1970s, IBM replaced its 360 series with the system/370 series that used only integrated circuit chips.

Fourth generation computers appeared in the late 1960s and exploited very large scale integration (VLSI) that contained thousands of components on very tiny silicon chips, greatly increasing performance with less cost. By the early 1980s, a silicon flake a quarter-inch on a side could hold a million electronic components, ten times more than in the 30 ton ENIAC and 30,000 times as cheap. Drawing the electric power of a bedroom nightlight instead of that of a hundred lighthouses, in some versions it could perform 200 times as many calculations per second as the ENIAC [38].

The history of the development of some of the earliest generations of electronic computers was described by Tropp [266] and Bernstein [22, 23].

1.3 Minicomputers, Microcomputers, and Multiprocessors

In the 1960s, when general purpose, higher level computers had evolved to perform a broad range of tasks, smaller special purpose minicomputers were developed to perform restricted sets of tasks with greater speed, economy, and convenience [79]. In 1962 the Laboratory Instrumentation Computer (LINC) was demonstrated by Clark and Molnar at the Lincoln Laboratory at the Massachusetts Institute of Technology (MIT), as a small, special-purpose computer that increased the individual researcher's control over the computer [65]. Waxman, then the executive secretary of the Computer Science Advisory Committee of the National Institutes of Health (NIH), arranged for a grant to construct, evaluate, and distribute 12 LINCs in 1963 to various computing research laboratories in the United States. Additional development of the LINC occurred at the University of Wisconsin by Rose, and at the University of Washington in St. Louis by Clark, Molnar, and Cox [186]. The Digital Equipment Company (DEC), founded in 1957 by Olsen, who had worked with Molnar and Clark at MIT, took over commercial production of the LINC machines [131]. The LINC was the first of a number of smaller, low-cost minicomputers to appear in the 1960s. Bell designed the first DEC Programmed Data Processor (PDP)-8; released in 1965, it helped popularize the term minicomputer [223]. In 1978 DEC introduced its VAX series of minicomputers; with more flexible and modular architecture, it was faster than the PDPs. In 1966 Hewlett-Packard introduced its Model 2116A minicomputer, more powerful than the LINC; by 1970 Hewlett-Packard was second only to DEC in the minicomputer market. Minicomputers were soon used for many medical applications because they outperformed the more expensive mainframe computers for specific input/output processing tasks, and demands at that time for processing large numerical calculations in clinical medicine were infrequent [127].

In 1970 Hyatt filed a patent application for a prototype microprocessor that used integrated circuits [159]. In 1971 Blankenbaker assembled what was considered by a panel of judges to be the first personal computer; 40 of his $750 Kenbak machines were sold [50]. The ALTO computer was developed in the early 1970s by Kay and associates at the Xerox Palo Alto Research Center (PARC) as a prototype personal computer with a graphical user interface (GUI) and an interactive programming language called Smalltalk. The ALTO had an operating system developed for its graphically oriented computer, and it used icons as symbols to represent files, documents, and programs. It also used a pointing device in the general form of a mouse for selecting programs, documents, and complex commands from menus of choices that could be shown by a cathode ray tube (CRT) display as a window into a much larger document or a database. PARC is also credited with inventing the laser printer in 1971 [81].

During the 1960s the central processing unit (CPU) could interpret and execute instructions stored directly in primary memory, in read only memory (ROM), and in random access memory (RAM). Later generation central processing units used complex instruction set computing (CISC). Such machines made extensive use of micro-programming, building instructions out of a series of micro-instructions stored in the ROM within the CPU [218]. CISC instructions usually required multiple clock cycles for machine execution, introducing potential inefficiencies. An alternative to CISC computing, known as reduced instruction set computing (RISC), was developed in the early 1980s by IBM and subsequently by others. RISC omitted the complex hardwired micro-programs of CISC, leaving only an efficient and essential set of instructions hardwired in the CPU. The RISC design required special language compilers that translated higher level languages into machine language code, and restructured the programs to run more efficiently. Although RISC processors used simpler instructions in place of fewer complex instructions, they usually provided improved performance through an increased processing speed [220].

The Intel company was formed in 1968 when Noyce left Fairchild Semiconductors to start an integrated circuit design and manufacturing company to develop a series of microprocessor chips. The power of a microprocessor is greatly influenced by the number of transistors it contains on a chip, by whether the transistors are connected to function in series or in parallel, by the scale of their integration, by the word size that governs the width of the computer's data path, and by the frequency of the electronic clock that synchronizes the computer's operations [265]. The central processing unit (CPU) of an electronic digital computer had previously been formed by combining a large number of individual components, while the CPU of a microcomputer consisted of one or more large scale integrated circuits on silicon chips. In 1969 J.M. Hoff Jr. fabricated at Intel the first CPU on a single chip; Intel then initiated a series of microprocessor chips that revolutionized the personal computer industry. The earliest chips functioning as central processing units had a small number of cores of transistors, with each core performing a task in series in assembly-line style; these were used for running operating systems, browsers, and operations requiring making numerous decisions. In 1970 Faggin designed Intel's first microprocessor, the Intel 4004, for use in calculators [185]. In 1973 Intel's 8080 microprocessor was introduced; it required only five additional circuit devices to configure a minimum system. The Intel 8748 was considered to be a microcomputer since it incorporated some read only memory (ROM) with its 8-bit microprocessor chips [261]. Further development in the 1970s led to large scale integration with tens of thousands of transistors on each chip. In 1975 Intel's 8080 microprocessor was the basis for the Altair 8800 that became the first commercial personal computer. The Intel 2008, an 8-bit microprocessor, required 50–60 additional integrated circuits to configure it into a minimum system; at that date it sold for $120. Introduced in 1980, the Intel 8088 chip contained 2,300 transistors and performed 60,000 operations per second (KOPS), or 0.06 million instructions per second (MIPS). In 1986 Intel's 80386 contained 750,000 transistors. In 1989 Intel's 80486 was a 32-bit processor that contained 1.2 million transistors; in 1992 its Pentium chip contained 3.1 million transistors; in 2002 its Pentium-4 had 55 million transistors. In 2006 Intel's dual-core chip contained 291 million transistors; in 2009 Intel released its chip containing nearly two billion transistors. In 2010 Intel released its Core i5 quad-core processors, and planned to add integrated graphics in a chip that contained 2.9 billion transistors in an area as small as a fingernail [105].

Johnson [142] reported that Intel was going beyond its traditional method of cramming more transistors onto a flat piece of silicon, in favor of building smaller chips in a three-dimensional array that put transistors closer together and enabled Intel to put 2.9 billion transistors on a chip about the size of a dime. Over this period of time the data path of commonly available microprocessors increased from 8 bits to 16 bits to 32 bits and then to 64 bits; the clock frequency increased from 8 to 66 MHz and higher. In 2011 Intel began to provide chips for Google's Android smartphones; and in 2012 Intel introduced a prototype smartphone that contained a tiny Intel microprocessor called Medfield [161]. Intel also introduced semiconductor random access memory (RAM) chips that soon replaced magnetic core memory for primary computer memory. Memory chips contained transistors in intersecting rows and columns, from which the bytes could be retrieved individually. This permitted the construction of a hierarchy of computers of different sizes. Memory chips also increased in their storage capacity and in their performance, in parallel with the development of increasingly powerful central processor chips.

Apple Computer Company was founded in 1976 by Jobs and Wozniak. Jobs was the designer and marketer of the Apple I machine in that year and the Apple II machine in 1977; Wozniak was the engineer who used the Motorola 6502 chip that had appeared on the market. The Apple Macintosh, introduced in 1984, was an innovative, compact, relatively portable, vertically designed computer with a built-in high resolution monitor; with floppy disk drives, a Motorola 68000 CPU chip, and 128-K bytes of RAM. The Macintosh had its own smalltalk-like operating system and provided some of the special features developed at the Xerox Palo Alto Research Center (PARC), including a mouse-like pointing device that allowed any displayed item to be selected; the ability to display symbols and icons representing files and documents; a bit-mapped graphical user interface; and support for applications with multiple windows of displays within displays. The Apple Macintosh computer became very popular within the educational profession because of its easy-to-learn, straightforward user interface; an estimated 120 million units were sold. In 1998 Apple launched the iMac; in 1999 it launched the iBook and entered the notebook market; in 2001 it launched the iPod and entered the mobile device business. In 2007 Apple launched the iPhone; an estimated 128 million were sold, and Apple was credited with transforming the mobile phone industry. In 2010 it launched its computer tablet, the Apple iPad; an estimated 28.7 million units were sold that year [54, 81, 183].

IBM's 5150 Personal Computer (IBM PC) was introduced in 1981. It used the Microsoft DOS operating system, the Intel 8088 chip, 16-K bytes of RAM, floppy disk drives, a variety of display monitors, and a detachable keyboard [295]. IBM's decision not to keep technical information about the PC confidential led to the appearance of many clones, not manufactured by IBM but having similar design and components, and performing identical functions. The IBM PC was rated in 1988 as the most successful personal computer design of the time [77].

Parallel processing multiprocessors were introduced in 1965 when Cray of the Control Data Corporation (CDC) designed the CDC 6600 machine with six computer processors working in parallel. The CDC 6600 in its time was the most powerful machine built [223]. In the late 1970s CDC built the Cyber 205, and Cray Research built the Cray-1; both had the ability to carry out many similar operations in parallel or concurrently on different aspects of a problem [160]. In the late 1990s parallel processing units were developed when multi-core processor chips became available. As the number of cores per chip increased, then transactional memory techniques evolved that allowed programmers to mark code segments as transactions; and a transactional memory system then automatically managed the required synchronization issues. Whereas a traditional CPU processed data sequentially, a parallel processing unit with multiple cores could divide large amounts of similar data into hundreds or thousands of smaller data collections that were then processed simultaneously.

Fung [109] defined computer graphics as image synthesis that takes a mathematical description of a scene and produces a two-dimensional array of numbers which serves as an image; this he differentiated from computer vision that is a form of image analysis that takes a two-dimensional image and converts it into a mathematical description. Graphics processing units, specialized microprocessors designed to rapidly process very large amounts of data, were increasingly used for high-definition video and for three-dimensional graphics for games. In 1999 Nvidia, a California-based company, marketed a single chip processor called GeForce 256 that functioned as a graphics processing unit (GPU), with numerous cores that simultaneously processed data in parallel and was capable of processing ten million polygons per second. In 2010 Nvidia had a product line called TESLA, with a software framework for parallel processing called CUDA; and marketed its NV35 GPU with a transistor count of about 135-million that could process very large calculations in 2 min that had previously taken up to 2 h. Parallel computing is more power-efficient than a processor chip built with several cores that compute one instruction at a time. Advanced Micro Devices (AMD), incorporated in 1969 in California, advanced as a producer of computer graphics chips when in 1985 it incorporated its ATI subsidiary that developed graphics controllers and graphics boards products. In 1991 AMD introduced its microprocessor family; in 1996 AMD acquired NextGen, a microprocessor company. In 2000 AMD was the first to break the 1-GHz – one billion clock cycles per second – with the AMD Athlon processor. In 2004 AMD demonstrated the world's first x86 dual-core processor. In 2009 it introduced its six-core AMD Opteron processor with a server platform that enabled advanced performance of the unified processor and chipset technology. In 2010 the AMD Opteron 6100 processor, a core package of two integrated circuits, contained a total of more than 1.8 billion transistors. In 2010 a GPU could have about three billion transistors, as compared to about one billion for a CPU.

Further advances continued in the development of multi-core transactional-memory chips for creating general-purpose, high-speed, parallel-processing computers. Combining Nvidia's graphics chips with Intel or AMD processor chips in a computer produced faster and more efficient data processing. By the end of 2010, Intel and AMD were the dominant manufacturers of 3.4 GHz computer processors, with Intel's high-end Core i7, and AMD's high-end Phenom II. The hybrid combinations of central processing units and embedded graphics processing units were called integrated graphics processors, high-performance units, or personal desktop supercomputers; they were expected to greatly increase computational efficiency and at a much lower cost [265].

Stanford Transactional Applications for Multi-Processing (STAMP) was developed by Minh [184] and associates at Stanford University to evaluate parallel processing with transactional memory systems by measuring the transaction length, the sizes of the read-and-write sets, the amount of time spent in transactions, and the number of re-tries per transaction. With increasing computer memory and data storage capabilities, databases rapidly evolved to store collections of data that were indexed to permit adding, querying, and retrieving from multiple, large, selected data sets.

1.4 Computer Operating Systems

The software most closely associated with a particular computer, usually provided by the computer manufacturer, the computer operating system controls the movements of all programs and data through the computer. It manages the execution of various applications programs; stores programs and data; allocates shared time to multiple concurrent users; operates the computer's peripheral input-output devices such as keyboards, disk drives, and printers; and manages data moving from storage to telecommunications lines and peripheral devices. The operating system often provides utility programs for disk maintenance, and diagnostic programs to determine causes of hardware and software malfunctions. Many operating systems are named with the acronym DOS, representing it as a disk operating system, as for example, Microsoft's MS-DOS.

In the 1940s the first computer operating systems were created for the early electronic digital computers; and they were sets of simple routines for data input and output, such as a program consisting of machine instructions for storing binary codes from a punched paper tape into successive memory locations; the entire operating system could consist of a few hundred machine instructions. In the 1950s operating systems for mainframe computers became larger and more complex; they ran in a batch mode, executing in rapid succession the programs submitted by many individual users. Because of the limited memory in many computers, functions of the operating system were divided so that input and output services needed by all programs were put into a kernel (or core set) that remained in the primary memory, while system utilities were retained in disk storage and read into main memory only when needed [86]. With the introduction of low-cost microcomputers, operating systems, like Kildall's Control Program for Microcomputers (CPM), were developed to work with many different computers [201, 213].

Time-sharing operating systems were conceived in the late 1950s by a group at MIT that developed Project MAC to support the new concept of time-sharing. Time-sharing operating systems could switch rapidly among several user programs, thereby giving the impression that the programs were being executed simultaneously [8]. Sponsored by the Department of Defense (DoD) Advanced Research Projects Agency (DARPA), the System Development Corporation (SDC) in Santa Monica developed an early time-sharing computer system that could accommodate 53 users simultaneously [190]. In the 1960s time-sharing systems were used on a number of commercial machines; higher-level operating-systems were developed for specific computers or for classes of computers. In the early 1960s the Burroughs Company used ALGOL for its operating system's programming language. In the late 1960s the MUMPS operating system was a special-purpose software package developed to support MUMPS language applications.

The UNIX operating system was developed in 1969 by Thompson, Ritchie, and McIlroy at AT&T Bell Laboratories. UNIX was attractive because it supported a number of powerful system utility programs that could be linked together in arbitrary useful sequences. It was a powerful time-sharing operating system that was multi-user (it could serve more than one user at a time), multi-tasking (it could run several applications at the same time), and had an open-architecture (it could be used by computers from different vendors). The Bell Laboratories C- language served as the basis for the UNIX operating system. UNIX became popular in the university setting because antitrust laws initially allowed AT&T to license the product for a nominal low fee [205]. By 1983 about 80 % of colleges that granted computer science degrees had adopted UNIX, and several versions of UNIX had evolved [131, 171]. In 1984, after AT&T's breakup, it was allowed by the courts to enter the computer business and sell the UNIX operating system. Able to run on a large number of different computers, singly or in a network, including IBM compatibles and Apple Macintoshes, UNIX became a major competitor for the powerful operating systems needed for networks of desktop computers, workstations, and mainframe computers. In early 1987 SUN Microsystems joined with AT&T to create a new version of UNIX with a graphical-user interface that used Internet protocols.

Control Program for Microcomputers (CP/M) was developed in 1974 by Kildall, the founder of Digital Research. The first operating system developed for 8-bit microprocessors, such as for the 8080-based computers, and subsequently for the

IBM PC series of personal computers, CP/M contained an important module called *BIOS* (Basic Input/Output Subsystem) that many applications programs and operating systems have continued to use to interface with their hardware components. By the end of the 1970s CP/M was used worldwide in more than 300 different microcomputers and in almost 200,000 installations [45, 150, 155, 205].

LINUX was released in 1989 by Torvalds, from the University of Helsinki, as an operating system that supported the functionality of UNIX. Made freely available to the public on the condition that its users would make public all of their changes, LINUX Online (http://www.linux.org/) provided a central location from which users could download source code, submit code fixes, and add new features. In 1999 Version 2.2 of the LINUX kernel was released and was shared by all LINUX distributors. The core component of its operating system supported multiple users, multitasking, networking, and Internet services, and some 64-bit platforms. In 1999 it already had more than 1,000 contributors and about seven million LINUX users, and it became a competitor to MS Windows [234].

The Smalltalk operating system, initially used in 1984 for the Apple Macintosh, provided a graphical user interface that permitted the use of displayed menus (lists of options available for selection) and icons (symbols representing options) from which the user could select items by using a mouse. Several versions of Apple Macintosh operating system were released in the 1990s, and in the 2000s the Apple Macintosh operating system and Microsoft Windows were the leading microcomputer operating systems.

Microsoft Disk Operating System (MS-DOS) was developed in the early 1980s when IBM needed an operating system for its new 16-bit 8088 microprocessor in its Personal Computer (IBM-PC). IBM contracted with Gates to develop the MS-DOS [82]. In the 1980s MS-DOS became the most widely used operating system in the nation for IBM- compatible personal computers. In the late 1980s Gates and associates independently developed an operating system called MS Windows; Gates separated from IBM, which continued the development of its IBM-OS/2 [18, 37]. In May 1990 Microsoft announced the MS-Windows 3.0 operating system; it employed a graphical user interface that allowed the use of displays within displays (from which it derived its name, *"Windows"*) and provided a mouse-pointer selector such as was used by the Apple Macintosh; it also had some networking capabilities. In 1994 a 32-bit Microsoft Windows 4.0 was introduced; and by the mid-1990s Microsoft Windows version 95 became the operating system most commonly used in personal computers [41]. Microsoft subsequently provided a series of major revisions with its MS Windows XP in 2001, MS Windows Vista in 2007, MS Windows 7 in 2009 [178], and Windows 8 in 2012.

1.5   Computer Programming Languages

Computer software includes the computer programs and related data that instruct the computer what to do and how to do it. Software includes computer operating systems, programming languages, computer applications, sets of programs and procedures with associated documentation, and all of the information processed by the computer. Wasserman [277] advocated computer software methodology to cover the entire development cycle, including transitional phases, and to validate throughout the cycle that system specifications were correctly fulfilled and user needs met. The term, computer software, is used in contrast to computer hardware, or those physical devices on which the software is run. Although advances in computer hardware were the basis for many innovations, it was the software that made the hardware usable for computer applications.

Computer programming languages can be defined as formal languages used by humans to facilitate the description of a procedure by the computer for solving a problem or a task that must be translated into a form understandable by the computer itself before it could be executed by the computer [119]. In 1943 Aiken used punched paper tape to enter instructions into the electro-mechanical Mark I computer to generate mathematical tables, and in 1946 ENIAC, the first electronic digital computer, used wiring diagrams showing how to set the machine's plug boards and switches to calculate ballistic trajectories needed during warfare. Programming errors were a common problem. In 1947, Hopper discovered a computer "bug" while she was working on the Mark II computer that suddenly stopped. A moth had become stuck in one of the computer's switches. She removed the bug with a tweezers and explained that she was "debugging" the computer, thus coining the term commonly used for correcting errors in programming [223].

Machine languages apply a series of binary numbers that address memory cells to store data. Computers can accept instructions in machine codes only by using the instruction sets with which they are designed. Machine language is the system of codes by which the instructions and the data must be represented internally. A programmer writing in a computer's low-level machine language uses machine instructions to address memory cells for storing data, uses accumulators to add and subtract numbers, and uses registers to store operands and results. Thus some codes represent instructions for the central processor (such as shifting the contents of a register 1 bit to the left or the right); some codes move the data from the accumulator into the main memory; some codes represent data or information about data; and some codes point to locations (addresses) in memory. Assembly languages (or assembly codes) were developed in the 1940s to reduce the tedium of writing in machine code. Computer programmers invented symbolic notations; instead of writing down the binary digits for each machine instruction, the programmer entered a short English word (such as "add" or "load") that would be translated automatically into the appropriate machine instructions. These English terms were more easily remembered than numerical instruction codes, and came to be called mnemonic (from the Greek, meaning "to remember") codes. Low-level languages used for writing programs to translate instruction mnemonics to machine executable binary codes were called assemblers and were generally written to meet the design requirements of specific computers. Programs that required extreme efficiency were often written in assemblers, since assembly language gave direct and efficient control over a program's operation.

Von Neumann was able to show that instructions for the computer could be stored in the computer's electronic memory and treated in the same manner as data by using an electrically alterable memory capable of storing both the program instructions and the data to be used in calculations. Previously, once a computer, such as the ENIAC, performed a specific sequence of calculations, its circuits had to be rewired for any other sequence [44]. Von Neumann's revolutionary design led to the ability to manipulate machine commands by arithmetic operations rather than by rewiring circuit boards. von Neumann demonstrated a programming language that stored instructions for the computer in the computer's electronic memory as numbers that could be treated in exactly the same manner as numerical data. For the first time logical choices could be made inside the machine and instructions could be modified by the computer [90]. Modern computer programming is usually considered to have begun at that time.

Composed of a set of statements based on a vocabulary of symbols, programming languages are either declarative (instructing the machine by listing the tasks to be completed) or procedural (instructing the machine about how to perform the tasks by listing the discrete steps to be taken). Different levels of programming languages evolved as each generation of computers required changes in programming. In the late 1950s, programming languages simulated as closely as possible the natural language that people use, employing English in the United States and using well-known English symbols as much as possible [84, 216]. Newer, more powerful programming languages abstracted sequences of machine-level instructions into conceptually useful operations that could be invoked with a single mnemonic command.

Algorithms commonly used in computer programming as a method for providing a solution to a particular problem or to a specific set of problems consist of a set of precisely stated procedures that can be applied in the same way to all instances of a problem. For complex problems, such as data mining, algorithms are indispensable because only procedures that can be stated in the explicit and unambiguous form of an algorithm can be presented to a computer [164].

1.5.1 Higher-Level Programming Languages

Unlike assembly languages, instructions to computers written in a higher-level language combined a greater number of machine-level operations into a single language command. Since the late 1950s most computer instructions have been written in higher-level languages, and some are even considered to approach automatic programming when the computer itself helps to prepare the program or code, thereby decreasing the amount of writing a programmer needs to do [158].

Compiler was a term first used in 1951 by Hopper, then at Remington Rand Univac, to describe her first translator program [259]. A compiler took the complete program written in the source code of the higher-level language and translated it into the machine-language code that was stored as an executable file in the computer. An alternative approach used an interpreter that scanned and parsed each line of the program-source code, and then interpreted and changed it into machine-language code each time it was used. Because they could be tested and changed as they were entered line by line, interpreted programs were easier to write and change. For an interpreted program to be executed, however, the interpreter had to be present in main memory, rendering it a potential source of heavy processing overhead. In contrast, once a program had been compiled, the compiler was no longer needed, resulting in faster overall performance.

With the development of higher level languages, where one English statement could give rise to many machine instructions, programs tended to be shorter and quicker to write, less prone to error, and able to run on different computers [84]. LISP (LISt Processing) language was developed in the late 1950s by McCarthy at the Massachusetts Institute of Technology (MIT) as a research tool to study artificial intelligence [3]. LISP is a high-level, interpreted language that uses lists as its only data structure for both programs and data. A list is any group or sequence of elements, called atoms, structured in a particular order and enclosed within parentheses [176]. LISP can manipulate any list of numbers, words, diseases, symptoms, symbols, deductions, and LISP statements; lists can be contained within lists. LISP was widely used by researchers in artificial intelligence because human thought involved more symbol manipulation than numerical calculations [152]. Several early medical expert-system programs, including MYCIN and INTERNIST-I, were originally written in LISP.

FORTRAN (FORmula TRANslator), an influential early high level programming language, was developed by Backus and associates at IBM in 1957 [259]. FORTRAN provided a compiler to replace the tedious coding of assembly language. FORTRAN continued to be widely used through the 1970s and 1980s, primarily because of its special capabilities for numerical calculations, and because many useful subroutines were developed over the years in FORTRAN. The standardization of FORTRAN facilitated the transfer of software among machines of different vendors and made FORTRAN extremely popular [33]. It soon became the standard language for scientific and engineering applications; by 1987 it was estimated that as much as one-fourth of the world's available machine cycles ran with code generated by some form of FORTRAN [84].

COBOL (COmmon Business-Oriented Language) is considered by some to have been invented by Hopper when she worked on the Mark I and UNIVAC computers in the 1950s [101]. COBOL was introduced in 1960 by a joint committee of computer manufacturers, computer business users, and government and academic representatives interested in developing a high-level programming language for business data processing that would use ordinary English statements and be usable by any computer. Because of the pervasiveness of business functions, COBOL became the most widely used programming language of the 1970s and 1980s [123]. Like FORTRAN, COBOL used a compiler and was not an interactive language. From the 1960s through the 1980s COBOL was used almost universally for the business and accounting functions in hospitals.

BASIC (Beginners All-purpose Symbolic Instruction Code) was developed in the early 1960s by Kemeny and Kurtz at Dartmouth, as a language modeled after FORTRAN, for introductory courses in teaching computer programming. BASIC is an interactive, interpretive language. The program is converted line-by-line into the computer's machine language; error messages are simple for students to understand, and program changes are easy to make and test. BASIC is relatively easy to learn and to use, and it became one of the most widely used high-level languages. The earliest BASIC program for microcomputers was developed in 1975 by Gates and Allen for the Altair computer; and on the basis of this product they founded Microsoft [110]. By the 1980s BASIC was available on almost every commercial personal computer.

APL (A Programming Language) was developed in the mid-1960s by Iverson at Harvard for mathematical computation using vectors and matrices. Whereas FORTRAN required definitions of arrays and operated on one element in a matrix at a time, APL uses symbols to execute these operations with minimal procedural definitions [28, 214].

ALGOL (Algorithmic Language) is a highly structured, compiled language that uses English-like instructions and conventional algebra terms in its statements [28]. ALGOL uses blocks of instructions in a modular fashion and allows assignment of variable values to be nested within other statements. In the early 1960s Burroughs used ALGOL as the system programming language for its B-5000 computer [254]. Although ALGOL was not widely used, it influenced the development of modern programming languages such as Programming Language One (PL/1), PASCAL, C- language, and Ada [33]. PL/1 was developed by a committee of IBM users in the early 1960s as a multi-purpose language that incorporated features of FORTRAN for scientific processing and COBOL for business and data-handling capabilities. Since the 1970s PL/1 has been used to develop several hospital information systems.

PASCAL, named after the seventeenth century mathematician, Pascal, was developed by Wirth in the late 1960s to teach and encourage structured programming. One of Wirth's goals was to develop a language that was independent of hardware [214]. Several medical decision-support programs were written in PASCAL. Versions of Pascal were used in the 1980s by Apple computers and the IBM 370 system; in the 1990s it was the basis for Oracle's language PL/SQL. The language Ada, was named after Ada Byron Lovelace, credited by some as the first computer programmer [94]. It was developed in the 1970s under a contract for the Department of Defense (DoD), and intended for use as a common standard language, independent of any hardware, for all DoD applications.

FORTH was developed by Moore in the late 1960s, and captured many features from ALGOL and LISP [188, 206]. FORTH was generally used for specialized scientific and manufacturing applications because it was "compact, fast, structured, extensible, and highly portable" [138].

The Massachusetts General Hospital Utility Multi-Programming System (MUMPS) was developed in 1966 by Barnett, Pappalardo, Marble, and Greenes in Barnett's Laboratory of Computer Science at the Massachusetts General Hospital

(MGH). MUMPS was created to implement the MGH modular hospital information system. The goal of the MUMPS system was to combine a simple yet powerful high-level language with an easy-to-use database management system [11]. The first publication describing MUMPS was by Greenes [118] and associates, who reported that MUMPS allowed a programming session to take the form of a conversational dialogue between the programmer and the computer terminal, thus minimizing the user's time in programming. Barnett [13, 14] described the important characteristics of MUMPS to be: (1) the language is interpretive, thus facilitating rapid development of new applications; (2) the language has powerful string-manipulating commands, facilitating the data management of the non-numerical data which make up the largest part of medical information; (3) the file structure is a sparsely-filled, tree-structured array where space is allocated only as needed allowing efficient use of disk storage space; (4) the method of storing data in this hierarchical storage array allows relative independence of access by the different modules (and thus relative independence of the development of modules) and yet easy exchange of data (thus facilitating the development of an integrated electronic medical record); and (5) a relatively large number of users can be supported simultaneously.

MUMPS became one of the most commonly used programming languages in the United States for medical applications. It was used to program COSTAR, a successful outpatient record system developed during the late 1960s and early 1970s, and became commercially available in 1969 when Pappalardo and Marble formed Medical Information Technology (Meditech). Because early versions of MUMPS were very popular and MUMPS was an interpretive language, the comparative merits of compilers and interpreters were often considered by early medical application developers [27, 42, 118]. Lewkowicz [165] noted that most MUMPS implementations used a version of compiled code that offered the advantages of an interpreted language without the associated overhead required in interpreting each line of code before execution. Accepted as a standard language in 1977 by the American National Standards Institute (ANSI), MUMPS joined COBOL, FORTRAN, and PL/1 as ANSI Standard Languages. In 1983 MUMPS had more than 4,500 installations around the world, and also by 500 or more users of microcomputers [273, 274]. By the end of the 1980s both the Department of Defense (DoD) and the Veterans Administration (VA) were installing nationwide MUMPS-based medical scientific and manufacturing applications, because of its advantages of being compact, fast, structured, extensible, and highly portable [138] In the 2000s the large medical multi-facility information systems at VA, DoD, and the Epic company's EpicCare were all MUMPS-based. Reviews of the early history and uses of MUMPS were published by Walters et al. [275] and by Blum and Orthner [31].

The C language was developed in the mid-1970s by Ritchie and Thompson at Bell Laboratories as a structured programming language that used block structures of statements similar to ALGOL and PASCAL; it produced efficient code that lent itself to systems programming. Used to program the UNIX operating system [149], the C language became popular because source code written in C would run on most computers and was used to implement object-oriented programming [170, 253].

The C++ language was invented by Stroustrup at AT&T Bell Laboratories in the 1980s as an extended version of the standard C language to further support object-oriented programming [252]. PERL was developed in 1987 with some of the features of C language; it was widely used for building Web-based applications, for interfacing and accessing database modules, for generating SQL queries, and for text processing [63].

GEMISCH (GEneralized Medical Information System for Community Health) was developed in 1969 by Hammond, Stead, and Straube at Duke University using a DEC minicomputer. An interactive, high-level, multi-user database management language, GEMISCH supported a variety of files and provided an extensive text string-manipulation program, mathematical and Boolean logic capability, and input- and output-control programs [126, 250]. Duke's The Medical Record (TMR) system was developed using GEMISCH programming language [248].

Smalltalk was a language developed in the early 1970s by Kay and associates at the Xerox Palo Alto Research Center (PARC), as a programming language to control simulations on their Alto computer [148, 258]. Alto's Smalltalk, with a built-in operating system and automatic storage management, became the basis for many features in the Apple Macintosh computer. It was an object-oriented language in which everything was an object, and objects communicated by sending messages to one another [3]. Each object was a collection of data and procedures which belonged to, and was an instance of, a class. Written instructions specified how instances of a class reacted when they received messages. Classes of objects could be moved from super-classes and between classes, and would inherit the attributes and variables of their instances. Smalltalk's graphical user interface (GUI) allowed users to use a mouse pointer to move displayed text and images [147] and provided a wide range of graphic objects for which special purpose applications could be developed [137].

PROLOG (PROgramming in LOGic) was originally developed in Europe and was made commercially available in the United States in 1984 [279]. Whereas earlier programs told the computer what to do by a series of explicit steps, PROLOG had pattern-matching capabilities and could be used to express logical relationships in a database as defined by rules, such as: if "A" and "B" are true, then "C" must also be true [237]. Used by researchers in artificial intelligence for advanced database retrieval methods and for processing natural language, PROLOG was the initial programming language used by the Japanese for their fifth generation, knowledge-based computer systems [100].

Structured Query Language (SQL) was developed in the early 1970s by Chamberlin [56] and Boyce at IBM, as a language designed for the query, retrieval, and management of data in a relational database management system, such as had been introduced by Codd [68]. In the 1980s the relational database design became dominant in industry; and versions of SQL were generally used to construct, manage, and query relational databases [269]. Ashton-Tate developed dBASE as a database management system for microcomputers; dBase II was used by the Apple computer and the IBM personal computer under Microsoft's DOS, and dBase III by UNIX. Java language was developed in the 1990s by Sun Microsystems as an object-oriented, high-level programming language. Used for a variety of operating systems, including Apple Macintosh, Linux, Microsoft Windows, and Sun Solaris, Java was acquired by Oracle when it bought Sun in 2010.

Markup languages began to evolve in the 1960s when Generalized Markup Language (GML) was developed by IBM to enable the sharing of machine-readable, large-project documents used in industry, law, and government. The term "markup" was introduced when revisions were written on the program's text document of instructions. In 1986 Standard Generalized Markup Language (SGML) was developed as an International Standards Organization (ISO) version of GML, and was used by industry and the Armed Services. In 1996 SGML began to be used for Web applications; in 1998 it was modified as Extensible Markup Language (XML) designed to provide a standard set of rules for encoding documents in machine-readable form, and to help simplify and support the usability of Web services. Hypertext Markup Language (HTML), with some features derived from SGML, was developed in 1990 by Berners-Lee while at CERN. Used by Web browsers to dynamically format text and images, HTML became the predominant markup language for describing Web pages and became an international standard in 2000.

Third generation languages were generally called imperative languages or procedural languages that required the use of imperatives (commands) in programming with consideration of computer addresses and storage schemes, and told the computer exactly how to take each step. Fourth generation languages were more directed to functional, non-procedural programming that allowed the programmers to concentrate on the logical purpose of the programs, and that told the computer what to do rather than how to do it. Specialized commercial applications programs were developed. For example, the Hypertext Preprocessor (PHP), an open source language for building Web applications, supports several databases and is used by Google and Facebook.

1.6 Computer Data Storage and Database Design

Data is processed by a digital computer as a collection of binary digits (bits), named after the binary code, 1 or 0. A byte is a set of 8 bits and is the basic unit of digital computing. A kilobyte (KB) is a thousand bytes, a megabyte (MB) a thousand KBs, a gigabyte (GB) a thousand MBs, a terrabyte (TB) a thousand GBs, a petabyte (PB) a thousand TBs, an exabyte (EB) a thousand PBs, a zettabyte (ZB) a thousand EBs, and a yettabyte (YB) a thousand ZBs.

Weinberger [278] defined information as a collection of data and estimated that the amount of digital information increased tenfold every 5 years. Frawley et al. [104] estimated that the amount of information generated in the world doubled every 20 months, and that the size and number of computer databases increased even faster. Noting the vast amount of data from computer-based sources, Enriques [98] estimated about 1.2 zettabytes of data were available in 2010 and this amount would be very much larger with the addition of genomic data.

Computer data storage devices are required for both the internal primary computer memory storage and for the external secondary storage of digital data. Secondary data storage in the early 1950s used magnetic tape drives for the writing and reading and the external storage of data, since reels of tape were low-cost, especially for backup data storage. Later in the 1950s magnetic hard disc drives were developed for storing digital data on rotating hard plastic discs with a magnetic covering. The drives were equipped with magnetic heads positioned to both write the data on, and read the data back from, the disc. The rotating disc had great advantages in that the user had the random access disc to quickly retrieve data at different locations on the disc, whereas the data on a tape could only be read sequentially. With the development of personal computers there evolved a variety of floppy disks made of a thin magnetic storage medium sealed in a rectangular plastic covering. Initially 8 in. in diameter, floppy discs next became 5.25 in., and then most commonly 3.5 in.; floppy disk drives were developed for each size to write and to read the data.

Optical secondary storage devices developed in the 1990s used a laser beam to record light in a spiral track on the surface of a disc that was usually in the form of a 4.7 or 5.25 in. compact disc (CD) as read only memory (CD-ROM). Optical disc storage devices were developed to be used as write once-read only (CD-R), and also for use as erasable-rewritable optical disc storage (CD-RW) [103, 228]. In the 1990s optical storage discs that were rewritable and/or erasable rapidly became the storage mode of choice. In the 2000s digital video drives (DVD) used red laser light and Blu-ray discs used a violet/blue light to both read and write (DVD-RW). Solid-state storage devices were used in the 2000s; with integrated circuits to store data and no moving parts, they were very quiet, portable, could read and write very fast, and used less power than hard discs. Universal Serial Bus (USB) flash drives (thumb drives) were small, portable, solid-state digital data storage devices with capacities of up to thousands of gigabytes. These consisted of a printed circuit board that carried the circuit elements, and USB connector to plug into a computer.

Computer-stored databases were considered by Coltri [73] to be one of the most important developments in software engineering, equivalent to the heart and the brain of a modern information system. Defined by Wiederhold [281, 283, 285] as collections of related data organized so that usable data could be extracted, databases were described by Frawley et al. [104] as logically integrated collections of data in one or more computer files, organized to facilitate the efficient storage, change, query, and retrieval of contained relevant information to meet the needs of its users. The functional and technical requirements for the development of efficient computer-stored databases were essential specifications. Coltri [73] noted that, although a single structural database model could initially allow for simpler coordination, operation, and reporting, designing a single database for successful querying became increasingly difficult as the database grew larger, became more complex with many functional relationships, and subsystem components required frequent changes in their data content. Moreover, as databases grew larger they often developed problems caused by excess redundant data.

Structural design of medical databases was substantially developed by Wiederhold at Stanford University [280–285]. Wiederhold emphasized that the effectiveness of a database depended on its relevance to its organizational purposes; and that a database management system was needed to control, enter, store, process, and retrieve the data. He advised that when using very large databases, it was helpful to apply automated methods for the acquisition, coding, storage, and retrieval of the desired data. In the 1950s with the early development of computers, users began to bring their work in batches to a central mainframe computer in order to be processed. The data were initially collected, entered, and merged into computer files stored on magnetic tape, and a file management system entered, stored, and retrieved the data. In the 1960s time-shared, mainframe computers that communicated by telephone lines to remote data entry terminals and printers allowed many users to process their data concurrently, and provided a relatively acceptable turn-around time for data services. Initially data were stored in computer databases on magnetic tape, but were soon moved to storage on random-access, magnetic disc drives, where they were organized in a manner more suitable for query and retrieval. However, at that time the high costs for computer storage greatly limited database capacities. In the 1970s with the emergence of magnetic, random-access disc storage, subsystem databases could be more readily merged into larger databases; this needed an integrating database management system. The retrieval of subsets of selected data from various databases required some re-organization of the stored data, as well as an index to the locations of the various data subsets. Attempts were made to design more efficient databases to make them independent of their applications and subsystems, so that a well-designed database could process almost any type of data presented to it. Terdiman [257] credited the development of microcomputer technology in the 1970s to many of the advances in database management systems.

In the 1980s microcomputers and minicomputers were increasingly used for small database systems, often called registries. As storage technology continued to become more efficient, and larger and cheaper storage devices became available, computer-based registries expanded their storage capacity for larger amounts of data and were generally referred to as databases. When huge storage capacity became available at a relatively low-cost, very large collections of data were often referred to as data warehouses. Helvey et al. [132] reported that in 1985 almost 100 medical online databases were available, distributed by a variety of information carriers, vendors and producers. The year of 1988 was called "the year of the database" by Bryan [49], who reported that more than 20 new or improved database management systems became available in that year. In 1989 the total number of computer-stored databases in the world was estimated to be about five million; although most of the databases were relatively small, some were huge, as was the 1990 U.S. census database comprising a million bytes of data [104].

Johnson [143] considered the data modeling designs that provided the conceptual schema for representing the information in clinical databases as important for large medical databases as their structural designs. He defined the conceptual schema for a database as a representation of all of the data types required to manage the data process, whether using a hierarchical, a relational, or an object-oriented structural database design, or a combination of database structural designs. While advising that the structural design of a database needed to provide rapid retrieval of data for individual users and to adapt to changing information needs of growth and of new technology, Johnson emphasized that its primary purpose was to implement the conceptual schema. To properly build a database, Johnson advised first developing a model of the database that defined its functional requirements, technical requirements, and structural design. The model needed to provide a formal description, a conceptual schema of all the data to be generated in the enterprise, and how all of the data were related. Thus the users of the database needed to fully define what they wanted the database and its database management system to do.

Hierarchical databases were considered by Coltri [73] to be the simplest and the earliest structural design used for medical databases. For a hierarchical database the connections between files, or between fields within files, needed to be defined at the start of the database. The data was organized in what was described as a "parent-child" relationship, where each "parent" could have many "children", but each "child" had only one "parent". Hierarchical data subclasses with inheritance of attributes could also appear in other databases, such as in relational and object-oriented databases. Coltri reported that the best known early example of a hierarchical structured, medical database was the one developed in the 1960s by Barnett [12, 1974a, b] and associates [118, 121].

Relational databases and their database management systems were developed in the 1960s for large, shared databases by Codd [66–69] while at the IBM Research Center in San Jose. Codd required that all data in a relational database be designed in the form of two-dimensional tables with uniquely labeled rows and columns. Every data element was logically accessible through the use of the names of its table and its column; data transformations resulted from following defined logical rules. In a relational database the data were organized into files or tables of fixed-length records; each record was an ordered list of values, with one value for each field. Information about each field's name and potential values was maintained in a separate metadatabase. The relational database model, because of its simplicity and power, soon became dominant in use; and in the 1970s Structured Query Language (SQL) was developed by Chamberlin and Boyce at IBM to construct, manage, and query relational databases (VanName [269]). SQL soon became the standard language used for programming relational databases. In 1979 a commercial relational database named ORACLE became available from the ORACLE Corporation, and in the 1980s Ashton-Tate developed dBASE for microcomputers [76]. Johnson [144] described an extension of SQL for data warehouses which enabled analysts to designate groups of rows that could be manipulated and aggregated into large groups of data, and then analyzed in a variety of ways to solve a number of analytic problems.

Multi-dimensional databases were developed as relational databases grew in size. Led by Online Analytic Processing (OLAP), commercial search-and-query programs designed for very large relational databases became available to provide answers to analytic queries that were multi-dimensional and used relational databases. OLAP generally stored data in a relational structured design, and used aggregations of data built from a fact-table according to specified dimensions. Relational database structures were considered to be multi-dimensional when they contained multiple attributes, such as time periods, locations, product codes, and other attributes that could be defined in advance and aggregated in hierarchies. The combinations of all possible aggregations in the database were expected to be able to provide answers to every query that could be anticipated of the stored data [69]. Connolly (1999) described a way of visualizing a multi-dimensional database by beginning with a flat two-dimensional table of data; then adding another dimension to form a three-dimensional cube of data called a "hypercube"; and then adding cubes of data within cubes of data, with each side of each cube being called a "dimension", resulting in a multi-dimensional database. Pendse [207] described in some detail the history of OLAP, and credited the publication in 1962 by Iverson of A Programming Language (APL) as the first mathematically defined, multi-dimensional language for processing multi-dimensional variables. Multi-dimensional analyses then became the basis for several versions of OLAP developed in the 1970s and 1980s by IBM and others; and in 1999 the Analyst module available in COGNOS was acquired by IBM. In the 2000s new OLAP derivatives were in use by IBM, Microsoft, Oracle, and others.

Object oriented databases were developed in the 1970s at the Xerox Palo Alto Research Center (PARC), and used the programming language Smalltalk [219]. Whereas traditional database programs represented the data and the procedures for manipulating the data separately, in an object oriented system the objects encapsulated both of these. Object oriented databases were designed to attempt to bring database programming and applications programming closer together, and treated the database as a modular collection of component data-items called objects. Members of an entity that belonged to types or classes of data with their own data and programming codes, objects incorporated not only data but also descriptions of their behavior and of their relationships to other objects. Using concepts such as entities, attributes, and relationships, objects could be members of an entity that belonged to types or classes with their own data and programming codes. Objects had an independent existence and could represent persons, activities, or observations, and were sufficiently independent to be copied into other programs. Attributes were properties that described aspects of objects; relationships described the association between objects. Objects were sufficiently modular and independent that they could be copied easily into other programs. An object-oriented database could serve a network of workstations in which one or more computers were designated as object servers that would supply applications programs with objects as needed to minimize workstation and server communications. By the late 1980s some database applications were programmed in object oriented languages that treated the database as a modular collection of component items called objects [85].

Connolly [76] described some relational variances for an object-oriented database in order to use Structured Query Language (SQL). Barsalou and Wiederhold [17] described their PENGUIN project that applied a three-layered architecture to an object-oriented database that defined the object-based data as a layer of data on top of a relational database management system, with a hypertext interface between the object-oriented database and the relational database that provided conceptual integration without physical integration. Their workstations were Apple personal computers; they used Apple's HyperCard program for their Macintosh computer to define and manipulate "stacks" of data corresponding to a relational database structure, with one field for each attribute, written in the Macintosh HyperTalk language to allow querying visual images that moved through a hypertext document.

Entity attribute value (EAV) databases were designed to help manage the highly heterogeneous data within medical databases, where over several years of medical care a single patient could accumulate thousands of relevant descriptive parameters, some of which might need, from time to time, to be readily accessible from a large clinical database that contained multiple relational tables. Dinu [87], Nadkarni et al. [191–196], and Brandt et al. [43] described the EAV database as an alternative to conventional relational database modeling where diverse types of data from different medical domains were generated by different groups of users. The term, EAV database, was generally applied when a significant proportion of the data was modeled as EAV even though some tables could be traditional relational tables. Conceptually, an EAV design used a database table with three columns: (1) Entity, that contained data such as the patient identification, with a time-stamp of the date-and-time of the beginning and end of each clinical event; (2) Attribute, that identified the event, such a laboratory test, or showed a pointer to a separate attribute table; and (3) Value, that contained the value of the attribute (such as the result of a laboratory test). A metadatabase was usually added to help provide definitions of terms, keys to related tables, and logical connections for data presentation, interactive validation, data extraction, and for ad-hoc query.

Metadatabases were developed to: (1) store metadata that are data describing the data contained in a database; (2) provide a data dictionary with definitions of terms and a list of coded data in the database with their codes; (3) serve as a thesaurus to recognize different terms that have similar meanings; and (4) provide a lexicon of standard, accepted, defined, and correctly spelled terms. A metadatabase contains associated relevant information to aid in the storage and retrieval of data in the database by providing linkages to other data items and files, keys to related tables, and logical connections for data presentation, interactive validation, data extraction, and ad hoc query, together with interfaces for any metadata additions or corrections.

Distributed database systems evolved in the 1970s with the introduction of lower-cost minicomputers and more efficient communication networks that brought computers closer to the users. In a distributed database system with a cluster of specialized subsystem databases, each subsystem collected and stored the data it generated in its separate database; a communications network provided linkages to an integrating central database for data entry and retrieval and linkages to other subsystem databases as needed (See also Sect. 3.4.3). Federated databases were developed to store large volumes of aggregated data in multiple partitions, or as functional-oriented databases that were logically interconnected. Directly accessible across multiple applications, they allowed multiple users to simultaneously access and query data in the various databases [73]. Data warehouses was the term applied to large, extended, central databases that collected and managed data from several different databases; as warehouses, they were capable of servicing the ever-increasing volume of patient data that were collected from the ever-changing and expanding medical technologies. As data warehouses grew larger they often developed partitions and data marts for specialized sub-sets of the data warehouse in order to better serve users with different functional needs [76]. When data warehouses were found to satisfy the needs of different users and to efficiently query large collections of data, this led to the development of online analytical processing (OLAP), and of translational data processing between multiple data warehouses.

Translational databases evolved in the late 1990s with more advanced designs of database management systems to: (1) optimize the translation, transformation, linkage, exchange, and integration of the increasingly voluminous collections of medical information that was becoming accessible from many large databases in multiple institutions that were located worldwide, by using wide area networks, the Internet, and the World Wide Web; (2) provide access to high-performance, super-computing resources; (3) facilitate the concurrent query, analyses, and applications of large amounts of data by multi-disciplinary teams; (4) encourage knowledge discovery and data mining, and support the transfer of new evidence-based knowledge into patient care; and (5) advance the use of biomedical computational methods. Since most data warehouses had been developed with database management systems that employed their own legacy and data-encoding standards, it usually required some reorganization and modification of their source data to be compatible with the data transferred from other different data warehouses before all could be merged into a single database schema. Thus it became necessary to develop translational database software.

Database managementsystems were designed to capture and process all of the data stored in the computer system, and to implement all of the functional requirements of the database [10]. Walters [272] considered the main contribution of database management science was to distinguish between what information should be stored in a system from how it should be stored. Wiederhold [283] defined a database management system as the hardware and software that controlled, stored, processed, and retrieved the data in the database. As defined by Blum [28, 29, 32], a database management system was software consisting of a collection of procedures and programs with the requirements for: (1) entering, storing, retrieving, organizing, updating, and manipulating all of the data within its database; (2) managing the utilization and maintenance of the database; (3) including a metadatabase to define application-specific views of the database; (4) entering data only once, even though the same data might be stored in other subsystems; (5) retrieving, transferring, and communicating needed data in a usable format, and having the ability to create inverted files indexed by key terms; (6) maintaining the integrity, security, and the required level of confidentiality of the data; and (7) fulfilling all management, legal, accounting, and economic requirements. Database management systems soon replaced the earlier file-based systems that often stored the same data in multiple files where it could be more difficult to retrieve and coordinate the data. Distributed database management systems involved the management of physically dispersed data in two or more databases located in different computers and used some means of communications for the distribution and exchange of the data. In large organizations, distributed database management systems were designed either as clusters of computers tightly coupled to a central large mainframe computer, or as loosely coupled in a distributed database system [172].

Cloud computing involves computing over a network, where a program or an application may run on many connected computers at the same time. It specifically refers to a remote group of computers commonly referred to as server, connected through a communication network such as the Internet, a local area network (LAN), or a wide area network (WAN). Any individual user who has permission to access the server can use its processing power to perform any computing task. Instead of needing a personal computer, the user can run an application or store data from anywhere in the world using the processing power provided by the server, which is connected to a network via the Internet or other connection. In common usage the term "cloud" is essentially a metaphor for the Internet; computer vendors have popularized the phrase "in the cloud" to refer to software sold remotely as a service through the Internet. Typically, the seller has actual energy-consuming servers which host products and services from a remote location, so end-users can simply log on to the network without installing anything. The major models of cloud computing services are generally known as "software services".

1.7 Computer Terminals, Data Input, and Data Output Devices

Data acquisition, input, retrieval, and data output are all important functions of a computer-based information system; and the various devices and computer terminals used to carry out these functions changed greatly with innovations in technology over recent decades. Typewriter keyboards for computer input accepted any combination of words and numbers, but required typing skills to be used efficiently; therefore most physicians did not find them acceptable for data entry. Typewriters were used by some as early computer data-output printers; at first they were restricted to printing only uppercase (capital) letters, but soon lengthy printouts were batch processed on higher-speed printers [168]. Tele-typewriters were among the earliest interactive computer devices that permitted a direct dialogue with users. However, since they could only accept typed alphanumeric input and could print only one character after another, they were soon replaced as data-input devices by visual display monitors equipped with typewriter-like keyboards. The earliest mode of directly entering data into a computer, punched paper cards were invented by Hollerith in 1882 [6, 276]. Hollerith's machine punched a hole into a paper card (the size of a dollar bill) in a specific location that corresponded to a unique digital code for each alphabet letter, each number, and each punctuation mark and selected symbol. Card readers sensed the holes in the punched cards using wires that brushed over the cards, making electrical connections through the holes to the metal plate under which the cards were passed [71].

Mark-sense paper cards were used by Schenthal [226, 227] to enter clinical data; these involved using a graphite pencil to make a mark on the card that was electrically sensed as a data input to the computer. Schenthal also used portable punch cards. Prescored portable punch cards could go directly from the user to a card-reader machine without intermediary keypunching. The card was placed in a card holder, and the holes for the appropriate items were punched in with a stylus. These cards were used by some for ordering laboratory tests and recording vital signs [7]. Premarked prepunched paper cards with specific data items for computer input were used to requisition clinical laboratory tests and to enter patients' responses in a questionnaire form [72]. Punched paper tape soon followed the use of punched cards. However both punched paper cards and paper tape became unnecessary for data input when keyboard devices, structured like a typewriter but with additional special-function keys, were directly connected to computers. Pressing a function key closed an electric circuit and sent a corresponding specific digital code to the computer.

Optically sensed marks on paper cards, forms, and pages with encoded data, readable by optical readers directly into the computer, appeared in the 1960s. Optically scanned cards were used to enter results from an ophthalmologic examination, including diagnoses and laboratory data [246]. At Baylor College of Medicine, optically read cards were developed and tested that coupled laser-imprinted cards to a computer for data input. Data in digital format were formed on a card with a milliwatt laser beam that placed 5-μm dimples on the specially treated surface of the card; a read-write device connected to a personal computer scanned in the medical information and displayed it on a screen [48]. Optically read cards were also developed by the Veterans Administration (VA) and tested with a specially designed workstation that provided the read-write, optical-card technology needed to service patient-care data for its VA Decentralized Hospital Computer Program [117].

In the late 1980s some medical information systems (MISs) began to pilot-test optical scanning and storage technology for medical record processing. Optical scanners converted paper records into bit-mapped images and stored these digitized files on optical disks with a huge storage capacity. High-resolution monitors attached to networked workstations permitted the viewing of the images of the paper records. By the end of the 1980s the available technology had advanced to provide a multimedia medical record. Using an Apple Macintosh microcomputer at Dartmouth-Hitchcock Medical Center, Shultz and Brown [229] developed a prototype MIS that processed and displayed text, images, animated sequences; allowed linkage to radiology and pathology images; and permitted the hearing of digitized heart sounds. The system drew information from multiple sources other than its own database, such as from a linked laser video disk and from other conventional databases. Friedman [106] foresaw as an important benefit of the computer-based patient record, new analytic capabilities to enhance the quality and efficiency of medical care by the creation of new databases that lent themselves to analyses. He called this process "informating" [after Zuboff [304]] rather than automating the medical record.

Matrix keyboards for structured data input became popular in the mid-1960s. Computer terminals used in some clinical laboratories and hospital nursing stations used matrix keyboards, such as the IBM 1092 terminal. Users entered data by pushing buttons located in rows; each button was identified by a preprogrammed format and the formats were structured by printed overlays placed on the keyboard. However, like other terminals that required a keyboard mode of entry, they were not acceptable to physicians even though technicians could easily be trained in their use.

Optical character readers (OCR), developed in the 1970s, could scan and input alphanumeric characters printed in standard fonts of type. Although handwriting was the most natural way for a physician to make notations in a patient's record, only hand-printed characters could be recognized by optical scanners. Optical character scanners contained light sensors that converted light into an electrical voltage that could be sensed by an electronic circuit. OCR recognized the shape of the characters by the contrast of light and dark areas created when light was reflected from the surface of the document, and converted the characters to a bit-map of pixels (picture-elements) representing the "on" (dark) areas or the "off" (light) areas. The OCR software matched each character with a pixel-by-pixel comparison to character templates stored in memory. As OCR technology advanced in the 1980s, it shifted to scanning pages of text and images by transforming the light reflected from the page into electrical voltages that were a function of the light intensity as, for example, a gray scale representing a range of shades between black and white. A bit-mapped graphic image of the page was sent to the computer where files of the digital data were created. Handheld, optical line scanners soon became available that could be used to guide the read-head along a line of text.

Barcode readers were developed in the 1980s as data entry devices to interpret black stripes printed on white paper or on white objects. The barcodes were read by passing a hand-held scanner over the stripes, or by passing the labeled items over a barcode reader. A commonly used method for reading barcode symbols was by assigning to each character (number, letter, or symbol) a unique combination of black bars and intervening white spaces. Barcode readers illuminated the printed code symbols with a bright light that was absorbed by the black bars and reflected back from the white spaces to a photo-detector. The scanner transformed the patterns of light and dark into patterns of electrical signals that were converted into standard codes for the alphanumeric characters, and transmitted them to the computer. Used in other industries for some time, optically read barcodes began to find applications in patient care in the early 1980s when barcode readers began to be used to identify patients' laboratory specimen containers. By the late 1980s barcodes began to be used for to identify hospital patients by reading patients' coded wristbands and also to identify patients' charts, blood-bank samples, laboratory test samples, and x-ray folders by reading the stripes on their labels [111].

For clinical applications that allowed the use of barcode labels, a wand barcode reader was connected to a computer or communicated to a computer via radio frequency transmissions. This was a much faster than manual typing, and more accurate. In the 1980s handheld, microcomputer-based, programmable terminals permitted data input by barcode reader keypads. In 1986 Monahan et al. [187] at the University Hospitals of Cleveland reported the use of handheld barcode readers for the automated entry of nurse identification, and of nursing diagnoses of patients' problems selected from a list of 61 possible diagnoses. Childs [61] described how a nurse with a handheld terminal with a barcode reader could read the patient's identification number from the code stripes on the patient's wrist band before giving a medication in order to verify that the patient was due to receive that specific medication at that time. When the computer identified matching bar codes, it authorized giving the medication and recorded the date and time. Hughes [136] described a portable handheld terminal with an optical barcode reader, a display for selecting menus and for presenting patient data, and a keypad for entering and requesting information; communications between the portable terminal and its base unit were by radio frequency transmission. With the implementation of electronic medical records, Willard [287] described how their use of barcodes facilitated data entry and decreased data-entry errors. In the 2000s digitized optical storage devices began to make feasible more accurate and sophisticated identification methods, such as the automated reading of fingerprints and facial photographs. Poon and associates [212] at Brigham and Women's Hospital in Boston credited the use of barcodes for decreasing error rates in the transcription of patient care orders and in the administration of drugs.

In the mid-2000s, hospitals began to use radio frequency identification (RFID) tags as an alternative to barcodes for identifying patients during medical procedures, identifying x-rays and specimens, managing inventory, and locating equipment and supplies. Each tag incorporated a very tiny microchip encoded with a unique identification number. When the RFID reader and tag were within the required proximity, the reader broadcast radio-frequency waves that were picked up by a tiny antenna connected to the chip, activating the chip's integrated circuit and causing it to transmit its encoded data by radio waves back to the reader; on receiving the tag's data, the reader communicated it to a computer database that reported back the desired identification data [1, 135]. When used in a hospital to collect data on staff workflow in an attempt to increase the efficiency and effectiveness of patient care, RFID was sometimes considered by nursing staff to be a form of surveillance and could create social-organizational unrest [102]. An RFID positioning system was used in outpatient clinics to monitor patients and staff behavior; patients carried transponders from check in to check out, and the staff wore transponders throughout the study period [247].

Sponsored by RAND Europe, Van Orange and associates [268] published a comprehensive review of the opportunities for, and the barriers to, the use of RFID in health care systems, including some cost-benefit analyses of its use in hospitals. They reported that the most promising RFID applications were for identifying and tracking patients, sensing for the monitoring of patients, and for the automatic collection and transfer of data. They cautioned that radio waves from RFID embedded devices could interact with other wireless hospital equipment and electronic devices and cause some devices to fail when in close contact, thus necessitating careful monitoring when used in intensive care units, emergency care units, clinical laboratories, and in other high-tech patient care areas.

Telephones were used as computer terminals as early as the 1960s. Allen [2] described a medical telecommunications project established by the Division of Computer Research at the National Institutes of Health (NIH). A standard 12-push-button, touch-tone telephone with an acoustic coupler was used for the input of numbers and letters. The user pressed combinations of numbers that were transmitted to a remote, time-shared computer. Voice output in this project was from an audio-response vocabulary of less than 200 words stored in the computer. A pharmacy in the NIH Clinical Center used a program for providing information on intravenous drugs. A more advanced voice-response system was developed by Friedman [108] and associates at the University of Wisconsin. Using a touch-tone input unit to a minicomputer connected to a time-shared mainframe computer, it provided audiotaped or synthetic voice-generating output. A standard touch-tone telephone acted as the input terminal to a minicomputer and controlled the audiotape unit by starting and stopping the tape at the beginning and end locations of the specific message. The voice synthesizer generated intelligible speech by producing the phonemes that served as the building blocks of words and phrases, and provided a limited amount of continuous speech. The system was used for taking a patient's branching medical history, and for supporting a variety of treatment consultation programs. Smith [245] and associates at Boston University Medical Center developed a telephone-linked computer system capable of communicating with patients by using a voice synthesizer. The system regularly communicated with a group of patients with hypertension who required repeated visits to the clinic to monitor their treatment, reaching each patient using a set of preprogrammed, voice-synthesized questions. The patient responded by pressing the appropriate keys on the keypad of a standard touch-tone telephone, and the system provided a set of appropriate preprogrammed responses for voice feedback to the patient. The system received and decoded the patient's keyed responses, recorded them in the patient's file, and printed out a report of the telephone interaction for the patient's physician.

Speech recognition for the direct entry of natural language text is a very desirable way for computer users to communicate by voice with a computer; but it required developing technology to provide speech recognition for data input to the computer. The use of medical transcriptionists was always popular with physicians, since dictating their notes to a person permitted them to use a familiar mode of communication, and transferred the task of data entry to clerical personnel. Although the need for free-text entry by automated speech-recognition systems was obvious, speech recognition by computer was very difficult. The speech patterns of people in different regions had nuances in sentence structure; voices varied between individuals; and the waveforms of two persons who spoke the same words appeared uniquely different on a display oscilloscope. Spoken words tended to run together, and vocabulary was relatively unlimited. The 1980s saw the development of some limited speech-recognition input modes for human-to-computer interfacing [286]. Systems in the late 1980s digitized the analog-wave-forms of the voice signals and stored the stream of digital data. Using a library of stored voice patterns recorded by the user, the system was "trained" to match the input speech-pattern to one in its library and to associate it with its text equivalent. These early systems required the user to pause between individual words or linked phrases. They were first employed by highly specialized clinical users, such as radiologists who for some common procedures often used a relatively limited and mostly predefined vocabulary with repetitive descriptive phrases, such as for reporting negative chest x-rays. The first Kurzweil voice-recognition systems could accept up to 1,000 individual words spoken directly into the computer with a pause between each word; and if the user "trained" the computer then it could accept a spoken phrase as if it were a single word. The entered words were immediately displayed for verification and editing [256]. By the end of the 1980s the Kurzweil system could recognize up to 10,000 words of a user after a suitable training period, yet recognition of continuous speech was still not reliable.

In the 1990s progress was made toward continuous speech recognition that used more complex statistical methods of associations between words; these systems were used by pathologists for whom the ability to perform hands-free data entry was a major benefit [20]. In the 2000s some speech recognition devices, such as Nuances' Dragon Naturally Speaking, could correctly recognize most commonly spoken words. Lacson and Long [154] described the use of a mobile phone to enter spoken dietary records into a computer, classified the words used for food items and food classifiers, and developed algorithms that allowed users to automatically document the spoken diet records for each patient in natural language text. Chase et al. [57] found that, although it was feasible to capture clinical information in natural language, the semantic complexity and the frequent use of acronyms and abbreviations presented challenges to machine-based extraction of semantic content. Pogue [211] noted that Nuance Communications had released each year a new version of Dragon NaturallySpeaking, and the amount of "training" of the program by reading a standard script was decreasing. Nuance hoped with its Medical Practice Edition that physicians could dictate directly into their patients' electronic medical records [182]. In the 2000s the transmission of visual and spoken English text became available on many smartphones. By the end of 2010 Apple's iPhone provided a personal voice assistant, called "Siri", that could respond to English spoken questions on social and commercial activities as did some Android smartphones using domain knowledge from the internet.

Handwriting recognition devices began to be developed in the 1980s. A stylus resembling a pen was used to write individual letters, numbers, and punctuation symbols on mobile digitizing tablets called pen-pads. These usually had a wire grid on the tablet as a receiving antenna and a coil of wire in the pen as the sending antenna. The coil sent brief pulses of radio waves that were received by the grid, thus functioning as radio direction finders to identify a precise location. An alternative method used a resistor decoding technology that pulsed a voltage from each of the four sides of the tablet, creating a voltage gradient across a thin metal film that induced a voltage inside the pen, and thereby identified its location. The individual characters were read by being compared to stored patterns that were displayed for editing and then stored in the computer. Reading continuous cursive handwriting was much more difficult. However, by the end of the 1980s mobile I-pads and pen-pads were being developed that could recognize inscribed individual characters, marks, or checks; these were being tested for simple applications, such as for charting the administration of medications.

Image input initially involved the entry only of any associated descriptive text, but by the 2000s information derived directly from digital images began to be integrated with its text. Shatkay et al. [236] described their method of extracting and downloading figures from XML published format. The figures were segmented into sub-figures that were classified by four image types (such as graphical, microscopy, electrophoresis, and others) and were then further clustered into sub-groups by 46 features. A Bayes' classifier was used to match images to a base training-group of known classified images.

Data input by a microcomputer was increasingly used for databases that needed an online interactive terminal with programs allowing data entry to a database management system. Blumenthal [36] described the software developed for a Radio Shack microcomputer to format and enter data into a research database at the University of Michigan, Ann Arbor.

Data output by computers in the 1940s used primarily punched paper cards and Teletype printers. In the 1950s line printers and dot-matrix printers began to be connected to computers. Every computer had a number of interfaces for printers, which received their signals from the computer's external bus. Each interface had a port consisting of a buffer, where the data to be printed was stored while the data was being printed. In 1961 the IBM Selectric typewriter became available. In the 1960s ink-jet printers appeared that formed images of characters made by pushing tiny drops of ink out of a nozzle on to the paper. In 1971 Centronics introduced the impact dot-matrix printer that generated patterns of dots in the shape of alphabet numbers and letters. A microprocessor stored the data transmitted from the computer and directed the firing of an array of tiny pins contained in the print head; and the pins pressed against the inked ribbon to imprint the characters on the paper; by the mid-1980s dot-matrix printers dominated the market. Electrostatic printers had been developed in the 1950s, and in 1973 Xerox produced its xerographic page printer. In 1975 IBM introduced the first laser printer that employed a laser beam controlled by a microprocessor to imprint microscopic dots, line-by-line, on one full page of paper at a time. By the end of the 1970s laser printers had set the standards for computer printers.

1.7.1   Display Terminals and Clinical Workstations

Clinical workstation was the term applied in the 1970s to powerful minicomputers designed to take advantage of network file-sharing and multitasking capabilities. In 1985 Blois [25] anticipated a physician's personal workstation that could exploit graphics and windows capabilities and support the clinical decision-making process. By the late 1980s personal microcomputers, designed to operate as stand-alone systems began to have enough power to replace minicomputers as workstations [222]. Soon clinical workstations with powerful microprocessors were linked together in local area networks (LANs), satisfying the online human-machine interface requirements of physicians and nurses and their need for fast response times, ease of use, and versatility.

Although the Apple Macintosh computer had provided a graphical user interface (GUI) since 1985, this technology was not applied to clinical workstations until the end of the 1980s. Workstations were then developed to use multimodal (multimedia) communication interfaces including keyboard data entry, high-resolution displays, a GUI with an on-screen pointer controlled by a hand device such as a mouse or trackball, multiple data and graphics display windows, full image retrieval, and basic voice input and output [145]. By the late 1980s hospitals began to use hand-held or semi-portable terminals as bedside and as on-site terminals to allow caregivers to enter patient data at the point of care. The patient's vital signs and the records of medications given to the patient were entered directly into the patient's computer-based record. Mobile terminals eliminated the paper charting process, allowing nurses more time for other nursing functions. By the end of the 1980s a medical information bus, a standardized connection that allowed any vendor's bedside technology to communicate with the medical information system (MIS) database, was being developed to take data from bedside and mobile terminals and integrate the data into the MIS database [91].

In 1984 McDonald [175] at the Indiana University School of Medicine reported a network of workstations connected to a central VAX 117/80 server. Each workstation carried all its own programs, tables, and medical records for several hundred patients. In addition to programs for prescribing medications, entering orders, and recording patient's diagnoses, each workstation provided medical information for generating flow sheets, executing reminder rules, facilitating ad hoc retrievals, and reporting facts about drugs, tests, and differential diagnoses. Tolchin [262] described the installation at Johns Hopkins Hospital (JHH) of several clinical workstations to support their expanding, networked, clinical information system. Consisting of Sun Microsystems equipment running UNIX and AT&T UNIX on personal computers, these workstations could access the minicomputer systems, as well as any server system in the JHH network. Schultz [230] at Dartmouth-Hitchcock Medical Center developed a clinical workstation that:(1) provided a uniform connection to multiple clinical subsystems, (2) operated each workstation independently although still as a part of the whole system, (3) was modifiable by the user as to its functions, (4) was linked to decision-support tools, and (5) had the ability to store a request for information that would be executed at a specified time (such as for automatically requesting and plotting daily electrolyte test values).

By the end of the 1980s clinical workstations were being developed by some large medical centers and for the multihospital information systems of both the Department of Defense and the Veterans Administration. Typical client/server computing systems were being designed so that the *client* workstation handled local data manipulation to meet individual user needs, and the *server* computer handled database functions, shared data and software, and provided backup and security. In the 1990s workstation terminals were developed to more efficiently support entry and retrieval of data, text, and images; these workstations had the abilities to communicate within the database-management system. Cimino and associates [64] at Columbia University in New York reported developing a prototype workstation. Built using Internet client-server architecture, it was used by their surgical staff to maintain patient lists, and to download and review their patients' clinical data including laboratory, radiology, and pharmacy; it also served a wide variety of other purposes including sign-out routines.

Video display terminals were greatly advanced by the end of the 1960s with their use in cathode ray tube (CRT) and television video display terminals which permitted direct interactive dialogue between the computer and the user. Data entry using display terminals involved three basic techniques: (1) Typewriter-type keyboard entry in which letters and numbers were individually entered; (2) List or menu selection in which preformatted phrases were entered by various input methods, such as by touching the screen or selector buttons, by using a light pen or a mouse or trackball; and (3) Function-key entry where multiple overlays determined the sets of data entered [240]. Although menu selection of displayed items or the use of overlays allowed using structured formats for data entry and minimized the need to acquire typing skills, they constrained the ability to quickly enter a complex or lengthy statement. Yet with such interactive display terminals, physicians and nurses began to use computer-based information systems without clerical intermediaries. Usually a physician interacted with a display terminal by first entering an identification code, and the display responded by showing the physician's name, the date and time of the interaction. Since most input transactions by the physician involved a single patient at a time, the physician entered the patient's name which then would be displayed on the computer, along with the patient's identification number and perhaps the hospital bed to which the patient had been assigned. The physician then might enter a diagnosis, a new examination finding, an order for some service such as a laboratory test, or other data. This information would be displayed back to the physician for verification and for correction of any errors. When approved by the physician as being correct, it would be stored in the patient's computer-stored record; a copy could be printed out if the patient also had a paper-based chart [242].

Graphic displays generated from the data in a patient's record were an important requirement for clinicians. Plotting graphically a set of variables, such as blood chemistry test results as they changed over time, was a useful way to monitor a patient's progress during an illness. Blum [35], working with the Time Oriented Database (TOD) developed at Stanford University, described the problems associated with the implementation of graphics on a display terminal without special graphics capabilities: (1) The cursor could move only left to right, top to bottom; thus graph positions had to be computed and stored before the graph was drawn; (2) Clinical activity tended to occur in bursts, so values usually distributed non-uniformly over a graph; and (3) Causal relationships typically involved more than two variables, creating the unmet need to display several variables and episodes in a single image. Most computer-based patient record systems generated flow sheets, displayed visually or printed out, as an efficient way of presenting large arrays of patient data over long periods of time. The limitations of the displays then available and the need for more flexible cursor control were not met until the 1980s, when graphical displays of patient data became readily available with the advent of terminals with graphical user interfaces.

Mouse selector devices, developed in the US and Germany in the 1960s were first used with computer graphical interfaces in Xerox PARC in 1972–1973, allowing the user to select and move data on a display not only up, down, and sideways, but also diagonally, with a greater selection choice than a displayed menu could provide. The mouse was held with one hand and rolled across a flat surface to direct its pointer on the screen; buttons were pressed on the mouse to control its activity. A microprocessor inside the mouse transmitted a packet of data when it detected a change in the position of the mouse or in the state of its buttons. A trackball was the equivalent of a stationary, turned-over mouse, and used the thumb, index, and middle fingers to manipulate the ball.

Display monitors developed in the 1970s permitted a user to enter data by directly interacting with the displayed screen. Some touch-sensitive screens used an optical system in which a user's finger interrupted crossing beams of infrared light, and the intersection of a vertical with a horizontal beam identified the location of the touch point. Other touch screens used a capacitance-sensing mechanism; when a user touched the screen, it changed the capacitance value of that particular area of the screen, but the finger was a relatively coarse data-selector device. More acceptable was the light pen that employed a light sensor in its tip that, when focused at a point on the display, sensed the screen's phosphor glow and located its position on an x-y axis. Keyboard selections from computer-displayed templates of structured data-sets began to be used for data entry, such as by physicians entering orders for medical procedures; for data output, such as by keyboard selections from computer displays of standard phrases that radiologists often used to report normal ("negative") x-ray examinations; or for routine statements, such as those commonly used in patients' discharge summaries.

In the 1970s computer terminals began to be located at the nursing stations in the hospitals, and some were placed in the outpatient clinics. In the 1980s some hospitals began to have computer terminals stationed at the patient's bedside. The ability of nurses to access the patient's computer-based record directly at the point of care was expected to improve the quality and documentation of nursing care at the bedside, and to save nursing time as well [249]. The first bedside terminals were "dumb" terminal extensions from a host computer. Later, "intelligent" or "smart" terminals appeared; these contained their own microcomputers with programs for transmitting (downloading) the patient record into the terminal for local data entry, and then returning (uploading) the updated record back to the central computer's database for permanent storage and for subsequent use at other terminals. Pesce [208] described the use of bedside terminals, which contained microcomputers that were interfaced by a local area network to the hospital-wide information system. Hospital personnel used display terminals with keyboards to select data from displayed menus of information; this allowed them to record directly into the computer, at the time of caring for the patient, the patient's vital signs, nursing observations, and the medications given. Printouts from a terminal located at the bedside could include graphs of the patient's vital signs and a variety of useful reports.

Structured data entry and reporting were credited by Johnson [140] to have been initiated by Slack et al. [243, 244], who used a Laboratory Instrument Computer (LINC) to allow patients to directly enter their medical history as responses to a series of individual questions displayed on the computer screen. Patients responded to each question by pressing a key on the keyboard corresponding to a response of "Yes", or a "No", or "I do not know", or "I do not understand". For a "Yes" response a second series of displays appeared with a second-level series of questions. Slack also employed open-ended questions, such as "What is your occupation?", and the patient typed in the response using the full keyboard. Greenes [120], and associates at Harvard Medical School, developed computer-generated, structured-output summaries of patient data acquired during ambulatory care visits, by selecting appropriate data-sets from a displayed menu of templates. The advances in entering and retrieving textual data and visual images by employing mobile communications technology are described in Sect. 1.7.

Visual displays of data output appeared at the end of the 1950s, and used a matrix of dots to form typewriter-like characters on oscilloscope screens. These were replaced in the late 1960s by cathode ray tube (CRT) displays in which an electron gun in the neck of the tube projected a beam of electrons that were emitted from the surface of the cathode and were pulled towards the anode that surrounded the bell of the picture tube. When the beam struck the front screen, which was coated on the inside with phosphors, this area of the screen briefly glowed. Varying the voltage on the anode modified the intensity of the brightness of the dot-of-light (a pixel) on the screen. The electron stream passed through an electromagnetic yoke, or a deflection device, on its way to the screen. The computer, by varying the strengths of the yoke's vertical and horizontal magnetic fields, deflected the electron beam and thereby generated and positioned visible characters anywhere on the phosphor display screen. The image was maintained as the monitor's local memory repeatedly scanned the display to refresh the phosphor glow. In the 1960s characters were formed on the screen by controlling the electron beam with short, line drawing movements or by a matrix of dots. A vector generator was added to draw lines by designating coordinate positions from one point to the next.

Raster-scan displays, such as were used in television tubes, began to be employed in the 1980s in personal computers. As the beam moved across the screen, line-by-line (raster), starting from the upper left corner to the lower right corner, its intensity varied from pixel to pixel and thereby generated an image on the screen. In the 1980s monitors for early microcomputers were mostly monochrome, with white letters on a black screen. By the mid-1980s color monitors usually used three separate electron guns to provide red, green, and blue colored signals striking appropriate triads of phosphor dots; and three dots in red, green, and blue colors made up a pixel. In the 1980s display monitors incorporated graphics microprocessor chips.

Flat-panel display screens were developed in the 1980s. Liquid-crystal displays (LCD) with flat-panel screens consisted of a matrix of twisted crystals sandwiched between two light polarizers. When a voltage was applied to a crystal, it untwisted and allowed polarized light to pass through, strike the rear polarizer, and be absorbed, making the addressed pixel look dark compared to the rest of the panel. The use of back lighting increased the contrast and readability of LCD displays. Gas plasma displays operated by exciting neon gas, or mixtures of neon and argon, by applying a voltage using a matrix of electrodes separated from the gas in a way to allow individual dots (pixels) to be activated. Electroluminescent (EL) displays consisted of a thin panel that contained a film of a phosphor that was sandwiched between a front, thin transparent film of a dielectric material similar to a semiconductor, and a back reflective dielectric material. By applying a voltage through a grid of electrodes, each pixel could be switched on; different phosphors were used to produce different colors.

Computer graphics generally refers to the technology that enters, processes, and displays graphs and pictures by digital computers; this requires complex programming. Programs from mathematical representations stored in the computer's memory generate the graphics displays. Three-dimensional objects require specialized complex representations of geometric shapes and patterns. Graphics displays are available as character-based, vector-based, or bit-mapped displays; bit-mapped displays are most suitable for digitized pictures. Graphic displays are often used when retrieving related large data sets from a medical database, such as the reports of panels of multiple laboratory tests collected over long periods of time. To aid in their interpretation, such data were often presented as charts and graphic displays, to make a patient's time-trend in data more easily used for clinical decision-making. Bull [51] noted that physicians could handle large amounts of data most easily and efficiently if the data were presented to them in the form of a graph. Connelly [75] also reported that computer-generated graphical displays for data aggregation and summarization could effectively convey the significance of laboratory results, since visual relationships portrayed by graphs and charts could be more readily grasped, and abnormal results and the degree of abnormality could be seen at a glance. As an example, Connelly cited the Technicon SMA-12 chemistry analyzer that used this type of display.

For some specialized clinical data-input functions that required the use of graphs, such as might be used when a patient was anesthetized, a digitizing graphics tablet was developed as the interface for computer record keeping during anesthesia management. Newbower et al. [197] described a graphics tablet that used magnetostrictive technology to detect the position of a special ball-point pen anywhere on its 11-by-11 in. active surface, representing 2,200 by 2,200 points. If a standard anesthesia record form was placed on the surface of the tablet and used as the routine paper anesthesia record, the entered information was automatically digitized, immediately interpreted, and in some cases displayed to the anesthetist; it could then be stored for subsequent hard-copy printout.

Radial graphic displays were used by Williams [289, 294, 295] for multiple test results that helped to support rapid pattern-recognition by the physician when examining the changes in the shape and skew of the displayed pattern of results. If all the test results were within normal limits, when the dots representing the test values were connected, a normal polygon would be formed with the number of sides corresponding to the number of test results. Abnormal test results would distort the polygon. For comparison both could be displayed on a radial arrangement with dots indicating the normal and the abnormal ranges. Williams believed that graphic radial displays were readily adaptable to enhance pattern recognition of the results of multiple tests, and effectively depicted temporal trends in a series of results. Cole [70] described the essential dimensions of a graphical display as its "integrality" and the "meaningfulness" its information design created by showing all essential data; for example, a radial graph usually presented more meaningful information than line graph. Computer graphics and digital image processing evolved as two different technologies aimed at different applications. Computer graphics were usually used for generating physical models, whereas digital imaging was used to capture pictures such as x-rays. Merging these two technologies was called *visualization*. In medicine, applications of visualization were applied to prosthesis design, radiation treatment planning, brain structure research, three-dimension modeling, and others.

With the advent of medical "expert" systems, data acquisition went from formatted and menu-based textual data entry to intelligent data entry. For example, a program at the LDS Hospital combined a centralized patient database and a medical knowledge base, and used these two databases to create data entry screens that fit the individual needs of the specific patient. The system also suggested procedures and treatments for the patient's problems [215].

In the 1970s computer terminals began to be located in medical offices and hospitals; in the 1990s mobile terminals became common place; and in the 2010s electronic health records linked to smartphones and electronic tablets became universal.

1.7.2 Mobile Terminals

By the late 1980s health care professionals began to use handheld or semi-portable terminals on-site to enter patient data at the point of care. Mobile cellular (cell) phones evolved in the 1990s. In addition to the usual telephone voice communication capabilities, they had key pads that allowed users to enter text, store frequently used numbers, send and receive text messages. Cell phones soon developed access to high-speed networks and to the Internet. Many cell phones had cameras and supported "Bluetooth" head sets for hands-free communications.

Smartphones were developed in the 2000s with electronic, computer-like operating systems. Powered by rechargeable lithium ion batteries that could be very small and light, they contained an electrolyte in which lithium ions passed from the cathode to the anode inside the battery, and then went out on a wire in an external circuit to provide electrical energy for the phone. Recharging the battery forced the ions back in the opposite direction to the original electrolyte. Broida [46] reported that some smartphone manufacturers were changing to induction charging of batteries that just required placing the phone on a special surface. Smartphones became available with computer operating systems in a variety of shapes and sizes and included small QWERTY keyboards; interfaces for mobile telephone, email, cameras and video; high-resolution display screens for graphics and images; and Universal Serial Bus (USB) capabilities to connect to computers. In 2003 Skype, a free-of-cost, mobile Internet service was introduced that allowed users of 3G mobile smartphones to communicate voice calls and images internationally. In 2005 YouTube inaugurated a wireless video-sharing, web-based storage on which users could upload, view, and share videos. Bought by Google in 2006, in 2010 YouTube provided more than two billion page views per day [122].

In 2007 the International Telecommunication Union (ITU) added WiMAX technology that included multiple wireless, broadband Internet services, including Skype, and Voice over Internet Protocol (VOIP) that delivered low cost broadband services. In 2010 Skype was acquired by Microsoft and became a dominant Internet provider of audio and video communications. The word, Skype, also began to be used as a verb. By the end of 2010 smartphones had evolved to provide capabilities for Web searching, connections to television, GPS navigation, and social networking; and they had introduced a variety of new applications such as Apple's Siri that used a voice-recognition program to let users answer emails by speaking, and to direct a variety of actions. In 2010 among leading manufacturers in the United States of 3G and 4G mobile smartphones were Apple's iPhone, Google's Android, Motorola's Droid X, and Microsoft Windows phone. Research-In-Motion's (RIM's) BlackBerry (made in Canada), HTC's Inspire (made in Taiwan), Samsung's Galaxy (made in Japan), and Nokia's Symbian operating system (made in Finland) were also among the leaders in the smartphone market in the United States. Among the leading wireless carriers were AT&T, Google, Sprint, t-Mobile, and Verizon [62].

In 2010 fourth generation (4G) wireless technology, some with Long Term Evolution (LTE) services, began to be marketed for smartphones, tablets, and laptops, offering between four and ten times faster performance than 3G networks, with peak speeds of 10 mbps or more. Able to service larger gigabyte loads at a lower cost, 4G technology provided mobile voice over Internet Protocol (VoIP) and was expected to offer higher-definition (HD) voice and three-dimensional video [180]. However, since 4G technology operated on different wireless frequencies than did prior 3G mobile phones, they required different connectivity technology. Sprint announced that advances in wireless communication made its WiMax 4G network up to ten times faster than its 3G service; and Wireless Gigabit (WiGi) Alliance was reported to provide faster transmission speeds of up to 6 gigabits-per-second [296]. The software development, HTML5, allowed offline storage of information and Internet utilities, and used markup programming that could add video to a Web page [189]. By the end of 2010 some smartphones, including those provided by Samsung and HTC, were powered with ultrafast, multi-core processors, using AT&T's 4G Long-Term Evolution (LTE) networks, and with large 4.5 in. displays [54, 153, 299]. In 2010 the Apple's iOS and the Google's Android operating system were the leaders for multimedia software applications in the mobile communications market [55]. Ellison [96] reported that the Verizon iPhone, to be released in 2011, would be competitive with the Apple iPhone. Microsoft announced its operating system for MS Windows 8 for release in 2012 was designed to better support mobile applications for smartphones, computer desktops, laptops, and for tablets [302].

Electronic tablets and digital notepads were introduced in the 2000s, equipped with electronic and wireless facilities similar to smartphones, but with larger screens that were better suited for displaying full text pages and videos. By 2010 electronic tablets with up to 9–10 in. diagonal display screens included Acer Iconia, Amazon Kindle Fire, Apple iPad, Asus Eee Pad, Barnes & Noble NOOK, Google Android, HTC Flyer, Lenevo ThinkPad, Motorola Xoom, Nokia, Samsung Galaxy, Sony Tab, Toshiba Thrive, and Vizio Tablet. Among the leaders in the electronic tablet market were Apple, Motorola, Toshiba, Acer, Samsung, and Dell. Apple released its Apple iPad 3 in 2012, and reported selling in the first quarter more than 35 million tablets in China alone [297, 300]. Intel was reported to be developing advanced technologies for a laptop hybrid called an ultrabook that would operate entirely on its microprocessors. By the late 2010s, laptop computers were replacing some desktop computers since computer laptops were smaller and, as a result, portable. However, laptops usually had smaller display screens and used rechargeable batteries as their power source. Serwer [235] noted that consumer preference for electronic tablets was replacing personal computers, and the preference for smartphones was revolutionizing the economy and disrupting all manners of businesses, including the laptop, personal computer, and electronic tablet businesses, as well as the social media, music, publishing, television, and advertising industries.

1.7.3   User Computer Interfacing

It was evident from the beginning that the acceptance of computer-based information systems by health professionals would depend on the computer terminals they would be using to enter and retrieve data. The computer terminal constituted the critical human-machine interface for users, since it allowed what could be described as something similar to a conversation mode [199]. However, a very serious problem was that humans and computers communicated in different languages. Researchers soon found it necessary to study carefully at least two factors that would significantly affect the user satisfaction with the system: (1) What kinds of "smart" computer terminals would the various health professionals be asked to use for entering and retrieving data? (2) How many terminals would be needed, and where would they be best located? Human factors certainly needed to be considered in order to select the computer terminals best suited for the various users of a medical information system [19]. For some users the human-machine interface controlled their major perception of the system.

Although clerical personnel could function fairly well using typewriter-type keyboards, many physicians were not trained to type. Physicians usually preferred voice dictation, although some would accept video display terminals with light-pen or mouse-pointer selectors for data entry and retrieval. Many systems supplemented the computer keyboards with special function keys. Some even modified their display screens by placing a vertical array of touch buttons along one side of the screen which allowed the selection of corresponding words or phrases from a variety of displayable menus. As an early example of the use of selector buttons, Seed [232] at Montefiore Hospital in New York City prepared a comprehensive set of checklists, and used a keyboard that had 30 buttons with labels at the left of each button. The labels also were projected by the display tube for each data set. The user entered data by pushing the button to the right of the desired label. The computer recognized the data entered by identifying which button had been pushed, and transmitted the data to the remote computer over telephone lines. Without typing any data, simply by making selections from the various menus, the user could generate the patient's record on the display screen and then print out a copy for the patient's paper-based office record [225].

It was evident that computer displays needed to have the flexibility to present data items that would meet the needs of a variety of users. Physicians wanted to use their personal order sets; they wanted test and procedure results presented in tables and trends. Also they wanted patient roster lists, patient records, and notification of alerts and alarms. Nurses needed check lists of procedures and medications to be given to their patients. Administrators wanted data on groups of patients for various analyses used for planning and budgeting. To customize data input terminals for health care professionals, different levels of complexity of video displays were developed for different degrees of user expertise. These were usually designed as orientation and training displays for first-time users, or as fully loaded data displays for experienced users. Custom-tailored displays with individualized content for frequent users could permit a full page of data to be entered with a few strokes of a finger, such as for a set of commonly used routine orders for a patient, sometimes referred to by physicians as their personal order set. The acceptable length of time for a computer to answer a query varied. For interactive terminals where physicians carried on a dialog with the computer, sub-second response times were necessary to complete the entry of a series of orders for a patient within an acceptable time. In the emergency room, a response to a query about an urgently sick patient might be needed within a few seconds, whereas a few days might be an acceptable wait for past-history information about a patient with a chronic or recurring condition.

As early as the mid-1960s, the Lockheed/Technicon hospital information system (HIS) used television-tube video terminals that displayed 24 rows of 40 double-sized characters, for use with a light-pen data selector containing a push-button switch; and also had a keyboard with additional function keys. Some physicians readily accepted this mode of computer interface for their hospital practice. In 1968 Siekert and associates at the Mayo Clinic reported on a test of the direct entry of medical orders by a group of 14 internists using Technicon terminals; the physicians responded that they thought computers would speed the retrieval of patient records, that the use of computers for such retrieval was inevitable, and that the computer reliability was sufficient [240]. The medical information system (MIS) at the NIH's Clinical Center also used an adaptation of the Technicon system with its television display terminals and push-buttons and light-pen selectors [99].

Barnett et al. [15] pointed out that the major need for an MIS was the development of acceptable mechanisms for the entry of information into the computer. He advocated using of online interactive terminals for information capture, because they permitted a high degree of quality control at the time of input, and because many kinds of information could be collected more efficiently by interactive techniques. Although Barnett's COSTAR used paper encounter forms for physicians to enter patient data for office visits, in 1970 Barnett's group described an operational system in the hypertension clinic of the MGH with terminals organized for a high degree of physician-computer interaction. The physicians used a CRT terminal located in the examining room that was connected to a time-shared computer system. Presented with a display of data items, the physicians selected a topic on which they wished to comment by touching a metallic strip overlying their choice on the display screen. The action of touching the display completed an electric circuit and caused a code to be transmitted to the computer that indicated the choice selected; and the computer display verified the item selected. When satisfied with the selections, the physicians proceeded to the next display frame and could choose history, physical examination, laboratory, or therapy. After entry of the data by the physician, the progress note was printed on a typewriter terminal [120].

The Kaiser Permanente medical information system (MIS) used cathode ray tube (CRT) visual display terminals with light pen selectors designed by Sanders Associates. The unit was capable of displaying approximately 1,000 characters in a vertical area about 7×10 in. It could display 20 lines with 52 characters on each line. Rather than having the long axis of the display horizontal, the Sanders display had its long axis vertical to make the displays look more like what physicians saw on the pages of the paper-based medical record. The user activated the system by inserting a user identification card into a reader on the terminal [242]. In the early 1970s, Control Data Corporation released their Digiscribe CRT display unit that required a user's finger to touch the screen or keyboard for data entry. Spectra Medical Systems used a color video display unit with light pen selector and a keyboard for data entry [9].

Williams et al. [290–293] at the University of Illinois Urbana Champaign developed his hospital information system called Program Logic for Automatic Teaching Operation (PLATO), using an interactive terminal with a touch-sensitive, plasma display screen designed with a 16×16 grid. When intersecting infrared light beams in the grid were intercepted by a user's finger, the computer recognized the position of the interruption. The terminal permitted input of data from a variety of visual displays programmed as frames, which automatically changed as terms were selected from each display. Called a displayed variable-phrase keyboard [58], this approach allowed the use of standardized language and terminology. The frame on the display screen was composed of vertical pages of terms and phrases. The selection of a term or phrase from one page resulted in the appearance of a second page of modifying terms. This process could be continued for five pages, resulting in the construction of a sentence. Although a relatively slow process, it provided the capability of generating common clinical phrases, such as those used in personal order sets and in much of the data entered in a physician's practice. The PLATO system provided interactive data entry for patient histories and for physicians' physical examinations of patients. Graphics displays of laboratory test results, problem lists, care plans, and progress notes were available either encoded or in natural language. The PLATO terminals were installed in several physicians' offices in the community, in the county blood bank, in a clinical pathology laboratory, and in the University of Illinois McKinley Student Health Service [59,60]. An unusual feature of Williams' system was the radial clocklike, polar-orientation display of patients' laboratory test results, which yielded distinctive patterns characteristic of specific disorders [289].

In the 1980s Friedman [107] concluded that the existing computer terminals failed to achieve acceptance because: (1) Many were poorly engineered and had frequent mechanical breakdowns; (2) They had typewriter keyboards rather than more specialized input modes; (3) Computer terminals often were placed in out-of-way locations; (4) Computer response time often was slow; (5) The physician was often required to take part in a long technical dialogue; and (6) Computer terminals were expensive. With the advent of microprocessors, more sophisticated methods were developed to minimize the need for typing by keyboard and to encourage the direct entry of data by the physicians and nurses. Womble et al. [301] described the use of a microprocessor-based terminal at Brooks Air Force Base, Texas, and reported that the microcomputer could fill the screen at a rate of 960 characters-per-second, or about ten times faster than prior terminals coupled to a host computer. The users' requests to the central database were stored on a floppy disk for retrieval at any later time if desired, either via the display or the printout.

In the early 1980s, several groups were testing interactive visual display terminals. Barnett's group evaluated microprocessors with video display terminals with 24 rows by 132 columns of characters and a mouse-type or touch-screen data selector. To facilitate computer-physician interaction, entry was in codable form for medications and laboratory test data, and in natural-language text for physical examination findings [177]. Ash [5] and associates developed a portable, self-contained microprocessor system that allowed patient data input, storage, retrieval, and printout in the examining room during the patient's office visit. A variety of function keys directed the computer program to the particular data-entry needs of the user; for example, the notation-problems function key permitted the entry by physicians and nurses of their progress notes, allowed linkage of data to the patient's problems, and facilitated generation of a problem-oriented record.

Esterhay et al. [99] compared three terminal systems operating in the early 1980s. One was Weed's Problem Oriented MIS (PROMIS), designed with the patient record as its primary focus. The PROMIS terminal displayed 24 rows by 80 columns of characters; every other row was sensitive to finger touch for selecting choices from a variety of frames of displayed functions such as "Prob List" (problem list), "Cur RX" (current treatment), and "Outst Test" (outstanding tests). Once entered, patient data would appear in the display and could be manipulated by the functions shown in the touch-selectable lines. The others compared by Esterhay were the Duke Hospital Information System and the NIH Clinical Center System, both designed to focus on the information needs of their hospitals. The Duke system used an IBM CRT display terminal with 24 lines of 80 characters each, a light pen, and a keyboard with programmed function keys; users could select from more than 1,000 display screens of pre-formatted items using the light pen for computer data entry or retrieval or enter data by the keyboard. The NIH system used a modified Technicon display terminal.

McDonald [175] developed a display in which a fixed data input form was shown on the screen. The user moved from field to field on the displayed form to enter data, similar to filling out a paper form; and this was considered better than when the user remained at a fixed point on the screen and the input questions moved up the screen. By the late 1980s, Blum and associates at Stanford University were developing a program called RADK that could automatically extract the useful information and produce summaries of patients' records [88]. Using time-oriented patient records from the ARAMIS rheumatology database, the program automatically extracted symptoms, physical examination findings, laboratory test results, descriptors, and diagnoses to generate a patient record summary; an interactive display allowed the user to review the summary data.

Streveler [251] evaluated the use of visual displays for clinical applications, and proposed the following principles for their design: (1) Minimize the number of eye fixations required to find the needed data; (2) Minimize the distance of the total eye movement path. (3) Minimize the number of changes in direction of the eye-movement path. (4) Minimize the number of wide eye movements required. Furthermore, well-designed displays should have positional, sequential, and semantic consistency as to content; that is, they should be consistent in format so that the same item (for example, the patient's name) was always located in the same place in the display; similar fields of data should be arranged in the same logical sequence; and data items and labels should be readily understood.

Elting [97] and associates compared the efficiency and accuracy of data entry achieved by two systems: (1) formatted screens that displayed lists of the data items (for example, patient name, or diagnosis code); after each item the user entered the appropriate data; and (2) prompted dialog that displayed menus from which the user selected the appropriate items to fit the patient's data They reported that neither system was consistently superior, and wide variation was demonstrated according to the type of data being processed. User preference was not predictive of superior performance for either entering or editing data.

Valenta [267] at the University of Illinois in Chicago used a Q-methodology to study physician acceptance of information technologies in the health care workplace. Finding that physicians could be categorized as (1) independently minded, self-motivated, and concerned, or (2) inexperienced and worried, Valenta recommended varying the amount of time to introduce physicians to new technologies and train them in their use. It was evident that computer displays needed to have the flexibility to present data items that would meet the needs of a variety of users.

1.8 Computer Communications

Computer-based information systems employ a variety of data communications technologies. London [172] described a cluster of computers as either loosely coupled as in a distributed database management system, or tightly coupled to a central computer. The wiring and switching methods originally used by public telephone networks were optimized for voice transmission, and this limited the transmission speed of data to a range between 300 and 9,600 bits-per-second (baud). A computer communicating with another computer over telephone lines required a modem (modulator-demodulator) to modulate the electronic pulses representing digital data into analog signals impressed on the telephone carrier signal. To receive the data, the analog audible signals needed to be demodulated back into the digital pulse form. Modems varied in their speed to transfer data. The number of times each second the line changed the signal was referred to as its modulation or baud rate.

Circuit switching was the usual mode public telephone systems used to transmit voice and data over long-distance telephone lines as a continuous stream. With this technique, once a data transmission was started, it would tie up the phone line during the entire time that one message was being sent, since the circuit could be broken only after all the data had been transferred. This was not well suited to many scientific applications, where bursts of data were often interspersed with periods of silence. For example, a scientist might transmit a batch of data characterizing a problem, then wait for the remote machine to return the answer. These periods of line idleness were costly and prevented others from using the circuits during the interim.

The theoretical basis for packet switching for computer communications on telephone lines was introduced in 1948 by Shannon, who considered digital bits as the fundamental units of information, and developed the transmission of messages in the form of closely spaced pulses that were equivalent to groups of digital bits [112]. That led to the development of pulse-code modulation and the use of pulsed digitized signals [210]. In 1964 Baran at the Rand Corporation used pulse-code modulation, and equipped each junction node in a distributed network that connected different computer sites with small, high speed, digital communications computers. The computer nearest the sender divided up the outgoing message into small packets of digital bits. Each packet was coded within its original message as to its sequence, where it came from and its recipient's address. In packet messaging, the packets were then routed as separate message blocks through intervening communications computers, so packets from one message might be routed over different accessible lines, or packets from different messages could be interweaved on one common transmission line. Finally, packets would arrive at the computer where they were addressed to go, and there the packets were then reassembled into the original message [151]. The receiving computer reassembled the message packets and reconstructed the message. The first modem transfer protocol program used by computers to send and receive data files by way of intervening communication computers was developed in 1977 by Christensen [179]. Thus with packet switching, multiple messages in the form of digital packets could be sent over one line. Digital packets soon replaced analog signals in telephone, radio, and satellite communications, and packet switching was eventually adopted by major wide area networks such as ARPANET, Telenet, and Tymnet [151]. Early computer hardware and software had to meet specific communications requirements, or protocols, for each remote system to be connected. Serial data transfer over an asynchronous line (where one wire carried all the data) had requirements for data transmission speed, the width of each datum, the start and stop signals used to control the flow of data between computers, data transfer methods, and error checking rules used for transmitting the data. The American Standard Code for Information Interchange (ASCII), established in 1967 as a binary, 8-bit code designed to represent all characters used in information exchange, was the most common standard used in the United States for serial data transfer.

Twisted pairs of wires were the early usual medium for data transmission by telephone lines, with a narrow bandwidth that was adequate for transmitting analog voice signals. Pairs of copper wires were twisted together to decrease interference between adjacent pairs of wires. Coaxial cables were later used for higher-speed wideband transmission; these were a single copper wire sheathed in plastic insulation and wrapped in metal or wire mesh for electromagnetic shielding.

Optical fibers, invented in the early 1950s, were glass fibers no thicker than a strand of human hair. In 1970 Corning Glass developed an optical fiber that could conduct light for at least 1 km [39]. Light signals traveled through the core of the fiber and were reflected back and forth from the core's boundary with the cladding; thus the fiber guided light rays along its length [78]. AT&T pioneered further development of optic fiber technology at its Bell Laboratories. However, telephone companies did not begin to offer services with fiber-optic lines until 1983. Analog voice or data signals were converted by an optic transmitter into pulses of light from a laser or a light-emitting diode flashing on and off at very high speeds. Amplifiers and repeaters were required in early fiber-optic systems to convert the attenuated light pulses to electronic signals, give them a boost of electric power, convert them back to amplified light pulses, and send them on through the next section of cable. Immune to electrical or magnetic interference, fiber optic lines provided cleaner, quicker, and more reliable transmission of text, voice, and images. The higher frequency of light carried more information than could telephone-wire voice signals. One single strand of glass fiber could carry 24,000 telephone conversations simultaneously, as compared to 4,000 conversations per pair of coaxial cables, or 24 for a pair of copper wires. By the late 1980s fiber optic technology had improved to the point that images could travel hundreds of kilometers without amplifiers or repeaters, using fibers transparent to conducting infrared light [89]. By the end of the 1980s fiber optic cables were rapidly replacing copper coaxial cables in telephone and communication services. This development spurred the creation of networks of integrated data systems. By the end of the 1990s fiber optic cables, some the thickness of fire hoses and packed with hundreds of thousands of miles of optical fibers, were laid everywhere including along the floors of the oceans; they carried phone,

Internet and Web traffic flowing from continent to continent, with speeds approaching that of light depending on their bandwidths and data capacity.

United States Senator Al Gore proposed a network of information superhighways linking the nation by fiber optic cables in the 1980s. Some broadband fiber optic networks began to be introduced into large medical centers by the addition of video channels to standard baseband LAN technology. This permitted linking text, voice, and video; transmitting data to and from minicomputers and laser printers; and communicating images to and from image scanners, digitized x-ray equipment, television monitors, and facsimile machines. In 1991 Senator Gore again proposed an information super-highways network linking the nation by fiber-optic cables, and the U. S. Congress passed the High Performance Computing & Communications (HPCC) Act. Dr. Donald A.B. Lindberg, in addition to then being the Director of the National Library of Medicine, became the first Director of HPCC's National Coordinating Office in 1992 [239].

Although it was important for networks to be concerned about the wires or cables that connected computers, it became even more important how the computers communicated data with each other – that is, the rules or protocols they used governing the format, response, time, message length, and error handling of messages. Orthner [202] pointed out that the data processing industry had minimized the use of the analog voice channels of the telephone industry and generally preferred to install coaxial cables; as a result there were myriad LANs, each with its own proprietary communications protocol. A decade later, Orthner et al. [204] described network protocols as required for the standardization of the variety of processes involved in data communication.

Communications standards for both the networks and for their transmission of data became essential requirements for the exchange of data between different computer systems. In the late 1970s the International Standards Organization (ISO) fostered the development of the Open Systems Interconnection (OSI) Reference Model. The ISO/OSI communications model used seven layers for the exchange of data between computers within network systems. Layer one, the physical layer, included interface hardware devices, modems, and communication lines, and the software driver for each communication device that activated and deactivated the electrical and mechanical transmission channels to various pieces of equipment. Layer two, the data-link layer, provided for transfer of blocks of data between data-terminal equipment connected to a physical link, and included data sequencing, flow control, and error detection to assure error-free communication. Layer three, the network control layer, provided routing and switching of messages between adjacent nodes in the network. Layer four, the transport layer, provided an end-to-end control of the transmission channel once the path was established. Layer five, the session-control layer, opened communications, established a dialogue, and maintained the connection including the control and synchronization for the transfer of messages between two computers. Layer six, the presentation layer, insured the message was transferred in a coded form that the receiving computer could interpret. Layer seven, the application-user layer, the only part of the system apparent to the user, provided services that facilitated data exchange between application processes on different computers [24]. Thus each of the seven ISO layers had a defined set of functions and a layer protocol that established the rules for exchange with the corresponding layer in another computer.

Vendors began to understand that open systems meant the strict adherence to the OSI standards. The connection and integration of LANs with other LANs required the development of (1) bridges that operated at layer two of the OSI seven-layer architecture and connected one LAN to another; (2) routers that operated at layer three and routed packets of data between dissimilar networks; and (3) gateways that operated at level seven and provided high-speed communications from a mainframe computer to a network. This ISO/OSI model had a great influence on the further development of large complex LANs. The Ethernet supported the first three levels of the OSI model to the level of the packet, and provided system software to perform the remaining four levels of converting logical messages to and from packets. IBM's System Network Architecture (SNA) supported all seven layers of the OSI model [28].

1.8.1   Computer Communication Networks

Computer communication networks evolved in the 1960s when large, time-sharing, host computers provided services to users located at different terminals with interactive access to the mainframe computer. In the 1970s the availability of minicomputers provided local data-processing capabilities to various work sites, and created the need for distributed data-processing systems. A variety of networking configurations were then developed to allow multiple users to have access to a common computing facility by using either: (1) direct tie-lines connecting distributed computers and/or terminals to a central host computer; (2) modems (modulator-demodulator devices) that modulated analog signals to digital codes, and back) connecting user's computers or terminals by telephone lines over a relatively wide geographic area; or (3) a local-area network (LAN) with cables connecting computers to one another [129].

Bandwidth measures the difference between the lowest and highest signal frequencies that a network can transmit, and determines the ability of networks to move data. Local area networks (LANs) transmit data either by baseband or broadband transmission. Baseband transmission directly encodes data as digital signals in a serial stream of formatted data packets on the network cable. Since only one transmission signal can be sent at a time, a baseband node can either send or receive, but cannot simultaneously do both. Broadband transmission allows multiple data signals to be present on the network line at the same time. In broadband transmission, the data packets are transmitted as analog signals that require high speed circuitry for analog-to-digital conversion, and vice versa. Broadband networks are more expensive, but can support many more users than baseband networks.

Network interface units, the controlling communications software functions, were moved in the 1980s from participating network nodes into the network itself which then contained its own computers. Thus any computer in the network had to communicate only with its network interface unit, which usually required a less complicated protocol and supporting software to be present on each participating node. Network models were one of the earliest organizational structures used for clusters of computers with distributed databases; they displayed pointers to link various data sets and procedures for manipulating them. Since the same data could reside in more than one database, a communications network was required to link such data. These early efforts led in 1971 to a Conference on Data Systems Languages (CODASL) that advocated a variant of the network model as a hierarchical form of database with a tree-like branching structure that, at the start of the database, defined connections between files [255].

Local area networks (LANs) typically connected on-site computers and peripheral devices, integrated departmental computing facilities, and connected local machines to a supporting computer center. By 1971 prototype LANs of distributed minicomputers were being proposed in a hospital environment [26]. Distributed computer systems limited the effect of the failure of one computer on the operation of the other computers. LAN communications were usually accomplished through one of two general methods. In the first, contention (or collision-detection) access each computer using the network had two connections, one for receiving data from, and one for sending data to, the network. Each node could send data only when no other message was being transmitted, so each computer had to listen for any traffic on the channel before sending. This method was used, for example, by Xerox's Ethernet [146]. The second, token-passing access, used an electronic signal of a packet of bits in a special pattern (token), that was passed from computer to computer in a ring or bus network. If a computer node had no message to transmit, it passed on the token. To transmit a message, a computer node retrieved a free token, held it while communicating, and sent the message specifying the destination address, and other computers checked the message as it passed by. IBM's PCNet and Datapoint's ARCnet used the token-passing method [129, 241].

Database integration on a LAN meant that the user who received a response to a query was unaware of where or how the data were stored. This technology involved either interfacing or integrating distributed heterogeneous data. The interfacing approach permitted exchange of data by building cross-reference tables, between each pair of physical computer files in two databases to be interfaced, which transformed or mapped one physical structure into the other as required; it allowed no technological controls over data integrity. Executive functions for interfacing could be defined in master data dictionaries used by all interfaced databases. The integrating approach permitted actual merging of data by employing a conceptual schema that was mapped to database structures as well as to user requirements. The schema standardized data by defining a consistent set of rules to be used for all data; integrated data by pulling together the data from multiple databases; assured data quality by enforcing data-integrity constraints; and maintained data independence by isolating data-structure changes from users' programs. A master data dictionary defined, described, and managed the schema and the transforms of the users' data [4].

Wide area networks (WANs) typically used public telephone lines for long-distance data transmission; and each analog message was transmitted in a continuous stream known as circuit switching, that would tie up the phone line during the entire time that one message was being sent. With packet switching, multiple messages in the form of digital packets could be sent over one line, and it soon replaced analog signals in telephone, radio, and satellite communications. The United States took the lead in the development of wide area computer networks for academic research.

Star networks appeared in the 1960s when local computers began to communicate with a central host, time-sharing computer; and usually used telephone lines as links radiating out from the host computer like spokes from a central hub. All communications on the network passed through the host computer to the users' terminals. The host computer rapidly shifted connections from terminal to terminal, giving each terminal user the illusion of having exclusive access to the host computer; however, if the central computer failed then all communication stopped.

Ring networks connected all computers in a loop, with each computer connected to two others. Each message passed around the circle in a single direction, it was received by the appropriate module, and was removed when it was returned to the original sender. Bus networks connected all computers via "drop-offs" from a two-way main line; and a message sent by any one computer traveled in both directions and could be received by all other computers. Bus local-area networks (LANs) were the most common at that time due to their lower cost, easy connectivity and expandability; they permitted broadcasting to all other computers, and were resistant to failures of any single computer.

By the mid-1980s communication specialists were planning a single, unified, Integrated Services Digital Network (ISDN) capable of tying together every computer and organization in the world. The goal was to provide a group of standards for worldwide, universal digital interconnectivity regardless of modality, for data, voice, and video, over ordinary telephone wires, to be potentially available from every telephone outlet [141]. ISDN allowed computers and telephones to communicate directly with each other and eliminated the need for modems. By the end of the 1980s, patchworks of ISDN in the United States showed that ISDN could successfully link existing equipment from multiple vendors. Orthner [203] described important advances for digital data communication systems that evolved in the 1980s–1990s: (1) time division multiplexed (TDM) systems that allowed several lower-speed digital communication channels to interweave onto a higher-speed channel; (2) the evolution of the Integrated Services Digital Network (ISDN) and the development of international standards to satisfy the needs for medical database systems and to provide users with universal, digital interconnectivity regardless of modality, including natural language text, voice, and three dimensional images; (3) the increasing use of broadband fiber optics for digital data communication; and (4) the evolving global use of wireless communications.

Wireless transmission of a spectrum of radio frequency signals provides the capability to have instant communications almost anywhere and is used for the transmission of radio, broadcast television, mobile phones, satellite data, and for a variety of Web services and devices. The radio wireless spectrum in the United States is regulated for specific frequency bands which are given maximum allowable power levels for their emissions by procedures that were developed prior to 1950 [231]. The range used by smartphones, ultra high-frequency television, and global positioning systems is in the 900–928 MHz frequency, where 1 Hz is one wave cycle-per-second. The commonly used rate of digital data transmission in a digital communication network is the megabits-per-second (mbits/s). Since the volume of data transferred is often measured in megabytes of data, and the network transfer rate and download speed of data are often measured in megabits-per-second; to achieve a transfer rate of 1 megabyte (1,024 kB) per-second, one needs a network connection with a transfer rate of 8 megabits-per-second.

Generation standards for mobile communications technology began to be defined in the 1980s by International Mobile Telecommunications (IMT) with the objectives of requiring each generation to offer significant advances in performance and capabilities as compared to the prior generation. Mobile cellular services initially used analog radio technologies, and these were identified as first generation (1G) systems. In 1985 the U.S. Federal Communications Commission (FCC) released several bands of the radio spectrum for unlicensed use; and the IEEE developed 802.11 standards for WiFi wireless networking technology. The term WiFi was applied to local area networks that were installed without wires for client devices in order to decrease the costs of network wiring. In the 1990s a variety of commercial, worldwide WiFi locations were operational, and led to the wide use of WiFi-enabled devices, such as personal computers, lap top computers, and mobile phones, to deploy local-area networks without any physical wired connections, and to subscribe to various commercial services and connect to the Internet. Digital second generation (2G) mobile technology was initiated and rapidly replaced analog 1G networks.

Third generation (3G) mobile technology was launched in 2001 in Japan, and in 2002 in the United States by Verizon Wireless. It delivered speeds of 0.4 mbps (megabits-per-second) to 1.5 mbps, about 2.4 times faster than by modem connections. 3G cellular phones also added functions such as video-conferencing, telemedicine, and global positioning system (GPS) applications that could enable a 911 call on a cell phone to inform the emergency responder of the location of the emergency caller.

In 2005 Sunnyvale, California, became the first city in the United States to offer citywide, free-of-cost WiFi service; by 2010 free WiFi services were offered at the airports in San Jose, San Francisco, and Oakland, California, (Bay Area News Group 06/22/2010), and free WiFi services became available in 6,700 Starbucks' coffee shops (TIME 06/28/2010). In 2010 WiFi service enabled wireless Voice over Internet Protocol (VOIP) to travel as data across the Internet. In 2011 an Internet Governance Forum (IGF) was organized under the auspices of the United Nations to construct a form of governance for the Internet. In 2012 the U.S. Congress authorized the Federal Communications Commission to sell unused or unlicensed wireless frequencies to mobile giants like AT&T and Verizon Wireless to open new frequencies, and connect mobile devices to new, long-range, next-generation, super

WiFi networks [124]. In 1998 the United States established the Internet Corporation for Assigned Names and Numbers (ICANN) to manage the Internet's address system. In the year 2000 all major existing cellular spectrum bands were made available; and that allowed using more multi-band radios, faster mobile phones, two-way text messaging and video transmissions. In 2012 ICANN was considering adding more generic top-level domains as the suffixes of Web addresses to the existing 22 that included .com and .org and .gov, and others.

In the 2000s Verizon initiated its Health Information Exchange, and other health care information technology vendors announced cloud computing services using Web-based technology that could communicate relatively secure and protected patient data between collaborating health care providers. The Wireless Gigabit (WiGi) Alliance reported an advance in wireless communication that provided faster transmission speeds of up to 6 gigabits-per-second [296]. A software development called HTML5 allowed offline storage of information and Internet utilities, and used markup programming for Web pages that could add video to a Web page [189].

Available in a variety of shapes, sizes, keyboards, and operating systems, mobile phones came with interfaces that provided telephone, email, screens for graphics and photos, connections to social networks (including Facebook, Flickr, and Twitter), and with 5–8 megapixel cameras.

1.8.2 The Internet and the World Wide Web

The 1957 launch of the Soviet satellite, Sputnik I, surprised the United States and prompted then President Eisenhower to create within the Department of Defense (DoD) an Advanced Research Projects Agency (DARPA) with an objective to develop computer and communications technology for defense purposes. In 1962 the first successful communications satellite, Telstar, was built, launched, and operated by Bell Laboratories; it relayed computer data and live television signals across the United States and to Europe. In 1970 the National Library of Medicine's Lister Hill Center began using satellite communications to send medical information to remote villages in Alaska. Telenet Communications Corporation, the first public packet-switching network, was initiated in 1972 by Bolt, Beranek, and Newman (BB&N); later it became a subsidiary of General Telephone and Electric (GTE) [229]. In the 1980s GTE's Telenet served more than half- million terminal users in and around 400 U.S. cities. Tymnet, an early competitor of Telenet, built a network with more capacity than its time-sharing business could fill. To use some of the excess capacity, Tymnet contracted to provide communications links between terminals installed in medical schools, and with the National Institutes of Health (NIH) to provide communication links between a computer and bibliographic databases in the National Library of Medicine (NLM). This arrangement worked out so well that other host computers were added to the network, which employed a variant of the packet-switching technology pioneered by ARPANET [74]. Earth orbiting satellites provided another alternative for communications between remote locations. The first successful active communications satellite, Telstar, launched in 1962, carried live television signals; the first commercial satellite, Intelsat I, was launched in 1965 [209]. By the end of the 1970s the fifth generation of the Intelsat satellites had been launched [92]. In the 1980s communication satellites were routinely used as an alternative means of transmitting information to remote locations.

ARPANET was created in 1966 when DoD's ARPA contracted with Bolt, Beranek and Newman (BB&N) in Cambridge, Massachusetts, to create a wide area network to link computers of different types in various colleges and institutions engaged in research for the DoD [151, 198]. In 1969 ARPANET began operations as the world's first interactive, computer-to-computer, packet-switching network [146]. Used to connect academic centers that conducted research for the DoD, ARPANET led to the evolution of the Internet and of the World Wide Web. By installing a communications minicomputer in each center to serve as a message router, DoD linked itself to the University of California in Los Angeles, then to Stanford Research Institute, to the University of California in Santa Barbara, the University of Utah, the Massachusetts Institute of Technology, and then to BB&N [198]. Whereas DoD previously had used a separate terminal for its communications with each academic center, ARPANET permitted all participating computer centers to be linked to any one terminal. By 1972 ARPANET was linked to 29 computer centers, and the basic technology developed for ARPANET was soon released for private commercial development. The national success of ARPANET soon led to expansion and the development of global inter-networking, greatly changing the means by which information could be communicated. Thus, with the advent of packet-switching networks, the boundary between computing and communicating, once sharply etched, became blurred [74]. In the 1980s ARPANET was a major component of a supernet. Called the Internet, it included the Computer Science Network (CSNET), which let academic computer scientists share computational resources and exchange email, and the National Science Foundation Network (NSFnet), which connected 60 major research centers in the United States [139].

Electronic mail (email) was first used in 1972 by Tomlinson, at Bolt, Beranek and Newman (BB&N) in Cambridge, Massachusetts, to transfer files from one computer to another; and the symbol @ was selected to identify an email address at BB&N. Email was rapidly accepted in their network and later was also used on the Internet [198].

Ethernet was developed in 1973 by Metcalfe and associates at the Xerox Palo Alto Research Center (PARC) in California as a local area network (LAN) that linked the 250 personal computers used on researchers' desks, and became one of the earliest coaxial cable networks for high-speed communications [134]. Tolchin et al. [263] reported that in 1985 the Johns Hopkins Hospital implemented an Ethernet communications network with coaxial cables attached to transceivers that coded and decoded the signals on the channel; communications servers connected terminals and remote printers to the host computer. Hammond et al. [128] described the use of the Ethernet after Xerox, Digital Equipment Corporation (DEC), and Intel joined together to define the strategy for their local area network. They used branching bus communications with coaxial cables optimized for high-speed (10-million bits-per-second) exchange of data between their data processing components, and interfaced a data communications controller between the computer data bus and the Ethernet to conform their data to the Ethernet format. Xerox licensed Ethernet to Metcalfe, who then started 3-COM (Computer Communication Company) to make hardware and software for Ethernet and other LANs; and Ethernet became the standard protocol for LANs. By 1974 many commercial networks were available, including AT&T's ISN, Control Data's CDCNet, Corvis Systems' Omninet, Datapoint's ARCnet, Digital Equipment's DECNet, IBM's SNA, and Wang's WangNet. In 1982 McNealy and associates developed the Stanford University Network (SUN) and initiated Sun Microsystems. Sun Microsystems revised the UNIX operating system for the Ethernet, and built Sun workstations with open standards so that every computer could be linked to any other computer anywhere in the LAN. In 1983 Novell, based in Orem, Utah, developed its Netware software for communication computers to function as database servers connected to personal computers; by the mid-1980s Novell Netware dominated client-server, personal-computer networks. In 1987 Cisco Systems developed data routers, with computers that would start, stop, and direct packets of information from router to router between networks. By 1989 about 5,000 computers at Stanford University were linked by a network similar in operation to ARPANET [233]. By the end of 1980s there were more than 75 LAN suppliers in the United States, and a 1988 survey reported 30 % of personal computer users were connected to LANs [134].

Transmission Control Protocol (TCP), sometimes referred to as the Transmission Control Protocol /Internet Protocol (TCP/IP) suite, was developed in 1975 to allow different packet-switching networks to inter-connect and to create networks of networks. TCP was responsible for ensuring correct delivery of messages that moved from one computer to another, while IP managed the sending and receiving of packets of data between computers (Connolly 1999). Lindberg [167] noted that the Internet Protocol Suite resulted from research and development conducted by the Defense Advanced Research Projects Agency (DARPA) in the early 1970s. After initiating the ARPANET, DARPA began to work on a number of other data transmission technologies. In 1972 Kahn joined DARPA, and in 1973 Cerf joined Kahn to work on open-architecture interconnection models with the goal of designing the next generation protocol for the ARPANET to more efficiently transmit and route traffic between end nodes. Their objective was to get a computer on the ARPANET and a computer on a satellite net and a computer on a radio net to communicate seamlessly with each other [125]. By locating all needed intelligence in the end nodes, it would then become possible to connect almost any network to the ARPANET. A computer served as a router to provide an interface to each network, and to forward packets of data back and forth between them. In 1974 while working at Stanford University, Cerf developed the first TCP specifications. In 1975 a two-network TCP/IP communication was completed between Stanford University and University College in London. In 1977 a three-network TCP/IP was conducted; and then other TCP/IP prototypes were developed at multiple research centers. In 1982 the U.S. Department of Defense declared TCP/IP as the standard for all military computer networking. In 1983 the migration to TCP/IP was officially completed; and by 1985 computer vendors initiated its commercial use [125].

The Internet emerged in 1986 when the National Science Foundation (NSF) initiated its network (NSFNET), and joined ARPANET and other networks to form the Internet. In 1986 a total of 2,308 Internet hosts had been registered [115]. In 1995 NSFNET terminated its funding of Internet, and awarded grants to regional networks so they could buy their own Internet connections. Soon the Internet could be accessed in a variety of ways, and became the term generally applied to the internetworking of networks. Browser programs, such as Mosaic and Netscape, allowed a user to download files from the Internet directly to their personal computers. In 1989 Case founded American Online (AOL), an Internet service provider (ISP), to furnish any user who had a computer with a modem connected to a telephone line, the interactive access to the worldwide use of email through the Internet. Major online computer services, including American Online (AOL), Compuserve, and others, began to offer complete Internet services. In the 1990s as personal computers began to connect to the Internet through television cables that could transmit data more than 100 times faster than the fastest modems, the communication of video became common [113]. In the 2000s the Web's support of email began to replace some modes of personal communications provided by postal mail and the telephone. Hartzband [130] observed that nothing changed clinical practice more fundamentally than the Internet, which transformed communications between doctor and patient, since it provided easily retrieved information to physicians for clinical decision support, and also to patients in search of self-diagnosis and better understanding of their diseases and prescribed therapies.

The National Library of Medicine (NLM) was frequently accessed in the 1980s using the Internet through Telnet, which facilitated wide distribution of NLM's computer resources and allowed Internet users access to the NLM databases as if they were using a terminal within the NLM [303]. A program called Gopher, originated at the University of Minnesota, was superficially similar to Telnet and also allowed access to a wide range of resources [113]. Soon NLM's MEDLINE became available to users through a nationwide network of many individual users and institutional users in government agencies, academic centers, hospitals, and commercial organizations. Its growth was remarkable. In 1997 alone, the NLM's MEDLINE, with PubMed and Internet Grateful Med, received requests for 75 million searches [169].

The Internet became global in the 1990s when Berners-Lee, a computer scientist at CERN, the European Particle Physics Laboratory in Geneva, Switzerland, devised a method for linking diverse Internet pages to each other by using a hypertext program that embedded software within documents to point to other related documents and thereby link non-sequentially stored information. Documents were stored on the Web using Hypertext Markup Language (HTML) and displayed by a Web browser that exchanged information with a Web server using the HTTP protocol. A user could find, link to, and browse related subjects by clicking on highlighted or underlined text, and then skip to other pages across the Internet. Berners-Lee assigned and stored a Universal Resource Locator (URL) address to each computer location on the Web, and used the Hypertext Transfer Protocol (HTTP) with TCP/IP developed for the ARPANET that allowed users to move around the Web and connect to any URL in any other location. He used Hypertext Markup Language (HTML) as the programming code to create hypertext links; thus, a user with a computer-pointing device, such as a mouse, could click on a high-lighted word and the links could transfer desired papers from one journal to another, display computer-based text, graphics, and images, and compile digital information from many sources.

In the 1990s the Internet could quickly and reliably deliver text, email, music, and images by employing a variety of digital communication technologies. By 1995 about 13,000 Web sites allowed public access. The User's Network (USENET) was available for discussion groups especially focused on medical subjects; and mailing list services commonly referred as listserv provided hundreds of medicine-related mailing lists covering all specialties in medicine. In 1998 the Web transmitted about five million emails each minute, and also began to be used by some physicians for providing consultations and patient education [40]. In 1999 private corporations and colleges sponsored the evolving Internet-2; and the Federal government supported the Next Generation (NG) Internet using fiber optic digital networks to develop the infrastructure for the information revolution that would allow the faster transfer of a mix of text, voice, and video.

World Wide Web (commonly referred to as the Web) was the name applied by Berners-Lee to the collection of URLs, an addressing system capable of linking documents on the Internet from one computer to another. The Web changed the usual two tier model (client-user, data processing server), to a three tier model (client-user, data processing applications server, database management server) over different distributed computers [21, 76, 139]. Whereas the Internet-based resources were often difficult for the non-expert to use, the Web supported an inexpensive, easy-to-use, cross-platform graphic-interface to the Internet. The most significant development that drove the rapid growth of the Web were the ease with which a user could successfully navigate the complex Web of linked computer systems of the Internet to access large online libraries with computer-mediated, inter-document links; and use general hypertext systems for reading and writing to form collaboration links, post messages, and conduct scientific or social networking. An international organization called the World Wide Web Consortium, composed of industry companies, government agencies, and universities, was formed to set Internet policies. By 2010 programmers at the Consortium had mapped 203 databases together using 395 million links [270]. In 1998, the Internet Corporation for Assigned Names and Numbers (ICANN) was created by the American Department of Commerce to generate, register, and control the suffixes for the domain names of information used on the Internet, such as ".com" or ".net" or ".org", and many others. Similarly, the Internet Assigned Numbers Authority (IANA) uses four numbers from 0 to 255, separated by dots, to uniquely identify every device attached to the Internet.

Browsers were generated in the 1990s to search and retrieve information resources on the Web. The combination of low-cost computers and packet switching in digital networks spawned a number of new companies. In 1993 Andreessen and associates at the University of Illinois Champaign Urbana developed a browser program called Mosaic to access and retrieve information available on the Web. In 1994 Clarke founded Netscape, using Mosaic as its Web browser and calling it Navigator, and developed software using the Web as a platform. In 1995 Gates added to Microsoft's Windows 95 its own Web browser called Internet Explorer. In 1994 Gosling at Sun Microsystems introduced JAVA software that could run applications on different computers regardless of their different operating systems, and could run on digital networks across the Internet. Portals to the Web, also called search engines, were developed to simplify searches for information or to locate material on the Internet by using indexes and directories of Web information; and allowed searches of Web pages by key words, phrases, or categories. Among the top browsers at this time are Microsoft Internet Explorer, Netscape Firefox, Google Chrome, Apple Safari, and Opera.

Social networks developed with the introduction of 3G and 4G smartphones and electronic tablets that provided text, acceptable voice and images, and Internet services; and resulted in the evolution of a variety of social networking media. In the 2000s the mobile phones became ubiquitous, and Web-based social networking sites became very popular. *Google* was founded in 1998 by Page and Brin, while students at Stanford University, and developed as a huge web-based warehouse with the goal to collect, store, and organize all of the world's information, from which one could search for any of the world's knowledge. It became very popular by collecting user-generated information; and by offering Web responses to queries based on a user-ranking algorithm of its stored contents. Google's Android operating system, and Apple's software, used Java programming; both became the leaders for multimedia software applications in the mobile communications market [55]. Google also developed an advertising business that sold lines of text linked to Web queries; and in 2010 Google reportedly processing several billion queries each day, and ran more than a million servers in multiple data centers [116]. By 2012 the Google database had more than 500 million people, places, and commonly requested items, and was able to provide a summary of related information with links to the main search results [166]. Google+ was offered as a social addition to Google's search services. Wolpin [298] observed that talking on the phone, the primary purpose for the invention of the cell phone, was now secondary to many other uses for the smartphone.

In 2010 there were several leaders in the consumer and social media accessed by smartphones and electronic tablets. LinkedIn was developed and used primarily by professionals and colleagues. Twitter allowed users to exchange text of up to 140 characters, called "tweets", for the quick exchange of brief news items. Friendster, founded by Abrams in 2002, is considered by some the first Web-based social networking site. By 2003 it had more than two million subscribers; however, in 2011 Friendster discontinued its social network accounts and limited itself to be a gaming site. My Space was launched in 2003 by Friendster users; and in 2004 was a Web's leading social networking site. Facebook, designed and launched in 2004 by Zuckerberg as a social web-based warehouse of everyone's identity, had become the world's largest social networking site by 2008 [299]. In 2010 Facebook was estimated to have 500 million active users in its online networking service despite its perceived laxness in protecting the privacy of personal data, a problem that became more evident from unsecured WiFi nets in peoples' homes. In 2006 the evolution of 3G cell phones and the popularity of message texting led to the launch of Twitter, that allowed users to type and broadcast 140-character text messages ("tweets") to their followers; and in 2009 it had nearly 45 million monthly visitors [299]. In 2009 Pinterest, a Palo Alto based group initiated an online scrapbook where users could "pin" images and other items of interest, and follow others; by the end of 2011 it had about 20 million users.

Conferences were initiated in 2004 to encourage Web 2.0, new collaborative Internet applications that expanded the use of the Web as a computing platform to include more than just searches, such as for running software applications entirely through a browser. Web 2.0 technologies increased user participation in developing and managing content to change the nature and value of information. Ekberg et al. [95] described a Web 2.0 system used for self-directed education of teenage diabetic patients in learning everyday needs of their disease. As increasingly broader communication services were provided to users over the Web, more audio and video services were developed for audio-video conferencing, such as by using Skype software; and for social networks such as for using Facebook and Twitter; and for photo sharing by using Flickr.

Prior to the Web a computer network had what was called a server, often a large mainframe computer that shared stored data files. After the establishment of the Internet and the World Wide Web, the term computer server was applied to a computer system that provided services to clients. The client-server model employed a communicating network that used the Web and the Internet Protocol (IP) to link a group of distributed data resources that functioned as one integrated data warehouse and could be shared by multiple clients. For patients' medical data this increased the risk of invasions of security and patients' data privacy.

Cloud computing is a term applied to the use of the Web by groups of computer servers, and is often represented in networking diagrams as a cloud; and tag clouds used tag-words as hyperlinks that led to collections of items associated with the tags. By using the Web, cloud computing enabled a client's computer applications to run off-site on the provider's (cloud) storage equipment and to link back to the client, thereby reducing the client's infrastructure costs by enabling the client to quickly scale the system up or down to meet changing needs, and to pay only for the services needed for a given time. The term cloud storage was generally applied to a group of servers or distributed data resources functioning as one integrated data warehouse that could be shared by multiple clients; and the concept was simply represented as storing the client's data online using a network of storage devices (servers) instead of storing it on the client's own hard drive. By the end of 2010 the Internet was a maze of thousands of servers and clients. Cloud storage services were provided by Microsoft Windows, Apple Mac OS, Google Android, Amazon Web services, and many others that allowed transferring files between computers, smartphones, and tablets. Barret [16] reported that Dropbox, developed by Andrew Houston, was storing on remote servers about 20 billion documents for four million client users with their 500,000 computers. When a user downloaded the Dropbox software to the user's computer, it created a folder for placing documents that the user wanted to access from the Web. However, the cloud storage of electronic patients' medical records did introduce new and potentially serious security and privacy concerns. Virtualization is a term sometimes used to describe moving data from a fixed storage site into a cloud. According to *The Economist* [260], *computing clouds* were essentially digital service factories that were global utilities accessible from all corners of the planet; as a "cloud of clouds," they offered three levels of service: (1) "Software as a Service" (SaaS) included Web-based applications; (2) "Platform as a Service" (PaaS) allowed developers to write applications for Web and mobile devices; and (3) "Infrastructure as a Service" (IaaS) allowed basic computing services that companies, like Amazon, used as their computer center. Lev-Ram [162] reported that Intel was developing cloud services that could work seamlessly on any device, allowing software developers to build applications using a standard set of tools. Intel's Cloud Builders program provided step-by-step guidance to companies that wanted to move data and services to the cloud; and Intel brought together a group of about 70 companies to develop cloud computing software and hardware standards. Soon IBM and other commercial vendors soon followed in offering cloud services.

The history of the early Internet and of the World Wide Web, and of their relationship to medical informatics has been described in some detail by Glowniak [113] and by Hafner and Lyon [125]. On reviewing the history of the ARPANET and the Internet, Shortliffe [238, 239] judged it to be one of the most compelling examples of how government investments led to innovations with broad economic and social impact.

1.9 Summary and Commentary

Blum [29] observed that in the 1940s a person was given a calculator and a set of formulae and was called a (human) computer. In the 1950s when an electronic device carried out the arithmetic functions of addition, subtraction, multiplication, and division, or the logical functions of *and*, *or*, and *not*, and was called a computer. However, with the development of digital computers they needed: (1) a central processing unit, and a primary main memory to hold the data being processed; (2) a program of instructions for processing the data, circuitry to perform arithmetic and logic operations and to control the execution of instructions; (3) peripheral equipment including secondary or auxiliary storage devices such as magnetic tapes and discs; data input devices such as keyboards, card and tape readers, and data input capabilities from secondary storage devices; and data output devices such as printers, displays, and plotters; and (4) communicating devices to receive and to transmit processed information.

These past eight decades have witnessed the transition from the end of the industrial age to the beginning of the information age. Computers evolved from expensive, slow, mainframe computers in the 1960s, to minicomputers with integrated circuits in the 1970s, to personal computers and local area networks in the 1980s, to the Internet and the World Wide Web using mobile smartphones and electronic tablets in the 1990s, to creating social networks and Web 2.0 in the 2000s, and to exploiting cloud computing and global networks in the 2010s.

The invention of the computer chip with its integrated circuits produced dramatic changes in computers, and was probably the most important event to usher in the information age. Although the computer's central processing unit was the basis for most early advances in informatics, it was the computer's software that provided the computer languages, programs, procedures, and documentation that made the hardware usable for applications. The first computer programs used the lowest level of machine codes for instructions to process data. Higher-level languages soon evolved to more efficiently program the increasingly powerful computers and to better meet the requirements of different users. By the 1980s many of the most commonly used programs were commercially available, and most computer users did little programming themselves. Noteworthy is the contribution of Barnett and associates [12] at the Laboratory of Computer Science at the Massachusetts General Hospital, who developed as early as the 1960s the language called MUMPS (Massachusetts General Hospital Utility Multi-Programming System) that provided an operating system, a database management system for handling large volumes of information, and an easy interactive mode for programmer-computer communication. MUMPS became one of the most common programming languages in the United States, used in the large medical information systems of the Department of Defense, the Veterans Administration, and some large commercial information systems.

Computer databases evolved with the development of computers and informatics technology. In the 1950s large mainframe, time-sharing computers were used for the earliest computer applications in medicine; most data were entered into the computer by punched cards and stored on magnetic tape or disc drives. The printed output was usually produced in batches. In the 1980s database technology and database management systems evolved as computer storage devices became larger and cheaper, computers became more powerful, more efficient computer programs were developed, and computer networks and distributed database systems were developed. Edelstein [93] noted that early users had to understand how and where the data were stored. Data could not be shared by different applications, resulting in much duplication of data and effort. Soon, however, computer systems were developed to permit the standardization of data access methods and to allow sharing of data.

Over time the complexity of computer applications greatly increased. More commercial software packages came to market, and software costs became a greater proportion of total computing costs. The development of efficient computer-stored databases was essential for many medical computing applications. Users found it more economical to obtain commercial application programs ("apps") packaged to perform commonly needed functions than to develop such programs themselves. Specialized commercial applications included databases, word processing programs, and spread sheets for tabular processing of numerical data; thus it became less necessary for the users of such software to know how to program a computer themselves. The amount of data available to computer users rapidly became so vast that Enriquez [98] estimated in 2010 there would be available about 1.2 zettabytes (a zettabyte is a trillion gigabytes) of data to users of translational medical databases, genomic databases, bibliographic data sources such as the National Library of Medicine, Google, cloud storage, and other data resources.

Computer communications moved from data transmission using copper wires to using fiber optic cables; and networks developed to join computers and users with worldwide, universal, integrated digital connectivity. For large medical information systems, an important innovation in the 1980s was the evolution of local, national, and worldwide high-speed communication networks. Using network technology a hospital could unite all the different computers throughout its various departments, even though the computers were located in geographically dispersed locations. Levy [163] noted that, although in the 1950s computers had introduced the "information age", it was not until the 1980s when microcomputers became absorbed into the popular culture of the United States, that computers became commonly accepted working tools. The increase in speed of computers was remarkable: a person could complete one calculation in about 150 s, ENIAC could complete 18 calculations per second (cps), UNIVAC could complete 190 cps, the IBM personal computer 250,000 cps, a 4G smartphone 36 million cps, and the iPad 2 can complete 1.7 billion cps.

The Defense Advanced Research Project Agency (DARPA), a research funding agent of the Department of Defense, contributed to the development of academic computer science departments at the University of California in Berkeley, Carnegie Mellon University, Massachusetts Institute of Technology, and Stanford University, among others. One of the most significant contributions of DARPA was its Advanced Research Agency Network (ARPANET) that led to the development of the global Internet [224]. In the 1990s the Internet made international communications with the use of computers commonplace. In the 2000s wireless mobile phones, the Internet, and the World Wide Web became the main modes used for local and global communications. Microsoft made computers easy for anyone to use; Facebook made video communication the basis of its social network. Laptops replaced desktop computers in consumer preference [235]. But it was the smartphone that revolutionized the economy and disrupted all manners of businesses, including the personal computer, the laptop, and electronic tablet businesses; the social media, music, publishing, television, and advertising industries; and health care services.

References

1. Albrecht K. RFID tag-you're it. Sci Am. 2008;299:72–7.
2. Allen SI, Otten M. The telephone as a computer input-output terminal for medical information. JAMA. 1969;208:673–9.
3. Amsterdamn J. Computer languages of the future. Pop Comput. 1983; 136–51.
4. Appleton DS. The technology of data integration. Datamation. 1985;31:106–16.
5. Ash SR, Mertz SL, Ulrich DK. The computerized notation system: a portable, self-contained system for entry of physicians' and nurses' notes. J Clin Eng. 1983;8:147–56.
6. Augarten S. Bit by bit: an illustrated history of computers. New York: Ticknor & Fields; 1984.
7. Ausman RK, Culliton EH, Graham TD, Slawson MR, Kehoe EJ, et al. Simplified input and output devices for patient data handling. Ann NY Acad Sci. 1969;161:749–55.
8. Bacon G. Software. Science (New York, NY). 1982;215:775–9.
9. Ball MJ. An overview of total medical information systems. Methods Inf Med. 1971;10:73–82.
10. Ball MJ, Collen MF, editors. Aspects of the computer-based patient record. New York: Springer; 1992.
11. Barnett GO. Computer-stored ambulatory record (COSTAR): US Department of Health, Education, and Welfare, Public Health Service, Health Resources Administration, National Center for Health Services Research; 1976.
12. Barnett GO, Souder D, Beaman P, Hupp J. MUMPS–an evolutionary commentary. Comput Biomed Res. 1981;14:112–8.
13. Barnett GO. Massachusetts general hospital computer system. In: Collen MF, editor. Hospital computer systems. New York: Wiley; 1974.
14. Barnett GO. The modular hospital information system. In: Stacy RW, Waxman BD, editors. Computers in biomedical research. New York: Academic; 1974. p. 243–5.
15. Barnett GO, Greenes RA, Grossman JH. Computer processing of medical text information. Methods Inf Med. 1969;8:177–82.
16. Barret V. Best small companies. Forbes. 2011;188:82–92.
17. Barsalou T, Wiederhold G. A cooperative hypertext interface to relational databases. Proc SCAMC. 1989;383.
18. Bender E. Presenting the future: what benefits will the OS/2 presentation manager bring and when? PC World. 1989;7:134–6.
19. Bennett WL. Terminal selection for an on-line hospital system. Proceedings of 24th national conference 1969. New York: ACM Pub P-69; 1969: p. 58–66.
20. Bergeron BP. Voice recognition: an enabling technology for modern health care? Proc AMIA Symp. 1996;802.
21. Berners-Lee T, Cailliau R, Luotonen A. The World Wide Web. Comm ACM. 1994;37:907–12.
22. Bernstein J. Profiles: The analytic engine-I. The New Yorker. 1963 (October 19); p. 58–96.
23. Bernstein J. Profiles: The analytic engine-II. The New Yorker. 1963 (October 26); p. 54–108.
24. Blaine GJ. Networks and distributed systems: a primer. Proc MEDINFO. 1983; 1118–21.
25. Blois MS. The physician's personal workstation. MD Comput. 1984;2:22–6.
26. Blois MS, Henley RR. Strategies in the planning of hospital information systems. J D'Infomatique Med. 1971;89–98.
27. Blum B. Design methodology. In: Orthner HF, Blum BI, editors. Implementing health care information systems. New York: Springer; 1989. p. 277–95.
28. Blum BI. A history of computers. In: Blum BI, editor. Clinical information systems. New York: Springer; 1986. p. 1–32.
29. Blum BI. Programming languages. In: Blum BI, editor. Clinical information systems. New York: Springer; 1986. p. 112–49.
30. Blum BI. A data model for patient management. Proc MEDINFO. 1983;83:748–51.

31. Blum BI, Orthner HF. The MUMPS programming language. In: Orthner HF, Blum BI, editors. Implementing health care information systems. New York: Springer; 1989.
32. Blum BI, Orthner HF. Clinical information systems. New York: Springer; 1986.
33. Blum BI. Information systems for patient care. New York: Springer; 1984.
34. Blum BI. An information system for developing information systems. AFIPS Natl Comp Conf. 1983;52:743–52. Arlington, VA: AFIPS Press.
35. Blum RL. Displaying clinical data from a time-oriented database. Comput Biol Med. 1981;11:197–210.
36. Blumenthal L, Waterson J. The use of a microcomputer as a front-end processor for data base management systems on large computers. Proc SCAMC. 1981;303–6.
37. Bonner P, Gralla P. OS/2 building for the future. PC Comput. 1988;1:76–88.
38. Boraiko AA. The chip: electronic mini marvel that is changing your life. Natl Geogr. 1982;162:421–56.
39. Boraiko AA. Fiber optics: harnessing light by a thread. Natl Geogr. 1979;156:516.
40. Borowitz SM, Wyatt JC. The origin, content, and workload of e-mail consultations. JAMA. 1998;280:1321–4.
41. Bott E. Inside windows 4.0. PC Comput. 1994;7:124–39.
42. Bowie J. Methods of implementation of the MUMPS global data-base. Inform Health Soc Care. 1979;4:151–64.
43. Brandt CA, Morse R, Matthews K, Sun K, Deshpande AM, et al. Metadata-driven creation of data marts from an EAV-modeled clinical research database. Int J Med Inform. 2002;65:225–41.
44. Brazier MA. From calculating machines to computers and their adoption by the medical sciences. Med Hist. 1973;17:235–43.
45. Brigham B. CP/M (computer operating system) summary guide for version 1.4 and 2.0. Glastonbury: Rosetta Stone; 1980.
46. Broida R. What features will smartphones have? Pop Sci. 2011;279:88.
47. Bronzino JD. Computerization concepts in the clinical laboratory. In: Bronzino JD, editor. Computer applications in patient care. Menlo Park: Addison-Wesley; 1982. p. 117–37.
48. Brown J, Vallbona C. A new patient record system using the laser card. Proc SCAMC. 1988;602–5.
49. Bryan M. The year of the data base. Pers Comput. 1988;12(1):100–9.
50. Bulkeley WM. Who built the first PC? Wall Str J. 1986 (May 14);31.
51. Bull BS, Korpman RA. The clinical laboratory computer system. Arch Pathol Lab Med. 1980;104:449–51.
52. Burks AR, Burks AW. The first electronic computer: the Atanasoff story. Ann Arbor: University of Michigan Press; 1989.
53. Burks AW, Burks AR. The ENIAC: first general-purpose electronic computer. 1981. MD Comput. 1994;12:206–12.
54. Caulfield B. The Steve Jobs economy. Forbes. 2011;188:16.
55. Caulfield B. Is Android vs. Apple like PC vs Mac? Forbes. 2011;188:44.
56. Chamberlin DD, Boyce RF. SEQUEL: a structured English query language. Proc 1974 ACM SIGFIDET (now SIGMOD) workshop on data description, access and control. 1974;249–64.
57. Chase HS, Kaufman DR, Johnson SB, Mendonca EA. Voice capture of medical residents' clinical information needs during an inpatient rotation. JAMIA. 2009;16:387–94.
58. Williams BT, Chen TT, Elston J, et al. The variable phrase keyboard and the clinical report. In: Hinman EJ, editor. Advanced medical systems: the 3rd century. Miami: Symposia Specialists Medical Books; 1977. p. 127–34.
59. Chen TT, Williams BT, Levy AH. Graphically enhanced medical information system network. In: Hinman EJ, editor. Advanced medical systems: the 3rd century. Miami: Symposia Specialists; 1977. p. 135–44.
60. Chen TT, Williams BT, Levy AH. A depository health-computer network. Inform Health Soc Care. 1976;1:167–78.

61. Childs BW. Bedside terminals: status and the future. Healthc Comput Commun. 1988;5:12–4.
62. Chiodo C, Hopkins B, Miles G. 101 essential apps for Android, Blackberry, and iPhone. PC World. 2010;28:91–8.
63. Chute CC, Crowson DL, Bluntrock JD, Crowson DL. Medical information retrieval and WWW browsers at Mayo. Proc AMIA. 1995;68–73.
64. Cimino JJ, Socratous SA, Grewal R. The informatics superhighway: prototyping on the World Wide Web. Proc SCAMC. 1995;111–5.
65. Clark WA, Molnar CE. The LINC: a description of the laboratory instrument computer. Ann NY Acad Sci. 1964;115:653–68.
66. Codd EF. Extending the database relational model to capture more meaning. ACM Trans Database Syst (TODS). 1979;4:397–434.
67. Codd EF. Further normalizations of the data base relational model. In: Rustin R, editor. Data base systems. Englewood Cliffs: Prentice-Hall; 1972. p. 33–64.
68. Codd EF. A relational model of data for large shared data banks. Commun ACM. 1970;13:377–87.
69. Codd EF, Codd SB, Salley CT. Providing OLAP (On-Line Analytical Processing) to user-analysts: an IT mandate. Technical report. San Jose, CA: Codd and Associates; 1993.
70. Cole WG. Integrality and meaning: essential and orthogonal dimensions of graphical data display. Proc SCAMC. 1993;404–8.
71. Collen M. A guide matrix for technological system evaluation. J Med Syst. 1978;2:249–54.
72. Collen MF. History of MHTS. In: Collen MF, editor. Multiphasic health services. New York: Wiley; 1978. p. 1–45.
73. Coltri A. Databases in health care. In: Lehmann HP, editor. Aspects of electronic health record systems. New York: Springer; 2006. p. 225–51.
74. Conlan RR. Understanding computers. Alexandria: Time-Life Books; 1986.
75. Connelly D. Communicating laboratory results effectively; the role of graphical displays. Proc AAMSI Cong. 1983;113–5.
76. Connolly TM, Begg CE. Database management systems: a practical approach to design. 2nd edition. New York: Addison-Wesley; 1999.
77. Consumer Reports. IBM clones. Consumer reports 1989 buying guide. 1989;53:308–12.
78. Cook JS. Communication by optical fiber. Sci Am. 1973;229:28–35.
79. Cox JR. Special purpose digital computers in biology. In: Stacy RW, Waxman BD, editors. Computers in biomedical research. New York: Academic; 1965. p. 67–99.
80. Crawford FR. Introduction to data processing. Englewood Cliffs: Prentice-Hall; 1968.
81. Crecine JP. The next generation of personal computers. Science. 1986;231:935–43.
82. Cringely RX. Accidental empires: how the boys of Silicon Valley make their millions, battle foreign competition, and still can't get a date. Reading: Addison-Wesley; 1992.
83. Davis M. The chip at 35. Pers Comput. 1983;7:127–31.
84. Davis RM. Evolution of computers and computing. Science. 1977;195:1096–102.
85. Dawson J. A family of models. Byte. 1989;14:277–86.
86. Denning PJ, Brown RI. Operating systems. Sci Am. 1984;251:94–130.
87. Dinu V, Nadkarni P. Guidelines for the effective use of entity-attribute-value modeling for biomedical databases. Int J Med Inform. 2007;76:769–79.
88. Downs SM, Walker MG, Blum RL. Automated summarization of on-line medical records; 1986.
89. Drexhage MG, Moynihan CT. Infared optical fibers. Sci Am. 1989;259:110–6.
90. Eamos C. A computer perspective. Cambridge, MA: Harvard University Press; 1973.
91. ECRI. Clinical information systems improve with new standard. Health Tech Trends. 1989;1:3–6.
92. Edelson BI, Pollack L. Satellite communications. Science. 1977;195:1125–33.
93. Edelstein SZ. Clinical research databases: a microscopic look. Proc SCAMC. 1981;279–80.
94. Edge RA, Marciniak TA. The ADA environment. Proc SCAMC. 1984;882–5.
95. Ekberg J, Ericson L, Timpka T, Eriksson H, Nordfeldt S, Hanberger L, et al. Web 2.0 systems supporting childhood chronic disease management. J Med Syst. 2010;34:107–17.

96. Ellison S. The dreamphone. Fortune. 2010;162:128.
97. Elting L, Lynn A, Bodey G. Human/computer interfaces: a randomized trial of data entry and editing formats. Proc SCAMC. 1988;459–62.
98. Enriquez J. The glory of big data. Pop Sci. 2011;279:31–5.
99. Esterhay Jr R, Foy JL, Lewis TL. Hospital information systems: approaches to screen definition: comparative anatomy of the PROMIS, NIH and Duke systems. Proc SCAMC. 1982;903–11.
100. Feigenbaum EA, McCorduck P. The fifth generation: artificial intelligence and Japan's computer challenge to the world. Reading: Addison Wesley; 1984.
101. Fenster JM. COBOL. Invent Technol. 2010;25:48–50.
102. Fisher JA, Monahan T. Tracking the social dimensions of RFID systems in hospitals. Int J Med Inform. 2008;77:176–83.
103. Francis B. PC back-ups optical understudy. Datamation. 1988;34:57–60.
104. Frawley WJ, Piatetsky-Shapiro G, Matheus CJ. Knowledge discovery in databases: an overview. AI Mag. 1992;13:57.
105. Friedel R. Transistor. Invent Technol. 2010;25:4344.
106. Friedman BA. Informating, not automating, the medical record. J Med Syst. 1989;13:221–5.
107. Friedman RB. Computers in medicine. In: Eden HS, Eden M, editors. Microcomputers in patient care. Park Ridge: Noyes Medical Publications; 1981. p. 90–5.
108. Friedman RB, Gustafson DH. Computers in clinical medicine, a critical review. Comput Biomed Res. 1977;10:199–204.
109. Fung J, Mann S. Computer vision signal processing on graphics processing units. Proc IEEE-ICASSP. 2004;5:93–6.
110. Gates B. The 25th birthday of BASIC. Byte. 1989;14:268–76.
111. Glazener TT, McDonald CJ. Putting doctors behind bars. MD Comput. 1986;3:29–33.
112. Gleick J. The unsplittable bit. Pop Sci. 2011;279:58.
113. Glowniak JV. Medical resources on the internet. Ann Intern Med. 1995;123:123–31.
114. Goldstine HH. The computer from Pascal to von Neumann. Princeton: Princeton University Press; 1972.
115. Goldwein JW, Benjamin I. Internet-based medical information: time to take charge. Ann Intern Med. 1995;123:152–3.
116. Gomes L. Attack of the freebies. Forbes 2010;185:42.
117. Gomez E, Demetriades JE, Babcock D, Peterson J. The department of veterans affairs optical patient card workstation. Proc SCAMC. 1991;378–80.
118. Greenes RA, Pappalardo AN, Marble CW, Barnett GO. Design and implementation of a clinical data management system. Comput Biomed Res. 1969;2:469–85.
119. Greenes RA. Medical computing in the 1980s: operating systems and programming language issues. J Med Syst. 1983;7:295–9.
120. Greenes RA, Barnett GO, Klein SW, Robbins A, Prior RE. Recording, retrieval and review of medical data by physician-computer interaction. N Engl J Med. 1970;282:307–15.
121. Grossman JH, Barnett GO, Koepsell TD, Nesson HR, Dorsey JL, et al. An automated medical record system. JAMA. 1973;224:1616–21.
122. Grossman L. The beast with a billion eyes. Time Magazine, Jan 30, 2012.
123. Gullo K. Steady as she goes. Datamation. 1987;33:37.
124. Gustin S. Wireless windfall. Time. 2012;179:11.
125. Hafner K, Lyon M. Where wizards stay up late: the origins of the internet. New York: Simon & Schuster; 1996.
126. Hammond WE. GEMISCH. A minicomputer information support system. Proc IEEE. 1973;61:1575–83.
127. Hammond WE, Lloyd SC. The role and potential of minicomputers. In: Haga E, Brennan R, et al., editors. Computer techniques in biomedicine and medicine. Philadelphia: Auerbach Publishers; 1973. p. 332–4.
128. Hammond WE, Stead WW, Straube MJ. Planned networking for medical information systems. Proc SCAMC. 1985;727–31.

129. Haney JP. Introduction to local area networks for microcomputers. Proc SCAMC. 1984;779–85.
130. Hartzband P, Groopman J. Untangling the web: patients, doctors, and the internet. N Engl J Med. 2010;362:1063–6.
131. Hassig L. Understanding computers, memory and storage. Richmond: Time-Life Books; 1987.
132. Helvey W, Brdlik M, Peterkin K. Online medical databases–1985: status and prognosis. Healthc Comput Commun. 1985;2:28.
133. Hodges A. Alan Turing: the enigma. New York: Simon and Schuster; 1983.
134. Hodges P. LAN growth surges. Datamation. 1989;36:32–6.
135. Hornyak T. RFID powder. Sci Am. 2008;298:68–71.
136. Hughes S. Bedside terminals: CliniCom. MD Comput. 1988;5(1):22–8.
137. Ingalls DH. Design principles behind smalltalk. BYTE Mag. 1981;6:286–98.
138. James JS. What is FORTH? A tutorial introduction. Byte. 1980;5:100–26.
139. Jennings DM, Landweber LH, Fuchs IH, Farber DJ, Adrion WR. Computer networking for scientists. Science. 1986;231:943–50.
140. Johnson KB, Rosenbloom ST. Computer-based documentation. In: Lehmann HP, Roderer N, Abbott P, editors. Aspects of electronic health record systems. New York: Springer; 2006. p. 308–28.
141. Johnson RL. Economic benefits of hospital system automation. US Healthc. 1989;6:38–40.
142. Johnson S. More and more of Moore's law. Intel is venturing beyond the co-founders old prediction with new chip technology. San Jose Mercury News. 2011.
143. Johnson SB. Generic data modeling for clinical repositories. JAMIA. 1996;3:328–39.
144. Johnson SB, Chatziantoniou D. Extended SQL for manipulating clinical warehouse data. Proc AMIA Symp. 1999;819.
145. Kahane SN, Goldberg HR, Roth HP, Lenhard RE, Johannes RS. A multimodal communications interface for endoscopy data collection with automated text report generation. Proc MEDINFO. 1986;26–30.
146. Kahn RE. Networks for advanced computing. Sci Am. 1987;257:136–43.
147. Kay A. Computer software. Sci Am. 1984;251:53–9.
148. Kay A. Microelectronics and the personal computer. Sci Am. 1977;237:230–44.
149. Kernighan BW, Ritchie DM. The state of C. Byte. 1988;13:205–10.
150. Kildall G. CP/M: a family of 8-and 16-bit operating systems. Byte. 1981;6:216–46.
151. Kimbleton SR, Schneider GM. Computer communication networks: approaches, objectives, and performance considerations. ACM Comput Surv (CSUR). 1975;7:129–73.
152. Kornfeld WA. Pattern-directed invocation languages. Byte. 1979;4:34–48.
153. Kowitt B. One hundred million Android fans can't be wrong. Fortune. 2011;164:93–7.
154. Lacson R, Long W. Natural language processing of spoken diet records. Proc AMIA Symp. 2006;454–8.
155. Larson J. The ins and outs of CP/M. Byte. 1981;6:268–82.
156. Larson R, Long W. Natural language processing of spoken diet records. Proc AMIA Ann Symp. 2006;454–8.
157. Ledley RS. A personal view of sowing the seeds. In: Blum BI, Duncan KA, editors. A history of medical informatics. New York: ACM Press/Addison-Wesley; 1990. p. 84–110.
158. Ledley RS. Introduction to digital computers and automatic programming. Biomed Electron IRE Trans. 1961;8:158–67.
159. Leibowitz MR. Profile: founding father Robert Noyce. PC/Comput. 1989;2:94–100.
160. Levine RD. Supercomputers. Sci Am. 1982;246:118–35.
161. Lev-Ram M. Intel's (latest) mobile comeback. Fortune. 2012;164:33–5.
162. Lev-Ram M. Intel's sunny vision for the cloud. Fortune. 2011;164:95–100.
163. Levy AH. Recent developments in microcomputers in medicine. Proc AAMSI. 1984;341–5.
164. Lewis HR, Papadimitriou CH. The efficiency of algorithms. Sci Am. 1978;238:96–109.
165. Lewkowicz J, Walters RF. Design of an advanced MUMPS programming environment. Proc SCAMC. 1986;336–43.

166. Liedtke M. Google search for knowledge. Bay Area News Group. 2012; C.1.2.
167. Lindberg D. The invention of the internet protocol suite. Personal communication. 2011.
168. Lindberg D. Electronic retrieval of clinical data. J Med Educ. 1965;40:753–9.
169. Lindberg D, Humphreys BL. Medicine and health on the internet: the good, the bad, and the ugly. JAMA. 1998;280:1303–4.
170. Linowes JS. It's an attitude. Byte. 1988;13:219–27.
171. Lockwood R. UNIX. Pers Comput. 1990;14:79–86.
172. London JW. A computer solution to clinical and research computing needs. Proc SCAMC. 1985;722–6.
173. Mackintosh AR. Dr. Atanasoff's computer. Sci Am. 1988;259:72–8.
174. McDonald C, Wiederhold G, Simborg DW, et al. A discussion of the draft proposal for data exchange standards. Proc IEEE. 1984;406–13.
175. McDonald CJ. The medical gopher: a microcomputer based physician work station. Proc SCAMC. 1984;453–9.
176. McGath G. A look at LISP. Byte. 1977;2:156–61.
177. McLatchey J, Barnett GO, McDonnell G, Piggins J, Zielstorff RD, et al. The capturing of more detailed medical information in COSTAR. Proc SCAMC. 1983;329–32.
178. Mediati N, Niccolai J. Microsoft introduces windows 8. PC World. 2011;15–6.
179. Meeks BN. Dialing up 1990. Byte. 1989;14:273–8.
180. Mies G. Best cell phones by carriers. PC World. 2010;28:38–40.
181. Miles WD. A history of the National Library of Medicine; the nation's treasury of medical knowledge. Washington, DC: US Government Printing Office; 1982.
182. Millard M. Dragon targets small practices with new speech technology. Health Care IT News, Jan 30, 2011.
183. Miller MJ. Apple's Macintosh. Pop Comput. 1984;3.
184. Minh CC, Chung J, Kozyrakis C, Olukotun K. STAMP: Stanford transactional applications for multi-processing. Workload Characterization. IISWC 2008. Proc IEEE Int Symp. 2008;35–46.
185. Mitroff S. Intel's first microprocessor turns 40. PC World. 2012;30:18.
186. Molnar CE, Clark WA. Development of the LINC. In: Blum BI, Duncan KA, editors. A history of medical informatics. New York: ACM Press/Addison-Wesley Pub. Co; 1990. p. 119–40.
187. Monahan ML, Kiley M, Patterson C. Bar code technology: its use within a nursing information system. Proc MEDINO. 1986;26–30.
188. Moore CH. The evolution of FORTH, an unusual language. Byte. 1980;5:76–92.
189. Mulroy J. Web 101: new site-design tools are coming. PC World. 2010;28:18.
190. Myer EP. A time-sharing multi-unit computing system. Ann NY Acad Sci. 1966;128:738–45.
191. Nedkarni PM. Management of evolving map data: data structures and algorithms based on the framework map. Genomics. 1995;30(3):565–73.
192. Nadkarni PM, Marenco L. Easing the transition between attribute-value databases and conventional databases for scientific data. Proc AMIA Symp. 2001;483–7.
193. Nadkarni PM, Brandt CM, Marenco L. WebEAV: automatic metadata-driven generation of web interfaces to entity-attribute-value databases. JAMIA. 2000;7:343–56.
194. Nadkarni PM, Marenco L, Chen R, Skoufos E, Shepherd G, Miller P. Organization of heterogeneous scientific data using the EAV/CR representation. JAMIA. 1999;6:478–93.
195. Nadkarni PM, Brandt C, Frawley S, Sayward FG, Einbinder R, et al. Managing attribute-value clinical trials data using the ACT/DB client-server database system. JAMIA. 1998;5:139–51.
196. Nedkarni PM, Cheung K-H. SQLGEN: an environment for rapid client–server database development. Comput Biomed Res. 1995;28:479–9.
197. Newbower RS, Cooper JB, Edmondson JE, Maier WR. Graphics-tablet for data-entry in computer-assisted anesthesia record-keeping. Proc SCAMC. 1981;139–42.

198. Newell A, Sproull RF. Computer networks: prospects for scientists. Science. 1982;215:843–52.
199. Nickerson RS. Man-computer interaction: a challenge for human factors research. Ergonomics. 1969;12:501–17.
200. Noyce RN. Microelectronics. Sci Am. 1977;237:62–9.
201. O'Malley C. The new operating systems. Pers Comput. 1986;10:181–5.
202. Orthner HE. New communication technologies for hospital information systems. In: Bakker AR, Ball MJ, Scherrer JR, Willem JL, editors. Towards new hospital information systems. Amsterdam: North-Holland; 1988. p. 203–12.
203. Orthner HF. Medical informatics: quo vadis? MD Comput. 1992;9(2):14–5.
204. Orthner HF, Scherrer JR, Dahlen R. Sharing and communicating health information: summary and recommendations. Int J Biomed Comput. 1994;34:303–18.
205. Pearlman D. How to choose an operating system. Pop Comput. 1984;3:148–50.
206. Pearson WR. Programming languages II. MD Comput. 1985;2:11–22.
207. Pendse N. OLAP omnipresent. Byte. 1998;23:1–2.
208. Pesce J. Bedside terminals: MedTake. MD Comput. 1988;5:16.
209. Pierce JR. Electronics: past, present, and future. Science. 1977;195:1092–5.
210. Pierce JR. Communications. Sci Am. 1972;227:31–41.
211. Pogue D. Talk to the machine. Sci Am. 2010;303:40.
212. Poon EG, Keohane CA, Yoon CS, Ditmore M, Bane A, et al. Effect of bar-code technology on the safety of medication administration. N Engl J Med. 2010;362:1698–707.
213. Pournelle J. The operating system jungle. Pop Comput. 1984;81–6.
214. Pournelle J. BASIC, computer languages and computer adventures. Byte. 1980;5:222–32.
215. Prokosch HU, Pryor TA. Intelligent data acquisition in order entry programs. Proc SCAMC. 1988;454–8.
216. Rapp W. Fourth generation languages. Comput Healthc. 1985;6:38–40.
217. Reid-Green K. History of computers: the IBM 704. Byte. 1979;4:190–2.
218. Robinson P. A world of workstations. Byte. 1987;12:251–60.
219. Robson D. Object-oriented software systems. Byte. 1981;6:74–86.
220. Rosch WL. Calculated RISC. PC Comput. 1988;1:172–88.
221. Rosen S. Electronic computers: a historical survey. ACM Comput Surv (CSUR). 1969;1:7–36.
222. Rubin C. Workstations: the personal computer alternative. Pers Comput. 1988;12:124–33.
223. Runyan L. The datamation hall of fame. Datamation. 1987;33:56.
224. Schatz W. United States computer research's basic dilemma. Datamation. 1989;35:44–7.
225. Schenker WJ. Physician-generated clinical records using a menu-driven, touch-panel microcomputer. Proc SCAMC. 1980;3:1405.
226. Schenthal JE. Clinical concepts in the application of large scale electronic data processing. In: Proc 2nd IBM medical symposium. New York: IBM; 1960.
227. Schenthal JE, Sweeney JW, Nettleton WJ, Yoder RD. Clinical application of electronic data processing apparatus: III. System for processing of medical records. JAMA. 1963;186:101–5.
228. Schipma PB, Cichocki EM, Ziemer SM. Medical information on optical disc. Proc SCAMC. 1987;732.
229. Schultz EK, Brown RW. The interactive medical record: a hypermedia prototype. Proc SCAMC. 1988;15–7.
230. Schultz EK, Brown RW. Graphmaker: a step in the design of a universal interface for a hospital information system. Proc SCAMC. 1989;675–8.
231. Sciences NN. Academies of calling all frequencies. NAS Infocus. 2010;10:1–2.
232. Seed JC. Restricted data formats. Ann N Y Acad Sci. 1969;161:484–526.
233. Segaller S. Nerds: a brief history of the internet. New York: TV Books, LLC; 1999.
234. Seltzer L. Software returns to its source. PC Mag. 1999;18:166–78.
235. Serwer A. Android calling. Fortune. 2011;164:8.

236. Shatkay H, Chen N, Blostein D. Integrating image data into biomedical text categorization. Bioinformatics. 2006;22:e446–53.
237. Shifman M, Jelovsek FR. Prolog: a language for programming medical logic. MD Comput. 1988;5:36–40.
238. Shortliffe EH. Networking health: learning from others, taking the lead. Health Aff (Millwood). 2000;19:9–22.
239. Shortliffe EH. The next generation internet and health care: a civics lesson for the informatics community. Proc AMIA Ann Symp. 1998;8–14.
240. Siekert RG, Hisey BL, Williams PE, Uber GT. A video terminal light-pen device for ordering medical tests. JAMA. 1968;206:351–6.
241. Simborg DW. Local area networks: why? what? what if? MD Comput. 1984;1:10–20.
242. Singer SJ. Visual display terminals in a hospital information system (HIS). Comput Biomed Res. 1970;3:510–20.
243. Slack WV, Hicks GP, Reed CE, Van Cura LJ. A computer-based medical-history system. N Engl J Med. 1966;274:194–8.
244. Slack WV, Peckham BM, Van Cura LJ, Carr WF. A computer-based physical examination system. JAMA. 1967;200:224–8.
245. Smith MB, Burke KE, Torgerson JS, Stollerman JE, Kern DC, et al. Logical and efficient conversation between patients and the telephone linked computer system. Proc SCAMC. 1988;463–7.
246. Spivey BE, O'Neill J. The use of optical scanning as a means of computer input in medicine. JAMA. 1969;208:665–72.
247. Stahl JE, Holt JK, Gagliano NJ. Understanding performance and behavior of tightly coupled outpatient systems using RFID: initial experience. J Med Syst. 2011;35:291–7.
248. Stead WW. A quarter-century of computer-based medical records. MD Comput. 1989;6:74–81.
249. Stefanchik MF. Point-of-care information systems: improving patient care. Comput Healthc. 1987;8:78.
250. Straube MJ, Hammond WE, Stead WW. The GEMISCH programming language. In: Orthner HF, Blum B, editors. Implementing health care information systems. New York: Springer; 1989. p. 384–95.
251. Streveler DJ, Harrison PB. Judging visual displays of medical information. MD Comput. 1985;2:26–38.
252. Stroustrup B. C++ users await next release. Byte. 1989;14:11–2.
253. Stroustrup B. A better C. Byte. 1988;13:215–8.
254. Taylor R. The computer: concept, development and problem environment. J Chronic Dis. 1966;19:333–48.
255. Taylor RW, Frank RL. CODASYL data-base management systems. ACM Comput Surv (CSUR). 1976;8:67–103.
256. Tello ER. Between man and machine. Byte. 1988;13:288–93.
257. Terdiman J. Ambulatory care computer systems in office practice: a tutorial. Proc AMIA. 1982;195–201.
258. Tesler L. The smalltalk environment. Byte. 1981;6:90–147.
259. Tesler LG. Programming languages. Sci Am. 1984;251:70–8.
260. The Economist. Tanks in the cloud. The Economist. December 29, 2010 (print version). Available at http://www.economist.com/node/17797794. Accessed August 9, 2015.
261. Titus JA. The impact of microcomputers on automated instrumentation in medicine. Advance in hardware and integrated circuits. Proc SCAMC. 1977;99–100.
262. Tolchin SG, Barta W. Local network and distributed processing issues in the Johns Hopkins Hospital. J Med Syst. 1986;10:339–53.
263. Tolchin SG, Arsenlev M, Barta WL, Kuzmak PM, Bergan E, et al. Integrating heterogeneous systems using local network technologies and remote procedure call protocols. Proc SCAMC. 1985;748–9.

264. Toole BA. Ada, the enchantress of numbers. Mill Valley: Strawberry Press; 1992.
265. Toong HD, Gupta A. Personal computers. Sci Am. 1982;247:86–107.
266. Tropp HS. The 20th anniversary meeting of the association for computing machinery: 30 August 1967. Ann Hist Comput. 1987;9:249–70.
267. Valenta AL, Wigger U. Q-methodology: definition and application in health care informatics. JAMIA. 1997;4:501–10.
268. Van Orange C, Schindler R, Valeri L. Study on the requirements and options for radio frequency identification (RFID) applications in health care. RAND Europe Rep. 2009;1–131.
269. VanName M, Catchings B. SQL-a database language sequel to Dbase. Byte. 1989;14:175–82.
270. Venkataramanan M. The database of databases. Pop Sci. 2011;279:56.
271. Verity J. The shifting shape of SNA. Datamation. 1985;93–112.
272. Walters RF. File structures for database management systems. MD Comput. 1987;5:30–41.
273. Walters RF. Developments and implementation of microcomputer MUMPS systems. J Med Syst. 1983;7:457–68.
274. Walters RF. Development of a micro MUMPS users group for the exchange of clinical applications. Proc SCAMC. 1980;3:1393–8.
275. Walters RF, Bowie J, Wilcox JC, Dayhoff RE, Reynolds SW. MUMPS primer, revised: an introduction to the interactive programming system of the future. MUMPS Users' Group; 1983.
276. Warner HR. Data sources. In: Warner HR, editor. Computer-assisted medical decision-making. New York: Academic Press; 1979. p. 6–101.
277. Wasserman AI. Software development methodologies and the user software engineering methodology. Proc SCAMC. 1982;891–3.
278. Weinberger D. Data, data everywhere. A special report on managing information. The Economist. 2010;3–19.
279. Weiner JL. The logical record keeper-prolog on the IBM. BYTE. 1984;9:125.
280. Wiederhold G. Databases, IEE computer, centennial issue. 1984; 17:211–23.
281. Wiederhold G. Databases for health care. In: Lindberg DA, Reichertz PL, editors. Lecture notes in medical informatics. New York: Springer; 1981. p. 1–75.
282. Wiederhold G. Modeling databases. Inf Sci. 1983;29:115–26.
283. Wiederhold G. Databases for ambulatory care. Proc AMIA Symp. 1982;79–85.
284. Wiederhold G, Walker MG, Blum RL. Acquisition of medical knowledge from medical records. Proc Benutzer-gruppenseminar Med Syst. 1987;213–4.
285. Wiederhold G. Database technology in health care. J Med Syst. 1981;5:175–96.
286. Wiersema M, McDonald CJ. Low-priced microcomputer voice-input boards. MD Comput. 1985;3:16–22.
287. Willard OT. Barcodes in a medical office computer system. Proc SCAMC. 1985;72–6.
288. Williams BT, Johnson R. Graphic displays. In: Williams BT, editor. Computer aids to clinical decisions, vol. II. Boca Raton: CRC Press; 1982. p. 170–8.
289. Williams BT, Foote CF, Galassie C, Schaeffer RC. Augmented physician interactive medical record. Proc MEDINFO. 1989;89:779–83.
290. Williams BT, Johnson RL, Chen TT. PLATO-based medical information system. Proc 1st Illinois conf medical information systems. Urbana, IL 1974;145–9.
291. Williams BT, Chen TT, Johnson R, Schultz DF. A terminal-orientated clinical record system. Biomed Comput. 1976;311–21.
292. Williams BT, Chen TT, Elston J, et al. The ariable phrase keyboard and the clinical report. In: Hinman EJ, editor. Advanced medical systems: the 3rd century. Miami, FL: Symposia Specialists Medical Books; 1977:127–34.
293. Williams BT, Chen TT, Schultz DF, Moll JD, Flood JR, Elston J. PLATO-based medical information system: variable keyboards. Proc 2nd Conf Med Inf Syst. 1975;56–61.
294. Williams BT. Computer aids to clinical decisions. Boca Raton, FL: CRC Press; 1982.
295. Williams G. A closer look at the IBM personal computer. Byte. 1982;7:36–66.
296. Williams M. Superfast wireless gigabit spec published. PC World. 2010;28:18.

297. Wingfield N. After iPhone sales bonanza in China, Apple's profit nearly doubles. New York Times. 2012;B1–2.
298. Wolpin S. The wild, wonderful, and wacky world of cell phones. Invent Technol. 2010;25:50–6.
299. Wolpin S, Winter I. Social networking. Invent Technol. 2010;25:52.
300. Wolverton T. Hoping Apple proves me wrong with iPad 3. Bay Area News Group. 2012.
301. Womble ME, Wilson SD, Keiser HN, Tworek ML. An intelligent terminal for access to a medical database. Proc SCAMC. 1978;517–23.
302. Wortham J, Wingfield N. Latest PC systems mimic mobile OS. Bay Area News Group. 2012; D2.
303. Zelingher J. Exploring the internet. MD Comput. 1995;12:100–8. 144.
304. Zuboff S. In the age of the smart machine: the future of work and power. New York: Basic; 1988.

Chapter 2
The Creation of a New Discipline

Morris F. Collen and Edward H. Shortliffe

Abstract The increasingly complex informatics technology that evolved since 1950 created a new domain of knowledge and a new professional discipline. In this chapter we discuss the foundations and evolution of the field of medical informatics, focusing on the role of publications, professional organizations, government, and industry in promoting the field's growth, success, and impact. The earliest reports on biomedical applications of computers began to appear at conferences sponsored by professional engineering societies as early as 1947. The English term, *medical informatics*, was successfully introduced at an international meeting held in 1974. Subsequently the range of topics and the field's scientific base have broadened, while academic informatics programs have been established at a growing number of institutions. The number of informatics articles published annually has grown rapidly, as have peer-reviewed informatics journals, the first two of which were launched in the 1960s. The first comprehensive medical informatics textbook (published in 1990) is now in its fourth edition. Starting in the 1960s, multiple organizations have been formed to focus on medical informatics; as their activities and influence increased, mergers followed, ultimately resulting in the creation of the American Medical Informatics Association (AMIA) in 1988. Other key players have included nursing, industry, academia, and the federal government, especially through the National Institutes of Health (NIH). More recently the field has been further nurtured at the federal level by the Office of the National Coordinator (ONC), which has championed the diffusion of electronic medical records, and the National Center for Advancing Translational Science (NCATS), which has funded clinical translational science awards and their supporting information systems.

Author was deceased at the time of publication.

M.F. Collen (deceased)

E.H. Shortliffe, M.D., Ph.D. (✉)
Arizona State University, Phoenix, AZ, USA

Columbia University, New York, NY, USA

Weill Cornell Medical College, New York, NY, USA

New York Academy of Medicine, New York, NY, USA
e-mail: ted@shortliffe.net

© Springer-Verlag London 2015
M.F. Collen, M.J. Ball (eds.), *The History of Medical Informatics in the United States*, Health Informatics, DOI 10.1007/978-1-4471-6732-7_2

Keywords Medical informatics • Biomedical informatics • Definitions • Professional organizations • Certification of professionals • Role of government • Academia-industry partnerships

The evolution of increasingly complex informatics technology created a new domain of knowledge and a new professional discipline. It increased physicians' use and dependence on technology, stimulated formal professional re-organizations and corporate re-orientation, and led to the development of new academic entities [145].

2.1 Naming the New Discipline

The earliest references in the scientific literature regarding the application of electronic digital computers to medicine appeared in bioengineering publications in the late 1950s. At that time the term bioengineering included all aspects of biology, engineering, and technology. A variety of names for this new discipline appeared over the next two decades, including generic terms, such as electronic data processing (EDP) or automatic data processing (ADP), and more medicine-specific names, such as medical computing, medical computer science, computer medicine, medical information processing, medical information science, medical software engineering, medical computer technology, and others. These terms were often used interchangeably – for example, medical information science with medical computer science – as though what was processed (information) and how it was processed (by computer) were similarly descriptive. In the early 1970s it became clear that there was a need to agree on a name for this new domain. To agree on the terms medicine and medical was not particularly controversial at the time, since any standard dictionary defined these terms as relating to or concerned with the research, teaching, and the practice of preventing, diagnosing, and treating diseases. However, over the years some professionals made it clear that they preferred the adjective health to medical, arguing that the discipline was as much about preserving health and preventing disease as it was about treating illness [31]. Harrison [77] observed that there was no single term in the English language to encompass the broad domain of knowledge that included computers, information, hardware, and software as applied in the fields of science, engineering, and technology, and he predicted that this knowledge domain would become a resource of unprecedented value.

Garfield [71] at the Institute for Scientific Information credited Mikhailov, at the Scientific Information Department of the Moscow State University, with first using for this purpose the Russian terms *informatik* and *informatikii*. The Russians had generally used the terms *informatsii* or *informatsiya* to mean information. Mikhailov used the term in his books entitled *Oznovy Informatiki* (*Foundations of Informatics*) and *Nauchnye Kummunikatsii ilnformatika* (*Scientific Communications and Informatics*), published in Russian in 1968 and 1976 respectively. In the second book, translated into English in 1984, he defined informatics as the scientific discipline that studied the structure and general properties of scientific information and the laws of all processes of scientific communication [125]. A search through DIALOG's *MIA International Bibliography* found that the term *informatics* first appeared in 1975 in the title of a Russian book as *informatika* [39]. The *Supplement to the Oxford English Dictionary* (1976) also credited the origin of the Anglicized word informatics to a translation from the Russian *informatika* and defined informatics as the discipline of science which investigates the structure and properties (not in a specific context) of scientific information, as well as the regularities of scientific information activity, its theory, history, methodology and organization. By 1987 the *Random House Dictionary* (1987) defined informatics as the study of information processing and computer science, also agreeing that the word informatics was a translation of the Russian *informatika* from the 1960s. It became clear that the English term informatics solved the need for a term to encompass the science, engineering, and technology for this new field, and it freed the field from all prior, more limited names and notions.

During the late 1960s, the French literature also used the terms *informatique de medecine*, or *informatique medicale*. University departments with these titles were established in the 1960s in France, Holland, and Belgium. In 1966 the term *applications de l'informatique a la medicine* was used in teaching a course by Pages and Grémy at Pitie Saltpetriere. In 1968 the Association pour les Applications de l'Informatique a la Medecine was created by Brouet et al. [54]. *Harrap's New Standard French and English Dictionary* (1979) defined the French term *informatique* as information processing and data processing and *informatique medicale* as medical computing. A search of the National Library of Medicine's MEDLINE found that articles in the French literature had first used the word informatique in 1968 [137]. Moehr [128] reported that, in Germany, computer science was called informatik from its very beginning in the 1960s. The German Society for Computer Science, Gesselshaft fur Informatik was founded in 1969. Peter Reichertz' division at the Hannover Medical School was called Medizinische Informatik from its beginning in 1969. In the 1970s the German literature also used the term *medizinische informatik* [185]. A 1975 article in the Polish literature referred to *informatyki medycznej* [34]. MEDLINE also cites the first article in Serbo-Croatian literature that used the term *medicinske informatike* [57].

Informatics, the English term, began to appear in the literature in the 1970s. An article in the French literature written in 1970 was translated into English as *Study of an Informatic System Applied to the Public Health Services* [78]. In 1970, the Organization for Economic Cooperation and Development (OECD), of which the United States was a member, considered trends and policy issues in computer-based databases and published in English *OECD Informatics Studies* [180]. The next article found that used the word informatics was published in 1972 in the Polish literature (in English) and was entitled *Informatics in Health Service* [106]. The combination of the terms, *medical* and *informatics*, first appeared in 1974 in three publications. Two were by Anderson, Pages, and Grémy, first, a book they edited that was published by the International Federation for Information Processing (IFIP) entitled *Medical Informatics Monograph Series, Volume 1, Education in*

Informatics of Health Personnel [9], and second, a paper on *Educational Requirements for Medical Informatics* [10]. Their paper appeared in a third publication, the *Proceedings of MEDINFO 1974, the First World Conference on Medical Informatics*, which Anderson, from Kings College London, co-edited with Forsythe. (For a full listing of MEDINFO Proceedings, see the back of this book). Anderson later wrote a personal note on the origin of the term *medical informatics*, in which he said that they had been searching for some time before 1974, as members of IFIP's Technical Committee No. 4 (which focused on information processing in health care), to find a suitable term for this subject area. Professors Pages and Grémy were interested in at least two aspects being represented in the final term – namely that, in French, *d'informatique* and *d'automatique* were terms used to cover medical information science or data processing. It was certain they had to find a new term and, after much discussion, they combined the two terms to form medical informatics, where the *inform* came from *d'informatique*, and the *atics* from *d'automatique*. They evidently intended the term to cover both the information and data parts as well as the control and the automatic nature of data processing itself [8].

Medical informatics was a term used freely in those historic 1974 publications, and some guidelines were formulated for a curriculum to teach medical informatics, but nowhere was this new term defined explicitly. In later discussions regarding the nature and definition of medical informatics, it evolved that medical informatics is a domain of knowledge that embraces all the following: medical data processing, medical information processing, medical computer science, medical information science, medical information systems, health care information systems, computer hardware and software; and all applications of computers and data processing by all health care professionals to the health care services, including health informatics, health care informatics, nursing informatics, dental informatics, clinical informatics, public health informatics. It also includes the basic concepts of the computer and information sciences that are fundamental to medical practice, to medical research, and to medical education. The first professional journal using this new term in its title appeared in April 1976, as *Medical Informatics – Medicine et Informatique*, edited by Anderson and Begon, and published by Taylor and Francis, Ltd (London). In Germany the first article written in English that used both of these terms was published in 1977, *Education in Medical Informatics in the Federal Republic of Germany* [95].

In 1977 Levy and Baskin [105] proposed that medical informatics be considered a basic medical science; and he defined medical informatics as dealing with the problems associated with information, its acquisition, analysis, and its dissemination in health care delivery processes. In the preliminary announcements distributed in 1977 for the Third World Conference on Medical Informatics, MEDINFO 80 in Tokyo, the program committee chair, Collen [43], defined the term medical informatics as the application of computers, communications, and information technology to all fields of medicine, i.e., to medical practice, medical education, and medical research.

Ten years after the historic conference in France that gave birth to the name medical informatics, many of the original European and American participants again met in order to consider further this new discipline [135]. Shortliffe [166] also emphasized that medical informatics included more than the applications of computers to medicine, since some in this field studied medical computing as a basic science subject (focused on methodology, technique, and theory development) rather than as a medical tool. At that conference, Shortliffe gave examples of studies in artificial intelligence that advanced medical information science yet would require extensive additional work for practical clinical application. The importance of computer communications was also emphasized at the conference by van Bemmel [187], who noted that medical informatics comprised the theoretical and practical aspects of information processing and communication, based on knowledge and experience derived from processes in medicine and health care. Reichertz [144], Moehr [128], and Haux [80] also offered definitions of medical informatics that emphasized dealing with the systematic processing of medical information, the use of appropriate methods and tools in information processing systems, and the study of medical information science. Blois [26] used the term *medical information science* to study and advance the theory and concept of medical information itself; and emphasized that the term, *informatics*, was broader than was the term *information science*, stressing that *informatics* included information engineering and technology. Blois [25] later drew further attention to the important distinction between information (the commodity with which thinking, analyzing, and decision making deal) and the computer (the tool for use in processing the commodity).

In 1985 the American Standards for Testing and Materials (ASTM), which had served as a catalyst in the United States for developing and publishing voluntary consensus-based standards for a variety of products and systems including computer-based systems, established a Subcommittee on Medical Informatics, with Gabrieli [68] as its chair. By the next year a committee of the Association of American Medical Colleges (AAMC), chaired by Myers, took the position that medical informatics combined medical science with several technologies and disciplines in the information and computer sciences, and provided methodologies by which these could contribute to better use of the medical knowledge base and ultimately to better medical care. The AAMC group defined medical informatics as a developing body of knowledge, and a set of techniques, concerning the organization and management of information in support of medical research, education, and patient care [124].

Greenes and Siegel [75], for the American College of Medical Informatics (ACMI), and Siegel, for the National Library of Medicine (NLM), reported a 1985 collaborative study undertaken by members of ACMI, assisted by NLM staff, to attempt to arrive at a definition for the content and scope of the field of medical informatics and the functions of the professionals in this field. They arrived at these descriptive summaries:

- Medical informatics may be considered to be composed largely of component disciplines, and the most important of these are computer science, decision science, statistics, library science, epidemiology, and the basic medical sciences;
- Medical informatics draws on those fields that are primarily viewed as basic sciences, including linguistics, mathematics, electrical engineering, and psychology;

- Medical informatics is used principally in the fields of clinical medicine, preventive medicine, public health, nursing, education, hospital administration, and health administration;
- The disciplines in which medical informatics is principally applied include: decision support, database management, knowledge management, image processing, simulation, and natural language processing.

They accordingly summarized the field with these component definitions:

- Medical informatics is the application of computer and information science to medicine and health services.
- Medical informatics is the field concerned with the properties of medical information: data, information, and knowledge.
- Medical informatics encompasses information science, information engineering and information technology used for medical practice, medical education, and medical research.

Based on these various definitions and summaries, the authors suggested that *medical informatics is the field concerned with the cognitive, information processing, and information management tasks of medical and health care and biomedical research, with the application of information science and technology to these tasks.*

Morris [129] studied the structure of the term medical informatics by analyzing the relationships between a set of NLM's MESH terms for information science and for information technology (IS/IT) in a retrieved set of journals from MEDLINE, published during 1955–1999. He concluded that the co-occurrence of indexed terms relating to these two words provided some complementary perspective on the structure of medical informatics as a field.

Lindberg's 1984 Long-Range Planning Committee for the National Library of Medicine also defined the term medical informatics as a field that seeks to provide the theoretical and scientific basis for the application of computers and automated information systems to biomedicine and health affairs. It also studies biomedical information, data, and knowledge and their storage, retrieval, and optimal use for problem-solving and decision-making. It touches on all basic and applied fields in biomedical science, and is closely tied to modern information technology, notably in the areas of computing and communications [107]. Blois and Shortliffe [24] also offered as the definition of medical informatics: *the rapidly developing scientific field that deals with the storage, retrieval, and optimal use of biomedical data, information, and knowledge for problem solving and decision making. It accordingly touches on all basic and applied fields in biomedical science, and is closely tied to modern information technologies, notably in the areas of computing, communications, and medical computer science.* Some questioned whether the term medical in medical informatics might be interpreted as referring only to physicians, so Ball et al. [13] suggested that the definition of medical informatics should explicitly be stated to include those informational technologies that concern themselves with the patient-care decision-making process performed by all health care practitioners, including physicians, nurses, dentists, and others. Stead [174] emphasized that the term medical, in medical informatics, did not just mean physicians but included all personnel in the health care arena. Bernstam et al. [22] defined medical informatics as the application of the science of information as data plus meaning to problems of biomedical interest.

Thus, the term medical informatics was broadened in its definition over the years to include not only the device (the computer), and what the device processed (information), but also all applications to medical science, medical research and development, medical education, and medical practice including such functions as clinical decision support [108]. In the 1980s and later, some also began to use the terms: clinical informatics [90], health informatics [127], nursing informatics [18], dental informatics [48] and also imaging informatics, public health informatics, and others. In academic settings, the first to be termed a Department of Medical Informatics in the United States was established at the University of Utah by Warner, who became the first Professor of Medical Informatics. The unit had started in the 1960s as a Department of Medical Biophysics but evolved over time and was the first to adopt the medical informatics terminology. The first Department of Computer Medicine had earlier been established at the Tulane University by Sweeney, who became the first Professor of Computer Medicine. The first Division of Clinical Informatics was established at the Harvard Medical School and its affiliates by Bleich and Slack, and was later formalized and led by Safran [154]. Shortliffe started a graduate degree program in medical information sciences at Stanford University in 1982, but within a few years had dubbed the academic unit that offered the degrees the Section on Medical Informatics.

With the growth of informatics methods applied to basic life sciences, and especially to the human genome project during the 1990s, a new term emerged that has been widely adopted: bioinformatics. Recognizing that the methods and issues in bioinformatics were very similar to those in medical informatics, the community sought to devise unifying terminology that would encourage the biological and clinical informatics communities to coexist, to share methods, and to tackle translational problems between the genetic and patient-care research environments. Academic units, in particular, began to adopt the term biomedical informatics by the turn of the new century, often including both bioinformatics and clinical informatics faculty and graduate students who worked either on biological, clinical, or translational problems. This inclusive term was gradually embraced and is increasingly accepted as the name for the field, supplanting medical informatics in many cases. With this change, the medical informatics term has come to be reserved by many in the field for disease- and physician-oriented informatics activities, with biomedical informatics referring to the broad basic discipline [97].

In 2012, the American Medical Informatics Association (AMIA) published a white paper in which they laid out the core competencies for graduate education in the field of *biomedical informatics* and offered the following definition: *the interdisciplinary field that studies and pursues the effective uses of biomedical data, information, and knowledge for scientific inquiry, problem solving, and decision making, motivated by efforts to improve human health* [97]. Although this new term for the field has gained increasing acceptance, in this volume we continue to use the long-established term medical informatics. Readers may wish to note, however, that the terminology and definitions are continuing to evolve, as they have throughout the history of the discipline.

2.2 The Diffusion and Integration of Informatics in Medicine

The beginning in the United State of what was to become known as medical informatics was attributed by Lindberg [108] to the initiation in 1879 of the *Index Medicus* by Billings. That same year Hollerith went to work for the U. S. Census Bureau, where Billings advised him to develop a method to use punch cards to count the census data. Major roles in the subsequent dissemination and the integration of this new field were played by biomedical publications; by professional bioengineering, medical, and nursing organizations; by commercial organizations; by federal agencies; and by academia. Some of those activities are summarized here.

2.2.1 The Role of Publications

As has been mentioned, *Index Medicus* was initiated by Billings in 1879, providing a bibliographic listing of references to current articles in the world's biomedical journals. A major contribution to medical informatics occurred when the National Library of Medicine (NLM) began to convert the Index Medicus to computer-based form with the printing of its 1964 edition, thereby implementing the first version of the Medical Literature Analysis and Retrieval System (MEDLARS). MEDLINE, the online version of MEDLARS, which supported search capabilities, was initiated in 1971.

Vallbona et al. [186] reported that an analysis of the Index Medicus regarding the number of papers on the subject of computers in medicine showed only 38 papers in 1960, 137 in 1961, 168 in 1962, 202 in 1963; and then an average of about 350 papers each year from 1964 to 1968. A search conducted in January 1986 by Parascandola at the NLM retrieved 2,506 MEDLINE citation titles between 1966 and 1984 using *medic* or *health* with *comput* (excluding articles in foreign languages). This study showed that on average only 35 new citations were added each year from 1966 to 1974. However, in 1975 the annual count of new citations abruptly increased, averaging 135 from 1975 to 1979; and then averaging 250 each year from 1980 to 1984 [136]. A similar search for these three words appearing anywhere in any journal article would have found perhaps several times as many articles and would have been more comparable to Vallbona's statistics. A later analysis by the NLM Technical Services Division yielded a total of 5,850 citations regarding the total of all articles in the general field of medical informatics in the published articles or proceedings for: (1) MEDINFO 1983, (2) Association for Medical Systems and Informatics (AAMSI) Congress 1984, (3) Symposium on Computer Applications in Medical Care (SCAMC) 1984, (4) in 12 months of issues of *Computers in Biomedical Research* (1983 and 1984), and (5) *Methods of Information in Medicine* (1984).

Although papers that described the use of analog computers had been published earlier, articles on applications of digital computers in medicine appeared first in engineering publications, then later in the biomedical engineering literature, and finally in medical journals. The first article found in the U.S. literature in which an electronic digital computer was reported to be used in any field of medicine appeared in the mid-1950s, written by Farley and Clarke [65] while they were at the Lincoln Laboratory at Massachusetts Institute of Technology (MIT). It dealt with simulation modeling to approximate various definitions of learning. The next article found was one written by Ledley [101], then at Johns Hopkins University, on digital computational methods in symbolic logic with examples in biochemistry. Soon after, Ledley and Lusted [100] published, in the journal *Science*, their classic article titled *Reasoning Foundations of Medical Diagnosis*. The lack of any published use of digital computers in medicine in the entire year of 1955 was evidenced by a comprehensive review article by Lusted [116] on progress in medical electronics. The term digital computers occurred only once at the end of the article, when mentioning the use of digital computers for large-scale data problems, without citing any references on this subject.

The few papers published in the second half of the 1950s on applications of digital computers to biomedicine were scattered in various specialized technical journals. They reported on studies with an electronic digital computer on cell multiplication in cancer [85], and on applications of an electronic digital correlator (which some people considered to be an analog device) to biomedical research in neurophysiology [20, 29].

The U.S. Air Force's Research and Development Command in Baltimore sponsored a series of conferences in 1956 and 1957 on applications of computers to medicine and biology [193]. By the early 1960s articles on how computers could be applied to clinical medicine began to appear regularly in some journals of the medical profession [23, 33, 44, 45, 47, 69, 114, 189].

The oldest informatics journal, *Methods of Information in Medicine*, was first published in 1961 in Germany by Schattauer Verlag, with Wagner as its founding editor. There was a half-century retrospective and celebration for this journal in Heidelberg in June 2011 [79]. *Computers in Biomedical Research* was the earliest US-based peer-reviewed journal in medical informatics, published by Academic Press, New York, beginning in 1967. It was edited by Warner at the University of Utah in Salt Lake City. Decades later, in 2001, this publication changed its name to the *Journal of Biomedical Informatics*. Other journals began to appear in the US after Warner's journal, including *Computers and Medicine* in 1972, edited by Harris and published by the American Medical Association (AMA) in Chicago. The *Journal of Clinical Computing* was also initiated in 1972, edited by Gabrieli in Buffalo and published by Gallagher Printing, New York. The *Journal of Medical Systems* appeared in 1977; it was edited by Grams at the University of Florida and published by Plenum Press, New York. *MD Computing*, initially published as

Medcom in 1983, was edited by McDonald at the University of Indiana and published by Springer-Verlag, New York. In 1985 a directory of journals and magazines in health informatics was prepared by Mackintosh [119]; it listed 42 such publications in the United States. In 1986 the *Journal of the American Medical Association (JAMA)* included for the first time medical informatics as a specialty in its annual review issue [108].

Books on medical computing began to appear in the United States in the 1960s, authored, for example, by Dixon [60], Sterling and Pollack [175]) Proctor and Adey [141], Ledley [102, 104], Atkins [11], Krasnoff [96], Taylor [178], and Lindberg [111]. Books that provided reviews of the accomplishments in the earliest decades of medical informatics included the *Use of Computers in Biology and Medicine* [104] and two volumes on *Computers in Biomedical Research* [171]. A review of early *Hospital Computer Systems* was edited by Collen [46]. *The Growth of Medical Information Systems in the United States*, a review of medical information systems in the 1970s was written by Lindberg [112].

Subsequent books on medical informatics topics are, of course, too numerous to summarize here. Particularly pertinent, perhaps, is the emergence, in 1990, of the first comprehensive modern textbook for the field, titled *Medical Informatics* [165]. Designed to emphasize the conceptual basis of the field (rather than specific applications or technologies) so that it would remain current for several years, the book helped to support the introduction of medical informatics courses in several medical schools and other university programs. Its success led to subsequent editions in 2000 and 2006, with the fourth and most recent version published in 2015, now under the title *Biomedical Informatics*, in [167].

The first book on *Computers in Nursing* was edited by Zielstorf and published in 1980 [198]. Reports on computer applications in nursing began to appear in the 1981 SCAMC Proceedings [30]. The International Medical Informatics Association (IMIA) introduced the term nursing informatics at the 1983 meeting of the IMIA Working Group on Nursing Informatics that was held in Amsterdam [18]. Five years later the first book on nursing with the term informatics in its title, *Nursing Informatics* [14], was published. Comprehensive reviews of the history of nursing informatics were edited by Weaver [192], Ball et al. [16, 12, 15, 17], and Saba and McCormack [152].

The first monograph on dental informatics was edited by Zimmerman et al. [199]. Dental informatics was advanced by the American Dental Education Association (ADEA); in the 2000s ADEA announced the book, *Dental Computing and Applications: Advanced Techniques for Clinical Dentistry*, by Daskalaki [50]. Programs for training in dental informatics became available from the Howard Hughes Medical Institute; and also in dental informatics research by the National Institute of Dental and Craniofacial Research (NIDCR) directed by Schleyer at the University of Pittsburg [159]. A department for the teaching of dental informatics was first established in the United States in 1986 as a division at the University of Maryland at Baltimore, with Craig as its first director [48]. In September 2009 the American Dental Education Association (ADEA) in its publication, *Dental Informatics Online Communications*, reported that the ADEA had established a

Dental Informatics Section. In 2009 the National Institute of Dental and Craniofacial Research (NIDCR) announced its initiation of a training program in the discipline of dental informatics [159].

In such a rapidly evolving discipline, where substantive advances often occurred within a single year, publications in traditional medical journals were often out-of-date, and books often described informatics technology that was already obsolete by the time the books were published. Accordingly, the timeliest articles on computer applications in medicine were often found in proceedings and transactions of meetings sponsored by professional and commercial organizations. The *Proceedings of the Symposium on Computer Applications in Medical Care* (*SCAMC*), published annually since 1977 (known as the *Proceedings of the AMIA Annual Symposium* since 1990), have been among the most comprehensive US resources for medical informatics research. (For a listing of these proceedings, see the appendices at the back of this volume.) A perusal of the first decade of annual SCAMC proceedings showed that these early issues addressed mostly computer hardware and software problems. In the second decade the preponderance of articles was related to database and to clinical decision-support applications. A similar analysis of the MEDINFO proceedings in 1983 and in 1986 [188] revealed that 17 % of the articles published in both years were related to computer hardware, software, and communications. Articles on medical information systems and databases decreased from 39 % in 1983 to 19 % in 1986. Those on processing clinical data from the clinical laboratory, radiology, and electrocardiography decreased from 36 % in 1983 to 10 % in 1986. Articles on computers used in therapy increased slightly from 3 % in 1983 to 5 % in 1986. Papers on medical research and education also increased slightly from 9 % in 1983 to 11 % in 1986. Articles on medical decision making increased the most, from 13 % in 1983 to 23 % in 1986. In the 1990s and 2000s, articles increasingly dealt with clinical decision support, clinical subsystems, clinical research and education, and Internet-supported translational databases.

Useful collections of articles for the first decade of computer applications to medical practice were also found in the July 31, 1964, issue of the *Annals of the New York Academy of Sciences*, entitled *Computers in Medicine and Biology*, and also in the *Journal of Chronic Disease*, Volume 19, 1966. The *Journal of the American Hospital Association* devoted its entire issue of January 1, 1964, to *Automatic Data Processing in Hospitals*. Several bibliographies of citations on various aspects of medical computing, some with annotations, were published in the 1950s and 1960s. The first extensive *Bibliography on Medical Electronics* was published in 1958 by the Professional Group in Bio-Medical Electronics of the Institute of Radio Engineers. This was followed in 1959 by Supplement I. In 1962, Knutson, at Remington Rand Univac in St. Paul, Minnesota, compiled and published an annotated *Bibliography of Computer Applications in Bio-Medical Research*. In 1963, Empey, at System Development Corporation in Santa Monica, California, compiled for the Association for Computing Machinery (ACM) *SIGBIO Newsletter* No. 1, *Computer Applications in Medicine and the Biological Sciences Bibliography*, and in 1967 ACM published in *Computing Reviews* a *Comprehensive Bibliography of Computing Literature*. In 1968 Robertson began to publish a series of *Computers in*

Medicine Abstracts. In 1984 the *MD Computing* journal began to provide annual listings of vendors of hardware and software for various medical applications [139]. Relevant articles published in these and in later decades are referred to in chapters later in this volume.

2.2.2 The Role of Bioengineering Organizations

A variety of organizations in the United States had significant roles in the diffusion and integration of informatics into medicine, including bioengineering organizations that applied informatics techniques to medical, nursing, and related health care problems; commercial organizations; federal agencies; and academic organizations.

The earliest reports on biomedical applications of computers began to appear at conferences sponsored by professional bioengineering societies. Many of the earliest computer applications involved the processing of clinical laboratory data, analog signals (such as electrocardiograms), and images (such as photographs and x-ray images). In 1947 the first Annual Conference on Engineering in Medicine was held, and in 1948 a group of bioengineers with interests in medical equipment held the First Annual Conference on Medical Electronics in New York City.

In 1947 the Association for Computing Machinery (ACM) was formed, and ACM established its Special Interest Groups (SIGs) in 1960 [146]. One of these was SIGBIO, in which the acronym BIO originally represented biomedical information processing. In 1966 ACM SIGBIO reorganized into the Society for Biomedical Computing, elected Barnett as its first president, and provided a forum in the early 1970s for presentations and proceedings articles on biomedical computing. Although SIGBIO and the Society for Biomedical Computing later became inactive for several decades, in 2010 ACM SIGBioinformatics was instituted with the aim of advancing computational biology and biomedical informatics, and to bridge computer science, mathematics, and statistics with biomedicine.

In 1951 the Professional Group in Bio-Medical Electronics (PGBME) of the Institute of Radio Engineers (IRE) was organized – the largest professional organization concerned with the broad area of biomedical technology and the engineering and physical sciences in the 1950s [160]. PGBME held a symposium on the applications of computers in biology and medicine at the annual IRE convention in 1957. It subsequently sponsored the Annual Conferences in Bio-Medical Electronics and published the *IRE Transactions on Medical Electronics* which, in the 1950s, was the main forum for papers on biomedical computing [118]. A 1955 review of the progress in medical electronics gave credit to the American Institute of Electrical Engineers (AIEE), later to become the Institute for Electrical and Electronic Engineers (IEEE), for sponsoring some of the earliest meetings on this subject [116].

The Rockefeller Institute sponsored a Conference on Diagnostic Data Processing in 1959 that was organized by Zvorykin and Berkley, and the proceedings of this conference were published in the *IRE Transactions* and contained a collection of papers that represented the state-of-the-science at that time [64].

In 1951 the IRE, AIEE/IEEE, and ACM, with the participation of the National Simulation Council, began to sponsor Joint Computer Conferences. At their Fall Joint Computer Conference in 1961, these professional associations formed the American Federation for Information Processing Societies (AFIPS). AFIPS continued to sponsor Fall and Spring Joint Computer Conferences until 1973, when it combined the two conferences into one large annual National Computer Conference, generally referred to as the NCC [66]. In time this conference disappeared, largely due to the growth of the field, the emergence of more specialized meetings, and the realization that a meeting that attempted to cover all of computer science research and application was impractical and unrealistic.

In 1968 five national engineering societies formed the Joint Committee on Engineering in Medicine and Biology (JCEMB). These societies were the Institute of Electrical and Electronic Engineers (IEEE), the Instrument Society of America (ISA), the American Society of Mechanical Engineers (ASME), and the American Institute of Chemical Engineers (AICHE). JCEMB soon comprised more than 20 organizations and it sponsored the Annual Joint Conferences on Engineering in Medicine and Biology (AJCEMB). The first volume of their conference proceedings was published in 1969, and contained several papers on computer applications in medicine.

In 1969 the Alliance for Engineering in Medicine and Biology (AEMB) was founded, with the intent to provide mechanisms whereby disparate professional workers and groups might collaborate effectively in dealing with issues of common concern involving medicine and the life sciences interacting with engineering and the physical sciences [74]. In the late 1960s the Engineering Foundation sponsored a series of conferences on engineering systems in medicine, focusing on multiphasic health testing systems, which resulted in the formation of the Society for Advanced Medical Systems (SAMS). By 1971 SAMS had joined the AEMB as an associate member; and then in 1974 as a full member; however, the ACEMB produced few articles on medical informatics. The Biomedical Engineering Society (BMES), the Association for the Advancement of Medical Instrumentation (AAMI), and the Health Applications Section of the Operations Research Society of America (ORSA) also provided some early articles on medical informatics.

The American Federation for Information Processing Societies (AFIPS) contributed to the evolution of medical informatics in the United States by serving as this nation's representative to the International Federation for Information Processing (IFIP). IFIP had many technical committees, some of which were active in medical computing. In 1974 IFIP's Fourth Technical Committee (TC-4) held its first MEDINFO Congress in Stockholm, which was so successful that TC-4 renamed itself the International Medical Informatics Association (IMIA). In 1988 IMIA became independent of IFIP, and had its own national representatives from most countries of the world. The US representative organization shifted from AFIP to AMIA shortly after AMIA was formed. Healthcare informatics was also a term used in 1983 by IMIA [41].

Many of the conferences and organizations mentioned in this chapter have been phased out, replaced, or renamed over time. Such is the nature of science and engineering, especially given the rapid evolution that we have witnessed in the last half-century. Today both the ACM and IEEE, which are now very large and strong organizations, have a significant presence with meetings and publications related to medical informatics topics. Some are jointly sponsored with organizations from the professional informatics community, and many medical informatics experts are active in ACM and/or IEEE as well as in AMIA and other informatics groups.

2.2.3   The Role of Medical Informatics Organizations

2.2.3.1   Medical Organizations

The publications cited above document that the earliest computer applications in any field of medicine were in medical research, medical education, and medical literature retrieval. Cardiologists and surgeons soon began to use computers for the monitoring of patients in intensive and coronary care units. Some of the earliest work in signal analysis was for the automated interpretation of electrocardiograms. Computers were soon used in automated clinical laboratory and multiphasic health testing systems, and were employed early in radiology and in pharmacy systems. In the 1960s some of the clinical specialties began to explore the use of computers for the processing of patient care information for outpatients in medical offices and for inpatients cared for in hospitals.

In the 1950s the American Hospital Association (AHA) and the Hospital Management Systems Society (HMSS) began to conduct conferences to acquaint hospital administrators with the potential of evolving hospital information systems (HISs). In 1961 HMSS became the Healthcare Information and Management Systems Society (HIMSS); in 1966 it affiliated with the American Hospital Association (AHA). However, about 25 years later in 1993, HIMSS separated from AHA and became an independent organization with its mission to lead healthcare transformation through the effective use of health information technology. In the 2000s HIMSS represented more than 38,000 individual members, more than 540 corporate members, and more than 120 not-for-profit organizations. It continues to conduct frequent national conventions and trade shows (typically drawing between 30,000 and 40,000 attendees) and distributes publications [83, 84].

By the late 1960s many large medical professional organizations had formed special committees and had sponsored conferences on computer applications related to their special medical interests. In April 1966 the American Medical Association (AMA) held a conference in Chicago on The Computer and the Medical Record, chaired by Yoder of Tulane University. In 1969 the AMA formed a Committee on the Computer in Medicine that was chaired by Parrott; this committee held its initial Conference on Computer Assistance in Medicine on November 20, 1969, in Washington, DC. In 1972 the AMA undertook a major activity regarding computer systems in medicine to try to increase physicians' awareness of the effects of computers on medical practice. In 1978 the AMA testified before the Congressional Subcommittee on Domestic and International Scientific Planning, Analysis, and Cooperation, supporting the use of computers in health care. At that time the AMA advocated that the primary thrust in the growing field of medical computer technology should remain in the private sector, and that any federal role should be to fund substantial research and development projects [76].

At least two other medically related professional organizations were playing an important role in the evolution of medical informatics by the 1980s. In 1983, Hogness, President of the Association of Academic Health Centers (AAHC), commissioned Piemme of George Washington University School of Medicine to write a document on the spectrum of medical informatics in the academic medical centers. Ball, from Temple University, joined in the effort, and the monograph, *Executive Management of Computer Resources in the Academic Health Center*, was published in January 1984 [1]. The publication discussed administration of computer resources as well as applications and resources in education, research, and patient care, forecasting how the future academic health center would function in an informatics-enriched world.

A second organization that played an important role in addressing early informatics issues during that period was the Association of American Medical Colleges (AAMC). By 1982 they had published a key document anticipating the implications of computer systems for managing information in academic medicine [122]. A few years later they published a monograph aimed at defining competencies for physicians in the twenty-first century, emphasizing, as one element, the role of computers and informatics in the future of clinical practice [2]. Continuing to study actively the role of computing in medical education [3], the association sponsored a Symposium on Medical Informatics: Medical Education in the Information Age in March 1985. Teams of academic leaders from 50 US and Canadian medical school met to consider the impact of advances in information science and computer and communications technologies on the clinical practice of medicine and education activities of the academic medical center [124].

2.2.3.2 IMIA and MEDINFO

As previously described, medical informatics, as an English term, became internationally accepted as a result of its use by the successful First World Conference on Medical Informatics: MEDINFO 74, which was held in Stockholm in August 1974 and then followed by a series of such international meetings on a triennial basis. The program committee chair of the historic first conference was Grémy from France; edited by Anderson and Forsythe [9, 10] from England, the proceedings included 194 papers, of which 42 (22 %) were from the United States. Of these 42, 10 were reports of hospital and medical information systems, with 6 of these reports describing the ground breaking Lockheed hospital information system installed in the El Camino Hospital in Mountain View, California. It is noteworthy that the term *informatics* appeared in the title of the proceedings of this congress but in only one paper, written by the MEDINFO proceedings editor, Anderson (1974) and associates.

MEDINFO 77, the Second World Conference on Medical Informatics, was held in Toronto in August 1977 and was again organized by IFIP's TC-4 (later to be known as IMIA). Schneider from Sweden was the program committee chair and the proceedings were edited by Shires and Wolf. MEDINFO 77 contained 199 papers, of which 53 were from the United States, and of these 15 dealt with medical information systems or medical records whereas 6 were on computer-aided clinical decision support.

MEDINFO 80, the Third World Conference on Medical Informatics, was sponsored by the newly named IMIA and was held in Tokyo; it was the first MEDINFO to have a significant US involvement. Collen from California was the program chair and the proceedings were edited by Lindberg (Missouri) and Kaihara (Tokyo). MEDINFO 80 contained 276 full papers, of which 51 (18 %) were from the United States, and of these 51 were on medical information systems; 6 were on diagnosis, decision support, or artificial intelligence. Still, in 1980, only four articles in these proceedings contained the term informatics, indicating that the new term for the field was slow to be widely embraced.

MEDINFO 83: the Fourth World Conference on Medical Informatics was held in Amsterdam. The program chair was Lodwick (Minnesota) and the proceedings were edited by van Bemmel (Netherlands), Ball (Pennsylvania), and Wigertz (Sweden). The MEDINFO 83 proceedings contained 318 full papers, of which 68 (11 %) were from the United States; of these 68 papers, 19 were on medical information systems and subsystems, 19 were on decision support and artificial intelligence, and 10 papers were on imaging. By this time the term informatics appeared in nine papers.

The next MEDINFO was the first to be held in the United States. MEDINFO 86: the Fifth World Conference on Medical Informatics took place in Washington, DC, in October 1986. Lindberg (NLM) was the organizing committee chair, van Bemmel (Netherlands) was the program committee chair, and Salamon (France) edited the proceedings. The widespread interest and support for medical informatics in the United States at that time was clearly evident by the relative ease with which Lindberg obtained the capital funding necessary to finance a MEDINFO. He formed a US Council for MEDINFO 86, which consisted of 12 US professional medical societies including the American Medical Association, American Society of Clinical Pathologists, and American Radiological Society; bioengineering societies (IEEE, ACM); and also medical informatics organizations (AAMSI, SCAMC). Each of these organizations provided a substantial loan which furnished the initial working capital; in addition, several donations and grants were received, the largest being from Kaiser Foundation Hospitals.

MEDINFO 89: the Sixth World Conference on Medical Informatics was held in 1989 in two parts: Part One took place as originally planned in November 1989 in Beijing. Part Two was held in December 1989 in Singapore, for those who could not or would not go to China following the Beijing Tiananmen Square student massacre of June 4, 1989. Manning (California) was the program committee chair for both parts of MEDINFO 89. By this time, despite the political challenges around the 1989 meeting, MEDINFO had become a successful and highly anticipated event that rotated to different cities every 3 years, generally adopting a cycle of Europe-North America-Asia in that order. IMIA member organizations now prepared bids to host the meeting and the process became quite competitive.

MEDINFO meetings continue until the present day, although they recently adopted a change to alternate year meetings starting in 2013. Meetings not previously mentioned include MEDINFO 92 in Geneva, Switzerland; MEDINFO 95 in Vancouver, British Columbia, Canada; MEDINFO 98 in Seoul, Korea; MEDINFO 2001 in London, UK; MEDINFO 2004 in San Francisco, California, USA; MEDINFO 2007 in Brisbane, Australia; MEDINFO 2010 in Capetown, South Africa; MEDINFO 2013 in Copenhagen, Denmark; MEDINFO 2015 in Sao Paulo, Brazil.

2.2.3.3 IHEA and IHEPA

In 1970 a meeting of users and providers of automated multiphasic health testing systems (AMHTS) took place in Washington, DC, chaired by Caceres from George Washington University's Medical Center. This meeting included a series of discussions of the value of AMHTS from both the financial and medical viewpoints, and it ended with the commitment to create an International Health Evaluation Association (IHEA) with the goal of supporting computer applications in health evaluation systems and in preventive medicine. In 1971, the first meeting of IHEA was held in Honolulu, Hawaii, chaired by Gilbert of the Straub Clinic and Pacific Health Research Institute. Gilbert was the inventor of the "carrel concept" of health testing which made AMHT practical for small size medical practices; he was subsequently elected the first President of IHEA. A collaboration with the Japan Society of AMHTS was also formed at this meeting, and IHEA moved toward the broader concepts of clinical preventive medicine and wellness.

In 1973 at its London meeting, IHEA decided to adopt a decentralized organizational structure to recognize and facilitate the international membership in IHEA. A central office in the US would remain to help coordinate the overall operations and meet ongoing U.S. requirements associated with the incorporation of the Association. Three regions were formed: Region I consisted of the United Stated (excluding Hawaii), Canada, and Latin America; Region II included Europe, Africa, and the Middle East; Region III included Asia and the Pacific region including Hawaii. Regions could then deal with local issues while still operating under the bylaws of IHEA. The collaboration of Region III with the Japan Society of AMHTS was also formed at this meeting. In 1973 the IHEA symposium in London was also faced with a major change in the support of AMHT in the United States when a severe economic recession terminated federal support for preventive medicine programs. The university-based programs and the USPHS demonstration and research centers for AMHT were phased out, the Staten Island Center funding was withdrawn, grant funding for the Massachusetts General Hospital Center program was eliminated, and legislation for Medicare reimbursement was withdrawn.

In 1974 the IHEA symposium was held in San Francisco, hosted by Kaiser Permanente (KP). Garfield [72] described his new ambulatory health care delivery model that provided the rationale behind KP's AMHT program, and Yasaka reported on the current status of health evaluation in Japan. In 1980 the IHEA symposium was held in Tokyo, in conjunction with the 1980 MEDINFO Congress, and joint meetings were also held with the Japan Society of AMHTS. After the 1984 IHEA meeting, a formal liaison was developed between the IHEA and the nascent American Association for Medical Systems and Informatics (AAMSI; see discussion below); the next two IHEA symposia were held in Washington, DC, in conjunction with MEDINFO in 1986 and with AAMSI in 1987. The 1988 symposium in Kailua-Kona, Hawaii, had sessions focused on health care workers such as dieticians, nurses, health educators, computer operators, laboratory technicians, x-ray technicians, and other technical support personnel. In 1988 Hinohara of Japan became the President of IHEA. In 1990 the Society for Prospective Medicine, an international organization dedicated to advancing the practice of disease prevention and health promotion, joined IHEA and the organization's name was changed to the International Health Evaluation and Promotion Association (IHEPA) in order to reflect more accurately the interest of this new larger organization. In 2000 the MJ group in Taiwan hosted the IHEA/IHEPA annual meeting in Taipei. In 2003, with the decreased support of multiphasic health testing systems in the United States, the last meeting in the United States for Region I of the IHEPA was held in Atlanta, Georgia, chaired by Blankenbaker of the University of Tennessee College of Medicine, Chattanooga. This meeting was opened with Lindberg, Director of the National Library of Medicine, as its keynote speaker, and it had presentations regarding automated multiphasic health testing programs from a variety of countries. In 2008, with the support of the MJ group in Taiwan, IHEPA's symposium was held in Beijing in collaboration with the Chinese Medical Association and the Chinese Society of Health Management. IHEPA subsequently held meetings in 2010 in Tokyo and in 2011 in Honolulu. In the 2010s, IHEPA Region III continued to be active in Asia, conducting bi-annual meetings with the support of its president, Hinohara of Japan, and its secretary, Shambaugh [161, 162] of Hawaii.

2.2.3.4   SCM, SAMS, and AAMSI

In 1967 the first professional organization in the United States with the primary goal of furthering technology systems in medicine, especially computer-based medical systems, was the Society for Advanced Medical Systems (SAMS). It held its first conference in July 1967 in Milwaukee, Wisconsin, and in 1968 SAMS was incorporated in the state of New York. SAMS had emerged from a series of Engineering Foundation Research Conferences sponsored by the Engineering Foundation of New York. These conferences were arranged by Devey of the National Academy of Engineering, originally to support the development of automated multiphasic health testing (AMHT) systems. The second conference was held in August 1968 at the Proctor Academy in Andover, New Hampshire [52]. At this Andover meeting, an organizational planning committee chaired by Davies from the University of Tennessee was initiated to form a professional society to focus on the evolving field of multiphasic health testing (MHT). The new organization, SAMS, cosponsored the next Engineering Foundation Research Conference which was held in August 1969 at the Deerfield Academy in Deerfield, Massachusetts, and defined this conference as SAMS' first annual meeting. Caceres of George Washington University was elected the first president of SAMS, and Davies the president-elect. On September 30, 1970, with the help of Hsieh of Baltimore's U.S. Public Health Service Hospital, SAMS offered a scientific program, and its Proceedings were later published [53]. Although SAMS' original major focus was multiphasic health testing systems, it soon expanded its activities to include all medical informatics systems.

Another early US professional organization that was committed primarily to medical informatics was the Society for Computer Medicine (SCM). On October 14, 1971, the charter meeting of the board of directors of SCM was held in Arlington, Virginia. SCM's first president was Jenkin from Lorton, Virginia; Sehnert, from Arlington, Virginia, was the president-elect. The first national meeting of SCM was held in Chicago in November 1971. These two organizations, SAMS and SCM, each had less than 500 members, and each held separate annual meetings in the 1970s. During this period, it became increasingly evident to the members, some of whom belonged to the boards of both organizations, that there was considerable duplication of effort for many common objectives. In 1980 during the MEDINFO 80 meeting in Tokyo, Ball from Temple University and then president of SCM, partnering with Bickel from the Armed Services and then president of SAMS, convened a joint ad hoc meeting of several members of their boards of directors to discuss their common interests and possible collaboration in future activities. It was unanimously agreed, in what was called the "Tokyo Accords", that it was timely to consider a merger of these two societies [92, 195]. A joint conference was held that became the 13th annual conference of SAMS with Kaplan as the SAMS conference co-chair, and the 11th annual conference of SCM with Jelovsek from Duke University as the SCM conference co-chair. This historic event immediately preceded the fifth annual Symposium on Computer Applications in Medical Care (SCAMC), held in November 1981 in Washington, DC (see discussion of SCAMC and AMIA below). The result of the merger of SAMS and SCM was a new professional organization with more than 700 members. It was incorporated in August 1981 in the state of Maryland. Although the names Association for Informatics in Medicine and American Medical Informatics Association had been proposed for this new organization, some of the SAMS founders wanted to retain the word systems in its title, so it was called the American Association for Medical Systems and Informatics (AAMSI). Kaplan was elected the first president of AAMSI for 1982; and Bauman of Danbury Hospital in Connecticut, became its president-elect [4].

Regional informatics meetings were also introduced during roughly the period when SAMS and SCM were active during the 1970s. For example, at the same time that the first MEDINFO was being hosted internationally in 1974, the University of

Illinois and the Regional Health Resource Center in Urbana, Illinois, with the support of the Champaign County Medical Society and several other organizations, initiated the First Illinois Conference on Medical Information Systems. Under the leadership of Williams, annual Conferences on Medical Information Systems, with published proceedings, were held in that state through 1980.

Initially in SAMS, and in AAMSI after the merger, Rickli of the University of Missouri-Columbia chaired an International Affairs Committee. In this role, he sought to offer a new US representative to IMIA. However, IMIA took the position that neither AAMSI nor any other US medical informatics organization was of sufficient size to satisfy IMIA's membership requirements. Accordingly, AFIPS continued to send a representative to IMIA, who during the early 1980s was Lindberg. He moved in 1984 from the University of Missouri to become Director of the National Library of Medicine, a position that he was to hold until 2015, making him historically the longest termed director of an NIH institute. With the advent of the American Medical Informatics Association (AMIA), discussed below, the United States had a single informatics organization that met IMIA's criteria for representation. AMIA promptly replaced AFIP as the US member organization for IMIA and AMIA's Ball became the U.S. representative to IMIA. Well known and respected in the international informatics community, in 1989 she became the president-elect of IMIA, and in 1992 assumed the role as the first American and the first woman president of IMIA.

In 1980 Emlet at Analytic Services in Arlington, Virginia, organized a meeting in Washington, DC, called the U.S. Committee for Computers in Health Care. Lindberg served as its chair; and he proposed that the group's name be the American Medical Informatics Association (AMIA). Lindberg formulated AMIA's goal to be to advance the field of medical informatics in the United States and that its organization should initially be composed of professional societies that should operate to facilitate their contributions to the growth of medical informatics [64]. Twenty-seven groups were represented at this meeting as clear evidence of the need in the United States for a better organization representing the various interests in medical informatics. However, since a large federation of varied societies was not an acceptable organizational model to many of the participants, this committee never met again. The AMIA name, however, had a certain appeal – inspired in part by its correspondence to the name of the international organization, IMIA – and its consideration recurred several times in the years that followed, as described below.

The enthusiasm of the MEDINFO 1980 Tokyo meeting resulted in the first conference held in the United States in May 1982 with the words medical informatics in its title. Organized by Collen in San Francisco, and sponsored by the Kaiser Foundation Hospitals, this meeting was called the First Congress of the American Medical Informatics Association (AMIA Congress 82). SCM, SAMS, IHEA, and others joined Kaiser as co-sponsors. The proceedings of the Congress were edited by Lindberg, Collen, and Van Brunt. Lindberg [109] noted in the foreword of these proceedings that, since the AMIA notion had been conceived during the MEDINFO 80 Congress in Tokyo, and due to the outstanding success of the MEDINFO meetings, it was decided to follow the MEDINFO model as much as possible and to initiate a similar annual congress in the United States. After holding its first annual conference in 1982 in Bethesda, MD, AAMSI took over the sponsorship of the AMIA Congress, renaming it the AAMSI Congress. Given the success and dominance of the SCAMC meetings each autumn in Washington, DC (see the discussion of SCAMC and AMIA below), AAMSI's best attended congresses were held on the West Coast every spring, starting in 1983, although they did also hold smaller East coast meetings in the autumn. The organization grew during the 1980s to a membership of about 1,000 and it supported a relatively large number of special interest professional specialty groups (PSGs) for its members interested in various medical computer systems and applications. AAMSI's International Affairs Committee acquired national representatives from many countries, yet, as mentioned, it was not accepted by IMIA as the official U.S. representative. In addition, AAMSI had continuing financial difficulties because its informatics conferences were relatively small and could not compete with the large and highly successful annual SCAMC conferences.

2.2.3.5   ACMI: Creation of an Elected College

In 1984, in response to the perceived need by specialists in this new field to achieve formal professional recognition, the American College for Medical Informatics (ACMI) was established. Its stated goal was the advancement of medical informatics and the recognition of experts in this field.

The College was initially created using an election process that assured that the founding fellows would be elected by their peers. In late 1983, five individuals (Blois, Collen, Lindberg, Piemme, and Shortliffe), seeking to initiate the college by electing 50 founding members, prepared a ballot of 100 names of leaders in the field and sent the ballot to all listed individuals. Every person on the list was considered to be a nominee for fellowship in the College and each one was asked to vote for 50 colleagues from among those on the list to become the founding fellows. In this way the initial set of 52 fellows was selected (three individuals were tied for the 50th place). The founding fellows then came together in San Francisco at the AAMSI meeting in May 1984. They incorporated the College, elected officers, and initiated a process through which the existing fellows would nominate and elect new fellows.

Blois, from the University of California in San Francisco (UCSF), was elected its first president, and Collen, at Oakland Kaiser Permanente (KP), was named president-elect. Piemme was elected initial Secretary, and he subsequently managed the corporation until the merger to form AMIA later in the decade. In those early days, ACMI fellows regularly met at the time of the spring AAMSI and the fall SCAMC conferences. During the fall, qualified nominees were listed on a mail ballot that was sent to the existing fellows. In the early years, nominees who were approved by at least half of the voting fellows became new College fellows. The election process was tweaked from time to time as the organization grew and new leaders tried to assure both a reasonable size of the college and a rigorous set of processes and criteria for the election of new members. By the end of the 1980s the College had about 100 fellows. The relatively quick acceptance of this new medical specialty by the medical profession was demonstrated by the election of some ACMI Fellows to Section I (Physical, Mathematical, and Engineering Sciences) of the Institute of Medicine (IOM) of the National Academy of Sciences (NAS). Cox and Collen were elected to the IOM in 1971, Flagle in 1978, Lindberg in 1985, Shortliffe in 1987, Kulikowski and Warner in 1988, Barnett and Lodwick in 1989, and others followed in the 1900s and 2000s, with about 50 ACMI Fellows elected to the IOM over the years.

ACMI continues to the present, although its organizational details have changed as described in the discussion of AMIA below. International fellows were added in recent years, and the number of fellows elected from the US and abroad now exceeds 300, with approximately 15–20 new fellows elected each year. Photographs of fellows elected through 1993 were published in the inaugural issue of the *Journal of the American Medical Informatics Association* (JAMIA) in January 1994, and photos and brief biographies of newly elected fellows are now published annually in JAMIA and made available on the AMIA web site.

2.2.3.6 AMIA and Its Conferences

The earliest large conference held in the United States that were dedicated entirely to medical informatics was the annual Symposium for Computer Applications in Medical Care (SCAMC). The meeting was initiated in 1977 by a group of interested individuals in the Washington, DC area. Never imagining the success that would occur, they held the first meeting in a small conference hotel in Arlington, Virginia, and drew 250 participants, with Orthner of the George Washington University Medical Center serving as the first program chair. After a second meeting in Arlington, annual attendance grew rapidly, forcing relocation in each of the next several years to larger facilities. SCAMC was incorporated in 1979, and the SCAMC board of directors delegated the organizing responsibilities for the symposia to its Executive Director, Piemme, under a contract with the Office of Continuing Medical Education at George Washington University, which Piemme directed. Much of the growth in the meeting was a result of the professionalism of the GWU organization, including its nationwide marketing of the meeting. Subsequently, the annual fall SCAMC was held, usually in Washington, DC, but occasionally in Baltimore, Maryland, with over 2,000 registrants attending each symposium throughout the 1980s. Each year's scientific program was directed by a different program chairperson selected by the SCAMC board of directors. The SCAMC program chair persons and the proceedings editors are all listed at the back of this book. The SCAMC programs were very successful in satisfying the interests of developers and users of computers for medical applications. During the 1980s the SCAMC proceedings, then published by the IEEE, were the most efficient resource for reviewing the current status of medical informatics' activities in the United States. The SCAMC organization, based in Washington, DC, was dedicated entirely to its annual symposia and was not a membership society. After the creation of the American Medical Informatics Association (AMIA) in 1989, AMIA took over the organization of the meeting, which became known as the AMIA Annual Symposium.

During 1986 and 1987 it became obvious to all involved that there was considerable overlap in the memberships of AAMSI, SCAMC, and ACMI (including among those sitting on their boards). Complaints arose from members who had to go to three different boards of directors' meetings and discuss similar objectives and problems. Many urged that a merger was worthy of consideration if professionals in medical informatics were to be appropriately served in this country. A series of meetings was held during those 2 years, bringing together corporate officers of AAMSI, SCAMC, and ACMI to try to arrive at an agreement for a merger. Finally, a joint meeting of 15 representatives of the three professional medical informatics organizations was held in July 1988 to plan to merge AAMSI, ACMI, and SCAMC into one organization, at last formally adopting the name that had been proposed in a variety of settings over the previous decade: the American Medical Informatics Association (AMIA).

AMIA was incorporated in November 1988 in the District of Columbia; and Lindberg was elected in 1989 as its first president. Letters of agreement were prepared by Lindberg between AMIA and the three merging organizations to ensure the perpetuation of the best features of each organization. Stead, the president of AAMSI, wanted AAMSI members automatically to become AMIA members and wanted the spring congress, the professional specialty groups, and the some sponsored medical informatics journals (included as membership benefits for AAMSI members) to be continued. Shortliffe, the president of SCAMC, wanted assurance that the annual fall SCAMC meetings would continue under AMIA's sponsorship (co-branded with the SCAMC name for at least 5 years). Warner, the president of ACMI, required that under AMIA's sponsorship the election of College fellows, and their ability to self-govern, would be continued in accordance with the provisions established by the fellows [7]. It was noted that the earlier use of the name *American Medical Informatics Association* and its *AMIA Congress 82* had not been incorporated, nor were the names copyrighted, so that somewhat simplified AMIA's more formal birth in 1989.

The purposes of AMIA, as stated in its articles of incorporation, were: to operate exclusively for charitable and education purposes, and to those ends to promote the use of computers in medical care (informatics) so as to advance health care; to sponsor conferences, workshops and symposia; to sponsor and/or publish journals, newsletters, and/or books; and to study, advance, and to promote the application of computers to the science and practice of medicine and the health sciences, to research and development in medicine, the health sciences, health sciences education, and the delivery of health care [6]. AMIA's board of directors developed plans in 1989 that included these goals:

- To expand the prior membership of AAMSI to several thousand; to continue the large annual fall symposia in Washington, DC, that had been conducted so successfully by SCAMC; and to extend the spring meetings annually held by AAMSI on the West Coast, eventually to rotate to additional other regions.

- To support ACMI as a functionally autonomous college within AMIA, and ask ACMI's fellows to support AMIA in achieving AMIA's goals.
- To continue the other worthy medical informatics activities of its predecessor organizations.

By the end of 1989 AMIA had completed its organizational mergers, had begun its national activities, had hired a full-time executive director, Mutnik, and had established its international interests by successfully proposing to IMIA that Ball become the official U.S. representative, representing AMIA.

AMIA's meetings have changed over the years, although the Annual Symposium, still held in the autumn and in Washington, DC, two out of every 3 years (on average), is now complemented by several other meetings. These include an annual ACMI Symposium (for ACMI fellows), a practice-oriented meeting known as iHealth, and, in lieu of the former AAMSI Spring Congresses on the West Coast, a Joint Summit on Translational Science conference, which combines complementary meetings on translational bioinformatics and clinical research informatics.

As AMIA grew in membership and influence, it became clear that the organization would benefit from a full-time leader drawn from the informatics profession. Then President of AMIA, Safran, proposed a change whereby AMIA would hire a full-time President and CEO and the former position of President (which was a part-time voluntary activity) would be renamed Chair of the Board of Directors. The Board recruited Detmer to be the first President and CEO, a role in which he served from 2004 to 2009. Subsequent Presidents and CEO have been Shortliffe (2009–2012), Fickenscher (2012–2013), and Fridsma (2014–present).

Starting in 2004, just as Detmer began his new position, there was growing interest in having AMIA play a role in defining and recognizing the professional role of clinical informatics practitioners. There followed a period of years during which this notion was explored and AMIA sought official recognition by formal medical organizations. This occurred when AMIA was elected to membership in the Council of Medical Specialty Societies (CMSS) and subsequently began to discuss the possibility of introducing subspecialty board examinations for physicians who worked as clinical informaticians. First Detmer, and subsequently Shortliffe, worked with the American Board of Preventive Medicine (ABPM) to develop the rationale, and a formal proposal, for the new subspecialty within the American Board of Medical Specialties (ABMS) [55].

Important pre-work had been done with support of the Robert Wood Johnson Foundation, leading to the publication of two key papers that defined the core competencies for clinical informatics practice and laid out the structure and content of formal clinical fellowships in the field. Safran [154] and Gardner [70] and associates defined the subspecialty of clinical informatics as using informatics concepts, methods and tools: (1) to assess information and knowledge needs of health care professionals and patients; (2) to characterize, evaluate, and refine clinical processes; (3) to develop, implement, and refine clinical decision support systems; and (4) to lead or participate in the procurement, customization, development, implementation, management, evaluation, and continuous improvement of clinical information systems, such as electronic health records and order-entry systems. In a companion article, Detmer [56] and associates described the tasks performed by clinical informaticians in four major knowledge and skills that clinical informaticians must master: (1) fundamentals; (2) clinical decision making and care process improvement; (3) health information systems; and (4) leadership and management of change.

The proposal for a new subspecialty was embraced by the ABMS and its component boards across the medical specialties, driven in part by Detmer and Shortliffe's arguments [56] that informatics was a valid area of clinical specialization for physicians and their prediction that 50,000 clinical informatics professionals would be needed in the US over the next decade, many of whom would also need to be trained as physicians. In September 2011 the American Board of Medical Specialists (ABMS) recognized clinical informatics as a medical subspecialty; with the certification of specialists based in large part on the set of core competences that had been developed and published by AMIA [121, 168]. The first board examinations were offered in October 2013 and almost 1,000 physicians took their boards in the first 2 years that they were offered.

Recognizing that not all clinical informaticians are boarded physicians, AMIA has also pursued an Advanced Interprofessional Informatics Certification (AIIC), intended to be made available to clinical informatics practitioners who are not eligible to take the ABMS board examination (e.g., non-boarded physicians or non-physicians). This certification option is intended to be offered in the next few years and will create a rigorous opportunity for nurses, pharmacists, dentists, PhDs, and other clinical informaticians to demonstrate their competency in a formal way.

2.2.4   The Role of Nursing Organizations

The term nursing informatics was introduced in 1977 at the first research state-of-the-art conference on nursing information systems that was held at the University of Illinois College of Nursing, coordinated by Werley and Grier Saba and Westra [150]. The nursing schools in the United States had established some courses in nursing informatics as early as 1978. Saba [151] organized the first national Nursing Special Interest Group on computer applications in nursing during the SCAMC held in 1982. In 1988, the University of Maryland at Baltimore initiated a graduate-level program entitled Nursing Informatics [81]. Saba (2011) and Westra published a detailed chronological listing of landmark events in nursing informatics from 1970 to 2010 and reported that, in the late 1970s, the National League of Nursing, the Public Health Service, the US Army Nurse Corps, and several university Schools of Nursing began to conduct conferences and workshops on computer applications in nursing. The NIH Clinical Center implemented one of the earliest clinical information systems in nursing practice.

In the 1980s, larger hospital information systems began to develop nursing sub-systems to document nurses' notes. Nurses were soon presenting more papers at informatics conferences and generating more nursing informatics publications. In 1983 the IMIA formed a Nursing Informatics Special Interest Group (IMIA/NI-SIG). Ball [16] emphasized that integrating computers into the practice of nursing was a challenge. The American Nurses Association (ANA) formed a Council on Computer Applications in Nursing (CCAN) and, in 1992, the ANA recognized nursing informatics as a specialty with a separate scope of practices, developed standards, and offered a certification examination. In 2004 the Nursing Informatics Working Group within AMIA initiated a listing of nursing pioneers who had helped to open a new area in nursing informatics and had provided a sustained contribution to the specialty. This listing and associated documentation is available from the National Library of Medicine (NLM) as the Nursing Informatics History Collection [153].

Ball [17], Skiba et al. [170], DuLong [62], Troseth [181, 182], and colleagues have all reported that a significant event occurred in 2005 for the nursing profession. At that time three million nurses made up 55 % of the health care work force in the nation. The event was a planning meeting, held at the Johns Hopkins University School of Nursing, to define the mission regarding what became known as Technology Informatics Guiding Educational Reform (TIGER). In 2006 a summit conference, co-chaired by Ball and Skiba and held at the Uniformed Services University of the Health Sciences in Bethesda, Maryland, developed a plan for TIGER to develop an initiative that would address nursing informatics in all health care settings, while focusing their efforts on collaborative issues that included standards and inter-operability, informatics competencies, education and leadership development, and the personal electronic health record. At the summit, they developed the notion of "Seven Pillars of the Tiger Vision" that included:

- Management and leadership that empowers and executes the transformation of health care
- Education toward knowledge development and dissemination for rapid deployment and dissemination of best practices
- Communication and collaboration of standardized person-centered technology-enabled processes across the continuum of care
- Informatics design of systems that support education and practice to foster quality and safety Information technology that is useable and standards-based
- Policy that is consistent, coalition-building, and achieves an ethical culture of safety
- Culture that leverages technology and informatics across multiple disciplines towards the goal of high quality and safety of patient care

Leading participants in the support of TIGER included nurse members of AMIA, HIMSS, and several nursing informatics associations. Ball et al. [17] observed that in 2010 nursing informatics was no longer an option for nurses, and that the time had come to leave manual information methods to the past.

2.2.5   The Role of Commercial Organizations

Although most of the research in medical computing in the United States was supported by federal government grants and contracts, private industry carried out much of the development of computer applications in medical care. Some outstanding examples were the early development of a hospital information system by Lockheed and Technicon, the development of computer-based automated blood chemistry analyzers by Technicon, the development of computer-based electrocardiogram systems by Hewlett-Packard and Marquette, and the development of computer-assisted tomography by several commercial vendors. Hardware vendors such as IBM and Technicon also helped to advance early research and development in medical computing by supporting periodic symposia.

The first annual IBM Medical Symposium was held in 1959 in Poughkeepsie, New York, presenting some of the earliest work on computer applications to medicine. These symposia were arranged by Taylor of IBM; and they continued for 10 years to be highly informative meetings for medical users of IBM computers. Beginning in 1965 in Ardsley, New York, Technicon's Whitehead sponsored a series of annual meetings on computer applications for Technicon equipment used in the clinical laboratory. McGraw-Hill Publications sponsored the First National Conference on Electronics in Medicine in 1969 in New York City. Some vendors directly supported the diffusion of medical informatics by making available substantial educational discounts for hardware or by contributing computers to support demonstration projects.

Some special interest groups of users of computer hardware and software were influential in the diffusion of medical informatics. Although user groups tended to be somewhat biased, they had an important educational role. User groups generally had as their objectives keeping the vendor of the hardware and software accountable to its users, providing input for product enhancement, and helping to write specifications for new product development [149]. In 1964 health industry users of IBM computers organized the Electronic Computing Health Oriented (ECHO) organization, which from that date held regular semiannual meetings. ECHO achieved a membership of 2,500 and shared the experiences of more than 1,000 hospitals [42, 87]. The Hospital Information Systems Sharing Group (HISSG) was formed in 1967. It was originally a users' group of the IBM Medical Information Systems Program (MISP), but the group became more diversified and expanded its membership and purposes to include any institutions having an interest in hospital information systems [184]. By the end of the 1980s a directory was published of 112 hardware and software user groups [51].

One of the most widely used early programming languages for medical applications, the Massachusetts General Hospital Utility Multi-Programming System (MUMPS), was developed in 1966. The MUMPS Users' Group (MUG) was formed in 1971, began its annual meetings in 1972, and grew to represent one of the largest groups of medical users of a specific programming language in the United States. MUG formed special interest groups, such as the MUG Education Committee, to provide MUMPS programming tutorials, to develop MUMPS training documents, and to provide computer-aided instruction programs in the MUMPS language [200].

An Apple medical users group was formed in 1980 to support the exchange of information among users of Apple computers [176]. In the 2000s the diffusion of electronic health records (EHRs) resulted in the development of a variety of user groups in AMIA and in other organizations.

Today there is a large and energetic health information technology (HIT) vendor community. As was mentioned earlier, the principal trade organization for HIT, HIMSS, has a large annual conference and trade show that has outgrown all but the largest of convention venues in the US. It and many of the vendor companies have also spread their influence to other parts of the world, both to sell products and to hold conferences. There are of course still important synergies between the corporate world and the medical informatics community, with industry adopting or licensing ideas and technologies that have been developed in research labs, hospitals, and other medical settings. Many people trained in the medical informatics community are now actively involved with rewarding roles in the HIT industry.

2.2.6   The Role of Federal Agencies and Academia

Prior to the 1940s, medical research in the United States was supported primarily by private funding and by philanthropic foundations and endowments [169]. In 1946 the U.S. Congress passed the Hospital Survey and Construction Act, generally referred to as the Hill-Burton Act, which through the mid-1970s provided tens of millions of dollars for hospital construction, renovations and replacements. The Act also laid the groundwork for the introduction of new technologies into hospitals. After World War II the early development of medical informatics was mainly supported by federal government grants and contracts. Brazier [29] reported that in 1955 only 25 universities in the United States had installed computers and only a few scientists were experimenting in their laboratories with prototype models of non-commercial computer designs. Saenger and Sterling [153] reported that the Medical Computing Center of the University of Cincinnati College of Medicine had purchased a Burroughs E 102 computer in 1958, and was the oldest medical computing center located solely within a college of medicine in the United States.

During the 1950s, the National Academy of Sciences (NAS) and the National Research Council (NRC) sponsored a survey, carried out by a committee chaired by Ledley, on the use of computers in biology and medicine. They found that a variety of biomedical research projects already employed computers [103]. In 1959 Senator Humphrey conducted hearings concluding that the time was appropriate for the federal government to increase the support of biomedical computing [88]. The National Institutes of Health (NIH) promptly initiated a two-pronged funding program: to support individual research and development projects for the use of computers in medicine, and to establish university-based biomedical computer centers. Lusted and Coffin [117] wrote that if a birthday were to be chosen for biomedical computing, the date of September 20, 1960, would be appropriate, because on that day the NIH Advisory Committee on Computers in Research was launched. Shannon, then the Director of NIH created the Advisory Committee with Hemphill as its Executive Secretary for the first year, followed by Waxman for the next 4 years. Lusted was its first chair person [191]. Lusted had already served since 1955 as a member, and then as the chair person, of the National Research Council Committee on the Uses of Electronic Computers in Biology and Medicine [118]. This Advisory Committee on Computers was given the basic function of a research study section to review grant requests dealing primarily with the problems of bio-medical computing in research [191]. It was this committee that was responsible for the initial funding of many of the leading academic centers in medical informatics in the United States; and was instrumental in moving many of the early applications of computers into medicine. Waxman [190] reported that the members of that committee shared high enthusiasm for their mission and, in the course of 2 years, they managed to grant more than $50 million. This work was chronicled in a four-volume book series entitled *Computers in Biomedical Research*, published by Academic Press between 1965 and 1974.

In 1962 Congress authorized an additional $2 million for NIH to make grants for a limited number of regional biomedical instrumentation centers. Among other criteria established by Director Shannon, these centers were to foster the sciences of biomathematics and biomedical electronics, with particular emphasis on the application of computers to biomedical problems [82]. In 1962 a separately budgeted Special Resources Branch was established in an independent Division of Research Resources (DRR) to provide funds for the establishment of computing facilities and of other widely applicable technological resources [73]. In addition, other NIH institutes, such as the National Institute of General Medical Sciences, supported projects involving the automation of research and of clinical laboratories, as well as the development of computer-aided diagnosis. The National Heart and Lung Institute supported projects on modeling cardiovascular and respiratory physiology, and on the automated analysis of the electrocardiogram. In 1966, before a U.S. Senate subcommittee hearing on health, Caceres [38] of the Medical Systems Development Laboratory of the Heart Disease Control Program in the NIH National Center for Chronic Disease Control, demonstrated the automated analysis of the electrocardiogram by a computer. By 1970 each of the National Institutes was involved with some development of biomedical computing, most notably the National Institute of General Medical Sciences, the National Heart and Lung Institute, and the National Institute of Neurological Diseases and Stroke [73].

In 1964 the NIH Advisory Committee on Computers in Research established the NIH Computer Research Study Section, with Warner as its chair person and Gee as its executive secretary, to review requests for NIH grants to support biomedical computer research. In 1970 the Computer Research Study Section became the Computer and Biomathematical Sciences Study Section, which was subsequently terminated in 1977 [110]. Gee [73], writing on the practices and policies of NIH at the time, stated that, with reference to biomedical computing, it was apparent that the NIH categorical institute structure was not particularly well suited for the provision of support for research tools that could be useful to all varieties of biological and medical scientists. It was argued that some new means needed to be found if the development of this important new field were to be encouraged.

Raub [143], the director of NIH's Life Sciences Computer Resources Program within the Division of Research Resources (DRR), defined the life sciences computer resources as those computer centers that were dedicated to serving a community of biomedical scientists within a given geographical region. In 1963, NIH initiated its sponsorship of life sciences computer resources and Surgeon General Terry established a New England regional, multicenter, $2.8 million research resources program, based at the Massachusetts Institute of Technology (MIT) and administered by the NIH Division of Research Facilities and Resources. The institutions that participated in this program included Boston University, Brandeis University, Brown University, Dartmouth College, Harvard University, Northeastern University, Tufts University, University of Connecticut, University of Massachusetts, and the Worcester Foundation for Experimental Biology [179]. By 1966 NIH supported a total of 48 centers in full operation, and the total annual support provided was over $8 million [143]. These general computing facilities were expected to conduct, and to afford opportunities for, research in computer technology in the biomedical sciences. They were also to make available to investigators in their institutions not only computer hardware, but also scientific and technical staff, to (1) assure optimal use of the hardware in the research and development of techniques and computer programs applicable to substantive research problems; and (2) provide instruction to both faculty and students in computer usage and programming. Gee [73] observed that the funding arrangements of these centers not only affected their economics, but also influenced their operational mode. As demands for computer utilization increased, most of the computing centers supplemented their grants with income from user fees. Subsequently, as the federal budget available for the support of computer facilities dwindled, the fee-for-service approach shifted a share of the financial responsibility to investigator-users of the facilities. These biomedical research computing centers further supported this development by emphasizing the importance of collaborative arrangements.

These NIH grants were instrumental in supporting many of earliest biomedical computing centers. In 1959 the Tulane University Biomedical Computer System was established, headed by Sweeney, who was (as previously mentioned) the first professor of computer medicine in the United States [158]. When asked what this title meant, he would jokingly reply that he treated sick computers [177]. In addition to providing biomedical statistical services, the Tulane group developed a computer data processing system for its medical clinic.

In 1959 the University of Michigan began to establish a biomedical data processing research center, equipped with an IBM 704 computer, and initiated a training program for its schools of medicine and public health with support from the U.S. Public Health Service and NIH [21]. In 1959, the Health Sciences Computer Facility at the University of California at Los Angeles (UCLA) was established with NIH support, with Dixon as its director. A primary functional emphasis of UCLA's computer facility was in statistics [32]. In 1961 Dixon published his first book on the *BioMedical Package* (BMDP), which was then a unique compilation of statistical packages to aid biomedical researchers in analyzing their data [60]. The UCLA center was lauded as a national resource in biomathematics [143]. In the 1960s the time-sharing UCLA computer facility, with an IBM 360/91 computer and graphics terminals, provided services to non-UCLA users for projects in genetic linkage, heart disease, tissue-typing studies, and in schizophrenia. In 1963 more than 100 medical research projects at UCLA were receiving support at the University's new Health Sciences Computing Facility – the nation's largest data processing center for medical research at the time [61]. In the 1960s and 1970s the computer center also supported projects in the UCLA School of Medicine and its hospital, notably Lamson's work on developing a hospital information system and in processing clinical-pathology textual data [183].

Warner began to use computers in 1956 for cardiovascular research. He reported his studies in computer-aided diagnosis in 1961, began to use computers for patient monitoring in 1969, and in the 1970s was developing the HELP hospital information system. Raub [143] praised the life science computer center established at the University of Utah in Salt Lake City, with Warner as its director, as a computer center without peer in the breadth and quality of its program in the health care field at that time. In 1986 Warner established at the University of Utah the first department of medical informatics in the United States, and Warner became the country's first professor of medical informatics.

In 1961 the Johns Hopkins Medical Computational Facility, supported by an NIH grant and headed by Shepard, was initiated as an extension of the university-wide computer center located at its Applied Physics Laboratory, directed by Rich [164]. It supported the evolution of a comprehensive medical information system at the Johns Hopkins Hospital. In 1964 the University of Minnesota's Health Sciences Center created a research and educational computer center, with Johnson as the principal investigator who received an NIH Health Computer Sciences Resource Grant [5]. In 1970 Ackerman was appointed Director of the Division of Health Computer Sciences and began to support a variety of health computing applications [28]. In 1964 biomedical computing centers were also operational at New York University [196] and at the University of Cincinnati College of Medicine [153]. Raub [143] cited the Washington University Computer Laboratories in St. Louis, Missouri, with Cox as its director, as the most advanced center concerned with the design and application of minicomputers in the health area. The senior professional staff of this resource, Clark and Molnar, MIT had designed and developed the LINC computer while at MIT, with some support from the Washington University program.

In 1966 Stanford University's research program, Advanced Computer for Medical Research (ACME), with Feigenbaum as director, Wiederhold as associate director, and Lederberg as chairman of its Computer Policy Committee, received a grant from NIH. With an IBM 360/50 computer, ACME soon supported about 200 medically related projects [49]. Raub [143] described the Stanford University computer resource as a unique time-sharing system, designed and implemented by resource personnel there; by 1971 it was in routine service to their entire biomedical community.

Yet as early as 1968 it was becoming clear that ACME did not have sufficient capacity to satisfy Feigenbaum and Lederberg's evolving project called DENDRAL, which was an approach to formal representation and predication of organic compound structures based on mass spectroscopy data [99]. The Stanford investigators therefore began to plan for a process to phase out the ACME computer and to replace it with a machine suitable for symbolic processing calculations. Their idea was to make the machine available for use by other, similarly minded researchers who were interested in applying the field of artificial intelligence in biomedicine. To do this would require a connection to the nascent ARPANET, which the Department of Defense (DOD) had supported to allow nationwide interconnectivity among DOD-supported computer research projects. Feigenbaum and Lederberg sought agreement from the DOD that they would permit an NIH-supported, medically oriented computer system to connect to the ARPANET. There was no precedent for connecting non-DOD machines, but the case was made, with help from NIH program officers. Thus the proposal for a new machine called for a community of medical AI researchers to share a single machine, using the ARPANET to access the computer from anywhere in the country. Eventually, in 1973, SUMEX-AIM (Stanford University Medical EXperimental Computer – Artificial Intelligence in Medicine) was established as a national resource funded by the Division of Research Resources [67]. The SUMEX-AIM computer project established criteria for other investigators to apply to use the machine at Stanford. It was an early demonstration of computer resource sharing within a national community, and it set a precedent for allowing non-military computers to connect to the ARPANET – a precedent that broadened over time until, by the mid-1980s, the ARPANET was managed by the National Science Foundation under a new name: the Internet. By the 1990s, it was opened up to commercial use and the government was no longer involved in running the Internet.

By 1982 the SUMEX-AIM network included computers not only at Stanford, but also at Rutgers University and the University of Pittsburgh. Computer scientists from these three universities and from the University of Missouri-Columbia joined in policy decisions and selection of research projects for computational support [109]. Funded by NIH's Biotechnology Resources Program in the Division of Research Resources, SUMEX supported a long-distance communications network with a user community comprising approximately 20 research projects. These spanned a broad range of biomedical application areas, including clinical diagnostic decision making, molecular structure interpretation and synthesis, cognitive and psychological modeling, instrument data interpretation, and the generalization of tools to facilitate building new knowledge-based, artificial intelligence programs. Early well-known clinical artificial intelligence programs were developed using the SUMEX-AIM resource, such as MYCIN [197], INTERNIST [126], and CASNET [194].

The National Institutes of Health (NIH) had their own computer center on its campus in Bethesda, Maryland, and in 1963 organized a systems programming group to meet the increasing demands within NIH for computing applications [37]. In 1964 the NIH computer center contained two Honeywell 800 computers [91]. In

1965 NIH established a Division of Computer Research and Technology (DCRT), with Pratt as its director, for intramural project development. The effort to provide computer services to the NIH began in 1966, using an IBM 360/40 computer for a small number of users [139]. NIH had adopted a plan that called for a multiplicity of small, medium, and large capacity machines to satisfy the existing and future needs of the NIH and related government agencies [93]. DCRT was rapidly expanded to include four large IBM 360/370 computers that shared a common library of computer programs and data, linked to peripherally located, medium-sized computers to serve the real-time, online computing needs of the NIH clinics and laboratories [140]. In 1961, NIH also began to support for-profit organizations through negotiated contracts, as distinguished from grants, to help to develop the biomedical electronics field [115]. The first program of this kind involved the introduction of the LINC computers to biomedical research laboratories [73]. In 1970, DCRT was the largest health computing facility in the nation [74]. In 1976, NIH operated two central computer facilities with four IBM 370 computers. In total, the NIH computer complement numbered approximately 130 machines, not including the machines in the independent computer resource at the National Library of Medicine [93].

Linvill [113] discussed the development of some early computer research complexes involving government, academia, health care, and industry, emphasizing how their creation and evolution was advanced by innovative military computing during World War II. Military computing during and immediately after the war had led to the location of teams of technical people in universities, working with the then available large computers. The Russian launching of Sputnik stimulated the invention of the transistor, produced the space race, and continued the active government and university collaboration. The effect of the federal government on the nation's ability to utilize computer electronics in the industrial as well as the defense sphere became evident as the industrial needs diverged from defense needs, soon greatly exceeding defense needs in magnitude. By the end of the 1980s, computer research centers had moved to industry and academia and a number of universities built major computer science centers with both industry and government support, including the Massachusetts Institute of Technology (MIT), University of California (UC) at Berkeley, California Institute of Technology, the Research Triangle Universities, the University of Minnesota, and Stanford University.

The Defense Advanced Research Projects Agency (DARPA), a research funding agent of the Department of Defense, also contributed to academic computer science departments, especially at the University of California at Berkeley, Carnegie Mellon University, Massachusetts Institute of Technology, and Stanford University. DARPA funded some basic research in artificial intelligence in the 1960s and 1970s, but changed its emphasis to applied research in the 1980s. One of the most significant contributions of DARPA was the previously mentioned development of ARPANET, or the Advanced Research Projects Agency Network [157].

In the 1960s, the U.S. Public Health Service through its Chronic Disease Division, supported some computer applications in multiphasic health screening systems and preventive medicine. The U.S. Congress established, under the Heart,

Cancer and Stroke Act of 1965, the Regional Medical Program (RMP) with Marston as its director. By 1967 there were 54 computer-based regional medical programs established, including clinical laboratory systems, clinical data collection studies, multiphasic screening systems, and tumor registries [147].

In 1968 within the Health Services and Mental Health Administration (HSMHA), the National Center for Health Services Research and Development (NCHSR&D), the earliest predecessor of what is today known as the Agency for Health Research and Quality (AHRQ) was organized, with Sanazaro as its director and McCarthy as its executive secretary. Sanazaro [156] described the purpose of NCHSR&D was to serve as the Federal focus for health services research and development, and its programs were directed to developing new methods, or improving existing methods of organizing, delivering and financing health services. Research and development, as formulated by NCHSR&D, was the process of identifying, designing, developing, introducing, testing, and evaluating new methods that met specified performance criteria under realistic operating conditions [155]. According to Raub [143], the differences in objectives and funding practices between NIH and NCHSR&D were that, whereas the NIH focused on health research and training, HSMHA and its NCHSR&D was primarily responsible for facilitating the delivery of health services, the improvement of hospital facilities, the institution of public health measures, and the like. As a consequence, whereas NIH tended to emphasize computer applications in basic research, clinical research, and medical education, NCHSR&D tended to sponsor computer applications in hospital automation and monitoring the critically ill.

To review grants for supporting research and development of medical computing, NCHSR&D established a Health Care Technology Program Advisory Council chaired by Flagle, and a Health Care Systems Study Section chaired by Collen, with Hall as its executive secretary. The Health Care Technology Program of the NCHSR&D was directed by Waxman, and its Medical System Development Laboratory was led by Caceres. NCHSR&D funded health services research centers, two of which had health care technology and information systems as their primary focus. One of these centers was at the Kaiser Foundation Medical Centers in Oakland and San Francisco and directed by Collen; the other was at the University of Missouri, Columbia School of Medicine, directed by Lindberg [156]. In addition to the health services research centers, the NCHSR&D initiated grants and contracts to fund a variety of information systems in the 1960s and 1970s. The status of its supported computer-based information systems at the peak of NCHSR&D support in 1969 and 1970, was summarized in a NCHSR&D report that mentioned some of the following projects as being operational and providing patient care functions: medical records projects, hospital information systems, clinical laboratory systems, x-ray information systems, physiological monitoring systems, pharmacy information systems, a multiphasic screening system, and patient interviewing projects. In its 1970 fiscal year, NCHSR&D's Health Care Technology Program funded 34 grants and 16 contracts for a total amount of about $6 million. The NCHSR&D further reported that between 1962 and 1970 more than $31 million was spent on projects sponsored by the Department of Health, Education, and Welfare (DHEW, which was later split into the Department of Health and Human Services and the

Department of Education). All of these involved the use of computers in the delivery of medical care. The NCHSR&D report concluded that the then available timesharing computing technology could not support the many divergent and data-rich requirements of services that existed in any relatively large hospital; and it predicted that networking computers could have more potential for the evolvement of a hospital information system than one very large machine [130]. In 1973 the NCHSR&D terminated its support for the development of medical informatics projects, shortening its name to the National Center for Health Services Research (NCHSR).

Under the direction of Rosenthal, NCHSR continued to fund research in the diffusion and evaluation of computer applications in health care. NCHSR supported the development and evaluation of: (1) hospital information systems including the Lockheed/Technicon MIS at the El Camino Hospital in California, and Weed's PROMIS at the University of Vermont [143]; (2) some ambulatory practice information systems including Barnett's COSTAR; (3) some clinical support systems including Seligson's YALE and Rappaport's Youngstown Hospital clinical laboratory systems; Lodwick's MARS radiology information system at the University of Missouri-Columbia, Baumann's Massachusetts General Hospital's radiology information systems; Caceres' and Piperberger's automated programs for interpreting electrocardiograms; and (4) automated patient monitoring systems and computer-based consulting systems including Cohen's METAPHOR and Shortliffe's MYCIN at Stanford University [168], and Warner's HELP program at the LDS Hospital [148].

In the 1970s the National Library of Medicine (NLM), which had been established in 1956 with authorization to provide a wide range of grant activities within DHEW, was the main support for training programs to provide the special education and experience for both pre- and postdoctoral individuals entering this field from medicine, as well as from computer-related disciplines [112]. In the 1980s the NLM, especially under its new director, Lindberg (who assumed the leadership role in 1984), became more active in the support of medical informatics through its extramural programs. In 1983 NLM initiated an Integrated Academic Information Management System (IAIMS) program to use computers and communication networks to transform a health institution's various information bases into an integrated system [132]. NLM sponsored a series of IAIMS symposia at which IAIMS progress reports were presented, including those from Johns Hopkins University, Harvard University, Baylor College of Medicine, University of Cincinnati, Columbia-Presbyterian Medical Center, Georgetown University, University of Maryland, and the University of Utah [35, 36, 121, 123, 133, 134]. NLM also initiated a Unified Medical Language System (UMLS) project to facilitate access to machine-readable information located in a variety of sources, including the scientific literature, factual databanks, knowledge-based expert systems, and computer-based patient records. UMLS brought together a number of participants to compile a database of biomedical terms that appeared in several different controlled vocabularies and classifications to form a metathesaurus that would establish relationships among terms from these different source vocabularies [89]. By 1989 approximately 10 % of NLM's budget was directly in support of medical informatics [131]. The NLM Medical Informatics Course, initiated in the 1980s and later renamed the

Biomedical Informatics Course, offered participants a week-long immersive experience in biomedical informatics taught by experts in the field. The course was held at the Marine Biological Laboratory (MBL) in Woods Hole, Massachusetts, for many years but in 2014 moved to Georgia Regents University (GRU).

Through the 1960s, large increases in the NIH budgets resulted in a great surge in medical research [163]. The decade of 1963 through 1972 was an extremely productive one for research and development of medical informatics in the United States, as parallel streams of substantial funds came from the NIH, the NCHSR&D, and the Regional Medical Program (RMP). NIH's growth was phenomenal, so much so that by 1965 NIH made up more than 37 % of the entire Federal health budget [19]. However, this percentage soon dropped with the growth of Medicare and Medicaid expenses. Furthermore, in the early 1970s during the Nixon administration, an abrupt curtailment of growth occurred in the NIH computer resources program. A decrease in NIH funding followed the death of Congressman Fogarty in 1968 and the retirement of Senator Hill in 1969, who together had aggressively led NIH support during the 1960s [163]. Raub [143] explained this decrease as reflecting the interaction of two basic forces: the overall slowdown in Federal Government research spending, and the rather cautious attitude on the part of the mainstream of the biomedical research community as to just how far the computer could penetrate this discipline. In the 1970s the increasing costs of medical care became a major concern of government and business. The Hill-Burton hospital grants program and the Regional Medical Program grants program were allowed to expire. The economic recession of the 1970s, accompanied by severe inflation and a rapid rise in utilization of medical services, led to an escalation of the costs of Medicare and of Social Security, which resulted in some condemnation of technology as the primary reason for the increased costs of medical care [172].

In his testimony in 1978 before a congressional committee, Lindberg [110] noted that although the National Institutes of Health (NIH) included the provision of medical information research in its overall mission, the NIH grant support typically terminated with the demonstration of the scientific success or failure of a project, which was usually given grant funds for less than 5 years. He argued that this time frame was usually not sufficient to develop a prototype commercial medical information system or even a subsystem. He also noted that there was not a systematic federal government plan for the deployment of the technology of medical information systems. Lindberg further pointed out that the most profound effect upon medical information systems was the introduction of the Medicare program that required hospitals to devote greatly increased resources to business-oriented office computing. Yet, even though these federal programs had created whole industries that offered computer-based support for third-party reimbursement payments, and despite a strong increase in demand for accounting-oriented information systems for hospitals and clinics, these developments were basically borrowed from the non-medical world and had little effect upon the development of the components of medical information systems. However, in the 1970s and later, the federal government did support the development of several large multihospital medical information systems.

2.3 Summary and Commentary

The beginning of medical informatics in the United States was attributed by Lindberg [108] to the initiation in 1879 of the *Index Medicus* by Billings – an observation that emphasizes that medical informatics is about more than computers, and that the science of information and knowledge management in medicine and biomedical research predated the development of computational technology. The subsequent diffusion and integration of informatics into medicine in this country was the result of many forces provided by bioengineering, medical, nursing, and commercial publications, organizations, federal agencies, and academia, all of which also influenced biomedical and health care professionals and their institutions.

As discussed, the earliest reports on biomedical applications of computers began to appear at conferences sponsored by professional engineering societies, arguably beginning in 1947 with the first Annual Conference on Engineering in Medicine. The English term, *medical informatics*, became internationally disseminated and ultimately accepted as a result of its use at the first International Congress for Medical Informatics, MEDINFO, in 1974. The American Medical Informatics Association (AMIA) was born in 1989 to promote the scientific base for the field, the use of computers in medical care, and the development of application of computers to support the science and practice of medicine and the health sciences [6].

In the 1960s and 1970s it seemed as though the U.S. Congress extended itself to do as much as possible to try to conquer important diseases, and several new institutes were added to NIH for this purpose. As part of this effort, Congress had authorized several streams of research support for biomedical computer applications. The National Institutes of Health (NIH) was the greatest contributor through its Division of Research Resources (DRR, with several NIH Institutes provided financial support for specialized computer applications), along with the National Library of Medicine (NLM), which supported both research and training programs in medical informatics. The Chronic Disease Division of the U.S. Public Health Service supported computer applications for health screening and preventive medicine. The National Center for Health Services Research supported many demonstration and evaluation projects, and the Regional Medical Program also supported some computer applications to patient care. The Department of Defense supported DARPA for research and the development of a multihospital information system for all of the medical facilities of its three armed services. The Veterans Administration supported the development of its own large multihospital information system. The Public Health Hospitals and the Indian Health Service also were independently developing their own multihospital information systems. NASA was developing remote health care projects for its staffed space missions. Whereas in the 1960s and 1970s federal government agencies had provided most of the funding for health research and development, in the 1980s industry began to support an increasing share of research and (especially) development in the United States. By the end of the 1980s, industry became the largest supporter [131].

By the 1980s the increasing expenditures for health care became a great national concern, and efforts to control the costs of care became a matter of high priority. In 1983 the Health Care Financing Agency (HCFA), today known as the Centers for Medicare and Medicaid Services (CMS), instituted for hospital patients a scheme of fixed Medicare payments by 468 diagnosis-related groups (DRGs) based on International Classification of Diseases (ICD) codes. In each hospital in the United States that accepted Medicare patients, this produced a rapid and often a major change in its hospital computer system, to allow collecting the data necessary to satisfy Medicare billing requirements. Since Medicare accounted for about 40 % of all hospital beds in use in the United States, it became clear in the 1980s that HCFA could be a powerful force in the diffusion of hospital information systems in this country. By the end of the 1980s, HCFA began to consider similarly requiring physicians to provide, in their claims for payments, the codes for the diagnoses of Medicare office patients, and the agency also explored the electronic processing and payments of claims. The Health Maintenance Organization (HMO) Act of 1973, loosely based on the Kaiser Permanente medical care program, led to a rapid increase in the number of prepaid group practice programs in the country. The rising costs of medical care, as well as the increased competition among medical organizations in the 1980s, produced a trend to the industrialization of medical care and the formation of medical conglomerates. This provided the stimulus for multi-facility medical information systems. The medical industry had become one of the largest in the United States. A 1988 *Market Directory of Computers in Healthcare* listed 750 vendors of medical computer systems, applications, and supplies [40]. In 1989 a compendium in the journal *MD Computing* listed almost 400 manufacturers or vendors selling more than 1,000 different medical computing products; most were designed for personal computers, and only about one-third were intended for clinical purposes [86].

Medical informatics gradually evolved over as health professionals learned to exploit the extraordinary capabilities of the electronic digital computer to meet their complex information needs. The first applications and articles on this subject appeared in the 1950s, and the number of publications rapidly increased in each of the following three decades. Medical informatics was identified as a new discipline in the 1970s, and it came to represent the broad field of computers, communications, information science, engineering, and technology as applied to medical practice, research, and education. Since its birth, medical informatics has gradually diffused throughout the United States (and globally), led by a few pioneers in the new field, supported by a relatively small number of professional organizations and universities, funded by federal grants and contracts, and pressured by the financing needs of increasingly expensive medical care. Blum [27] categorized the 1950s as phase 0, when most computer-based biomedical applications were for processing signals, images, and laboratory tests; and called the 1960s phase 1, when computers began to find some applications to patient care. Blum considered phase 2 to begin in 1975 when medical informatics began to mature, with more applications to clinical information systems and clinical decision support [27].

Compared to the acceptance of the automobile for transportation and the telephone for communication, the acceptance of computers in medicine has been relatively slow. By the 1950s automobiles and telephones were among the day-to-day tools of physicians. Starr [172] credited the telephone and the automobile with the greatest improvements in the productivity of medical practitioners. According to Starr, physicians were among the first to use the telephone in the late 1870s to connect their offices with local drug stores for ordering patients' prescriptions and to communicate with patients requesting house calls. Ford put out the first Model T automobile in 1908, and a Chicago dentist is said to have purchased the first Model A Ford on the market in 1927 [98]. In the early 1900s, the *Journal of the American Medical Association* reported that automobiles were already generally accepted by medical professionals as their usual mode of travel; they enabled doctors to cut in half the time required for house calls. In addition, they made it easier for patients to visit physicians in the doctor's offices [94]. Clearly, the automobile and the telephone quickly and dramatically affected the way the medical profession provided patient care. The automobile was much more efficient than the horse in transporting the busy physician to his home, office, and hospital. The telephone was more efficient than was the postal mail in getting urgent messages to and from the physician. As we have mentioned, Hollerith was working on punched cards for the 1880 census at roughly the same time that Bell was beginning to market the telephone. The great automobile race was held in 1895 from Paris to Bordeaux and back. But it became evident in the latter half of the twentieth century that physicians were much slower to adopt the computer than they had been with either the telephone or the automobile.

Although the personal computer began to diffuse rapidly into doctors' offices in the decade of the 1980s, by the end of the 1980s the computer was not yet a day-to-day tool of physicians. It did not significantly affect patient care services or alter visibly the quality or costs of medical care. Given the need to finance increasingly expensive medical care, one could have expected that the potential of the computer to increase the performance of health care professionals, to increase the quality of medical care, and to decrease the costs of care would stimulate a more rapid diffusion of medical informatics for patient care in the remainder of the 1990s. In the 2000s the federal government began to support the diffusion of electronic medical records and the expansion of translational medical information systems, in part to accelerate the use of a technology that many had viewed as important and inevitable for over a decade [59, 58].

References

1. AAHC. Executive management of computer resources in the academic health center. Washington, DC: Association of Academic Health Centers; 1984.
2. AAMC. The GPEP report: physicians for the twenty-first century: report of the panel on the general professional education of the physician and college preparation for medicine. Washington, DC: Association of American Medical Colleges; 1984.

3. AAMC. Association of American Medical Colleges. 1985. Annual report 1984–1985. 2015.
4. AAMSI News. 1982; 1.
5. Ackerman E, Gatewood LC, Connelly D, Hamann R. Distributed capacity networks for clinical information processing. Biosci Commun. 1976;2:293–305.
6. AMIA. Articles of incorporation, article 3. Washington, DC: American Medical Informatics Association; 1988.
7. AMIA. Minutes of incorporator's meeting, attachments 2, 3, 4. Wahington, DC: AMIA; 1988.
8. Anderson J. Personal communications to M Collen. 1986.
9. Anderson J, Gremy F, Pages JC. Educational requirements for medical informatics: results of the first international survey. Proc MEDINFO. 1974;1974:207–11.
10. Anderson J, Gremy F, Pages JC. Education in informatics of health personnel: a study and recommendation by an international working group (WG 4.1.) set up by the International Federation for Information Processing. Amsterdam; 1974.
11. Atkins H. Proc. progress in medical computing. London: Elliott Medical Computing; 1965.
12. Ball M, Douglas JV, Walker HP. Preface. In: Ball MJ, Douglas JV, editors. Nursing informatics: where caring and technology meet. New York: Springer; 2011.
13. Ball M. Integrating information systems in health care. In: Bakker AR et al., editors. Towards new hospital information systems. Amsterdam: Elsevier; 1988. p. 39–44.
14. Ball MJ, Hannah KJ, Jelger UG. Nursing informatics: where caring and technology meet. New York: Springer-Verlag; 1988.
15. Ball MJ, Douglas JV, Walker PH, DuLong D. Nursing informatics: transforming nursing. In: Ball MJ, Douglas J, Walker P, editors. Nursing informatics: where technology and caring meet. London: Springer; 2011. p. 5–12.
16. Ball MJ, et al. Nursing informatics: where caring and technology meet. 2nd ed. New York: Springer; 1995.
17. Ball MJ, et al. Nursing informatics: where caring and technology meet. 4th ed. New York: Springer; 2011.
18. Ball MJ, Hannah KJ, Browne JD. Using computers in nursing. Reston: Reston Publishing Co; 1984.
19. Banta HD, Behney CJ, Sisk JS. Toward rational technology in medicine: considerations for health policy. New York: Springer; 1981.
20. Barlow JS. An electronic method for detecting evoked responses of the brain and for reproducing their average waveforms. Electroencephalogr Clin Neurophysiol. 1957;9:340–3.
21. Bartels R, Moore FF. Practical considerations in establishing a biomedical data processing research center. In: Proc 3rd IBM symp. Endicott, NY: IBM. 1961. p. 153–63.
22. Bernstam EV, Smith JW, Johnson TR. What is biomedical informatics? J Biomed Inform. 2010;43:104–10.
23. Best WR. The potential role of computers in medical practice. JAMA. 1962;182:994–1000.
24. Blois MS, Shortliffe EH. The computer meets medicine: emergence of a discipline. In: Shortliffe EH, Perrault L, editors. Biomedical informatics. Reading: Addison-Wesley; 1990. p. 3–6.
25. Blois MS. The effect of hierarchy on the encoding of meaning. Proc SCAMC. 1986:73–80.
26. Blois MS. Information and medicine: the nature of medical descriptions. Berkeley: University of California Press; 1984.
27. Blum BI, Lenhard Jr RE, McColligan EE. An integrated data model for patient care. IEEE Trans Biomed Eng. 1985;32:277–88.
28. Borass BA. Applications programming in a health services computing center. Proc ACM Annual Conf 1971:613–21.
29. Brazier MA. From calculating machines to computers and their adoption by the medical sciences. Med Hist. 1973;17:235–43.
30. Brennan PF. Nursing at SCAMC: have we done what we said we were going to do? Proc SCAMC. 1984:597–600.

31. Breslow L. Health care versus medical care: implications for data handling. In: Laudet M, editor. Proc of an international symposium. London: Taylor and Francis; 1977. p. 69–75.
32. Britt PM, Newton CM. A case for functionalization of large computing centers. Proc ACM Annu Conf 1971:357–8.
33. Brodman K, Erdmann AJ, Goldstein LS. Interpretation of symptoms with a data-processing machine. AMA Arch Intern Med. 1959;103:776–82.
34. Brodziak A, Suchan L. The introduction of medical informatics: our experiences. Pol Arch Med Wewn. 1975;54:233–41.
35. Broering NC, Hendrickson GL. Integrated academic information management systems: introduction. Bull Med Libr Assoc. 1986;74:235–7.
36. Broering NC, Potter J, Mistry P. Linking bibliographic and information databases: an IAIMS prototype. Proc AAMSI. 1987:169–73.
37. Brunelle RH. Systems programming at a biomedical computing facility. Ann N Y Acad Sci. 1966;128:731–7.
38. Caceres CA. Computers in biomedicine. In: Dickson JFB, editor. Future goals of engineering in biology and medicine. New York: Academic; 1969.
39. Cardarov S. Terminolgicen Recnik po Informatika. Naujcnoj iTexniceskoj Informacii 1975.
40. Cardiff Publishing. Fifth annual market directory of computers in healthcare. Englewood: Cardiff Pub. Co; 1988.
41. Childs BW. Healthcare informatics. 1989. p. 6.
42. Childs BW. ECHO and its board. Health care comput and communic. 1985. p. 32–43.
43. Collen MF. Foreword. In: Proceedings: AMIA congress. 1982. p. 82.
44. Collen MF. Computers in preventive health services research. In: 7th IBM medical symposium. Poughkeepsie, NY: IBM. 1965. p. 331–44.
45. Collen MF. Machine diagnosis from a multiphasic screening program. In: Proc of 5th IBM medical symposium. Endicott, NY: IBM. 1963. p. 1–23.
46. Collen MF. Automated multiphasic health testing. In: Collen MF, editor. Hospital computer systems. New York: Wiley; 1974. p. 274–94.
47. Collen MF, Rubin L, Neyman J, Dantzig GB, Baer RM, Siegelaub AB. Automated multiphasic screening and diagnosis. Am J Public Health Nations Health. 1964;54:741–50.
48. Craig JF. Personal communications to M Collen. 1989.
49. Crouse L, Wiederhold G. An advanced computer for real-time medical applications. Comput Biomed Res. 1969;2:582–98.
50. Daskalaki A. Dental computing and applications: advanced techniques for clinical dentistry. Dental informatics online communications. 2009.
51. Datamation International. User group directory. 1988; 34:25–48.
52. Davies DE. AAMSI'S forebearers. AAMSI News. 1985;4:1–2.
53. Davies DE. The first ten years of the society for advanced medical systems. In: Hinman E, editor. Advanced medical systems: an assessment of the contributions. Miami: Symposia Specialist; 1979. p. 125–33.
54. Degoulet P. The French term Informatique Medicale. Personal Correspondence to M Ball 2010.
55. Detmer DE, Shortliffe EH. Clinical informatics: prospects for a new medical subspecialty. JAMA. 2014;311:2067–8.
56. Detmer DE, Lumpkin JR, Williamson JJ. Defining the medical subspecialty of clinical informatics. JAMIA. 2009;16:167–8.
57. Dezelic G. Modern medical documentation and the role of medical informatics in solving its problems (author's transl). Lijec Vjesn. 1979;101:521–4.
58. Dick RS, Steen EB, Detmer DE. The computer-based patient record: an essential technology for health care. Revised Edition. Washington, DC: National Academy Press; 1997.
59. Dick RS, Steen EB, Detmer DE. The computer-based patient record: an essential technology for health care. Washington, DC: National Academy Press; 1991.

60. Dixon WJ. BMDP computer program manual. Los Angeles: UCLA; 1961.
61. Dixon WJ, Britt PM. Health sciences computing facility, UCLA, 1959–79. In: Blum B, Duncan K, editors. A history of medical informatics. New York: Addison-Wesley; 1990. p. 76–83.
62. DuLong D, Ball MJ. TIGER: technology informatics guiding education reform: a nursing imperative. In: Weaver CA et al., editors. Nursing and informatics for the 21st century. 2nd ed. Chicago: Healthcare Information and Management Systems Society and American Medical Informatics Association; 2010. p. 17–24.
63. Eden M. Storage and retrieval of the results of clinical research. Proc IRE Trans Med Electron (ME-7). 1960:265–8.
64. Emlet HE. Minutes of initial meeting of the U.S. Committee on computers in health care. 1980.
65. Farley BG, Clark W. Simulation of self-organizing systems by digital computer. IRE Trans Inform Theory. 1954;4:76–84.
66. Forest RB. NCC at the crossroads. Datamation. 1986. p. 169–72.
67. Freiherr G. The seeds of artificial intelligence: SUMEX-AIM. Rockville: National Institutes of Health; 1980.
68. Gabrieli ER. Standardization of medical informatics (special issue). J Clin Comput. 1985;14:62–104.
69. Galler BA. Value of computers in medicine. JAMA. 1960;174:2161–2.
70. Gardner RM, Overhage JM, Steen EB, Munger BS, Holmes JH, Williamson JJ, et al. Core content for the subspecialty of clinical informatics. JAMIA. 2009;16:153–7.
71. Garfield E. Informatics and the future of biomedical education curricula. Curr Contents. 1986;4:3–5.
72. Garfield SR. The delivery of medical care. Sci Am. 1970;222:15–23.
73. Gee HH. Organization and influence in biomedical computing. Rocquencourt: Journee d'Informatique Medicale; 1970. p. 437–50.
74. Goodman L. New activities for AEMB. Memo. AEMB J. 1972; 5 Oct 1972.
75. Greenes RA, Siegel ER. Characterization of an emerging field: approaches to defining the literature and disciplinary boundaries of medical informatics. Proc SCAMC. 1987:411.
76. Hampton HP. Oversight hearings/computers in health care. Special Report. Comput Med 1979; 8:1–6.
77. Harrison AJ. Common elements and interconnections. Science. 1984;224:939–42.
78. Hatton AJ, Perdrizet S, Burghard G, Petitjean R. Study of an informatic system applied to the public health services. Bull Inst Natl Sante Resch Med. 1970;25:427–36.
79. Haux R. Special issue celebrating 50th anniversary. Methods Inf Med. 2011;50:487–555.
80. Haux R. On medical informatics. Methods Inf Med. 1989;28:66–8.
81. Heller BR, Romano CA, Damrosch SP, McCarthy MR. A needs assessment for graduate specialization in nursing informatics. Proc SCAMC. 1988:337–42.
82. Hemphill FM, Shannon JA. Medical research potentials in the light of modern data processing. In: Proc 3RD IBM med sym. Endicott, NY: IBM. 1961. p. 9–19.
83. HIMSS Analytics. Essentials of the U.S. hospital IT market. Chicago: Health Information Management and Systems Society; 2011.
84. HIMSS Legacy Workgroup. History of healthcare management and systems society. Chicago: HIMSS; 2010.
85. Hoffman JG, Metropolis N, Gardiner V. Digital computer studies of cell multiplication by Monte Carlo methods. J Natl Cancer Inst. 1956;17:175–88.
86. Hoffman T. The 6th annual medical hardware and software buyers guide. MD Comput. 1989;6:334–77.
87. Huesing SA, ECHO. Past, present and future. US Healthc. 1988;5:30–2.
88. Humphrey H. Senate hearing on the U.S. government and the future of international medical research. Jul 1959.
89. Humphreys BL, Lindberg DAB. Building the unified medical language system. Proc SCAMC. 1989:475–80.

90. Jenkin MA. Clinical informatics: a strategy for the use of information in the clinical setting. Inform Health Soc Care. 1984;9:225–32.
91. Juenemann HJ. The design of a data processing center for biological data. Ann N Y Acad Sci. 1964;115:547–52.
92. Kaplan B, ed. Computers in ambulatory medicine. In: Proc Joint Conf of SCM and SAMS. Washington, DC. 1981.
93. Kastner V, Pratt AW. Resourcing. Comput Methods Prog Biomed. 1976;5:189–205.
94. King LS. The automobile makes an impact. JAMA. 1984;251:2352–5.
95. Koeppe P. Education in medical informatics in the Federal Republic of Germany. Methods Inf Med. 1977;16:160–7.
96. Krasnoff SO. Computers in medicine; a primer for the practicing physician. Springfield: Thomas; 1967.
97. Kulikowski CA, Shortliffe EH, Currie LM, Elkin PL, Hunter LE, Johnson TR, et al. AMIA board white paper: definition of biomedical informatics and specification of core competencies for graduate education in the discipline. JAMIA. 2012;19:931–8.
98. Lacey R. Ford, the men and the machine. Boston: Little, Brown; 1986.
99. Lederberg J. How DENDRAL was conceived and born. In: Blum B, Duncan K, editors. A history of medical informatics. New York: Addison-Wesley; 1990. p. 14–44.
100. Ledley RS, Lusted LB. Reasoning foundations of medical diagnosis; symbolic logic, probability, and value theory aid our understanding of how physicians reason. Science. 1959;130:9–21.
101. Ledley RS. Digital computational methods in symbolic logic, with examples in biochemistry. Proc Natl Acad Sci U S A. 1955;41:498.
102. Ledley RS. Medical diagnosis and medical-record processing. In: Ledley RS, editor. Use of computers in biology and medicine. New York: McGraw-Hill; 1965. p. 418–95.
103. Ledley RS. Report on the uses of computers in biology and medicine. National Research Council. 1960.
104. Ledley RS. Use of computers in biology and medicine. New York: McGraw-Hill; 1965.
105. Levy AH, Baskin AB. Clinical computing-1977. J Med Syst. 1977;1:361–74.
106. Ligezinski P. Informatics in health service. Pol Tyg Lek. 1972;27:1735–9.
107. Lindberg D. NLM long range plan. Report of the board of regents. 1987. p. 31.
108. Lindberg D. Medical informatics/computers in medicine. JAMA. 1986;256:2120–2.
109. Lindberg D. Computer networks within health care. In: Peterson H, Isaksson A, editors. Communications networks in health care. Amsterdam: North Holland; 1982. p. 109–20.
110. Lindberg D. Impact of public policy on the development, adoption, and diffusion of medical information systems technology. Washington, DC: U.S. Govt. Printing Office; 1978.
111. Lindberg D. The computer and medical care. Springfield: CC Thomas; 1968.
112. Lindberg DAB. The development and diffusion of a medical technology: medical information systems. In: Medical technology and the health care system: a study of the diffusion of equipment-embodied technology. Washington, DC: National Academy of Science; 1979. p. 201–39.
113. Linvill JG. University role in the computer age. Science. 1982;215:802–6.
114. Lipkin M, Engle RL, Davis BJ, Zworykin VK, Ebald R, Sendrow M, et al. Digital computer as aid to differential diagnosis: use in hematologic diseases. Arch Intern Med. 1961;108:56–72.
115. Lusted LB. Summary of discussions on medical data centers. In: Proc 3rd IBM Med Sym. Endicott, NY: IBM. 1961. p. 203–13.
116. Lusted LB. Medical progress: medical electronics. N Engl J Med. 1955;252:580–5.
117. Lusted LB, Coffin RW. An automated information system for hospitals and biomedical research laboratories. Chicago: Year Book Pub, Inc; 1967.
118. Lusted LB. Computers in medicine: a personal perspective. J Chronic Dis. 1966;19:365–72.
119. Mackintosh DR. Directory of publications in health systems and informatics. Washington, DC: AAMSI; 1985.

120. Manos D. Clinical informatics becomes a board-certified medical subspecialty. Healthcare IT News. 2011.
121. Matheson N. Symposium: integrated academic information management systems (IAIMS) model development. Bull Med Libr Assoc. 1988;76(3):221–67.
122. Matheson NW, Cooper JA. Academic information in the academic health sciences center: roles for the library in information management. J Med Educ. 1982;57:1–93.
123. Matheson NW. Introduction. Bull Med Libr Assoc. 1988;76(3):221.
124. Myers HD. Medical education in the information age. Proc Sym Med Inform. Washington, DC: Assoc Am Med College, 1986.
125. Mikhailov, AIC. Scientific communications and informatics. Arlington: Information Resources Press; 1984.
126. Miller PL. ATTENDING: a system which critiques an anesthetic management plan. Proc AMIA. 1982: 36–40.
127. Milsum JH, Laszlo CA. From medical to health informatics. Methods Inf Med. 1983;23:61–2.
128. Moehr JR. Personal communication to M Collen. 1988.
129. Morris TA. Structural relationships within medical informatics. Proc AMIA 2000: 590–4.
130. NCHSR&D. Summary of grants and contracts active in fiscal year 1970. Rockville: HEW, NCHRSR 1970.
131. NIH. National institutes of health data book. Bethesda: NIH; 1990.
132. NLM extramural programs: NLM grant activities fact sheet. 1984.
133. NLM News. Second IAIMS symposium emphasizes health sciences education. NLM News. 1986;41:1.
134. NLM: Planning for integrated academic information systems. Proc NLM symp 1984. Bethesda: NLM; 14 Oct 1984.
135. Pages JC, Levy AJ, Gremy F, Anderson J. Meeting the challenge: informatics and medical information. New York: Elsevier Science; 1983.
136. Parascandola J. Personal communication to M Collen. 1986.
137. Pardon N. Informatique and occupational medicine. Arch Mal Prof. 1968;29:699–701.
138. Polacsek RA. The fourth annual medical software buyer's guide. MD Comput. 1987;4:23.
139. Pratt AW. Medicine and linguistics. Proc MEDINFO. 1974: 5–11.
140. Pratt AW. Progress towards a medical information system for the research environment. In: Fuchs G, Wagner G, editors. Sonderdruck aus Krankenhaus-Informations system. New York: Schattauer; 1972. p. 319–36.
141. Proctor LD, Adey RW. Proc. automatic data processing of electrocardiography and electroencephalography. Washington, DC: NASA; 1964.
142. PROMIS Laboratory. Automation of the problem-oriented medical record. NCHSR&D Research Digest Series 1977; DHEW Pub No (HRA). p. 77–3177.
143. Raub WF. The life sciences computer resources program of the National Institutes of Health. 1971. p. 693–700.
144. Reichertz PL. Medical informatics – fiction or reality? Methods Inf Med. 1980;19:11–5.
145. Reiser SJ, Anbar M. The machine at the bedside: strategies for using technology in patient care. New York: Cambridge University Press; 1984.
146. Revens L. The first twenty-five years: ACM 1947–1962. Commun ACM. 1972;15:485–90.
147. RMP proceedings. Conference workshop on regional medical programs. 1968.
148. Rosenthal G. NCHSR&D research report: computer applications in health care. Washington, DC: DHEW Pub. No. (PHS 79–3251); 1979.
149. Rothschild K. The age of influence. Datamation. 1988;34:18–24.
150. Saba VK, Westra BL. Historical perspectives of nursing informatics. In: Saba V, McCormick K, editors. Essentials of nursing informatics. 5th ed. New York: McGraw-Hill; 2011.
151. Saba VK. Introduction. Proc SCAMC. 1982: 515.
152. Saba VK, McCormick K. Essentials of nursing informatics. New York: McGraw-Hill, Medical Pub. Division; 2011.

153. Saenger EL, Sterling TD. Design and operation of a medical computing center. Ann N Y Acad Sci. 1964;115:591–9.
154. Safran C, Shabot MM, Munger BS, Holmes JH, Steen EB, Lumpkin JR, et al. Program requirements for fellowship education in the subspecialty of clinical informatics. JAMIA. 2009;16:158–66.
155. Sanazaro PJ. Federal health services R & D under the auspices of the National Center for Health Services Research and Development. In: Flook E, Sanazaro PJ, editors. Health services research and R&D in perspective. Ann Arbor: Univ of Michigan Health Adminstration Press; 1973. p. 150–83.
156. Sanazaro PJ. National center for health services. Res Dev Dig. 1969;1:1–12.
157. Schatz W. United States computer research's basic dilemma. Datamation. 1989;35:44–7.
158. Schenthal JE, Sweeney JW, Nettleton W. Clinical application of electronic data processing apparatus: II. New methodology in clinical record storage. JAMA. 1961;178:267–70.
159. Schleyer T. Dental informatics: the right time to invest in training and research? Dental Tribune. 2009.
160. Schwan HP. Bio-medical electronics past and present. Biomed Electron IRE Trans. 1961;8:234–8.
161. Shambaugh V. MJ Clinics in Asia. Personal communication. Mar 2012.
162. Shambaugh V. The origin of the International Health Evaluation and Promotion Association (IHEPA). 2010.
163. Shannon JA. Federal support of biomedical sciences: development and academic impact. J Med Educ. 1976;51:1–98.
164. Shephard RH. Plans for developing a computational facility at the Johns Hopkins Medical Institutions. In: Proc 3rd IBM med symp. Endicott, NY: IBM. 1961. p. 191–6.
165. Shortliffe EH, Perreault L. Medical informatics: computer applications in health care. Reading: Addison-Wesley; 1990.
166. Shortliffe EH. The science of biomedical computing. In: Pages J, Levy A, Gremy F, Anderson J, editors. Meeting the challenge: informatics and medical education. New York: Elsevier Science; 1983. p. 3–10.
167. Shortliffe EH, Cimino JJ. Biomedical informatics: computer applications in health care and biomedicine. London: Springer Science + Business Media, LLC; 2015.
168. Shortliffe EH, Detmer DE, Munger BS. Clinical informatics: the emergence of a new profession. In: Finell JT, Dixon BE, editors. Clinical informatics study guide: text and review. London: Springer; 2015.
169. Shortliffe EH. Computer-based medical consultations, MYCIN. New York: Elsevier; 1976.
170. Shryock RH, Arnau M. American medical research: past and present. New York: Arno Press; 1980.
171. Skiba DJ, DuLong D, Newbold SK. TIGER collaboratives and diffusion. In: Ball M, Douglas J, Walker P, editors. Nursing informatics. 4th ed. London: Springer; 2011. p. 35–50.
172. Stacy RW, Waxman BD. Computers in biomedical research. New York: Academic; 1965.
173. Starr P. The social transformation of American medicine. New York: Basic Books; 1982.
174. Stead WW. A window on medical informatics. Proc SCAMC. 1987: 3–5.
175. Sterling T, Pollack S. MEDCOMP: handbook of computer applications in biology and medicine. Cincinnati: University of Cincinnati; 1964.
176. Stoneburner LL. APPLE medical users group international. Proc SCAMC. 1980;3:1399–400.
177. Sweeney JW. The role of a computer center in biomedicine. In: Proc 5th IBM symp. Endicott, NY: IBM. 1963. p. 5–18.
178. Taylor R. The computer: concept, development and problem environment. J Chronic Dis. 1966;19:333–48.
179. Terry LT. News release. HEW, NIH Division of Research Facilities and Resources. 1963.
180. Thomas U. OECD informatics studies. Computerized data banks in public administration. 1971.
181. Troseth M. The TIGER initiative. In: Saba VK, editor. Essentials of nursing informatics. New York: McGraw-Hill; 2006.

182. Troseth MR. The TIGER initiative. In: Saba VK, McCormick K, editors. Essentials of nursing informatics. New York: McGraw-Hill; 2011. p. 633–40.
183. Turner WA, Lamson BG. Automatic data processing in hospitals: a powerful new tool for clinical research. Hospitals. 1964;38:87–90.
184. Tvedness JA. HISSG: leading the way. MUG Q. 1983;12:3.
185. Uberla K. Medizinische informatick. Neue Munch Beitr Gesch Med. 1978;7–8:629–33.
186. Vallbona C, Spencer WA, Levy AH, Baker RL, Liss DM, Pope SB. An on-line computer system for a rehabilitation hospital. Methods Inf Med. 1968;7:31.
187. Van Bemmel J. The structure of medical informatics: bibliography on educational courses at the Free University, Amsterdam. Inform Health Soc Care. 1984;9:175–80.
188. Van Bemmel J, Shortliffe EH, Salamon R, Blum B, Jorgensen M. Medical informatics: from art to science. Proc MEDINFO 1986; Foreword p. vii–xv.
189. Warner HR. A mathematical approach to medical diagnoses: applications to congenital heart disease. JAMA 1961:177(3):173–6.
190. Waxman BD. Planting the seeds: personal observations. In: Blum B, Duncan K, editors. A history of medical informatics. New York: ACM Press; 1990. p. 111–5.
191. Waxman BD. Public health service support of biomedical computing. In: Proc of the 3rd IBM Medical Symposium. Endicott: IBM; 1961. p. 199–202.
192. Weaver CA. Nursing and informatics for the 21st century: an international look at practice, trends and the future. Chicago: Healthcare Information and Management Systems Society; 2006.
193. Weinrauch H, Patishall E. The air force and applications of computers to medicine and biology. Mil Med. 1958;3:178–80.
194. Weiss S, Kulikowski CA, Safir A. Glaucoma consultation by computer. Comput Biol Med. 1978;8:25–40.
195. Williams B. Tokyo Accords. Enclosure 1 minutes of SAMS board of directors meeting. 30 Oct 1980.
196. Woodbury MA, Tick LJ, Cady LD. The biomedical computing section in a general-purpose computing laboratory. Ann N Y Acad Sci. 1964;115:609.
197. Wraith SM, Aikins JS, Buchanan BG, Clancey WJ, Davis R, Fagan LM, et al. Computerized consultation system for selection of antimicrobial therapy. Am J Health-Syst Pharm. 1976;33:1304–8.
198. Zielstorff RD. Computers in nursing. Wakefield: Nursing Resources; 1980.
199. Zimmerman JL, Landesman HM, Bilan JP, Stuffelbeam D, Ball MJ, Bydalek RO. Study of computer applications in dental practice. Dent Clin N Am. 1986;30:731–8.
200. Zimmerman JL, Achtenberg J, Sherentz DD. Education in computing: the MUMPS user group example. Proc MEDINFO. 1980;80:358–61.

Part II
Direct Patient Care

Chapter 3
Development of Medical Information Systems (MISs)

Morris F. Collen and W. Ed Hammond

Abstract By the late 1960s, mainframe-based hospital information systems (HISs) had been developed that could integrate patient data in a single database. In the 1970s, minicomputers made it possible to link the subsystem databases for clinical subspecialties and ancillary services to the mainframe and integrate patient data into the patient records stored there. In the 1980s, microcomputer-based systems that had evolved independently for specialized services became subsystems of larger medical information systems with an integrating central database management system. Storage grew cheaper; registries became databases; databases became data warehouses; and secondary clinical databases were developed. The recognition that databases were equally as important for querying and retrieving data as for documenting care lead to addressing issues of terminologies and other data standards. The fact that much data was unstructured led to the development of natural language processing (NLP) for retrieving and understanding unstructured data. In the 1990s, patient care data expanded in volume and complexity, and innovative clinical information systems offered hospitals and clinics new capabilities. From the 1990s on, the impact of the Internet and the Web grew, enabling global exchange of clinical data and medical knowledge. In the 2000s, distributed information systems allowed physicians using clinical workstations to enter orders and retrieve test results across multiple medical center databases. In the 2010s, federal support greatly increased the use of computer-based patient records. Global wireless communications with cloud storage for translational networks evolved that linked data warehouses in collaborating medical centers nationally and offered mobile e-health care for individual patients.

Keywords Hospital information systems • Computer-based patient records • Interoperability • Data integration • Database managementsystems • Data standards • Clinical databases • Clinical information systems • Medical information systems • Terminologies

---

Author was deceased at the time of publication.

M.F. Collen (deceased)

W. Ed Hammond (✉)
Duke Center for Health Informatics, Duke University, Durham, NC, USA
e-mail: William.hammond@duke.edu

© Springer-Verlag London 2015   123
M.F. Collen, M.J. Ball (eds.), *The History of Medical Informatics
in the United States*, Health Informatics, DOI 10.1007/978-1-4471-6732-7_3

From the 1950s to today, when people went to see a physician, the doctor asked about the patient's medical problems and obtained the patient's medical history. The physician then recorded the patient's physical examination findings and arrived at a preliminary diagnosis. Usually the physician would order laboratory or diagnostic tests, documented as part of the encounter, to confirm the preliminary diagnoses. The physician frequently would prescribe a medication or other treatment. The patient might then be scheduled for a return visit to evaluate the outcome of the treatment.

This chapter describes the development, evolution, and diffusion of Medical Information Systems (MIS) in the United States. A number of factors have influenced the course of development of MISs including exponential growth in technology, changing reimbursement models, explosive expansion of knowledge, new kinds of data to be recorded, advancements in connectivity, a wealth of programming languages and database models, and finally a wealth of developments of applications from home-grown to major commercial vendors. The period is best described as one of constant change.

Moore [246] described the medical care system as being predominantly informational, in that it depended largely on the acquisition, storage, and interpretation of information by both the patient and the doctor. Although the basic kinds of information that pass directly between the patient and the physician differed little between the 1950s and the 2010s, there were substantial changes in the methods of collecting, storing, retrieving, and using medical information. Moreover, there was a much greater volume of information captured as a result of many innovations both in diagnostic technology (for example, in automated laboratory testing and radiology image scanners) and in therapeutic technology (for example, new antibiotics and more organ transplants). Furthermore, the complexity of information processing was greatly increased by fundamental changes in the organization and financing of medical practice, such as by health maintenance organizations (HMOs) with multi-hospital organizations that received a fixed payment per-person per-month for specified medical services rather than for fees-for-services provided; insurance reimbursement programs such as Medicare payments for patient care by coded diagnosis-related groups (DRGs); and an increasing interest of government policy makers in supporting and monitoring the costs and effectiveness of patient care services. By 2010 the provision of patient care in the United States had several dimensions of linkages and integration of patient care information, including local integration of information within a hospital or an outpatient clinic; vertical integration of information between affiliated hospitals and medical offices; and horizontal integration among associated hospitals, clinics, and community health and welfare support groups.

Information systems were described by Ledley and Lusted [194] as consisting of three essential parts: a system for documenting and organizing the information in a file; a method for locating in this file the information on a specific subject; and a method for keeping the information in the file up to date. Collen [73] defined a medical information system as one that used electronic data processing and communications systems to provide on-line processing with real-time responses for patient data within one or more medical centers that included both hospital and outpatient services. Lindberg [206] defined a MIS as a set of formal arrangements by which information concerning the health and health care of individual patients were collected, stored, and processed in computers.

In the 1950s with the introduction of computers into health care, medical practitioners began to speculate about the development and use of computer-based medical information systems (MISs). Physicians began to bring batches of their patient data to a central computer to be processed. Patient care data were initially collected, entered, and merged into computer files that were stored on magnetic tape; and file management systems were developed to enter, store, and retrieve the data. In the 1960s time-shared, mainframe computers that communicated by telephone lines to remote data entry terminals and printers allowed many users to process their data concurrently; and also provided a relatively acceptable turn-around time for many computer services. Patients' data that were initially stored in computer databases on magnetic tape were soon moved to storage on random-access, magnetic disc drives; and were then better organized in a manner more suitable for query and retrieval of the data. However, at that time the high costs for computer storage greatly limited database capacities.

By the mid-1960s solid-state integrated circuits in third-generation computers began to satisfy some of the technical requirements for MISs. Spencer and Vallbona [311] had optimistically concluded that with the available technology and with the proper functional requirements and technical design, the following areas of medical practice should soon be open to improvement by computers: patients' records, medical diagnosis, laboratory testing, patient monitoring, hospital communications, and utilization of hospital services and facilities.

In the 1970s as clinical support subsystems evolved for the clinical laboratory, radiology, pharmacy and for other clinical services, most developed their own separate subsystem databases. With the availability of random-access disc storage, the development of the modern electronic patient record began; since subsystem databases could be more readily merged into larger databases, which then needed an integrating database-management system. The retrieval of subsets of selected data from various subsystem databases required some re-organization of the stored data; and also needed an index to the locations of the various data subsets. Attempts were made to design more efficient databases to make them independent of their applications and subsystems, so that a well-designed database could process almost any type of data presented to it, and satisfy the functions of a patient record. Terdiman [317] credited the development of microcomputer technology in the 1970s with many of the advances in database management systems in that decade.

In the 1980s minicomputers and microcomputers were increasingly used for small database systems. As storage technology continued to become more efficient, and larger and cheaper storage devices became available, then computer-based registries expanded their storage capacity for larger amounts of data and were then generally referred to as databases. When huge storage capacity became available at a relatively low cost, very large collections of data were then often referred to as data warehouses. The year of 1988 was called the year of the database by Bryan [45] who reported that more than 20 new or improved database-management systems became available in that year. In 1989 the total number of computer-stored databases in the world was estimated to be about five million; and although most of the databases were considered to be relatively small, some were huge, such as the 1990 U.S. census database comprising a trillion bytes of data [102].

3.1 MIS Diffusion in the United States

The introduction and diffusion of medical information systems in the United States was always considered by many to be much too slow. Best [30] raised the question in the early 1960s, that if the computer was going to do so much good for medicine, why the delay in its introduction? His answer at that time was that computers were too expensive, the input-output devices were not adequate, and that suitable software was yet to be developed. In 1965 Summerfield [315] listed in the United States 73 hospital and office information system projects and 28 clinical support systems projects for clinical laboratories and pharmacies. Barnett [20] reviewed the status of ten developing hospital information systems (HISs), one outpatient information system (OIS), three clinical laboratory systems, and one multiphasic health testing system. A 1967 survey reported that 568 hospitals in the United States had computers, of which less than 20 % had computer applications in patient care or in medical research [225]. In 1968 a questionnaire survey with responses from approximately one-half of the 2,400 hospitals surveyed, found that 50 % of the hospitals with more than 200 beds used computers, whereas only 14 % of the hospitals with less than 200 beds had computers [139]. Barnett [20] also observed that the most widely implemented application of computers to patient care was for the electronic processing of clinical laboratory data. Caceres [47] reported that one-fourth of the users of computers in health care services were in hospitals with more than 250 beds, one-fourth were in state or city health departments, one-fourth in employee health screening or group practice programs, and one-fourth in medical research.

Galbraith [123] cautioned that the successful development of sophisticated complex technology required a heavy investment of capital; they needed to be designed and guided by sophisticated technologists; and they involved a great lapse of time between any decision to produce and the emergence of a marketable product. Flagle [99] also warned of the seriousness of the challenge when he emphasized that it must be recognized if the hopes of a comprehensive health service system were to be fulfilled, the enormity of the communications and analysis tasks demanded the full potentials of communication and computing technology. Flagle [100] further commented on the obstacles to overcoming the complex technology in the health field, since the processes of direct patient care did not meet the requirements for simple mechanization. He believed that industry needed to have adequate incentives to engage and invest in technological product development and have access to a clinical setting for development and testing. An additional problem was the necessity to overcome the absence of consistent policies, standard plans, and definitions. Further, the practices in medical care left industry without adequate specifications for functional and technical specifications.

Lindberg [209, 212] noted that the maximum progress was made in implementing a MIS when:

- There was enthusiastic endorsement of attempts to introduce computers into a medical setting on the part of the medical and administrative authorities of the institutions.
- The technical computer group reported directly to the institution's highest-level administrative authority but had no hospital direct line authority.
- There was adequate financial support for the venture.
- Each member of the group did the job for which they were best suited. It was the proper role of the medical group to make medical judgments and to leave technical decisions to computer people. The reverse was also true.

Lindberg [210] was one of the earliest to analyze the reasons for computer failures and successes in the first decade. He questioned why after almost 10 years of attempts, few computer applications had survived; an even smaller number actually performed medical service functions without the parallel operation of former manual systems; and in no case could one yet say that medical care of ill patients actually depended upon a computer or an information system. Lindberg observed that medical people had been extremely slow to spell out in a cohesive and organized form the conditions under which they wished to work with an information system. The lack of significant successes of computers in medicine had been the result of a consistent "over-sell" of capability on the part of manufacturers and computer enthusiasts. Lindberg concluded that this brought a feeling of uncertainty to physicians that the manufacturers and system analysts did not understand what medicine needed; that computers could not actually do something for, rather than with, the physician; and there were only a specified number of tasks in medical practice which one must program for the computer. Lindberg proposed that none of these assumptions were true, but rather that computer-engineering experts had little understanding of the complex problems of a medical office or of a hospital practice. Developers had consistently underestimated the complexity of the problems, and MISs could not be well built unless they were defined with a physician as the continuing major contributor and user of the information.

Barnett [25] questioned why government and industry had already spent millions of dollars implementing MISs with little payoff, and he concluded that much of the frustration in building such systems was due, at that date, to violations of what he referred to as his "ten commandments":

- It was essential to know what one wanted to do even though most elements of the health care delivery system did not have a well defined set of objectives, much less a defined pattern of information flow.

- Construct a modular system, since given the chaotic state of the typical hospital operation, the conflicting governing power structure, the rapid changes in manpower utilization, and the available computer technology, it was impossible at this date to construct a total MIS.
- Build a system that can evolve in a manageable way. Once subsystems have been developed and are operational, it is much easier to see how to build the next system and its interconnections; and the system must be capable of being expanded without requiring redesign or reprogramming.
- Build a system that allows easy and rapid programming, development, and modification, since it is characteristic of a MIS that the objectives and specific procedures will change with time.
- Build a system that has a consistently rapid response time to queries, and is easy for a computer-illiterate person to use.
- Have duplicate hardware systems to assure a reliable backup operation, and when the system does fail it should do so without loss of data.
- Build and implement the system as a joint effort with real users in a real situation with real problems, since the best critics are those who use the system.
- Consider the costs and benefits of the system.
- Acquire a commitment of continuing support from the administration and the organization.
- Be optimistic about the future, be passionate in your commitment, but always be guided by a fundamental skepticism and do not confuse future potential with present reality [25].

Lamson [191] also offered some general principles that he believed were associated with successful computer applications in hospitals:

- Develop computing competence within the hospital staff; set attainable goals with realistic time tables;
- Use a modular approach;
- Avoid dependence on complex manual interfaces such as handwritten manual records;
- Avoid creating increases in local work in order to achieve longer-term and more broadly based efficiency; and
- Avoid confining general communication solutions to isolated segments of the hospital; and select the initial and subsequent applications guided by maximum cost-effectiveness.

From a series of case studies in the 1960s, Collen [72] similarly found that during that decade a number of hospitals in the United States had tried to implement a MIS, but in 1972 there was not yet a single successfully completed total MIS. He cited the following five major reasons for their failure:

Most commonly the failure was due to a suboptimal mix of medical and computer specialists in the project staff who consisted of well-motivated physicians who had little experience with computers and computer and system experts who had little experience with medical practice. The extreme difficulty with intercommunicating the highly technical and complex aspects of these two disciplines usually resulted in the computer staff underestimating the vast medical needs. Most organizations grossly underestimated the large amounts of money and time involved in implementing a total MIS, so there was an inadequate commitment of capital for long-term development. Some projects were terminated after 3–5 years because several million dollars had already been spent and the system was still far from being completed.

A sub-optimized systems approach was frequently used and several projects failed because they had successfully implemented one or more subsystem components for the administration, for hospital bed-census, patient scheduling, for the clinical laboratory and pharmacy and then wanted to integrate all the subsystems into an MIS. At that point, they discovered serious incompatibilities between the various modules that would require major reprogramming at prohibitive costs to achieve an integrated patient database; and these projects then usually continued the individual subsystem modules as independent computer-based units. At the other extreme were some projects that began with the global systems approach to implement a total MIS, but the sheer enormity of such an approach had not yet found anyone with the necessary vast resources capable of successfully following that course.

Unacceptable computer terminals were a prime reason why many of the early MIS projects were never implemented. The first systems required physicians and nurses to use keyboard-type, typewriter-like terminals. It was soon established that physicians would not accept such means for communicating with the computer, and for these systems the clerical personnel had to take over the process of data entry.

An inadequate management organization was an occasional cause of failure. Several projects in the United States were initiated in smaller hospitals with inexperienced medical management, and they terminated after having completed an administrative-business type of system. Large technological systems tended to commit an organization to a relatively fixed goal for a number of years. Since an investment in an MIS was usually a heavy one, a poor technical judgment could be disastrous. Later Collen [75] added that for a MIS with a medical database management system, the situation was further aggravated by the lack of standardization of medical data and medical practice, and the difficulties of demonstrating the cost-effectiveness of the MIS.

Davis [83] described what he considered to be three fundamental problems in developing a MIS at that time.

- As there were yet no operational, comprehensive MISs, there was little realistic insight or understanding of their full potential, and there was not a broad base of support or demand for such large and expensive systems. This lack of demand translated into a lack of long-term commitment of resources, and insufficient capital necessary to construct such complex technological systems over the needed long development time.
- Medical practice was diverse, dynamic, and non-standardized. Physicians were unable to state objectively a set of standards or specifications to a sufficiently explicit degree suitable for computer design and programming.

- The high costs of equipment, the poor reliability for 24-h, online uninterrupted use, and inflexible terminal devices made the use of these systems awkward, undependable, and difficult to cost justify [84].

Baker and Spencer [12] emphasized the need for a MIS to be readily transferrable, since there would not be a major effect on the health care system unless medical information systems could be transferred successfully to various sites. To meet the cost-effectiveness requirement of potential host sites, they recommended that a transferrable information system should be demonstrably beneficial in terms of cost-effectiveness; well defined to facilitate determination of the procedure changes involved in implementing the automated system; compatible with the available resources that supported any other computer processes at the host site; and consistent with the institution's long-term goals for automation. They proposed that for an MIS to accommodate the local conditions of various sites, a transferrable MIS had to have adequate and variable scope to be applicable to a class of problems; computer programs written in a popular language that could be used on a variety of machines, with the transferability of software in the context of the available hardware at the host site; fast transaction rates which were determined not only by computer speeds but also by the efficiency of the algorithms that processed the messages and generated the responses, since a user of interactive terminals had a set of expectations about the time required to perform a particular task; and acceptance of the system by users, and that depended not only on what the system did but also on how the operations were carried out.

Rockart [285] noted that successful implementation of a system depended on the match between the collection, processing, and output of the information system with the process model held by the system user. He advocated that medical information systems should be more concerned with medical, as opposed to administrative, aspects of the delivery of medical care. Yet he pointed out that few systems analysts had medical training of any sort, so difficulties in conversations with physicians were many.

Jenkin [168] reported that a review of successful MISs at the time indicated that design concepts to ensure the necessary generality, flexibility, and ease of use vital to their acceptance included the following requirements:

- The input data, which involved the area of human-machine interaction, had to be accurate. To capture any significant amount of clinically useful information the system had to support the logic paths of the medical practitioner; and this support could be assured only through the practitioner's direct involvement at the time of medical content development. Jenkin also noted out that for each and every system action, an input transaction had to be generated. Since in the clinical situation these usually originated with the physician, it was also most efficient to have the physician generate and verify the input transcriptions.
- The database management system had to be independent of its applications. The data had to be storable and retrievable independent of user or application.
- The clinical environment required more of a capability for message handling and file management, rather than of computing power. It was extremely important to

have the ability to handle various transactions using many different devices; and to connect each transaction, independently of the device involved, to the appropriate application program.

Giebink and Hurst [126] described 29 medical computing projects at 19 sites, with their beginning dates from 1963 to 1972. These included five stand-alone hospitals, eight hospitals with outpatient clinics, three prepayment health plans or group practices, one community clinic, and one hospital with outpatient and community clinics. Of the 29 projects, 25 had electronic medical records, 24 were for patient care applications, 23 for diagnostic or consultation assistance, 20 for research, 9 for appointment scheduling, 8 for signal analysis (electrocardiography or electroencephalography), 7 for history taking, 5 for clinical support services (laboratory, radiology, or pharmacy), and 2 for multiphasic screening. The objectives given for these 29 projects included improve quality of patient care (13 sites); improve utilization of skilled personnel (10 sites) and improve efficiency (8 sites). Principal funding came from the U.S. Department of Health, Education and Welfare and, in some instances, from private foundations. The health care delivery organization itself rarely completely sponsored its medical computing work. In projects that had been in existence for more than 2 or 3 years, the institution sponsored a part of the cost of the information system. Some projects evolved from research projects to operational capability with the research funded by the government; and the system then funded entirely by the receiving institution after the government funding terminated. They also reported that many of the vendor-sponsored MISs planned or initiated in the late 1960s were extinct in the 1970s and served as testimony to the difficulties of implementing computer-based information systems for health care delivery. In 1975 they saw a gradual evolution of successful medical computer applications rather than a sharply escalating growth pattern. Medical computer applications that met operational criteria were rare except for their routine business applications; and computer-based medical records were usually abstracts of more complete paper-based patient records maintained in hard copy form. They also listed as major developmental or operational problems such items as: poor response time, poor system reliability, high machine down-time, unreliable terminals, bad data storage disks, power failures, poor telecommunications, problems with telephone lines, difficulties in interfacing with other automated applications, lack of physician agreement and standardization on data content, high costs of equipment, inadequate resources, and badly designed software.

Henley and Wiederhold [148] and associates reviewed 17 operational OISs in the United States. They found that most of the computer equipment in actual productive use was about 10 years old. They concluded that one reason for long lead times was the sequential process of the systems development effort. When computers were new, they required initial work in basic software development to make them suitable for computer medical applications development, which took time; and then integration of the applications services into the ongoing health care environment took even more time.

In the 1970s the clinical support systems for the laboratory, radiology, electrocardiology, and pharmacy readily incorporated computers, and these specialties soon radically changed the practice of medicine. However, the diffusion of medical computing into the general clinical specialties was much slower. Lindberg [214] commented on the rate of adoption of non-clinical applications, which he called relatively simple grade-one innovations. He noted that by the mid-1970s more than 85 % of all U.S. hospitals used computer systems or services in connection with their patient billings, collections, and third-party reimbursement functions; and the rate of adoption of computers in hospitals for such purposes was not slower than for industry in general. By 1976, 2.7 % of all general purpose conventional computers within the U.S. were owned by medical and hospital services; and this compared with 2.9 % which were owned by the transportation and carrier industry, and 2.7 % which were owned by the printing and publishing industry. Lindberg [205] also reported that in 1976 less than 200 U.S. hospitals had MISs which included significant amounts of indirect patient care activities; and less than 100 of these MISs rendered direct clinical care services.

Van Brunt [322] suggested that the requirements for an integrated computer-based patient record were so difficult to meet that it limited the development of a MIS. Although it was a limiting factor in MIS development, he advised that arguments for the standardization of medical procedures and information needs were overemphasized; and that greater flexibility and sophistication were needed in the arena of collation, of communication, and of the reporting of clinical data.

The Office of Technology Assessment (OTA) of the U.S. Congress reported in 1977 that major problem areas for developing MISs were: (1) the great variability in medical care and the lack of rules specifying what information should be entered in the medical record; (2) unresolved technical problems to satisfy health professionals' needs for data entry and retrieval; and (3) lack of long-term commitment of capital, which had been provided by private industry, by the federal government primarily by the National Center for Health Services Research and Development (NCHSR&D), and by the medical care institution involved. Expenditures by NCHSR&D for grants relating to MISs had decreased from a high of $4.6 million in fiscal year 1974 to $3.3 million in fiscal year 1976 [267].

Friedman [114] and Gustafson also observed that the overall influence of computers on health care delivery in the mid-1970s was smaller than had been expected; and they gave four reasons for this delay:

• The physician-computer interaction was not successfully accomplished; and a main impediment to successful physician-computer communications was that many computer user terminals were poorly engineered resulting in frequent mechanical breakdowns. The computer terminals were expensive, and were often placed in out-of-the-way locations, making them inconvenient to operate, and useless for rapid access to data retrieval; and the computer response time was often too slow for busy physicians. To obtain information from the computer, the physician was usually required to take part in a long technical dialog that often required knowledge of special passwords, codes, or computer languages.

- The physicians were often not provided with computer-based medical applications that exceeded their own capabilities. Whereas in other fields, the computer was often used to perform tasks previously incomprehensible to a human, in health care delivery the computer applications often merely duplicated the physician's actions.
- Another major impediment to the successful utilization of computer technology in medicine and health care was the difficulty in proving a significant positive effect on patient care by cost-effectiveness studies. It had not been demonstrated that physicians could make better, or less costly decisions because of computer use.
- Computer applications were not always easily transferred from one institution to another.

Friedman [113] also advised that, to be successful, developers of MISs needed to solve the problems of computer-physician interaction; develop software that exceeded the physician's capabilities; demonstrate a significant clinical benefit; develop easily transferable programs; conduct research in a change-oriented manner; and learn from mistakes on earlier computer systems.

In contrast to the computer applications in the clinical laboratory and radiology, where the added costs for computer processing could be included in the charges for these procedures, neither a medical information system nor its computer-based patient record were directly chargeable or reimbursable as specific procedures or as identifiable services to patients. Willems [333] wrote that financing methods figured prominently in technology diffusion; and that in contrast to fee-for-service reimbursement, prospective reimbursement for medical services forced health care providers to weigh alternatives, and to choose among them within the financial constraint of their budgets. As a result, one expected greater emphasis on cost-reducing technologies under prospective-payment programs than under retrospective cost-reimbursement programs.

In his testimony before a Congressional Committee, Lindberg [208] attributed some of the slow diffusion of medical computing applications to the lack of longer-term support from the National Institutes of Health (NIH). Although in the 1960s and 1970s NIH did support many research and developmental projects in medical informatics, most of these were for less than 5 years of funding, which was not a sufficient time to develop a prototype MIS. Furthermore, he was critical of the great effect that the Medicare reimbursement system had on diverting hospital funds into the development of accounting systems for claims reimbursement, rather than into patient care applications. He advocated a federal interagency approach for the management of MIS development and diffusion, recommending that the National Library of Medicine (NLM) take the role of lead agency to orchestrate these activities. However, Lindberg [207] noted that there was a limit to the role of NIH in the support of the development and diffusion of MISs, in that the NIH support always terminated once the scientific success of the project had been declared; and this was not usually consistent with the time frame needed to bring a MIS to the stage of even a prototype commercial system, and to provide for the transition of the system to a

self-sustaining basis. Lindberg [206] again wrote on the barriers to the development
and diffusion of MIS technology; and provided a comprehensive review of the then
existing literature. He proposed four grades of complexity of MIS technology: simple functions like accounting; more complex tasks such as automated electrocardiogram analyses; highly complex functions like computer-based patient records; and
new models of an existing function such as the computer-based medical record.

Lindberg asserted that barriers to diffusion of MISs were sociological and behavioral as well as technological; and that two kinds of technical barriers had been
encountered: those typical of any newly evolving technology enterprise, and those
more specific to the medical environment. With respect to the latter, he was critical
of medicine having an administrative pattern of "balkanization," with social barriers
that slowed its adaptability by the health professions. Lindberg [206] further asserted
that nothing about the computer techniques used in MISs made these systems fundamentally different from the computer systems used in nonmedical fields; but there
were two special nontechnical barriers inherent in the medical application; and
these were limitations in the state of medical knowledge about illness and health,
and limitations in the state of medical systems management.

Whereas in the 1960s MIS development was limited by computer power and
storage capacity, by the late 1970s it was evident that further MIS utility would
depend on developing software that more fully satisfied physician needs. By the end
of the 1970s, Levy et al. [198, 199] and Lindberg [206] concluded that although the
advent of microprocessors had greatly advanced the hardware support for MISs,
especially for OISs in ambulatory care, that further growth for HISs would depend
more heavily on software development. Blum [40] agreed that the 1970s had introduced computers with very large-scale integration (VLSI) which had produced
computers of great reliability, small size, and low cost; and had produced applications that were previously impractical but had now become cost-effective. However,
during this phase it became clear that the most expensive component in a MIS had
become the cost of software development. Blum considered 1975 to be a watershed
year since computer technology was finally able to support the information processing requirements of the medical community.

Ball [16] reported on a survey conducted in 1980 of what was called Class-B
MISs that integrated interdepartmental and specialty services in hospitals. Ball further divided the Class-B group into Level 1 systems that provided primarily administrative functions with some reporting features for laboratory or pharmacy and
Level 2 systems, which provided a patient care record and clinical and nursing services functions. She found that in 1980 at least 18 vendors in the U.S. were marketing and selling Level 1 systems, and approximately 500 Level 1 systems had been
installed in U.S. hospitals since 1974. Five of 18 vendors marketing Level 1 systems
were also marketing a Level 2 system. Ball [15] listed some other barriers: vendors'
tendency to oversell; unrealistic expectations of recipients: perceived threats to traditional procedures; insufficient medical profession involvement: a desire to
improve old systems rather than to shift to new approaches; and fear of the unknown.

Van Brunt [320] reflected why, in the 1970s, so few operating medical service
applications had been fully integrated into the patient care process. He considered

the development of computer-based clinical medical applications to be an evolutionary process because of the nature of the medical record and the uses of medical information; the problems of data collection, with the sources of medical data being large in number and the validity of the data uncomfortably variable; and the important problem of inaccurate or unrealistic expectation of what could be achieved over short periods of time. He urged providers of care to become more involved in the processes of planning, developing, and implementing clinical information systems.

Hanmer [142] suggested that the diffusion of medical computing technology could be represented by an S-shaped curve with four stages of growth: (1) Introduction, when only a few pioneers used the innovation; (2) Trial, when a bandwagon effect created a broad-based demand; (3) Consolidation, when growth resulted in system problems and cost concerns; and (4) Maturity, when a balance developed with acceptable efficiency for the user and the system.

Hanmer concluded that technologies that had diffused rapidly and were in stages 3 or 4, were those used in well-defined medical informatics specialties such as in radiology, clinical laboratory, and cardiology. Since physicians tend to practice in single medical specialties, Hammer thought that it was not surprising to see that specialty-specific technologies most readily fitted the existing communications patterns [125].

Lindberg [206] also believed that the success of the specialized computing systems for radiology, laboratory, and cardiology occurred because they required fewer conceptual changes and offered more immediate benefits. He wrote that the MIS innovations expected to have the slowest rate of diffusion and acceptance would be those that had to substitute a new conceptual model of the complex activity in question and simultaneously attempt to automate that activity. Lindberg [213] added that benefits from MIS usage that pertained to the long-term benefits for the patients, the institutions, and for the profession were difficult to appreciate for the individual physicians who came in contact with the MIS.

Hodgdon [157] gave his reasons for resistance to implementing MISs were that in the pre-implementation period, change was opposed because of satisfaction with the status quo, a basic mistrust of computer systems or a fear of the new or unknown, a threat to vested interests or job security or status, or a perception of the system as being inadequate or being implemented too fast. After installation resistance to the system existed because there were unrealized positive expectations, the system performance appeared to be inferior to the old system, the system was confusing or disruptive, some strained social interpersonal relationships had developed, or the system served as a scapegoat for unrelated problems.

By the early 1980s more reports appeared suggesting that obtaining user acceptance of an MIS, especially by physicians, was becoming more important than further improving the technology. Brown and associates [16] proposed four guidelines for improving the acceptance of an MIS: (1) user involvement, since systems were created to serve people, rather than vice versa; (2) system design and implementation that adequately represented nontechnical interests in the technical aspects of system design; (3) management that recognized that systems could not be imposed on an environment but must be imbedded in it, and that users must be made to feel that a system was theirs; (4) educational programs that aimed at user acceptance and user competence.

Shortliffe [304] also emphasized the importance of the education of physicians in medical computing to ensure better future acceptance of MISs by physicians. An interesting incentive for the physicians' use of a MIS was offered by Watson [312] from the Boston Center for Law and Health Sciences: that courts might impose liability on providers for patient injuries caused by the absence of medical computers even where the custom of most other providers would not have required computer use.

Naisbitt [254] described three stages of technological development that readily applied to the development of MISs. In the first stage, the new technology or innovation followed the line of least resistance; that is, it was applied in ways that did not threaten people, thereby reducing the chance that it would be rejected. Thus, in medicine, computers were first used for business and accounting functions. In the second stage, the technology was used to improve or replace previous technologies. For example, microcomputer-based word processors replaced typewriters. In the third stage, new directions or uses were discovered that grew out of the technology itself. In radiology, computer-based imaging devices created inventions not previously imagined. Naisbitt suggested that computer technology was to the information age what mechanization was to the industrial revolution; that it was a threat because it incorporated functions previously performed by workers; and when new technology was introduced to society, there needed to be a counterbalancing human response or the technology would be rejected; and the more high technology was present, the more the need for human touch.

Kwon [189] reported in 1983 that almost 90 % of the nation's 5,987 short-term, acute-care general hospitals were using computers, with about 80 % of the computer use was said to be for administrative purposes. Further, only about 10 % of the hospitals used more than 50 % of their computer capacity in the clinical area. Ball [17] analyzed a questionnaire given to 900 private-practitioner physicians enrolled in a postgraduate course of continuing medical education and reported that half responded that they saw no immediate use for a computer in their hospital or private practice. Of those who did respond that they used a computer, about one-half of the applications were for accounting and billing and about one-fourth were for scheduling, planning, and statistical functions. Less than 10 % used the computer for patient records and patient care functions.

Glaser and associates [127] presented a model of the relationships of a MIS and a health care organization that proposed that a MIS affected not only its users but also the organization as a whole and that some of these effects might be entirely unintended. A MIS could produce personnel changes, centralize decision-making, and affect the social structure of the health care organization. They stated that the MIS should fit the users' information, psychological, social, and task needs. If the technical system ignored the organization's social system, the MIS might not fit with other systems and, even if accepted, might lead to a less effective organization.

Grams [136] reported that U.S. hospitals spent $4.1 billion, or about one-percent of their operating budgets, for data processing. More than 30,000 physicians were then using personal computers for their practices. Linton [215] categorized physician users in three types: type 1 was the adventurer who enthusiastically embraced the computer and who developed new ways to use the computer; type 2 was the pragmatist who comprised the largest user category and had little interest in the computer except as a tool to achieve an objective; and type 3 was the recalcitrant – dissenter, gainsayer, or conservative, a steadfast non-user of computers. With reference to user psychology and temperament, Linton forecasted that in all probability, no matter how great the technological successes, there were frontiers that would never be crossed by present lines of computer technology.

Fineberg [96] proposed ten factors that influenced the adoption or abandonment of a medical technology, all of which applied to some degree to a MIS:

- The prevailing theory and accepted explanations for empirical phenomena appeared to have a strong influence on the acceptance of new ideas and might delay the acceptance of ultimately proved innovations.
- Attributes of the innovation enhanced diffusion to the extent that they were easy to use, required little effort to learn, imposed little change in practice style, were highly remunerative and satisfying, and had no clinically worthy competitors.
- An innovation that solved an important clinical problem and was seen as highly pertinent to practice was likely to be adopted more readily than an otherwise equally attractive innovation that addressed a less pressing or pertinent situation.
- The presence of an advocate who promoted the innovation often contributed to the successful diffusion of new practices.
- Many studies of diffusion sought to explain adoption in terms of physician attributes, such as their technical skills, demographic characteristics, professional characteristics, socio-metric status, and attitudes toward innovation.
- The practice setting was a factor, since physicians in group practices appeared to adopt innovations more rapidly than physicians in solo practice. The size and teaching status of hospitals appeared to influence hospital acquisition of equipment.
- The decision-making process that involved more people was likely to require a longer time to come to a conclusion.
- Environmental constraints and incentives, such as regulatory agencies and medical care insurers, exercised direct and indirect control over the diffusion of many medical practices.
- Conduct and methods of evaluation could act directly on the perception of physicians. It could influence experts who in turn influenced physicians, or it could influence the policy decisions of regulatory bodies or of third-party payers and hence alter the environment in which medical practice decisions were made.
- Channels of communication could influence the rate of diffusion. Studies of how doctors learned about new medical practices, based on physician surveys, found

that medical journals, discussion with colleagues, and continuing education were each regarded as important sources, with journals most consistently cited as high in importance.

Kling [185] published an extensive analysis of the social aspects of computing and wrote that, although computers were commonly viewed as a tool, they should more accurately be looked on as a package that included social, in addition to technical, elements. He noted that computer-based systems could increase the influence of those who had access to the technology and can organize data to their advantage and understand computer use. Markus [222] expanded on Kling's publication and presented three reasons for resistance to using MISs: (1) Some people resisted MISs because it was their human nature to resist all change; (2) Poor system design resulted in technical problems and thus tended to cause resistance to acceptance; and (3) Interactions between MIS and the organization, such as when the MIS tended to alter the balance of power by increased centralized control, and this also increased resistance to user acceptance.

During the 1980s Anderson and Jay [4, 7] at Purdue University and Methodist Hospital of Indiana conducted extensive studies on the effects of physician attitudes on the acceptance and diffusion of medical computing applications. They observed that the adoption of much of the emerging medical technology was highly influenced by the relationships that physicians form with their mentors and later with their peers. Rather than the flow of communication and influence being a simple process of going from opinion leaders to followers, they concluded that the diffusion process involved a network of interconnected individuals who were linked by patterned flows of information. Diffusion involved a mutual process of information sharing and influence over time that resulted in relative homogeneity among subgroups that were socially integrated. From their study of a large hospital staff with a MIS, they found that physicians significantly influenced one another's decisions, and the physician's location in the professional network affected other physicians' perceptions and practice behavior. Physicians in the central location of the professional network were relied on by their colleagues to provide them with information on new developments. They concluded that the physician's position in the consultation network significantly influenced the rates of adoption and diffusion of new computer technology [3, 4, 9]. Subsequently, they reported that once physicians formed initial attitudes and practice patterns involving computer-based clinical information systems, their attitudes were likely to persist. Their studies indicated that physicians' attitudes toward the use of computers for patient care, and the frequency with which the physicians used a MIS in practice were highly stable over a 3-year period [3, 6]. Anderson and associates [5] also demonstrated that influential physicians could be identified and deliberately used to increase the use of personal order sets to enter orders into a MIS. Anderson's group confirmed by many studies that the successful implementation of clinical computer-based systems depended heavily upon physicians' valuation of these systems.

Logan [217] also studied physicians' attitudes toward MISs and concluded that MISs would not be useful to many practitioners until the intuitive part of medical reasoning could be converted to knowledge-based rules within the design of MISs. He contended that all MIS developers believed firmly that the long-term advantages of computer-assisted diagnoses and of the automation of patient records outweighed the short-term disruptions that came with their adoption. Logan alleged that the perceived threats to professional autonomy from standardization of medical terminology as federal interference, was an important consideration for innovators in determining the acceptability of MISs. Friedman [103] considered the control of the development of a MIS by physician users to be so important that he advised a large hospital that implemented a MIS to establish a physician as its Medical Information Director. Greer [138] at the University of Wisconsin studied the diffusion of new medical technologies used primarily for specialized procedures such as in intensive neonatology care, and found that for such technologies their initial diffusion was problematic and controversial, as these were closely associated with their early developers whose skills and teaching were important to their reception and diffusion.

Kaplan [175] observed that it was important to understand and be sensitive to the symbolic potency of the computer, since it had implications for MIS acceptance. She believed that differences of perception of a MIS indicated more about differences in the perceiver than they did about inherent characteristics of the computer; thus the computer functioned as a sort of Rorschach test. Kaplan [176] completed a comprehensive dissertation on her studies of the generally prevailing concept that there had been a lag in the diffusion of computers in medicine, as compared to the adoption of computers in industry and agriculture. Like others, she found that for administrative, business, and accounting applications, and for clinical laboratories and imaging services, there had not been a lag but rather a rapid acceptance and diffusion. It was with special reference to the adoption of the more complex, physician-directed applications that she wrote later on the barriers she perceived to the application of computers to medicine when she referred to the so-called lag in the applications of computers in medicine. Before the mid-1960s computer use was thought to lag with respect to its potential for research. From the mid-1960s to the early 1970s it was seen to lag with respect to its potential in patient care. Since the early 1970s computers were considered lagging with respect to their use in rationalizing the health care system. Kaplan [174] summarized what she perceived as the barriers to medical computing and grouped them into four general areas: (1) barriers of insufficiency, including lack of funding, technology, staffing, training, and effort; (2) barriers of poor management, including difficulties of interdisciplinary teams, planning, and approach, and lack of attention to human factors and methodologies; (3) barriers inherent in medicine, including insufficient medical knowledge, and the difficulty of translating medical knowledge into a form suitable for computing and institutional constraints; and (4) physician resistance.

Kaplan concluded that the most significant attribute of the majority of these barriers to MISs was that they were extrinsic to medical computing. This certainly was true with regard to the financing of MIS applications. For example, computer-based patient records for procedures not reimbursable by third-party payers of health insurance were more difficult to finance, in contrast to computer tomography (CT) scans which were reimbursable procedures, and the payment for CT scans by insurers supported their rapid diffusion. Similarly, the diffusion of automated clinical laboratory analyzers that processed groups of tests was rapid as a result of their reimbursement of costs by insurers. On the other hand, a programmed battery of automated multiphasic procedures for health testing was not reimbursed by insurers in the United States that led to its demise, in contrast to the rapid diffusion of automated multiphasic health testing in Japan where it was an insured, reimbursable health care benefit.

In the 1980s some persistent intrinsic medical problems did continue, for example, the continuing lack of support for MISs by health care professionals and the lack of standardization of medical practice and medical information [74]. At the end of the 1980s there were few MISs operational in the United States that provided the basic required patient care functions described in Sect. 3.1. In 1988 Childs [57] listed 40 vendors that in the first four decades of developing MISs, had entered and then left the business. In 1988, the fifth edition of the Computers in Healthcare Market Directory listed 750 vendors of computer systems and supplies available to the health-care industry. In 1989, a vendors' survey reported 30 vendors for HISs and applications, 105 vendors for office management and ambulatory systems, and 15 vendors for medical record systems [158]. Childs [56] reported that systems vendors had done well with the development of some departmental subsystems; however, few vendors had put their departmental systems together into a fully operational integrated MIS; and advised that MIS components should all be connected on-line and operated in real-time so the user perceived a total integrated MIS.

Although federal agencies had as yet done little to coordinate the early development of MIS technology, the National Library of Medicine (NLM) in the 1980s established its Unified Medical Language System (UMLS) and its Integrated Academic Information Management Systems (IAIMS) programs. At the end of 1989, the Institute of Medicine (IOM) established a Committee to Improve the Patient Record, recognizing that the patient computer-based record was the core of a successful MIS. This committee was to examine the problems with existing patients' medical record systems and to propose actions and research for these systems' improvement and diffusion in light of new technologies [53]. The IOM published its recommendations in 1991 [87]. In the 2010s the Federal government initiated its support of computer-based patient records in physician offices and outpatient clinics for ambulatory patients. Commercial organizations like EPIC, McKesson and Cerner began to implement large MISs. By 2012 OISs, HISs, MISs, and MHISs were becoming commonplace in the United States (see Chaps. 4, 5, and 6).

3.2   Functional and Technical Requirements of a MIS

Every medical care organization had structural and functional requirements for each organizational level, and the MIS for the total patient care system comprised the aggregate structures and functions of all of its subsystems. As a result, the higher the level of organization, the more complex became its total information system due to the larger range of structural and functional variations, with an increasing number of possible connections among information subsystems. That, in turn, permitted the evolution of higher and more varied forms of MIS structure and function. Thus, the development of an information system for a hospital was more complicated than that for a physician's office or even that for a group of physicians within a clinic. Similarly, a multi-facility information system for a large medical care organization that consisted of multiple hospitals and clinics was more complex than an information system for a single hospital, especially with regard to its information communications requirements. It soon became evident that it was necessary to plan carefully for both the function (that is, what the information system was to do) and the structure (that is, how the system was to be technically designed and built) to ensure that all information subsystem modules worked together properly.

Through these decades the goals and objectives evolved for a MIS; and these generally included the use of computers and communications equipment to collect, store, process, retrieve, and communicate relevant clinical and administrative information for all patient care activities and clinical functions within the hospital, its outpatient clinics, its clinical support services, and any affiliated medical facilities. In addition to providing administrative and clinical decision support, a MIS needed to have the capabilities for communicating and integrating all patient data collected during each patient's lifetime of care from all the information subsystems in a medical care program. Such a MIS also was expected to improve the quality and decrease the cost of medical services. It was also expected to be flexible enough to scale for increasing numbers of patients and for expansion of its system components. The overall goal of every MIS is generally stated to be the improvement of patient care. To accomplish this goal, MIS users first had to develop detailed requirements for its functionality. That is, the future users of the MIS had to first define exactly what they wanted the MIS to do for the users to be able to improve patient care. They then gave these functional requirements to computer technologists, thus permitting these technical experts to develop a set of design specifications for the MIS and for the computer hardware, software, and communications that would satisfy the users' functional requirements. Then the MIS could be purchased or developed and installed in the medical facility.

Lindberg [214] described the degrees of difficulty for the development of MISs in the grades of their complexity. The easiest was the automation of a simple function such as providing a patient's billing for services. The more difficult was the automation of a more complex function such as collecting and storing a patient's medical history. The very difficult was constructing a very complex function such as a medical database, and the most difficult was developing the highly complex medical information and database-management system for a hospital. Starr [312] had aptly ranked the hospital to be the most complex organizational structure created by man. Ball [16] also recognized the complexity of MISs and classified them according to their functionality:

- Class A MISs were individual stand-alone medical systems that addressed the specific requirements of single departments or clinical specialties, such as laboratory systems or family practice systems.

- Class B MISs included those that crossed inter-departmental and specialty boundaries by a network that transmitted orders between patients' services and clinical departments.
  - Class B, Level 1 systems were those primarily oriented to administrative functions.
  - Class B, Level 2 systems were administratively based, but also provided some clinical and nursing services.
- Class C MISs used the patients' records as their database, and fully integrated and supported clinical, nursing, and ancillary systems.

Functional requirements for a MIS, as early as the 1950s were recognized to be very different from those of information systems for other industries. Ledley and Lusted [195] defined the functional requirements for any information service to be: (1) keeping the information current had to be fast and easily accomplished; (2) easily locating past and current information on any included topic; (3) looking up the desired information had to be fast, be mechanically simple, easy to use, and require no special skill; and (4) making the desired information readily available to the user.

Blum [38] wrote that the requirements of a MIS could be described as a set of interactions between processes and data. He designed a data model with its components and the relationships between the components; namely, the patients to be treated, the associated clinical data, medical orders, and the treatment sequences. Lindberg [214] noted that a MIS had many dimensions and that its functional requirements depended on:

- the type of population served (such as adults or children);
- the type of institutional setting (such as an office, clinic, hospital, or medical center), general or specialized services);
- medical service area (such as outpatient ambulatory care, hospital inpatient care, clinical laboratory, intensive care);
- data elements collected (patient identification, diagnoses, past hospitalizations);
- functions performed (such as patient record retrieval, direct patient monitoring);
- system users (patient's physician or nurse, medical consultant, hospital administrator);
- method of financing (such as fee for service or by reimbursement of payments for health insurance claims.

Flagle [98] also offered as general requirements for a MIS completeness of all required data elements; timeliness of operations to permit appropriate responses; reliability of processing information without error; economy in information handling; and operability and retrievability in useful form. Lindberg [204] further offered these basic functional requirements for a MIS: careful medical measurements over the life of an individual should be made, recorded, and monitored; the lifelong patient's medical record should be complete and in machine-readable format if it is to be useful; and the general accessibility to relevant medical knowledge should be extended through linkages to literature citations and information retrieval systems.

A medical information system (MIS), whether processing data from hospital inpatients or from office outpatients has to be able to identify and register each patient, record the date and time of the patient visit or of the care transaction; collect, store, process, and integrate the data in a patient record that will be usable by health care professionals; support the decision-making processes involved in patient care; communicate and provide capabilities for data linkages to other medical sites when necessary for the transfer of any patient care data.

Every MIS had to support clinical service functions for patients on a continuous 24-h basis and to capture at source and to store in each patient's record the following categories of data:

- the essential information for the patient's identification data (ID), medical history and physical examination findings
- physicians' progress notes, diagnoses, and orders
- physicians' consultations
- pathology and surgery reports
- nurses notes; clinical laboratory test results
- x-ray and electrocardiogram reports
- drugs administered either in the hospital and dispensed in the outpatient pharmacies
- records of any other ancillary services such as dietary and physiotherapy [73, 169].

Functional requirements of MISs varied to some extent in different practitioners' offices and in different hospitals, in accordance with the logistics of data collection as well as in the scope, volume, and rate of the data captured. When seen in a physician's office, patients were mostly ambulatory and were usually well enough to use self-administered questionnaires to enter a part of their own medical past histories in their record. These ambulatory patients then usually went to clinical laboratories and/or radiology services. Their reports for these services were sent to their physicians to be filed in the patient's record. Hospitals had sicker patients who were mostly confined to their beds; so their laboratory specimens usually were collected at their bedside. Their paper-based hospital charts were kept at the hospital nursing stations. Sicker inpatients required larger volumes of data to be processed faster, so their more severe functional requirements required more powerful, faster computers with greater data storage capacity.

Whereas physicians and nurses needed information on their individual patients, administrators of clinics and hospitals needed information on the operation of the medical facility as a whole. Therefore, every MIS had to support such basic administrative functions as scheduling patients' appointments, processing and storing patients' records; supporting procedures for monitoring and ensuring the quality of patient care; and information on utilization of services for management decision making. Among the first computer applications usually installed in either a hospital or a medical office are its business functions, such as maintaining financial accounts, billing its patients or health insurance agencies, processing payrolls, maintaining employee records, keeping inventories, ordering and paying for supplies and services; and sometimes needing to access a patient's record to obtain demographic data. Blum [36] noted that a MIS also supported administrative functions by modifying the workflow through reduced redundancy of information processing, by reassigning clerical tasks that had normally been performed by health care professionals, and by improving the timeliness of transmitted information once it had been recorded. These changes in workflow resulted in more rapid access to information, reduced the number of errors since the system could be programmed to reject unreasonable inputs and to query questionable entries, and provided access to new functions, such as resource utilization, that could not be monitored as easily in a manual setting.

In 2010 the functional requirements of a computer-based, electronic patient record (EPR) within a MIS had to be designed to satisfy the needs of all its primary and secondary users. The EPR was usually the most complex requirement of any component of a MIS. For any clinical research purposes, users of the secondary data sets needed to have access to subsets of patient data located in the primary patient records and be subject to satisfying all of the regulations for maintaining privacy and confidentiality of the patient data.

Blum [36, 39] advised that the definition process for the functional requirements of a MIS was concluded when there was a full and detailed statement that fully satisfied all of the MIS objectives. The completion of the definition of the functional requirements usually resulted in a decision to build the MIS either "in-house" or, more commonly, to issue a request for proposals from commercial vendors to build it. To satisfy the functional requirements of a MIS, the computer technologists had to select hardware, software, and communication devices to fit the design for the organization of the database to be able to contain all the data for all the users of the MIS. Then they had to design and develop an electronic patient record (EPR) and a database management system that could collect all the patient data from all various physical sites; generate integrated patient records in various formats as desired by their professional users; provide readily retrievable data at various sites; have the capability of providing the information as needed to support decision-making processes at the various care sites; and be able to provide communication linkages to external databases as needed. Finally, the MIS had to be able to service all the needed applications and subsystem components, and be capable of adding enhancements when needed.

Technical requirements of a MIS needed to be developed to satisfy all of the complex functional requirements of a MIS. Computer scientists and engineers had to select the appropriate hardware, software and computer applications. They needed to fit the design for the organization of the database, the computer-stored patient record, to contain all the data for all the users. They had to develop a database management system that could collect all the patient data from various physical sites; generate integrated patient records in various formats as desired by professional users; be readily retrievable at various sites; have the capability of providing the information as needed to support decision making processes; and provide communication linkages to external databases as needed. They had to develop a MIS that could:

- Have adequate computer power for processing and storing large volumes of patient data, for identifying and linking individual patient's data and integrating the data into individual electronic patient records
- Process and retrieve the large amounts of natural language narrative text in the medical records
- Transmit data among a variety of different MIS subsystems
- Provide terminals for communicating with the system that were acceptable to demanding health professionals
- Protect both the data and the system from unauthorized access
- Be flexible in design so that it could change frequently to meet requirements for new types of data from technology innovations and changing legislative mandates.

According to Greenes [137], the technical requirements of a MIS included being able to: process text as well as numeric data; permit highly interactive, non-computational use, often by relatively unskilled users; contain complex databases that demand multilevel tree or tabular representation of relations; provide multi-user access to shared databases; provide support for specialized input devices, such as devices for rapid data acquisition in an intensive care unit, devices that collect images for radiology, light pens, mouse pointers, and graphics tablets; have flexible output capabilities, such as displays, printers, and plotters; and perform symbolic reasoning and handle artificial-intelligence applications.

By the mid-1960s solid-state integrated circuits in third-generation computers had begun to satisfy some of the requirements for MISs, and some early users, such as Spencer and Valbonna [311] optimistically concluded that with the available technology and with the proper functional requirements some components of a MIS could be developed, as was demonstrated in their technical design. However, it soon became evident that a medical information system (MIS) was an extremely complex integration of multiple subsystems that could include a hospital information system (HIS) and an outpatient information system (OIS), and an electronic patient record system (EPR). The HIS and the OIS could contain a separate or combined administration information system (AIS), a clinical information system (CIS) and several clinical support systems (CSSs); and might even include a clinical decision support system (CDSS). The administration information system (AIS) could include its own subsystems since almost every clinical action initiated a transaction for the administrative, business and accounting functions; and in addition an AIS was responsible for patient registration, scheduling, admission and discharge; and for other patient-processing activities. The term clinical information system (CIS) was used for the component of a MIS that was related to the direct care of patients. A CIS could have many modules (subsystem components) called clinical departmental systems or clinical specialty system; and these usually included the patient care services for general medicine and its clinical subspecialty systems for cardiology, pulmonology, nephrology, and others; for general surgery, orthopedics, urology, and others; for obstetrics and gynecology, for pediatrics, psychiatry, and others; for an intensive care unit (ICU), an emergency department (ED), and others. Clinical support systems (CSSs) included the clinical laboratory (LAB), pathology (PATH), radiology (RAD) and other imaging specialties; electrocardiography (ECG), pharmacy (PHARM), and other support systems; and all of these provided the essential patient care services to patients in the offices, clinics, and hospitals. The clinical support systems (CSSs) were relatively independent functionally, but were essential to the MIS, In addition, affiliated care facilities might include rehabilitation or nursing care services [39]. The computer-based electronic patient record (EPR), the basic information repository for every component of a MIS, has its own functional and technical requirements. Another critical requirement for a MIS is a communications network since it is the principal means for initiating, transferring, and completing much patient care information.

Blois [33] wrote that consideration of the elements underlying the design of information systems for physicians' use also had to take into account the nature and structure of physicians' personal medical knowledge and the ways in which they draw upon this in the course of practice, the structure and availability of the sources which they can draw upon for information, and the technological capabilities (the "state of the art") of information support tools. The computer-stored electronic patient record (EPR) needed to be considered as an essential and most complex component of a medical information system (MIS). Blum [36, 37] advised that based on his experience, the distribution of effort in the development of a MIS was generally 40 % of the effort was for analysis and design, 20 % for implementation, and then 40 % was for validation and correction of errors and deficiencies of the MIS.

3.3 Approaches to Developing MISs

Several approaches evolved for the design of a MIS to satisfy its functional requirements [251]. The total systems approach was developed in the 1960s and employed a single integrated computer-stored database with all patient data from all MIS modules electronically stored in one integrated computer database. Some duplicate patient data sets and most internal departmental processing data, such as those generated within the clinical laboratory, usually were still retained for a limited time in the distributed databases of various MIS sub-system modules. As the volume and the variety of data in computer-based patient records increased, it became increasingly difficult to find and retrieve specific items or sets of data stored in one large central database. The modular systems approach for developing a MIS evolved in the 1970s with the arrival of low-cost minicomputers that were followed by even lower-cost microcomputers in the 1980s. Patients' records began to be processed and stored in these relatively cheap computers with their direct random-access disks, resulting in various distributed databases that required using a distributed database management system [163]. This change produced the need to collate functionally all of each patient's data into a single electronic medical record readily usable by clinicians, either through interfaced or integrated systems. Interfaced computers managed their own files, and copies of their data were exchanged or transmitted between systems. Integrated subsystems shared a common, central medical database [81]. The utility concept was introduced by Kastner and Pratt [178]. It was compatible with either the total or the modular approaches and was conceived as a hierarchically organized hardware-software configuration comprised of small, medium, and large capacity computers. The aggregate of computers permitted the MIS to serve as a computer utility that used the various capacities for the different data-handling tasks that were required by the users and was an updated variation of the former time-sharing systems.

In comparing the total and the modular approaches, Lindberg [206] wrote that some believed that all elements of a MIS needed to be designed initially, and some believed that the total system must inevitably result from an aggregation of functioning subsystems. Lindberg called the former approach holistic in which the computers and procedures were applied to a total system design. He called the latter approach cumulative where the ultimate system was the aggregate of all subsystem modules. Greenes [137] compared the total and the modular approaches, and he favored the modular systems approach as better accommodating a diversity of applications. It was more flexible to change, had more effective data control through only local access, had higher reliability because a local computer failure did not bring down the whole system, and was most responsive to local user needs. However, he believed that the total systems approach better incorporated mainstream computing provided by the software that was available in 1983, and that it provided better database integration. Van Brunt [321] offered that the primary difference was that the total systems approach required that all data for each individual patient be maintained in a single, continuously updatable, chronologically ordered data set. The advantages of this approach were that it lent itself to improved data quality control, more efficient computer system utilization, more efficient inter-subsystem data communication, and better control of confidentiality of patient data. In practice, with either a total or modular approach, the various subsystem modules had to be brought into the system in some desired sequence. Only a few organizations followed a total systems approach to developing a medical information system with physically integrated patient records. In practice, with either a total or modular approach, the various subsystem modules had to be brought into the system in some desired sequence.

Since the total systems approach required a long-term strategic plan for the entire MIS, this plan usually included the early installation of a separate computer-stored medical record module that provided an integrated medical database, to which all the other modules and subsystems were connected as they were added. An example of this approach was the system at Kaiser Permanente in the 1960s. Only a few organizations followed a total systems approach to developing a medical information system with physically integrated patient records. In practice, with either a total or modular approach, the various subsystem modules had to be brought into the system in some desired sequence.

In the 1970s MISs usually acquired one application or module at a time as it became available; and initially each module had its own database. As a result, when the patient administration (PAD) module was available, then the patient's identification data resided in the PAD computer's database. When the clinical laboratory (LAB) module was installed, then the laboratory test results were stored in the LAB computer's database, along with sufficient PAD data to identify the patient. When the pharmacy system (PHARM) module was installed, all the prescription data were stored in the PHARM computer's database, along with sufficient PAD data to identify the patient. Similarly, when the other modules (order entry, results reporting, radiology, and so forth) were added, the locally collected patient data usually resided in the separate databases that were created for each module. If the central computer was large enough, it might contain some of these subsystem databases. In these early MISs with several separate modules, the physicians and nurses usually had to enter their requests for the patient's laboratory data in a terminal connected to the LAB computer system. Then, a separate request for the patient's medications would be entered into the terminal connected to the PHARM computer system. Similarly, separate terminals would need to be used for any remaining modules. Thus, the nurses had to use a cluster of several separate terminals, each requiring that they enter the same patient identification data to obtain the desired data for one patient from the various separate databases. The installation of a separate integrating medical record database was usually not considered until several clinical information modules were already operational.

The majority of MIS developers in the 1970s undertook a modular approach, because, as advocated by Barnett [24], it had the advantages of technical feasibility, easier achieving of organizational agreement, lower start-up costs, greater reliability, more rapid achievement of a useful system, greater flexibility for change and expansion, and greater potential for transferability. However, Barnett [24] cautioned that three areas of possible weakness in the modular approach were an inefficient use of computer hardware, fragmentation of management, and increased difficulty in creating an integrated patient medical record – but that was achievable in any system since the integration of medical data did not require that all the data, whatever the source, reside on the same physical storage device or even in the same computer. Barnett advised that the critical requirement for an integrated medical record system was the ease and timeliness with which the user could access any or all parts of the information, independent of the type of information and independent of the source of collection, but the provision of such access required a powerful database management system. He stated that a plan to employ separate computer modules might make it difficult either for any single module to assume an increasing number of functions or for different modules to exchange data. To prevent this problem, Barnett [24, 26] also advised that those who managed a modular system needed to give particular attention to the selection of computer hardware and software in order to assure that the programming language would be powerful enough to permit the development of modules of different types of functions within the same software system and that the file structure would allow the form of the data storage to be virtually independent of the source of the data.

Thus in those early decades, most MISs installed separate subsystem modules as they were developed either in-house or purchased from vendors; and the usual result was a distributed database system with each module having its own database. Accordingly, there evolved the need to design such distributed database systems in which each module could have its own separate database, with the databases for all modules being connected by a communications network so that a user in one module could access any data in any other database in the entire network, as though the data were all stored in the user's module. Thereby the system could provide a functionally (virtual or logically) integrated database that constituted the patient's electronic record; yet it was not necessarily apparent to the user where the data were collected or processed. However, every time the same sets of data were requested by the health care professionals there still remained the problem of transferring, retrieving, and collating all the data for each patient from all the subsystem databases in a distributed system.

An early example of a software solution to the data integration problem in a modular MIS was the development of the Massachusetts General Hospital Utility Multi-Programming System (MUMPS) by Barnett's group. In 1965 Barnett and associates reported on the development of a time-sharing, remote-access computer system with terminals and communications for the use of hospital personnel, providing access to a computer-based medical record [21, 22]. Barnett described the integrated MGH system in 1974 as having four functionally equivalent computer systems on which the various modules were implemented [23]. Since all of these systems operated under MUMPS, it was not apparent to the user of any application programs which particular subsystem was being used [24]. Three of these subsystems used Digital Equipment Corporation (DEC) PDP-9 machines, and the fourth used a newer PDP-15. Since Barnett used compatible hardware and software throughout his MIS, he avoided the problem of interfacing any incompatible subsystems.

Hammond [140], Stead, and their associates at Duke University developed a generalized, online, DEC PDP minicomputer-supported information system with a different software approach. They called their operating system GEMISCH. GEMISCH was composed of programs which perform specific tasks as defined by the tables. User programming consisted of the creation of appropriate tables entered through an interactive editing and file-handling system. The user-oriented source files were converted into machine-oriented operating files, and these operating files were combined with the system programs to form a GEMISCH operating system. Another example of the cumulative modular approach in an organization that installed information subsystems, one at a time; and then connected them together with a communications network that integrated patient databases to provide a usable patient record, was in the MIS developed at the Johns Hopkins Hospital.

It soon became evident that if MISs were to be used efficiently and were to be acceptable to health care professionals, they needed to include an integrating database management system that could generate an integrated patient record.

Most early MISs had been implemented either by the installation of separate modules that had been developed in-house or by the purchasing of acceptable vendor-provided modules. The usual result was a distributed data processing system, with each module having its own database. There evolved the need to design distributed database systems in which each module could have its own separate database, with the databases for all modules connected by a communications network so that a user in one module could access any data in the entire network exactly as though the data were all stored in the user's module. Thereby the system could provide a functionally (virtual or logically) integrated database output that constituted the patient record, yet it would not necessarily be apparent to the user where the data were collected or processed. Even though most users of such a distributed MIS would be unaware of whether the clinical information system was distributed or integrated, there still remained the problem of transferring, retrieving, and collating all the data for each patient from all the databases in a distributed system every time the same sets of data were requested by the health care professionals. If MISs were to be efficient and acceptable to health care professionals, it soon became evident that distributed databases needed an integrating database management system that could generate an integrated patient database. Such a system required that all patient data be entered into the MIS only once, even though some data might be replicated in different subsystem files (such as was required for the patient identification data) and all data for one patient could be retrieved by a physician in any desired collated format from one terminal in any module of the MIS, even though the data had been collected in several subsystem modules.

To permit the integration of information among all of its subsystems, a MIS also required some degree of standardization of the data terms in its database. Although standardization could decrease information content by discouraging richness of language variations, it clearly facilitated information transfer and communication. Individual departments within a hospital often had unique internal information processing requirements (such as for the processing of tests and procedures in the different laboratories), and these had to be accommodated. A standard data dictionary, a meta-database, also became necessary to define data elements entered in the common database with validation rules for accepting new terms as they were continually added by innovations in medicine.

3.4 Natural Language Processing (NLP)

In the 1950s the clinical data in the medical records of patients in the United States were mostly recorded in natural, English language. This process was commonly done by physicians when recording their notes on paper sheets clipped in the patient's chart. Data recording was for the patient's medical history and physical examination, for reporting specialists' interpretations of x-ray images and electrocardiograms, and for the dictated descriptions of special medical and surgical procedures. Such patients' data were generally recorded by healthcare professionals as hand-written notes or as dictated reports that were then transcribed and typed on paper sheets. These sheets were then collated in paper-based charts. These patients' medical charts were then stored on shelves in the medical record room. The process of manually retrieving data from patients' paper-based medical charts was always cumbersome and time consuming.

In the 1960s when computer-stored medical databases began to be developed, it was soon recognized that a very difficult problem was how to process in the computer in a meaningful way, the large amount of free-form, English-language textual data that was present in almost every patient's medical record; most commonly recorded in patients' histories, in dictated surgery-operative reports, in pathology reports, and in the interpretations of x-rays and electrocardiograms. In some clinical laboratory reports, such as for microbiology, descriptive textual data was often required and had to be keyed into the computer by the technologist using a full-alphabet keyboard or by selecting codes or names for standard phrases from a menu that could be entered using specially designed keyboards or by selecting from a visual displayed menu [218, 308, 334].

So, one of the most frustrating problems for developers of an electronic medical information system (MIS) was how to process in a meaningful way the free-form, English language text in patients' records. What was needed was a natural language processing (NLP) program that could interact with the computer in ordinary English language. Certainly, fluent English language is markedly different from a formal, structured computer language. Computers readily surpassed humans at processing strings of numbers or letters; however, people find it more effective to communicate with each other using strings of words. It soon became evident that the large amount of free text used in patients' records was not present because physicians were unnecessarily verbose, since they usually wrote relatively sparse notes. Rather, adequate documentation of the patient care process created a major problem for a computer-based medical information system because narrative English text required more storage space than did numbers, it was often difficult to interpret and was often difficult to retrieve.

It became evident that the development of natural language processing (NLP) programs was essential, since textual data was generally unstandardized and unstructured, was often difficult to interpret, required special computer programs to search and retrieve, and required more storage space than did digital numbers or letters. To help overcome these problems, English-language words and phrases were often converted into numerical codes, and coding procedures were developed to provide more uniform, standardized agreements for terminology, vocabulary, and meaning. These were followed by the development of computer programs for automated encoding methods and then by special query and retrieval languages for processing textual data. In machine translation of data, the purpose of recognizing the content of an input natural-language string is to accurately reproduce the content in the output language. In information retrieval these tasks involved the categorization and organization of the information content for its use by others in a variety of situations. However, since for the automatic processing of medical textual data the required well-formed syntactical language was rare, syntactic/semantic language programs needed to be developed.

Pratt [273] observed that the data a medical professional recorded and collected during the care of a patient was largely in a non-numeric form and in the United States was formulated almost exclusively in English language. He noted that a word, a phrase, or a sentence in this language was generally understood when spoken or read, and the marks of punctuation and the order of the presentation of words in a sentence represented quasi-formal structures that could be analyzed for content according to common rules for the recognition and validation of the string of language data that was a matter of morphology and syntax. The recognition and the registration of each datum and of its meaning was a matter of semantics, and the mapping of the recognized, defined, syntactical and semantic elements into a data structure reflected the informational content of the original language data string. These processes required definition and interpretation of the information by the user.

Natural language processing began to evolve in the 1980s as a form of human-computer interaction. There are many spoken languages in the world; this book only considers English language text, and uses NLP to represent only natural (English) language processing. NLP was defined by Obermeier [261] at Battelle Laboratories, Columbus, OH, as the ability of a computer to process the same language that humans used in their normal discourse. He considered the central problems for NLP were how to enter and retrieve uncoded natural-language text and how to transform a potentially ambiguous textual phrase into an unambiguous form that could be used internally by the computer database. This transformation involved the process of combining words or symbols into a group that could be replaced by a code or by a more general symbol. Different types of parsers evolved which were based on pattern matching, on syntax (grammar), on semantics (meaning), on knowledge bases, or on combinations of these methods. Hendrix [146] at Stanford Research International (SRI), described the complex nature of NLP as:

- the study of sources of lexical knowledge that is concerned with individual words, the parts of speech to which they belong, and their meanings,
- syntactic knowledge that is concerned with the grouping of words into meaningful phrases,
- semantic knowledge that is concerned with composing the literal meaning of syntactic units from the semantics of their subparts,
- discourse knowledge that is concerned with the way clues from the context being processed are used to interpret a sentence, and
- domain knowledge that is concerned with how medical information constrains possible interpretations.

Clearly NLP had to consider semantics since medical language is relatively unstandardized. It has many ambiguities and ill-defined terms and often has multiple meanings of the same word. Wells [329] offered as an example of semantically equivalent phrases: muscle atrophy, atrophy of muscle, atrophic muscle, and muscular atrophy. In addition NLP had to consider syntax or the relation of words to each other in a sentence, such as when searching for strings of words such as "mitral stenosis and aortic insufficiency", where the importance of the ordering of these words is evident since the string, "mitral insufficiency and aortic stenosis", has a very different meaning. Similarly, the phrase "time flies for house flies" made sense only when one knew that the word "flies" was first a verb and then a noun. Inconsistent spelling and typographic errors also caused problems with word searches made by a computer program that exactly matched letter-by-letter. Pryor [280] also observed that the aggregate of data collected by many different health-care professionals provided the basic information stored in a primary clinical data-base and to accurately reflect their accumulated experience required that all of their observations had to be categorized and recorded in a consistent and standardized manner for all patients' visits. To facilitate the retrieval of desired medical data, Pryor advocated that a clinical database needed to incorporate a coded data-entry format. Johnson [170] also considered structured data-entry and data-retrieval to be basic tools for computer-assisted documentation that would allow a physician to efficiently select and retrieve from a patient's record all data relevant to the patient's clinical problems; and also to be able to retrieve supplementary data from other sources that could be helpful in the clinical-decision process; and to be able to enter into the computer any newly acquired data, and then generate a readable report.

Sager and associates [292–295, 297], at New York University made substantial contributions to natural language processing (NLP) in the late 1970s when they initiated their Linguistic String Project (LSP) that extracted and converted the natural language, free-text narrative from patients' medical records into a structured database. They also addressed the problem of developing a query program for retrieval requests sent to the database. Story [314] described the LSP's early approach to NLP as first recognizing the time-dated information such as dates and times of clinical events found in the text of patients' hospital discharge summaries and then computing from that information the ordering of the times of the recorded medical events. For example, data used in patients' discharge summaries included birth dates, admission and discharge dates, dates and times of any recorded patients' symptoms, signs, and other important clinical events. Sager [292, 295] further described their LSP process for converting the uncoded natural-language text that was found in patients' hospital discharge summaries into a structured relational database. In a relational database, the query process had to search several tables in order to complete the full retrieval. So for a query such as, "Find all patients with a positive chest x-ray", the program executed a query on one table to find the patients' identification numbers and then another query on another table to find those patients reported to have positive chest x-ray reports. Whereas earlier attempts at automating encoding systems for text dealt with phrases that were matched with terms in a dictionary, this group first performed a syntactic analysis of the input data, and then mapped the analyzed sentences into a tabular format arrangement of syntactic segments in which the segments were labeled according to their medical informa-tion content. Using a relational structured database, in their information-format table, the rows corresponded to the successive statements in the documents and the columns in the tables corresponded to the different types of information in the statements. Thus their LSP automatic-language processor parsed each sentence and broke the sentence into syntactic components such as subject-verb-object. They then divided the narrative segments into six statement types: general medical management, treatment, medication, test and result, patient state, and patient behavior; and it then transformed the statements into a structured tabular format. This transformation of the record was suitable for their database-management system, and it simplified the retrieval of a textual record that when queried was transformed back to the users in a narrative form.

Sager [299] described in some detail their later approach to converting unstructured free-text patient data by relationships of medical-fact types or classes (such as body parts, tests, treatments, and others); and by subtypes or sub-classes (such as arm, blood glucose, medications, and others. Their LSP information-formatting program identified and organized the free text by syntactic analysis using standard methods of sentence decomposition and then mapped the free-text into a linguistically structured, knowledge base for querying. The results of tests for information precision and information recall of their LSP system were better than 92 % when compared to manual processing. In 1985 they reported that their medical-English lexicon that gave for each word its English and medical classification which then numbered about 8,000 words [220]. Sager (1986) reported that they had applied their methods of linguistic analysis to a considerable body of clinical narrative that included patients' initial histories, clinic visit reports, radiology and pathology reports, and hospital discharge summaries. They successfully tested their approach for automatic encoding of narrative text in the Head-and-Neck Cancer Database maintained at that time at the Roswell Park Memorial Institute. Sager [299] reported their LSP had been applied to a test set of asthma patients' health-care documents. When subjected to a SQL retrieval program, the retrieval results averaged for major errors only 1.4 %, and averaged 7.5 % for major omissions. Sager [298] further reported using Web processing software to retrieve medical documents from the Web, and by using software based on Standard Generalized Markup Language (SGML) and Hypertext Markup Language (HTML), they coupled text markup with highlighted displays of retrieved medical documents.

McCray [228] at the National Library of Medicine (NLM) described the medical lexicon as the embodiment of information about medical terms and language, and it served as the foundation for natural language processing (NLP). McCray proposed that the domain knowledge combined with lexical information and sophisticated linguistic analysis could lead to improved representation and retrieval of biomedical information and facilitate the development of NLP. McCray et al. [230] studied the nature of strings of words found in the NLM's UMLS Metathesaurus and studied their usefulness in searching articles in the NLM's MEDLINE database. Their studies indicated that the longer the string of words, for example more than four words, the less likely it would be found in the body of the text and therefore less likely to be useful in natural language processing. Grams [135] reviewed the design specifications for databases that stored natural language text (including graphs, images, and other forms of non-digital information that were collected from reference sources such as journals and text books), and could display the requested information in a user friendly, natural language format. Grams concluded that such a database required a companion meta-database that defined terms, and provided a thesaurus for data that was acquired from different sources. Carol Friedman [105], after many years of work developing a natural language processing (NLP) system, concluded that although encoded medical data was necessary for its accurate retrieval, much of the data in patients' records were recorded in a textual form that was extremely diverse. The meanings of words varied depending on its context, and the patients' records were usually not readily retrievable. So efficient NLP systems were essential for processing textual data, but these systems were very difficult to develop. They required substantial amounts of relevant knowledge for each clinical domain in which they were employed.

Friedman et al. [102, 107, 108] reviewed and classified some of the approaches to NLP developed in the 1980s. They classified NLP systems according to their linguistic knowledge:

- Pattern matching or keyword-based systems that were variations of the keyword-in-context approach in which the text was scanned by the computer for combinations of medical words and phrases, such as medical diagnoses or procedures and used algorithms to match those in a terminology or vocabulary index, and, when identified, would be translated automatically into standard codes. These were relatively simple to implement but relied only on patterns of key words, so relationships between words in a sentence could not readily be established. This approach was useful in medical specialties that used relatively highly structured text and clinical sub-languages, such as in pathology and radiology.
- Script-based systems combined keywords and scripts of a description or of a knowledge representation of an event that might occur in a clinical situation.
- Syntactic systems parsed each sentence in the text, identified which words were nouns, verbs, and others, and noted their locations in the sequence of words in the sentence. These were considered to be minimal semantic systems, where some knowledge of language was used such as syntactic parts of speech. So simple relationships in a noun phrase might be established but relationships between different noun phrases could not be determined, and it would require a lexicon that contained syntactic word categories and a method that recognized non-phrases.
- Semantic systems added definitions, synonyms, meanings of terms and phrases, and concepts. Semantic grammars could combine frames to provide more domain-specific information. Semantic systems used knowledge about the semantic properties of words and relied on rules that mapped words with specific semantic properties into a semantic model that had some knowledge of the domain and could establish relationships among words based on semantic properties and could be appropriate for highly structured text that contained simple sentences.
- Syntactic and semantic systems included stages of both of these processes and used both semantic and syntactic information and rules to establish relationships among words in a document based on their semantic and syntactic properties.

- Syntactic, semantic, and knowledge-based systems included reference, conceptual, and domain information, and might also use domain knowledge bases. These were the most complex NLPs to implement and were used in the most advanced NLP systems that evolved in the 1990s and the 2000s.

In the 1990s Friedman, Cimino, Hripcsak and associates at Columbia University in New York reported developing a natural language processing (NLP) system for the automated encoding and retrieval of textual data that made extensive use of UMLS. Their model was based on the assumption that the majority of information needs of users could be mapped to a finite number of general queries, and the number of these generic queries was small enough to be managed by a computer-based system but was too large to be managed by humans. A large number of queries by clinical users were analyzed to establish common syntactic and semantic patterns. The patterns were used to develop a set of general-purpose, generic queries that were then used for developing suitable responses to common, specific, clinical information queries. When a user typed in a question, their computer program would match it to the most relevant generic-query or to a derived combination of queries. A relevant information resource was then automatically selected, and a response to the query was generated for presentation to the user. As an alternative, the user could directly select from a list of all generic-queries in the system, one or more potentially relevant queries, and a response was then developed and presented to the user. Using the NLM's UMLS Metathesaurus they developed a lexicon they called A Query Analyzer (AQUA) that used a Conceptual Graph Grammar that combined both syntax and semantics to translate a user's natural language query into conceptual graph representations that were interpretations of the various portions of the user's query. The result could be combined to form a corporate graph that could then be parsed by a method that used the UMLS Semantic Net. Starting with identifying the semantic type that best represented the query, the parser looked for a word in a sentence of the given domain, for example, "pathology", that could be descended from this type and then looked for semantic relations this word could have with other words in the sentence. The algorithm then compiled a sublanguage text representing the response to the query [67, 68, 171].

Hripcsak and associates [162] described developing a general-purpose NLP system for extracting clinical information from narrative reports. They compared the ability of their NLP system to identify any of six clinical conditions in the narrative reports of chest radiograms and reported that the NLP system was comparable in its sensitivity and specificity to how radiologists read the reports. Hripcsak [161] reported that the codes in their database were defined in their vocabulary, the Medical Entities Dictionary (MED), which is based on a semantic network and serves to define codes and to map the codes to the codes used in the ancillary departments, such as the clinical laboratory codes. Hripcsak [161] also compared two query programs they used. The first, AccessMed, used their Medical Entities Dictionary (MED) and its knowledge base in a hierarchical network, with links to defining attributes and values. The AccessMed browser looked up query terms by lexical matching of words that looked alike and by matching of synonyms, and it then provided links to related terms. The second, Query by Review, used a knowledge base structured as a simple hierarchy; and provided a browser that allowed a user to move to the target terms by a series of menus. Hripcsak compared the recall and precision rates of these two programs to gather the vocabulary terms necessary to perform selected laboratory queries, and reported that Query by Review performed somewhat better than AccessMed but neither was adequate for clinical work.

Friedman and associates [106, 110, 111] at Columbia University in New York made substantial contributions to natural language processing (NLP) with the development of their Medical Language Extraction and Encoding (MedLEE) system that became operational in 1995 at Columbia-Presbyterian Medical Center (CPMC). Their NLP program was written in a Prolog language that could run on various platforms and was developed at CPMC as a general purpose NLP system. Friedman described the MedLEE system as composed of functionally different, modular components (or phases), that in a series of steps each component processed the text and generated an output used by the subsequent component. The first component – the preprocessor – delineated the different sections in the report, separated the free-form textual data from any formatted data, used rules to determine word and sentence boundaries, resolved abbreviations, and performed a look-up in a lexicon to find words and phrases in the sentences that were required for the next parsing phase. It then generated an output that consisted of lists of sentences and corresponding lexical definitions. The parser phase then used the lexical definitions to determine the structure of each sentence, and the parser's sentence-grammar then specified its syntactic and semantic structures. The phrase-regularization component then regularized the terms in the sentence, re-composed multi-word terms that had been separated, and then contiguous and non-contiguous lexical variants were mapped to standard forms. The last phase – the encoder – associated and mapped the regularized terms to controlled vocabulary concepts by querying the synonym knowledge base in their Medical Entities Dictionary (MED) for compatible terms. MED served as their controlled vocabulary that was used in automated mapping of medical vocabularies to the NLM's Unified Medical Language System [101, 342]. MED was their knowledge base of medical concepts that consisted of taxonomic and other relevant semantic relations. After using MED's synonym knowledge base, the regularized forms were translated into unique concepts, so that when the final structured forms of the processed reports were uploaded to their Medical Center's centralized patient database, they corresponded to the unique concepts in their MED. The output of the structured encoded form was then suitable for further processing and interfacing, and could be structured in a variety of formats, including reproducing the original extracted data as it was before encoding, or presented in an XML output, that with Markup language could highlight selected data. In their Medical Center the output was translated into an HL7 format and transferred into its relational medical database. All computer applications at their Medical Center could then reliably access the data by queries that used the structured form and the controlled vocabulary of their MED. Hripcsak et al. [162] evaluated the performance of the MedLEE system for 200 patients with six different medical diagnoses and who each had chest x-rays. They found that their NLP system's final performance report was the same as that of the radiologists.

Friedman [112] reported extending a WEB interface to MedLEE by using a WEB browser, or by direct access for processing patients' records using their Uniform Resource Locator (URL). She and her associates [107, 108] described further development of the MedLEE system as one that analyzed the structure of an entire sentence by using a grammar that consisted of patterns of well-formed syntactic and semantic categories. It processed sentences by defining each word and phrase in the sentence in accordance with their grammar program. It then segmented the entire sentence at certain types of words or phrases defined as classes of findings that could include medical problems, laboratory tests, medications, and other terms which were consistent with their grammar. Next, it then defined as modifiers, qualifiers and values such items as the patient' age, the body site, the test value, and other descriptors. For the first word or phrase in a segment that was associated with a primary finding that was identified in their grammar, an attempt was made to analyze the part of the segment starting with the left-most modifier (or value) of the primary finding. This process was continued until a complete analysis of the segment was obtained. After a segment was successfully analyzed, the remaining segments in the sentence were processed by applying this same method to each segment. The process of segmenting and analyzing was repeated until an analysis of every segment in each entire sentence was completed. Friedman [108] described some additional changes to MedLEE system that allowed five modes of processing:

- The initial segment included the entire sentence, and all words and multi-word phrases needed to be arranged into a well-formed pattern;
- The sentence was then segmented at certain types of words or phrases, and the process was repeated until an analysis of each segment was obtained;
- An attempt was made to identify a well-formed pattern for the largest prefix of the segment;
- Undefined words were skipped; and
- The first word or phrase in the segment associated with a primary finding was identified. The left-most modifier of the finding was added, and the remaining portion was processed using the same method.

The MedLEE system was initially applied to the radiology department where radiologists were interpreting their x-ray reports for about 1,000 patients per day. The radiologists dictated their reports that were generally well structured and composed mostly of natural-language text. The dictated reports were transcribed and entered into their Radiology Information System and then transferred into the clinical database of their Columbia Presbyterian Medical Center (CPMC) Clinical Information System. The automated reports of 230 chest x-rays were randomly selected and checked by two physicians and showed a recall rate of 70 % and a precision of 87 % for four specified medical conditions. In another evaluation of more than 3,000 sentences, 89 % were parsed successfully for recall, and 98 % were considered accurate based on the judgment of an independent medical expert. Friedman [108] also reported that most medical NLP systems could encode textual information as correctly as medical experts, since their reported sensitivity measures of 85 % and specificity measures of 98 % were not significantly different from each other. The Medical NLP systems that were based on analysis of small segments of sentences rather than on analysis of the largest well-formed segment in a sentence showed substantial increases in performance as measured by sensitivity while incurring only a small loss in specificity. NLP systems that contained simpler pattern-matching algorithms that used limited linguistic knowledge performed very well compared to those that contained more complex linguistic knowledge.

Zeng and Cimino [343] evaluated the development of concept-oriented views of natural-language text in electronic medical records (EMRs). They addressed the problem of information overload that often resulted when an excess of computer-generated, unrelated information was retrieved after clinical queries were entered when using EMRs. They compared the retrieval system's ability to identify relevant patient data and generate either concept-oriented views or traditional clinical views of the original text and reported that concept-oriented views contained significantly less non-specific information. When answering questions about patient records, using concept-oriented views showed a significantly greater accuracy in information retrieval. Friedman [107] published an analysis of methods used to evaluate the performance of medical NLP systems and emphasized the difficulty in completing a reliable and accurate evaluation. They noted a need to establish a "gold reference standard", and they defined 21 requirements for minimizing bias in such evaluations.

The extension of MedLEE to a domain of knowledge other than radiology involved collecting a new training body of information. Johnson and Friedman [172] noted that the NLP of discharge summaries in patients' medical records required adding demographic data, clinical diagnoses, medical procedures, prescribed medications with qualifiers such as dose, duration, and frequency, and clinical laboratory tests and their results. In addition the system must be able to resolve conflicting data from multiple sources and be able to add new single- and multi-word phrases. All data must be found in an appropriate knowledge base. Barrows [28] also tested the application of the MedLEE system to a set of almost 13,000 notes for ophthalmology visits that were obtained from their clinical database. The notational text that is commonly used by the clinicians was full of abbreviations and symbols and was poorly formed according to usual grammatical construction rules. After an analysis of these records, a glaucoma-dedicated parser was created using pattern matching of words and phrases representative of the clinical patterns sought. This glaucoma-dedicated parser was used and compared to MedLEE for the extraction of information related to glaucoma disease. They reported that the glaucoma-dedicated parser had a better recall rate than did MedLEE, but MedLEE had a better rate for precision; however, the recall and the precision of both approaches were acceptable for their intended use. Friedman [105] reported extending the MedLEE system for the automated encoding of clinical information in text reports in to ICD-9, SNOMED, or UMLS codes.

Friedman and associates [109] evaluated the recall and precision rates when the system was used to automatically encode entire clinical documents to UMLS codes.

For a randomly selected set of 150 sentences, MedLEE had recall and precision rates comparable to those for six clinical experts. Xu and Friedman [338] described the steps they used with MedLEE for processing pathology reports for patients with cancer:

- Identify the information in each section, such as the section called specimen;
- Identify the findings needed for their research project;
- Analyze the sentences containing the findings, and then extend MedLEE's general schema to include representing their structure;
- Adapt MedLEE so that it would recognize their new types of information which were primarily genotypic concepts and create new lexical entrees;
- Transform the reports into a format that MedLEE could process more accurately, such as when a pathology report included multiple specimens it was necessary to link reports to their appropriate specimen. To minimize the modifications to MedLEE, a preprocessing program was also developed to perform this function.
- Develop a post-processing program to transform the data needed for a cancer registry.

Cimino [64] described a decade of use of MED for clinical applications of knowledge-based terminologies to all services in their medical center, including clinical specialty subsystems. Cao [51] reported the application of the MedLEE system in a trial to generate a patient's problem list from the clinical discharge summaries that had been dictated by physicians for a set of nine patients, randomly selected from their hospital files. The discharge summary reports were parsed by the MedLEE system and then transformed to text knowledge-representation structures in XML format that served as input to the system. All the findings that belonged to the preselected semantic types were then extracted, and these findings were weighted based on the frequency and the semantic type. A problem list was then prepared as an output. A review by clinical experts found that for each patient the system captured more than 95 % of the diagnoses and more that 90 % of the symptoms and findings associated with the diagnoses.

Bakken and associates [14] reported the use of MedLEE for narrative nurses' reports, and compared the semantic categories of MedLEE with the semantic categories of the International Standards Organization (ISO) reference terminology models for nursing diagnoses and nursing actions. They found that all but two MedLEE diagnosis and procedure-related semantic categories could be mapped to ISO models, and suggested areas for extension of MedLEE. Nielson and Wilson [256] at the University of Utah reported developing an application that modified MedLEE's parser that, at the time, required sophisticated rules to interpret its structured output. MedLEE parsed a text document into a series of observations with associated modifiers and modifier values. The observations were then organized into sections corresponding to the sections of the document. The result was an XML document of observations linked to the corresponding text. Manual rules were written to parse the XML structure and to correlate the observations into meaningful clinical observations. Their application employed a rule engine developed by domain experts to automatically create rules for knowledge extraction from textual documents. It allowed the user to browse through the raw text of the parsed document, select phrases in the narrative text, and then it dynamically created rules to find the corresponding observations in the parsed document.

Zhou [346] used MedLEE to develop a medical terminology model for surgical pathology reports. They collected almost 900,000 surgical pathology reports that contained more than 104,000 unique terms. The model that had two major patterns for reporting procedures beginning with either 'bodyloc' (body location) or 'problem.' They concluded that a NLP system like MedLEE provided an automated method for extracting semantic structures from a large body of free text and reduced the burden for human developers of medical terminologies for medical domains. Chen et al. [54] reported a modification in the structured output from MedLEE from a nested structured output into a simpler tabular format that was expected to be more suitable for some uses such as spreadsheets.

Lussier et al. [219] reported using BioMedLEE system, an adaptation of MedLEE that focuses on extracting and structuring biomedical entities and relations including phenotypic and genotypic information in biomedical literature. This application was used for automatically processing text in order to map contextual phenotypes to the Gene Ontology Annotations (GOA) database that facilitates semantic computations for the functions, cellular components and processes of genes [223]. Lussier described the PhenoGo system that can automatically augment annotations in the GOA with additional context by using BioMedLEE and an additional knowledge-based organizer called PhenOS in conjunction with MeSH indexing and established biomedical ontologies. PhenoGo was evaluated for coding anatomical and cellular information and for assigning the coded phenotypes to the correct GOA PhenoGo was found to have a precision rate of 91 % and a recall rate of 92 %.

Chen et al. [55] also described using MedLEE and BioMedLEE to produce a set of primary findings (such as medical diagnoses, procedures, devices, medications) with associated modifiers (such as body sites, changes, frequencies). Since NLP systems had been used for knowledge acquisition because of their ability to rapidly and automatically extract medical entities and findings, relations and modifiers within textual documents, they described their use of both NLP systems for mining textual data for drug-disease associations in MEDLINE articles and in patients' hospital discharge summaries. They focused on searching the textual data for eight diseases that represented a range of diseases and body sites and for any strong associations between these diseases and their prescribed drugs. BioMedLEE was used to encode entities and relations within the titles and abstracts of almost 82,000 MEDLINE articles, and MedLEE was used to extract clinical information from more than 48,000 discharge summaries. They compared the rates of specific drug-disease associations (such as levodopa for Parkinson's disease) found in both text sources. They concluded that the two text sources complemented each other since the literature focused on testing therapies for relatively long time-spans, whereas discharge summaries focused on current practices of drug uses. They also concluded that they had demonstrated the feasibility of the automated acquisition of medical knowledge from both biomedical literature and from patients' records. Wang and associates [323] described using MedLEE to test for symptom-disease associations in the clinical narrative reports of a group of hospitalized patients and reported an evaluation on a random sample for disease-symptom associations with an overall recall rate of 90 % and a precision of 92 %. Borlawsky and colleagues [41] reviewed semantic-processing approaches to NLP for generating integrated data sets from published biomedical literature. They reported using BioMedLEE and a subset of PhenoGo algorithms to extract, with a high degree of precision, encoded concepts and determine relationships among a body of PubMed abstracts of published cancer and genetics literature, with a high degree of precision.

3.4.1 Standards for Medical Data, Data Exchange, Terms, and Terminologies

To overcome the problem of unstructured narrative text, whenever possible, English language words were usually converted into shorter language codes and their interpretation involved uniform agreement of vocabulary and meaning. The encoding and processing of English language text imposed the need for using standard medical terms and also required standard rules for the aggregation and communication of the data. Ease of retrieval required the development of special query and retrieval programs.

Medical data standards for the transfer, exchange, and interoperability of data were essential. The need to have standardized sets of data was especially important for users of electronic patient records (EPR) obtained from different vendors and for public health and governmental agencies that collected health statistics, monitored morbidity and mortality of population groups, and studied the use and costs of health care services [250]. As a result, in the early 1970s uniform, basic, minimum data sets were published for hospital patients [80], for ambulatory patients [201], and for health care plan patients [86]. By the late 1970s many governmental agencies were pressing for legislation requiring the use of standard data sets for reporting patient care services [166]. In the 1980s, under chairman Breslow, uniform Minimum Data Sets were published by the National Committee on Vital and Health Statistics (NCVHS) for hospital discharge data [79], for long-term health care data [302], and for ambulatory care data [335]. However, even in the late 1980s, patients' records were still mostly hand written and paper-based and did not readily lend themselves to uniform data sets or to the transmission of their data to other sites. Although it became possible to search and retrieve computer-stored text by matching desired words in standard data sets, it was much simpler to search and retrieve by using numbers and letters. Thus, to facilitate storage and retrieval of English terms, they were usually represented by numerical codes; yet the efficient transfer and combination of text required standardization of terms and of terminology.

Medical data standards for data interoperability began to be developed in 1983. McDonald [231, 234, 237] provided a review of the early history of medical standards development. Those standards addressed what items of data should be included in defining an observation, what data structure should be employed to record an observation, how individual items should be encoded and formatted, and what transmission media should be used. Formal attempts to improve the standardization of medical data were carried out by collaborating committees, such as the subcommittees on Computerized Systems of the American Standards for Testing Materials (ASTM), the oldest of the nonprofit standards-setting societies and a standards-producing member of the American National Standards Institute (ANSI) [287]. The ASTM technical subcommittee E31.12 on Medical Informatics considered nomenclatures and medical records [118]. In 1988 ASTM's subcommittee E31.11 on Data Exchange Standards for Clinical Laboratory Results published its specifications, E1238, for clinical data interchange, and set standards for the two-way digital transmission of clinical data between different computers for laboratory, for office, and for hospital systems. As a simple example, all dates for years, months and days should be recorded as an eight-character string, YYYYMMDD. Thus the date, January 12, 1998, should always be transmitted as 19980112 [10, 11].

Since the exchange of clinical data between different MIS databases required the use of standard terms, in 1983 standards for the transmission of clinical data between computers began to be developed [237]. The proposed standards addressed what items of information should be included in defining an observation, what data structure should be employed to record an observation, how individual items should be encoded and formatted, and what transmission media should be supported. The Medical Data Interchange (MEDIX) P1157 committee of the Institute of Electrical and Electronics Engineers (IEEE), formed at the Symposium on Computer Applications in Medical Care (SCAMC) in 1987, was also developing a set of standards based on the International Standards Organization (ISO) application-level standards for the transfer of clinical data over large networks from mixed sources, such as from both a clinical laboratory and a pharmacy, for both intra- and inter-hospital data exchange. Linkages of data within a hospital were considered to be tight, synchronous linkages and between hospitals were assumed to be loose asynchronous [288].

McDonald [231, 235] emphasized the need for clinical data interchange standards that became essential when computer-based electronic medical records (EPRs) became technically feasible and created a need to integrate all of the various formats and structures of clinical data from the computer-based clinical laboratory system, the radiology system, pharmacy system, and from all of the medical specialty computer-based subsystems such as the intensive-care unit and emergency department.

Health Level 7 (HL7), an international organization whose membership included computer vendors, hospital users, and healthcare consultants, was formed in 1987 to develop interface standards for transmitting data between medical applications that used different computers within hospital information systems with the goal of creating a common language to share clinical data [307]. HL7 communicates data as a sequence of defined ASCII characters that are hierarchically organized into segments, fields, and components. The Open Systems Interconnection (OSI) model was the starting point for HL7 interface standards for transmitting data between applications in hospital information systems. The message content of HL7 conforms to the International Standards Organization (ISO) standards for the applications level seven of the Open Systems Interconnection (OSI) model, and hence its name. The HL7 Version 2 family of standards was influenced by the ASTM 1238 Standard. Version 2 standards use the same message syntax, the same data types, and some of the same segment definitions as ASTM 1238 [232–234].

HL7 expanded its activities in the 1990 and became an ANSI-accredited Standards Developing Organizations (SDOs). HL7 has collaborated with other SDOs to develop standards, specifications and protocols for the interoperability of hospitals clinical and administrative functions. HL7 created its Reference Information Model (HL7 RIM) in 1995 as a basis for developing model-based Version 3 standards. The goal was to provide improved standard vocabulary specifications for the interoperability of healthcare information systems and improved representation of semantic, syntactic and lexical aspects of HL7 messages. Bakken [14] described some activities of the HL7 Vocabulary Activity Committee related to vocabulary domain specifications for HL7-coded data elements and for its guidance in developing and registering terminology and vocabulary domain specifications including those for HL7 RIM. In 2004 HL7 released its draft standards for the electronic medical record that included direct care functions, including care management and clinical decision support; supportive care functions, including clinical support, research, administrative and financial functions; and information infrastructure functions of data security and records management [97]. Benson [29] provides a detailed history of the development of HL7.

Medical terminologies are systemized collections of terms used in medicine to assist a person in communicating with a computer. They require developing and using standard definitions of [266, 319]:

- terms that are units of formal language such as words or numbers;
- entities that are units of reality, such as human body sites, population groups, or components of a system or of an organization such as the radiology department in a hospital;
- codes that are units of partitions, groups of words, letters, numbers, or symbols that represent specific items, such as medical diagnoses or procedures;
- nominal phrases that are units of natural language; and
- concepts that are representations of thoughts formed in the mind, that are mental constructs or representations of combined things, objects, or thoughts.

Chute [62] reviewed in some detail the evolution of healthcare terminologies basic to medical encoding systems and how its history went back several centuries. Current terminologies and methods for encoding medical diagnoses and etiologies, and procedures began in the 1940s by the World Health Organization (WHO), who undertook the classifying and codifying of disease diagnoses by systematic assignment of related diagnostic terms to classes or groups. The WHO took over from the French the classification system they had adopted in 1893 that was based primarily on body site and etiology of diseases [95].

International Classification of Diseases (ICD) published under the WHO sponsorship was in its sixth revision in 1948. In the 1950s medical librarians manually encoded ICD-6 codes for diagnoses and procedures. In the 1960s ICD-7 codes were generally key punched into cards for electronic data processing. The International Classification of Diseases, Adapted (ICDA) was used in the United States for indexing hospital records, and was based on ICD-8 that was published in 1967. Beginning in 1968 the ICDA began to serve as the basis for coding diagnoses data for official morbidity and mortality statistics in the United States. In addition, the payors of insurance claims began to require ICDA codes for payments; and that encouraged hospitals to enter into their computers the patients' discharge diagnoses with their appropriate ICDA codes. The ninth revision, ICD-9, appeared in 1977; and since ICD was originally designed as an international system for reporting causes of death, ICD-9 was revised to better classify diseases. In 1978 its Clinical Modification (ICD-9-CM) included more than 10,000 terms and permitted six-digit codes plus modifiers. ICD-9-CM also included in its Volume III a listing of procedures. Throughout the three decades of the 1980s, 1990s, and 2000s, the ICD-9-CM was the nationwide classification system used by medical record librarians and physicians for the coding of diagnoses. The final versions of the ICD-9 codes were released in 2010 (CMS-2010), and ICD-10 codes were scheduled to be used in the U.S. in 2014.

Current Medical Terminology (CMT), created by Gordon [132] and a committee of the American Medical Association, was an important early contribution to the standardization of medical terminology. Their objective was to develop an alphabetical listing of terms with their definitions and simplified references. The first edition of CMT was published in 1962, with revisions in 1964 and 1965 [131]. Current Medical Information and Terminology (CMIT) was an expanded version of CMT in 1971 to provide a distillate of the medical record by using four-digit codes for descriptors, such as symptoms, signs, laboratory test results, x-ray and pathology reports [129, 130]. CMIT also defined diagnoses terms that were a common deficiency of SNOP, SNOMED, and ICD as all lacked a common dictionary that precisely defined their terms. As a result, the same condition could be defined differently in each and be assigned different codes by different coders [147].

An important benefit from using a common dictionary was to encourage the standardization of medical terms through their definitions and thereby facilitate the interchange of medical information among different health professionals and also among different medical databases. Since the data stored in patients' records came from multiple sub-system databases such as from pathology, laboratory, pharmacy, and others, some standards for exchanging data had to be established before they could be readily transferred into a computer-based, integrated patient record. Since CMIT was available in machine-readable form, it was an excellent source of structured information for more than 3,000 diseases. It was used by Lindberg [212] as a computer-aid to making a diagnosis in his CONSIDER program, for searching CMIT by combinations of disease attributes, and then listing the diseases in which these attributes occurred.

Current Procedural Terminology (CPT) was first published in 1967 with a four-digit coding system for identifying medical procedures and services primarily for the payment of medical claims. It was soon revised and expanded to five-digit codes to facilitate the frequent addition of new procedures [94]. Subsequently, the American Medical Association provided frequent revisions of CPT, and in the 1970s and 1980s, CPT-4 was the most widely accepted system of standardized descriptive terms and codes for reporting physician-provided procedures and services under government and private health-insurance programs. In 1989 the Health Care Financing Organization (HCFA) began to require every physician's claim for payment of services provided to patients seen in medical offices to include ICD-9-CM codes for diagnoses, and to report CPT-4 codes for procedures and services [286].

The Standard Nomenclature of Diseases and Operations (SNDO), a compilation of standard medical terms, by their meaning or by some logical relationship such as by diseases or operations, was developed by the New York Academy of Medicine and was published by the American Medical Association in 1933. It was used in most hospitals in the United States for three decades. SNDO listed medical conditions in two dimensions: by anatomic site or topographic category (for example, body as a whole, skin, respiratory, cardiovascular, etc.) and by etiology or cause (for example, due to prenatal influence, due to plant or parasite, due to intoxication, due to trauma by physical agent, etc.). The two-dimensional SNDO was not sufficiently flexible to satisfy clinical needs; its last (5th edition) was published in 1961.

The Systemized Nomenclature of Pathologists (SNOP), a four-dimensional nomenclature intended primarily for use by pathologists, was developed by a group within the American College of Pathologists led by Wells and was first published in 1965. SNOP coded medical terms into four TMEF categories: Topography (T) for the body site affected; Morphology (M) for the structural changes observed; Etiology (E) for the cause of the disease; and Function (F) for the abnormal changes in physiology [329].

Thus a patient with lung cancer who smoked cigarettes and had episodes of shortness of breath at night would be assigned the following string of SNOP terms: T2600 M8103 (bronchus, carcinoma); E6927 (tobacco-cigarettes); F7103 (paroxysmal nocturnal dyspnea) [276]. Complete, as well as multiple, TMEF statements were considered to be necessary for pathologists' purposes [133]. The result of these applications was the translation of medical text into the four fields (T, M, E, and F) as listed in the SNOP dictionary. The successful use of SNOP by pathologists encouraged Cote, Gantner, and others to expand SNOP to attempt to encompass all medical specialties. In the 1960s pathologists generally adopted the use of SNOP, as it was well suited for coding data for computer entry when using punched cards. In the 1970s it was the basis for the development of computer programs to permit automatic SNOP encoding of pathology terms [273, 274, 276].

The Systemized Nomenclature of Medicine (SNOMED) was first published in 1977 (SNOMED 1977). In addition to SNOP's four fields of Topography (T), Morphology (M), Etiology (E), and Function (F), SNOMED contained three more fields: Disease (D) for classes of diseases, complex disease entities, and syndromes, which made SNOMED as suitable for statistical reporting as the ICD; Procedure (P) for diagnostic, therapeutic, preventive, or administrative procedures; and Occupation (O) for the patient's occupational and industrial hazards [77, 124].

Some reports compared SNOMED and ICD and advocated SNOMED as being superior for the purposes of medical care and clinical research, since ICD was designed primarily for statistical reporting and its codes were often too general to identify specific patient problems. In addition SNOMED defined the logical connections between the categories of data contained in the final coded statement; and SNOMED codes could be used to generate ICD codes, but not vice versa [134].

The Systemized Nomenclature of Medicine Reference Terminology (SNOMED-RT) was also developed by the College of American Pathologists (CAP) to serve as a common reference terminology for the aggregation and retrieval of health care information that had been recorded by multiple individuals and organizations [313]. Dolin [89] described the SNOMED-RT Procedure Model as providing an advanced hierarchical structure with poly-hierarchies representing super-types and sub-types relationships; and that included clinical actions and healthcare services, such as surgical and invasive procedures, courses of therapy, history taking, physical examinations, tests of all kinds, monitoring, administrative and financial services.

SNOMED Clinical Terms (SNOMED-CT) was developed in 1999 when the similarities were recognized between SNOMED-RT and the National Health Service of the United Kingdom that had developed its own Clinical Terms Version 3 that evolved from the Read Codes CTV3. SNOMED-CT is a comprehensive multi-lingual medical terminology for atomic sites, organisms, chemicals, symptoms, diagnoses, and other such concepts. Spackman [309] reported on 3 years' use of this clinical terminology and described changes in SNOMED-CT that included removing duplicate terms, improving logic definitions, and revising conceptual relationships. The Lister Hill Center of the National Library of Medicine (NLM) identified a subset of the most frequently used problem list terms in SNOMED-CT and published it as the Clinical Observations Recording and Encoding List (CORE) Subset of SNOMED CT. The CORE Problem List Subset is updated four times a year, and in 2012 contained about 6,000 concepts (NLM Problems and Services 2012).

Problems with inconsistencies in the various medical terminologies soon became apparent. Ward [324] described the need for associations of health care organizations to be able to maintain a common database of uniformly coded health outcomes data; and reported the development of the Health Outcomes Institute (HOI) with their uniquely coded, medical data elements. In 2004 the National Health Information Infrastructure (NHII) was initiated to attempt to standardize information for patients' electronic medical records (EMRs). It recommended the standard terminologies for EMRs to be the Systemized Nomenclature of Medicine (SNOMED), and the Logical Observation Identifiers Names and Codes (LOINC). The National Cancer Institute (NCI) developed the Common Data Elements (CDEs) to define the data required for research in oncology [259].

The convergence of medical terminologies became an essential requirement for linking multiple databases from different sources that used different coding terminologies. In 1960 Medical Subject Headings (MeSH) vocabulary file was initiated by the National Library of Medicine (NLM) to standardize its indexing of medical terms and to facilitate the use of its search and retrieval programs. MeSH was developed primarily for the use of librarians for indexing the NLM's stored literature citations, and was NLM's way of meeting the problem of variances in medical terminology by instituting its own standard, controlled vocabulary. However, MeSH was not designed to serve as a vocabulary for the data in patients' medical records. MeSH is a highly structured thesaurus consisting of a standard set of terms and subject headings that are arranged in both an alphabetical and a categorical structure, with categories further subdivided into subcategories; and within each subcategory the descriptors are arranged hierarchically. MeSH is the NLM's authority list of technical terms used for indexing biomedical journal articles, cataloging books, and for bibliographic search of the NLM's computer-based citation file.

In 1987 the NLM initiated the development of a convergent medical terminology with its Unified Medical Language System (UMLS) that included a Semantic Network of interrelated semantic classes and a Metathesaurus of interrelated concepts and names that supported linking data from multiple sources. UMLS attempted to compensate for differences in terminology among different systems such as MeSH, CMIT, SNOP, SNOMED, and ICD. UMLS was not planned to form a single convergent vocabulary but rather to unify terms from a variety of standardized vocabularies and codes for the purpose of improving bibliographic literature retrieval, and to provide standardized data terms for computer-based information.

Humphreys [164, 165], at NLM, described UMLS as a major NLM initiative designed to facilitate the retrieval and integration of information from many machine-readable information sources, including the biomedical literature, factual databases, and knowledge bases. Cimino and Barnett [66] studied the problem of translating medical terms between four different controlled terminologies: NLM's MeSH, International Classification of Diseases (ICD-9), Current Procedural Terminology (CPT-4), and the Systemized Nomenclature of Medicine (SNOMED). When a user needed to translate a free-text term from one terminology to another, the free-text term was entered into one system that then presented its list of controlled terms, and the user selected the most correct term. If the user did not recognize any of the presented terms as a correct translation then the user could try again. It was recognized that an automatic translation process would be preferable for the conversion of terms from one system to another. They created a set of rules to construct a standard way of representing a medical term that denoted semantic features of the term by establishing it as an instance of a class, or even more specifically of a subclass that inherited all of the required properties. They developed an algorithm that compared matches of a subset of terms for the category of "procedures," and reported that matches from ICD-9 to the other terminologies appeared to be "good" 45 % of the time, and that when a match was "suboptimal" (55 % of the time) the reason was that ICD-9 did not contain an appropriate matching term. They concluded that the development of a common terminology would be desirable.

Cimino [96] and associates at Columbia University also addressed some of the inconsistencies in terms in different terminologies, and emphasized the necessity for a controlled, common medical terminology that was capable of linking and converging data from medical applications in different hospital departmental services, from different patient-record systems, and also from knowledge-based systems and from medical literature databases. They proposed as criteria for a controlled medical terminology:

- domain completeness, so it did not restrict the depth or breadth of the hierarchy;
- non-redundancy, to prevent multiple terms being added for the same concept;
- synonymy, to support multiple non-unique names for concepts;
- non-vagueness, each concept must be complete in its meaning;
- non-ambiguity, each concept must have exactly one meaning;
- multiple classification, so that a concept can be assigned to as many classes as required;
- consistency of views, in that concepts in multiple classes must have the same attributes in each concept; and
- explicit relationships, in that meanings of inter-concept relationships must be clear.

Cimino [65] further added that it was desirable that controlled medical vocabularies should:

- provide an expandable vocabulary content;
- be able to quickly add new terms as they arise;
- be able to change with the evolution of medical knowledge;
- consider the unit of symbolic processing to be the concept, that is the embodiment of a particular meaning;
- have terms that must correspond to only one meaning and meanings must correspond to only one term;
- have the meaning of a concept be permanent, but its name can change when, for example, a newer version of the vocabulary is developed; and
- have hierarchical structures, and although a single hierarchy is more manageable, polyhierarchies may be allowed;
- support that multipurpose vocabularies may require different levels of granularity; and
- allow synonyms of terms, but redundancy, such as multiple ways to code a term, should be avoided.

Cimino [63, 65, 67] applied their criteria for a convergent terminology to their Medical Entities Dictionary (MED) that they developed for their centralized clinical information system at Columbia University. MED included subclassification systems for their ancillary clinical services, including the clinical laboratory, pharmacy, and electrocardiography. MED was a MUMPS-based, hierarchical data structure, with a vocabulary browser and a knowledge base. Since classes of data provided within their ancillary systems were inadequate for the MED hierarchy for both the multiple classification criteria and for its use in clinical applications, a subclassification function was added to create new classes of concepts. By the mid-1990s MED contained 32,767 concepts; and it had encoded 6 million procedures and test results for more than 300,000 patients.

Mays and associates [224] at the IBM Watson Research Center in Yorktown Heights, New York, described their K-Rep system based on description logic (DL) that considered its principal objects of representation to be concepts, such as laboratory tests, diagnostic procedures, and others; and that concepts could include subconcepts, such as the concept of a chemistry test could include the sub-concept of a serum sodium test, and thereby enabled an increased scalability of concepts. They considered conceptual scalability to be an enhancement of system scalability; and their strategy allowed multiple developers to concurrently work on overlapping portions of the terminology in independent databases. Oliver and associates [264, 265] reported the formation of the InterMed Collaboratory that consisted of a group of medical informaticians with experience in medical terminology with the objective of developing a common model for controlled medical vocabularies.

A collaborative group from the Mayo Clinic, Kaiser Permanente, and Stanford University developed Convergent Medical Terminology in the late 1990s. The objective was to achieve a convergence of some different existing terminologies to better support the development of informatics applications and to facilitate the exchange of data using different terminologies. They had found that some medical terminologies, such as SNOMED International and ICD-9-CM, used a hierarchical structure that organized the concepts into type hierarchies that were limiting since they lacked formal definitions for the terms in the systems and did not sufficiently define what a term represented or how one term differed from another [48]. Building on the experience with the K-Rep system described by Mays [224], they developed a convergent medical terminology they called Galapagos that could take a collection of applications from multiple sites and identify and reconcile conflicting designs and also develop updates tailored specifically for compatibility with locally enhanced terminologies. Campbell and colleagues [49] further reported their applications of Galapagos for concurrent evolutionary enhancements of SNOMED International at three Kaiser Permanente (KP) regions and at the Mayo Clinic. They found their design objectives had been met, and Galapagos supported semantic-based concurrency control and identified and resolved conflicting decisions in design. Dolin [88] and associates at KP described the Convergent Medical Terminology as having a core comprised of SNOMED-CT, laboratory LOINC, and First DataBank drug terminology, all integrated into a poly-hierarchical structured, knowledge base of concepts with logic-based definitions imported from the source terminologies. In 2004 Convergent Medical Terminology was implemented in KP enterprise-wide and served as the common terminology across all KP computer-based applications for its 8.4 million members in the United States. Convergent Medical Terminology served as the definitive source of concept definitions for the KP organization. It provided a consistent structure and access method to all computer codes used by KP, with its inter-operability and cross-mappings to all KP ancillary subsystems. In 2010 KP donated the Convergent Medical Terminology to the National Library of Medicine for its free access.

Chute and associates [61] introduced the notion of a terminology server that would mediate translations among concepts shared across disparate terminologies. They had observed a major problem with a clinical terminology server that was used by clinicians to enter patient data from different clinical services was that they were prone to use lexical variants of words that might not match their corresponding representations within the nomenclature. Chute added as desirable requirements for a convergent medical terminology:

- word normalization by a normalization and lexical variant-generator code that replaced clinical jargon and completed abbreviated words and terms,
- target terminology specifications for supporting other terminologies, such as SNOMED-RT or ICD-9-CM, that were used by the enterprise,
- spell-checking and correction,
- lexical matching of words against a library of indexed words,
- semantic locality by making visible closely related terms or concepts,
- term composition that brought together modifiers or qualifiers and a kernel concept, and
- term decomposition that broke apart complex phrases into atomic components.

3.4.2 Encoding Medical Text

Encoding text greatly simplified the search and retrieval of textual data that was otherwise done by matching letters and numbers; so when English language terms were replaced by numerical codes, then the textual data could be represented and entered into the computer in a readable, compact, and consistent format. The disadvantages of encoding natural language terms were that users had to be familiar with the coding system, codes had a tendency to reduce the flexibility and richness of textual data and to stereotype the information, and codes required updating and revisions for new terms or they could become obsolete [283, 284]. Yet the process of coding was an important early method used for natural language processing (NLP); and manual encoding methods often used special-purpose, structured and pre-coded data-entry forms.

Ozbolt [268] reported testing manual auditors for their reliability and validity for coding standard terms they had collected from a set of 465 patients' medical care records that were submitted by nine hospitals. Manual auditors identified almost 19,000 items in these patients' records as representing statements of patients' medical problems, patients' outcomes from care, and patient-care problems; and they found that their set of standard terms and codes matched 99.1 % of these items. They concluded that this was a useful demonstration that medical terminologies could meet criteria for acceptable accuracy in coding, and that computer-based terminologies could be a useful part of a medical language system. Hogan and Wagner [159] evaluated allowing health care practitioners to add free-text information to supplement coded information and to provide more flexibility during their direct entry of medications. They found that the added free-text data often changed the meaning of coded data and lowered data accuracy for the medical decision-support system used with their electronic medical records (EMRs).

Chute [62] reviewed in some detail the evolution of healthcare terminologies basic to medical data-encoding systems, and how its history went back several centuries. Current terminologies and methods for encoding medical diagnoses began in the 1940s by the World Health Organization (WHO), who undertook the classifying and codifying of diseases by systematic assignment of related diagnostic terms to classes or groups. The WHO took over from the French the classification system they had adopted in 1893, and was based primarily on body site and etiology of diseases [95].

Automated encoding of text by computer became an important goal since the manual coding of text was a tedious and time-consuming process and led to inconsistent coding. Efforts were soon directed to developing NLP software for automatic encoding by computer, and that needed standardized terminology and rules for coding, aggregating, and communicating textual data. Bishop [31] defined its requirements to be: a unique code for each term (word or phrase), each code needed to be defined, each term needed to be independent, synonyms should be equitable to the code of their base terms, each code could be linked to codes of related terms, the system should encompass all of medicine and be in the public domain, and the format of the knowledge base should be described completely in functional terms to make it independent of the software and hardware used. It was also apparent that the formalized structuring and encoding of standardized medical terms would provide a great savings of storage space and would improve the effectiveness of the search and retrieval process for textual data. Automated data encoding, as the alternative to manual encoding, needed to capture the data electronically as it occurred naturally in a clinical practice, and then have a computer do the automated data encoding. Tatch [316], in the Surgeon General's Office of the U.S. Army, reported automatically encoding diagnoses by punching paper tape as a by-product of the normal typing of the clinical record summary sheet. The computer program operated upon actual words within selected blocks, one word at a time, and translated each letter in the word into a unique numeral; the numeral was matched to an identification table and an identity code was appended to the numeral. Based on a syntax code, the numerals were added one-at-a-time, until a diagnostic classification was determined. The diagnostic code related to the final sum was retrieved from computer memory and added to the clinical record summary.

Demuth [85] described some of the earliest approaches that had been used to develop automated text encoding systems included a language-based system that matched English words against a dictionary, and if a match or an accepted synonym was found, it was then assigned a code. This approach also included a knowledge-based or expert system that included the domain of knowledge recorded by experts for whom the particular data system was intended; and the expert system attempted to mimic the reasoning and logic of the users. Hierarchical, tree-based, decision systems tried to automate human reasoning and logic by using simple queries and responses; and the decision-tree design mandated the nature and order of the questions to be asked, and how they were to be answered. Demuth concluded that an automated coding system had to possess characteristics of both a language-based and a knowledge-based system in order to provide the feedback necessary to help a medical records professional arrive at the correct codes.

Pratt [275] at the National Institutes of Health (NIH), reported the automated encoding of autopsy diagnoses using the Standard Nomenclature of Pathology (SNOP). He noted that in the creation of a computer-based, natural language processing (NLP) system, it was necessary to provide for the morphological, syntactic, and semantic recognition of the input data. He used SNOP as his semantically organized dictionary; and noted that SNOP was divided into four major semantic categories: Topography (T), Morphology (M), Etiology (E), and Function (F). He further defined additional semantic subcategories and morphemes (the smallest meaningful parts of words) to permit the successful identification of word forms that were not found in the SNOP dictionary, and also to help in the recognition of medical synonyms. He developed parsing algorithms for morphological, syntactic, and semantic analyses of autopsy diagnoses; and he developed a computer program which, when given as input a body of medical text, produced as output a linguistic description and semantic interpretation of the given text [277, 278].

Whiting-O'Keefe and associates [332] at the University of California in San Francisco reported a system that automatically encoded patients' data from their medical records. A computer program was developed that extracted partially encoded patient data that had been gathered by the Summary Time Oriented Record (STOR) system for ambulatory patients and converted it to fully encoded data. The primary display of the STOR system was a time-sequenced flow sheet. Much of the data captured was structured, which could be viewed as a form of partial data coding, and this approach made the automated- encoding system feasible. Their coding program allowed a user to develop a set of coding specifications that determined what data and how the data in the STOR database was to be coded. In July 1983 the first machine-encoded data was passed from the STOR system to the ARAMIS database.

Gabrieli et al. [120] developed an office information system called "Physicians' Records and Knowledge Yielding Total-Information for Consulting Electronically" (PRAKTICE) for processing natural language text in medical records [119, 121]. Gabrieli developed a computer-compatible, medical nomenclature with a numeric representation, where the location of a term in a hierarchical tree served as the code. For example, the diagnosis of polycythemia was represented by 4-5-9-1-2, where 4 = clinical medicine, 4-5 = a diagnostic term, 4-5-9 = hematologic diagnostic term, 4-5-9-1 = red cell disorder, and 4-5-9-1-2 = polycythemia [121]. He also developed a lexicon that contained more than 100,000 terms. He used his system for processing medical text; and described his method as beginning with a parser that recognized punctuation marks and spaces, and then broke down each sentence into individual words while retaining the whole sentence intact for reference. Each word was numbered for its place in the sentence, and then matched against his word lexicon, and given a grammatical classification (noun, verb, etc.) and a semantic characterization (grouped among 'clue' medical words, modifiers, or others). The program then looked for any words near to the medical term that might be modifiers altering its meaning (usually adjectives). Thus, the term "abdominal pain" might be preceded by a modifier such as "crampy abdominal pain." The remaining words were then analyzed for their relationship to the other words in the sentence.

Powsner and associates [271] at Yale University reported on their use of semantic relationships between terms by linking pairs of related terms to try to improve coding and retrieving clinical literature. They found that defining semantic relationships for certain pairs of terms could be helpful; but multiple semantic relationships could occur in the clinical literature that was strongly dependent upon the clinical specialty. In the 1990s and the 2000s more advanced NLP systems were developed for both the automated encoding and the automated querying of uncoded textual medical data.

3.4.3   Querying Medical Text

The approaches to automatic encoding of textual data led to the development of methods for the automated retrieval of encoded textual data (structured) and then for the much more difficult process of automated retrieval of uncoded textual data. The earliest retrieval of unstructured textual data functioned by the matching of words and phrases within the text. This process based on the key-word-in-context (KWIC) search [181], led to a pattern matching of word strings [340]. Early automated query systems attempted to match document word with a similar word in their own data dictionary or lexicon. If no direct match was found the system then searched for a synonym listed in their lexicon that could be accepted by the user. Ideally what was needed was a natural-language processing (NLP) system that could automatically interact with the computer while using English language text. The approach of matching words and phrases was useful for processing some highly structured uncoded text; however, this method still ignored the syntax of sentences and thereby missed the importance of the locations of words within a sentence and of the relations between words.

Hersh [149] reviewed the evolution of natural language processing (NLP) for information retrieval systems and noted that they were among the earliest medical informatics applications. He defined information retrieval systems as systems to catalog and provide information about documents. Querying a medical database involved accessing, selecting, and retrieving the desired data was an essential function for a medical database. This process usually required transforming the query so it could be executed by the computer by using special programs to retrieve the selected data. This process required developing standards for the uniform collection, storage, and exchange of data. Blois [32] emphasized that special programming languages were required to reach into a database and draw together desired subgroups of patients' data, and then to specify the desired operation to be performed on the data. Blois proposed that the detailed needs of such retrieval languages could be met by using a form composed on the screen (query-by-form), by a series of selections from a displayed "menu" of terms or phrases, or by the use of a natural-language, front-end, computer program that converted a question expressed in English into a formal query language and then execute it by the computer database-system programs. Broering [43] noted that without computer help, users had to develop their own sets of rules to search, retrieve, and reconcile data from multiple databases. As the numbers of databases increased, it became much more difficult to manage all of the different rules between databases, so automated programs for querying data became a necessity. Hersh [149] observed that in 1966 when the National Library of Medicine (NLM) launched its MEDLINE, it initially required specially trained users and a several-week turn-around time for a response to a mailed search statement. In 1997 NLM announced its Web-based MEDLINE and PubMed with easy-to-use interfaces.

The ability to query natural language text was essential for the retrieval of many textual reports of clinical procedures and tests, of physicians' dictated surgery operative reports, pathology reports, x-ray and electrocardiogram interpretations, and for some clinical laboratory reports such as for microbiology that often required descriptive textual data rather than numeric data [196, 218, 334]. Eden [92] noted that as medical databases increased in size, it took more time to conduct a search by the method of querying by key words. It was obvious that there was a need to develop computer programs that could efficiently conduct automatic query and search programs for textual data in databases.

One of the earliest programs for the search and retrieval of data for medical research was developed in 1959 by Sweeney and associates at the University of Oklahoma. It was called General Information Processing System (GIPSY). GIPSY was designed to permit the user, without any additional programming, to browse through the database, to pose complex queries against any of the stored data, and to obtain answers to ad-hoc inquiries from the assembled information. GIPSY was used at the University of Oklahoma as the primary support in projects concerning analysis of patients' psychiatry records [2]. Nunnery [260] reported that in 1973 GIPSY was modified for use by health professionals. The program was renamed "Medical Information Storage System" (MISSY) and used for some epidemiological studies. In 1982 a microcomputer-based system called MICRO-MISSY, with more statistical procedures, was written in Microsoft BASIC and used CP/M operating system. In the 1960s a relatively simple method for entering and retrieving uncoded textual data without encoding the data was to enter words, phrases, or sentences into a computer and then retrieve such text by entering into the computer the exact matching of letter-by-letter, or word-by-word, or phrase-by-phrase (KWIC). In the 1960s an early way of applying this KWIC method was by using an IBM Magnetic Tape/Selectric Typewriter (MT/ST) that was interfaced to a magnetic tape drive connected to a digital computer. Robinson [282] used such a system to enter narrative surgical-pathology reports. At the time of the transcription, the MT/ST system permitted the information to be entered into the computer by the typewriter, and the computer program then matched each word against a standard vocabulary. The program also identified new or misspelled words for editing.

In the early 1960s Barnett and associates at the Massachusetts General Hospital (MGH) implemented their laboratory information system, and in 1971 they developed their Computer-Stored Ambulatory Record (COSTAR) system. In 1979 they developed the Medical Query Language (MQL) that was used to query their databases that were programmed with the MGH Utility Multiprogramming System (MUMPS) language. They structured the narrative textual data, such as commonly found in physicians' progress notes, by using an interactive, conversational technique with a predetermined branching structure of the data and using a fixed vocabulary. The user entered the query by selecting the desired items from a list on a display screen [27]. MQL was used for the retrieval and analysis of data from their COSTAR ambulatory patients' records. A MQL query was made up of a series of statements, and each statement began with a keyword. MQL queries could be indefinitely long or could be broken down into a series of sub-queries with each designed to accomplish some portion of the total problem. The statement was scanned and passed on to a parser that matched the scanned symbols to rules in the MQL grammar. The program then executed the search. MQL permitted non-programmer users to submit complex, branching-logic queries that could be intricate and indefinitely long and could be broken down into a series of sub-queries, each designed to accomplish some portion of the total problem. MQL had capabilities for cross-tabulation reports, scatter plots, online help, intermediate data storage, and system maintenance utilities [247, 305, 328]. Murphy [252] reviewed 16 years of COSTAR research queries that used MQL to search a large relational data warehouse, and reported that MQL was more flexible than SQL for searches of clinical data.

In the early 1960s Warner and associates at the University of Utah LDS Hospital developed a clinical database, Health Evaluation through Logical Processing (HELP), which they used for patient care, clinical decision support, and clinical research. They stored the patient care data in sectors organized in groups dealing with specific subsets of potential medical decisions. They developed a query program to search and format the requested data. To permit a rapid, interactive response-time, their query functions were run on a microcomputer that communicated with their central computer system. The HELP database was also used for alert reports from their laboratory, pharmacy, and radiology subsystems [145]. Ranum [281] described their NLP approach to radiology reports that were typically presented in a typewritten format. They had formerly created a list of common x-ray reports from which the radiologist selected and checked the one most appropriate for a patient's x-ray, or had the option of entering by text a different report, They developed a knowledge-based, data-acquisition tool they called Special Purpose Radiology Understanding System (SPRUS) that operated within their HELP system and contained knowledge bases for common conditions, beginning with frames of data for 29 pulmonary diseases. Haug and associates [144] described their further development of NLP for chest x-ray reports with a new system they called Symbolic Text Processor (SymText) that combined a syntactic parser with a semantic approach to concepts dealing with the various abnormalities seen in chest x-rays, including medical diseases, procedural tubes and treatment appliances. The program then generated output for the radiologists' reports to be stored in the patients' medical records. Warner [326] described their multi-facility system as one using a controlled vocabulary and allowing direct entry of structured textual data by clinicians.

In 1962 Lamson [192] at the University of California, Los Angeles, reported entering surgical pathology diagnoses in full English language text into a computer-based, magnetic-file storage system. The information was keypunched in English text in the exact form it had been dictated by the pathologists. A patient's record was retrieved by entering the patient's name or identification number, and a full prose printout of the pathologist's diagnosis was provided. To avoid manual coding, Lamson collected 3 years of patients' data into a thesaurus that related all English words with identifiable relationships. His computer program matched significant words present in a query and then retrieved patients' records that contained those words. In 1965 his patients' files contained about 16,000 words and his thesaurus contained 5,700 English words. His thesaurus contained hierarchical and synonymous relationships of terms. For example, the program would recognize that "dyspnea" and "shortness-of-breath" were acceptable synonyms [167]. He recognized that more programming would be necessary to provide syntactic tests that could help to clear up problems of a syntactic nature. Lamson, working with Jacobs and Dimsdale from IBM, went on to develop a natural-language retrieval system that contained a data dictionary for encoded reports from surgical pathology, bone-marrow examinations, autopsies, nuclear medicine, and neuroradiology, with unique numeric codes for each English word [263]. Patients' records were maintained in master text files, and new data were merged in the order of patients' medical record numbers. A set of search programs produced a document that was a computer printout of the full English text of the initial record in an unaltered, unedited form. However, Lamson recognized that more programming was necessary to clear up both semantic and syntactic problems.

In 1963 Korein and Tick at New York University Medical Center designed a method for storing physician's dictated, narrative text in a variable-length, variable-field format. The narrative data were then subjected to a program that first generated an identifier and location of every paragraph in the record. The program then reformatted the data on magnetic tape with the data content of the document converted into a list of words and a set of desired synonyms. On interrogation the program would search for the desired words or synonyms, and then would retrieve the selected text. This technique of identifying key words served as a common approach to retrieving literature documents [186–188].

Buck [46], in Lindberg's group at the University of Missouri at Columbia, described their program for retrieving patients' records from computer files that included the coded patients' discharge diagnoses, surgery reports, surgical pathology and cytology reports, and the interpretations of electrocardiograms and x-rays. The diagnoses files were stored on magnetic tape in a fixed-field format and processed by an IBM 1410 computer system. Queries were entered from punched cards containing the code numbers of the diagnoses to be retrieved. The computer searched the magnetic-tape files that in 1966 contained more than 500,000 patients' records for the diagnoses and then identified the medical-record numbers of the patients' records that contained the desired diagnoses. Lindberg [212] also developed a computer program called CONSIDER that allowed a query from a remote computer terminal to search, match, and retrieve material from the Current Medical

Terminology knowledge database that contained definitions of more than 3,000 diseases. The CONSIDER program was interactive in that it allowed the user to retrieve lists of diseases, matched by Boolean combinations of terms and sorted in a variety of ways, such as alphabetical, by frequency, or other method. The CONSIDER program accepted a set of signs, symptoms, or other medical findings and then responded by arraying a list of names of diseases that involved the set of medical findings that had been specified. Blois and associates [35] at the University of California-San Francisco expanded the program and called it RECONSIDER that was able to match diseases by parts of disease names or by phrases within definitions. Using a DEC 11/70 minicomputer with the VAX UNIX operating system, they were able to search inverted files of encoded text of Current Medical Information and Terminology (CMIT) 4th edition as the knowledge base. They concluded that RECONSIDER could be useful as a means of testing other diagnostic programs [34, 35]. Nelson and associates [255] at New York State University at Stony Brook tested various query strategies using the RECONSIDER program and reported they were unable to determine a strategy that they considered to be optimal. Anderson [8] further modified the RECONSIDER program to use it for differential diagnoses and added a time-series analysis program, an electrocardiogram signal analysis program, an x-ray images database, and a digital image analysis program.

In the 1960s commercial search and query programs for large databases became available, led by Online Analytic Processing (OLAP) that was designed to aid in providing answers to analytic queries that were multi-dimensional and used relational databases [71]. Database structures were considered to be multidimensional when they contained multiple attributes, such as time periods, locations, product codes, diagnoses, treatments, and other items that could be defined in advance and aggregated in hierarchies. The combination of all possible aggregations of the base data was expected to contain answers to every query, which could be answered from the data. Chamberlin and Boyce [52] at IBM developed the Structured Query Language (SQL) in the early 1970s (as a language designed for the query, retrieval, and management of data in a relational database-management system such as had been introduced by Codd [70]. However, Nigrin [257] noted that in general, clinicians and administrators who were not programmers could not themselves generate novel queries using OLAP or SQL. Furthermore, Connolly [76] advised that querying a relational database with SQL required developing algorithms that optimized the length of time needed for computer processing if there were many transformations for a high-level query with multiple entities, attributes, and relations. He also described a way of visualizing a multi-dimensional database by beginning with a flat file of a two-dimensional table of data. He then added another dimension to form a three-dimensional cube of data called a hypercube. He next added cubes of data within cubes of data with each side of each cube called a dimension. The result represented a multi-dimensional database. Pendse [269] described in some detail the history of OLAP and credited the publication in 1962 by Iverson of A Programming Language (APL) as the first mathematically defined, multidimensional language for processing multidimensional variables. Multidimensional analyses then became the basis for several versions of OLAP developed by IBM and others in the 1970s and 1980s. In 1999 the Analyst module in Cognos was developed and was subsequently acquired by IBM. By the year 2000 several new OLAP derivatives were in use by IBM, Microsoft, Oracle, and others.

In 1970 McDonald and associates at the Regenstrief Institute for Health Care and the Indiana University School of Medicine began to develop a clinical database for their Regenstrief Medical Record System (RMRS). Much of the clinical data was filed in a manually coded format that could be referenced to the system's data dictionary. This approach permitted each clinical subsystem to specify and define its data items. Data were entered by code, or by text that had been converted to code. The RMRS had a special retrieval program called CARE that permitted non-programmers to perform complex queries of the medical-record files. CARE programs also provided quality of care reminders, alert messages, and recommended evidence-based practice guidelines [236, 238].

Myers and associates [253] at the University of Pennsylvania reported a system in which a pathology report was translated into a series of keywords or data elements that were encoded using arbitrarily assigned numbers. While the typist entered the text of the pathology report using a typewriter controlled by a paper-tape program, the data elements were automatically coded, and a punched paper tape was produced as a by-product of the typing. The report was then stored on either magnetic tape or on a disk storage system. Karpinski and associates [177] at the Beth Israel Hospital in Boston described their Miniature Information Storage and Retrieval (MISAR) System, written in the MUMPS language for their PDP-15 computer and designed to maintain and search small collections of data on relatively inexpensive computers. MISAR was planned to deal with summaries of medical records in order to abstract correlations of clinical data. It was a flexible, easy-to-use, online system that permitted rapid manipulation of data without the need for any additional computer programming. A principal advantage of MISAR was the ease with which a small database could be created, edited, and queried at a relatively low cost. In 1972 Melski, also at the Beth Israel Hospital in Boston, used MISAR for eight registries, each consisting of a single file divided into patients' records. Each record was divided into fields that could take on one or more values. MISAR stored its patients' records in vertical files that were arranged in order of the data items as they were collected. The data were also reorganized in inverted files by data items (for example, by laboratory chemistry sodium tests) in order to be able to rapidly perform searches and manipulate simple variables. Soon the system was expanded to MISAR II with an increase in speed and able to serve simultaneously up to 22 user-terminals and to accommodate interactive analyses of multi-center studies and of large clinical trials. They were impressed with this improved capability of using a convenient terminal to rapidly perform complex searches and analyses of data from a computer database [239].

In 1973 Weyl and associates [330] at Stanford University Medical Center developed their Time Oriented Databank (TOD) system that was designed as a table-driven computer system to record and analyze medical records. The TOD system consisted of more than 60 programs, which supported data entry and data update, file definition and maintenance, and data analysis functions. The TOD system was used on a mainframe computer for the ARAMIS database. In 1982 the TOD system converted to a microcomputer-based version called MEDLOG [193].

Enlander [93] described a computer program that searched for certain pre-established key words in each diagnosis sentence according to a hierarchical structure that was based on the four-digit SNOP codes. As a test when this mode was applied to 500 diagnostic sentences, the automated key-word search then encoded about 75 % of the sentences. In the clinical information system at Kaiser Permanente in Oakland, California, Enlander used a visual-display terminal equipped with a light-pen pointer to select and enter a diagnosis, and the SNOP-coded diagnosis was then automatically displayed.

In 1976 a group at the Harvard School of Public Health developed a generalized database management system called MEDUS/A, for the kinds of data generated in the clinical-care process and also used for clinical research. Its principal mode of data acquisition and display was by the use of user-written, interactive questionnaires and reports [245]. In 1977 MEDUS/A was used at Harvard School of Public Health for a study that used data from patients with diabetes mellitus. MEDUS/A was also used for another study using data from patients with coronary artery disease. King [182, 183] reported that MEDUS/A enabled nonprogrammers to use their databases and customize their data entry, support their data queries, generate reports, and provide statistical analyses. A second version of MEDUS/A was written in Standard MUMPS language [128]. In 1983 a statistical package was added called GENESIS.

In 1976 the Division of Research Resources of the National Institutes of Health (NIH) sponsored the development of a clinical information system called CLINFO for data entry, query, retrieval, and analysis. It was developed by a consortium of computer scientists at the Rand Corporation and a group of clinical investigators at Baylor College of Medicine, University of Washington, the University of Oklahoma, and at the Vanderbilt University. Lincoln [202] at the Rand Corporation and the University of Southern California described the early CLINFO system that was used for a test group of leukemia patients. In a single, small, interactive, user-oriented system, it provided the integration of the schema, the study data file, the components designed for data entry and retrieval of time-oriented data, and a statistical analysis package. These units had been programmed separately, but their usefulness was increased by their integration. The Vanderbilt group that participated in the development of CLINFO reported on their first 5-years of experience with its use by more than 100 clinical investigators. They found that the positive and successful experience with the use of the CLINFO system was due to its set of functions directed towards data management and data analysis. They stated that CLINFO was a friendly, easy-to-use, computer tool, and that it eliminated for its users the operational problems that often had been associated with their shared central-computer resources [173, 221]. The CLINFO consortium reported a series of CLINFO-PLUS enhancements written in the C language. The system then consisted of about 100 systematically designed and closely integrated programs. A clinical investigator could specify for the computer the types of data being studied and then enter and retrieve the data in a variety of ways for display and analysis. The investigators communicated with the system by means of simple English-language word-commands, supported by a number of computer-generated prompts. The system was designed for a clinical investigator with no expertise in computing. The investigator was not required to acquire any knowledge of computing in order to use the system [318, 331]. By the end of the 1980s CLINFO was widely used for clinical research in the United States. In 1988 the NIH Division of Research Resources (DRR) listed 47 of its 78 General Clinical Research Centers as using CLINFO for multidisciplinary and multi-categorical research [258].

Some of these research centers also used a program similar to CLINFO called PROPHET that was developed in the early 1980s by Bolt, Beranek and Newman in Cambridge, Massachusetts. PROPHET allowed the use of interactive, three-dimensional graphics designed more for the use of biomedical scientists than for clinical investigators. McCormick and associates [226] in the Medical Information Systems Laboratory at the University of Illinois in Chicago described their design of a relational-structured, clinical database to store and retrieve textual data, and also pictorial information such as for computer tomography, automated cytology, and other digitized images. Their Image Memory was incorporated into an integrated database system using a PDP 11/40 minicomputer. They predicted that an image database would become a normal component of every comprehensive medical database-management system that included digital-imaging technology.

With the increasing need to be able to efficiently query larger and multiple databases, it became evident that more efficient programs were needed for querying uncoded textual data. The need was to replace the usual KWIC approach where the user would query narrative textual data by selecting what were judged to be relevant key words or phrases for the subject that the user wanted to query. The program would then search for, match, and retrieve these key words or phrases in the context in which they were found in a reference knowledge source. One approach was to expand the number of key words used to query the knowledge source in the hope those additional terms in a phrase or a sentence would allow the user to apply some semantic meaning since most English words have several meanings. This approach might improve the recognition and matching of the users' information needs and lead to better retrieval performance. In addition to query programs that permitted investigators to search and retrieve uncoded textual data from clinical databases by entering user-selected key-words or phrases, more sophisticated programs began to be developed to assist the investigator in studying medical hypotheses. More advanced NLP systems added knowledge bases to guide the user by displaying queries and their responses, and employing rules and decision trees that led to the best matching code. Although the search for matching words in a knowledge base made their retrieval easier, it was still difficult to search for and retrieve exact, meaningful expressions from text, since although it was easy to enter and store and match words, it was not always easy for the retriever to figure out what they had meant to the one who had originally entered the words into the knowledge base. Blois [33] explained the problem by saying that computers were built to process the symbols fed to them in a manner prescribed by their programs, where the meaning of the symbols was known only to the programmers, rarely to the program, and never to the computer. Consequently one could transfer everything in the data except its meaning. Blois further pointed out that the available codes rarely matched the clinical data precisely, and the user often had to force the data into categories that might not be the most appropriate. Some advanced automated NLP programs used machine-learning programs with algorithms that applied relatively simple rules such as, "if-then," to automatically "learn" from a "training" knowledge base that consisted of a large set of sentences in which each had the correct part of speech attached to each word. Rules were generated for determining the part of speech for a word in the query based on the nature of the word in the query, the nature of adjacent words, and the most likely parts of speech for the adjacent words. Some processes used more complex statistical methods that applied weights to each input item and then made probabilistic decisions and expressed relative certainty of different possible answers rather than of only one. Machine-learning programs would then need to be tested for their accuracy by applying them to query new sentences.

Doszkocs and associates [90] at the National Library of Medicine noted that rapid advances had occurred in automated information-retrieval systems for science and technology. In the year 1980 more than 1,000 databases were available for computerized searching, and more than 2-million searches were made in these databases. In the 1980s a variety of other approaches were developed for searching and querying clinical-research databases that were linked to patient care databases. Kingsland's [184] Research Database System (RDBS) used microcomputers for storing and searching a relatively large number of observations in a relatively small number of patients' records. Shapiro [303] at the Medical University of South Carolina developed a System for Conceptual Analysis of Medical Practices (SCAMP) that was able to respond to a query expressed in natural language. Words in free-text, rather than in codes, were used, such as "Which patients had a prolapsed mitral valve?" The program parsed the request that was expressed in English. It looked up relevant matching words in a thesaurus and passed linguistic and procedural information found in the thesaurus to a general-purpose retrieval routine that identified the relevant patients based on the free-text descriptions. Miller's System 1022 could access and query relational databases [244]. Dozier [91] used a commercial Statistical Analysis System (SAS) database. Katz [179] reported developing the Clinical Research System (CRS) that was a specialized, database-management system intended for storing and managing patient data collected for clinical trials and designed for the direct use by physicians.

Porter [270], Safran [289], and associates [290, 291] at the Boston's Beth Israel Hospital, the Brigham and Women's Hospital, and the Harvard Medical School, in 1964, expanded the Paper Chase program into a program called ClinQuery that was designed to allow physicians to perform searches in a large clinical database. ClinQuery was written in a dialect of MUMPS and was used to search their ClinQuery database, which contained selected patient data that was de-identified to protect patient's privacy. The data was transferred automatically every night from the hospital clinical information systems.

Adams [1] compared three query languages commonly used in the 1980s for medical-database systems:

- The Medical Query Language (MQL) that was developed by Barnett's group with an objective of query and report generation for patients using the Computer-Stored Ambulatory Record (COSTAR), and MQL was portable to any database using the MUMPS language. At that date COSTAR was used in more than 100 sites worldwide, with some carrying 200,000 patient records online.
- The CARE System that was developed by McDonald's group, with a focus on surveillance of quality of ambulatory patient care and contained more than 80,000 patients' records. CARE was programmed in VAX BASIC running on a DEC VAX computer.
- The HELP (Health Evaluation through Logical Processing) System that was developed by H. Warner's group, with a focus on surveillance of hospital patient care was implemented on a Tandem system operating in the Latter Day Saints (LDS) hospitals in Utah.

Adams reported that the three programs had some common properties, yet used different designs that focused on the specific objectives for which each was developed. Adams concluded that each was successful and well used.

Broering and associates [42, 43] at Georgetown Medical Center described their BioSYNTHESIS system that was developed as a NLM IAIMS research project. The objective of the project was to develop a front-end software system that could retrieve information that was stored in disparate databases and computer systems. In 1987 they developed BioSYNTHESIS/I as a gateway system with a single entry pointing into IAIMS databases to make it easier for users to access selected multiple databases. BioSYNTHESIS/II was developed to function as an information finder that was capable of responding to a user's queries for specific information and to be able to search composite knowledge systems containing disparate components of information. The system therefore had to be capable of functioning independently with the various knowledge bases that required different methods to access and search them.

Hammond [141] reported that a program called QUERY was written to permit users to access any data stored in Duke's The Medical Record (TMR) database. The program could access each patient's record in the entire database or in a specified list of records and carry out the query. The time for a typical query run, depending on the complexity of the query, was reported to require 4–6 h on a database containing 50,000–100,000 patients. Prather [272] reported that by 1990 the Duke group had converted their legacy databases into relational-structured databases so that personal computers using the SQL language could more readily query all of the patients' records in the TMR clinical databases. By 1995 they had accumulated 25 years of patient data.

Frisse [116], Cousins and associates [78] at Washington University School of Medicine described a program they developed to enhance their ability to query textual data in large, medical, hypertext systems. As the amount of text in a database increased, they considered it likely that the proportion of text that would be relevant to their query would decrease. To improve the likelihood of finding relevant responses to a query, they defined a query network as one that consisted of a set of nodes in the network represented by weighted search terms considered to be relevant to their query. They assigned a weight to each search term in the query network based on their estimate of the conditional probability that the search term was relevant to the primary index subject of their query; and the search term's weight could be further modified by user feedback to improve the likelihood of its relevance to the query. Searches were then initiated based on the relative search term weights; and they concluded that their approach could aid in information retrieval and also assist in the discovery of related new information. Frisse [115] emphasized that information relevant to a task must be separated from information that is not considered relevant, and defined the relevance of a retrieved set of documents in terms of recall and precision. Frisse defined recall as the percentage of all relevant items in a collection retrieved in response to a query and defined precision as the percentage of items retrieved that were relevant to the query. He defined sensitivity as the percentage of true positives that were identified; and specificity as the percentage of true negatives that were identified. He also noted that if the query statement were widened by including an additional search term using the word, "or", then one was more likely to retrieve additional items of interest but was also more likely to retrieve items not relevant to the specific query. Also, if one increased the number of constraints to a query by using the word, "and", then one would retrieve fewer items but the items retrieved were more likely to be relevant to the expanded query.

Levy [200] described an approach to NLP that was used at that time in the Veteran's Administration (VA). Commercial Natural Language Incorporated (NLI) software was the NLP interface that allowed English queries to be made of the VA database. Software links between the NLP program and the VA database defined relationships, entities, attributes, and their interrelationships, and queries about these concepts were readily answered. When a user typed in a question, the NLP processor interpreted the question, translated it into an SQL query and then responded. If the query was not understood by the NLP system, it then guided the user and assisted in generating a query that could be answered.

Das and Musen [82] at Stanford University compared three data-manipulation methods for temporal querying by the consensus query representation, Arden Syntax, SQL, and the temporal query language, TimeLineSQL (TLSQL). They concluded that TLSQL was the query method most expressive for temporal data. They built a system called Synchronus that had the ability to query their legacy SQL databases that supported various data time-stamping methods. O'Connor [262] also noted that querying clinical databases often had temporal problems when clinical data was not time-stamped, such as when a series of laboratory test reports did not provide the time-intervals between the tests. They developed a temporal query system called Tzolkin that provided a temporal query language and a temporal abstraction system that helped when dealing with temporal indeterminacy and temporal abstraction of data.

Schoch [300] compared four commercial NLP systems that were reported to be used for searching natural-language text in MEDLINE: FreeStyle (FS) from Lexis-

Nexis; Physicians Online (POL); Target on Dialog (TA) from Knight-Ridder; and Knowledge Finder (KF) available from Aries only on CD-ROM. In one day in 1995, 36 topics were searched, using similar terms, directly on NLM's MEDLINE, and the first 25 ranked references from each search were selected for analysis. They found that all four systems agreed on the best references for only one topic. Three systems – FS, KF, and TA – chose the same first reference, and POL ranked it second. The 4 searches found 12 unique references with all concepts matching. Clinical experts often based the evaluation of NLP systems on comparing their individual outputs for completeness of recall and for accuracy in matching of specified criteria and sometimes as compared with the "gold-standard" of manual output. However, given a set of criteria, human evaluation was often found to be more variable in its results than computer evaluation.

Conceptual approaches to querying large, complex medical databases were developed in the 1990s and were based on combining the characteristics of the query subject and creating a conceptual model for the search, rather than just using key words and phrases. From this approach, ontologies of concepts and relationships of medical knowledge began to be developed. Chute and associates [60] at the Mayo Clinic in Rochester, Minnesota, reported updating their legacy 4.6 million, paper-based, patient record Master Sheets that dated back to 1909. With the addition of their newer electronic clinical database, their researchers were confronted with more than 200 clinical specialized databases that resided on various hardware and used a variety of software. They needed to interface these disparate databases on a spectrum of platforms to many types of workstations using a variety of browsers. To meet these problems and facilitate the retrieval of their stored medical information, they introduced Web protocols, graphical browsers, and several versions of Hypertext Mark-up Language (HTML) to link to their computer server. They also used the high-level language, Perl, which supported SQL interfaces to a number of relational-structured databases. They used Perl interfaces for dynamically generated HTML screens. They also observed the legal need for maintaining the security and confidentiality of patient data when using the Web.

Hersh [149–155] and associates at Oregon Health Sciences University outlined their requirements for clinical vocabularies in order to facilitate their use with natural language processing (NLP) systems for their electronic medical records. The requirements should include lexical decomposition to allow the meaning of individual words to be recognized in the context of the entire sentence; semantic typing to allow for identification of synonyms and their translation across semantic equivalence classes; and compositional extensibility to allow words to be combined to generate new concepts. They addressed the problem of accessing documents with desired clinical information when using the Web with its highly distributed information sources. They reported developing an information retrieval system called SAPHIRE (Semantic and Probabilistic Heuristic Information Retrieval Environment). SAPHIRE was modified from NLM's UMLS Metathesaurus, which had been created by NLM to allow translation between terms within different medical vocabularies. SAPHIRE provided a Concept-Matching Algorithm that processed strings of free text to find concepts and then mapped the concepts into a semantic-network structure for the purposes of providing both automated indexing and probabilistic retrieval by matching the diverse expressions of concepts present in both the reference documents and in the users' queries. For the purpose of indexing, each textual document was processed one sentence at a time. Its concepts were weighted for terms occurring frequently, thereby designating a term's value as an indexing concept. In retrieval the user's query was processed to obtain its concepts, which were then matched against the indexing concepts in the reference documents in order to obtain a weighted list of matching documents. To formulate a search with SAPHIRE, the user entered a free-text query and received back a list of concepts, to which the user could delete or add concepts. The search was then initiated. A score was calculated summing the weights for all the concepts, and the concepts with highest scores were ranked for first retrievals. Hersh [152, 153] reported a series of modifications to their concept-matching, indexing algorithm to improve the sensitivity and specificity of its automated retrievals. He also completed some evaluations of recall and precision of automated information-retrieval systems compared to traditional key-word retrieval using text-words, and suggested that it was uncertain as to whether one indexing or retrieval method was superior to another. Spackman and Hersh [310] evaluated the ability of SAPHIRE to do automatic searches for noun phrases in medical record discharge summaries by matching terms from SNOMED and reported matches for 57 % of the phrases. They also reported evaluating the ability of two NLP parsers, called CLARIT and the Xerox Tagger, to identify simple noun phrases in medical discharge summaries. They reported exact matches for 77 % and 69 %, respectively, of the phrases.

Hersh [155] also reported developing CliniWeb, a searchable database of clinical information on the Web that provided a database of clinically-oriented Universal Resource Locators (URLs), an index of URLs with terms from the NLM's MeSH vocabulary, and an interface for accessing URLs by browsing and searching. He described problems due to Web databases being highly distributed and lacking an overall index for all of its information. CliniWeb served as a test bed for research into defining the optimal method to build and evaluate a clinically oriented Web resource. The user could browse the MeSH hierarchy or search for MeSH terms using free-text queries and then rapidly access the URLs associated with those terms. Hersh [150] noted that SAPHIRE could query a database in seven languages other than English by using a dictionary based on the multilingual aspects of the NLM's UMLS Metathesaurus. He also observed that in addition to the NLM, other health related federal agencies used the Web for dissemination of free information, including the Centers for Disease Control and Prevention (CDC), the Food and Drug Administration (FDA), and the National Cancer Institute (NCI). Zacks [341] and Munoz [249], also working with Hersh, studied a variety of search strategies for retrieving medical review articles from Web hypertext medical documents. He found a great variation in their sensitivity and specificity for accurately retrieving review articles on clinical diagnosis and therapy and noted that the more complex strategies had higher accuracy rates. Price [279], also associated with Hersh, described developing Smart Query that could provide context-sensitive links from the electronic medical record (EMR) to relevant medical-knowledge sources. Smart

Query could help the clinician find answers to questions arising while using a patient's EMR.

Cimino et al. [67] reviewed some methods for information retrieval reported in the 1990s. Some methods were used to provide the retrieval of medical information from multiple sources such as from clinical databases and from medical bibliographic resources, and some used NLM's Unified Medical Language System (UMLS) for retrieving medical information by online bibliographic searches and then integrating the information into their clinical databases. They concluded that additional work was needed to better understand the information needs of different users in different settings. The work needed to satisfy those needs through more sophisticated selection and use of information resources, translate concepts from clinical applications to information resources, and better integrate the users' systems. They noted that although early database management systems allowed only their own data applications to be accessible from their own computer terminals. As they developed more advanced approaches, they sought to integrate outside information sources at the application level so that patient data could be used for realtime literature retrieval. An instant of this application might be when an abnormal laboratory test raised questions that could be answered by a search of medical literature.

In 1998 physicians at Vanderbilt University Hospital began to use their locally developed, computer-based, free-text summary report system that facilitated the entry of a limited data summary report for the discharge or transfer of patients. They reported that two datasets were most commonly used for these summaries: (1) patients' treatment items that comprised summaries of clinical care, in addition to patient's awareness and action items; and (2) care coordination items that included patients' discharge and contact information and any social concerns. They recommended formalizing and standardizing the various clinical specialty data patterns to reduce the variability of the summary sign-out notes and to improve the communication of patient information [50]. Zeng and Cimino [343] evaluated the development of concept-oriented views of natural-language text in electronic medical records (EMRs). They also addressed the problem of "information overload" that often resulted when an excess of computer-generated, but unrelated, information was retrieved after clinical queries were entered when using EMRs. They compared the retrieval system's ability to identify relevant patient data and generate either concept-oriented views or traditional clinical views of the original text; and they reported that concept-oriented views contained significantly less non-relevant information; and when responding to queries about EMR's, using concept-oriented views showed a significantly greater accuracy in relevant information retrieval.

Hogarth and associates [160] at the University of California in Davis introduced Terminology Query Language (TQL) as a query language interface to server implementations of concept-oriented terminologies. They observed that terminology systems generally lacked standard methodologies for providing terminology support, and TQL defined a query-based mechanism for accessing terminology information from one or more terminology servers over a network connection. They described TQL to be a declarative language that specified what to get rather than how to get it, and it was relatively easy to use as a query language interface that enabled simple extraction of terminology information from servers implementing concept-oriented terminology systems. They cited as a common example of another query language interface, SQL, for relational databases. TQL allowed the data structures and names for terminology-specific data types to be mapped to an abstract set of structures with intuitively familiar names and behaviors. The TQL specification was based on a generic entity-relationship (E/R) schema for concept-based terminology systems. TQL provided a mechanism for operating on groups of 'concepts' or 'terms' traversing the information space defined by a particular concept-to-concept relationship, and extracted attributes for a particular entity in the terminology. TQL output was structured in XML that provided a transfer format back to the system requesting the terminology information.

Seol et al. [301] noted that it was often difficult for users to express their information needs clearly enough to retrieve relevant information from a computer database system. They took an approach based on a knowledge base that contained patterns of information needs. They provided conceptual guidance with a question-oriented interaction based on the integration of multiple query contexts, such as application, clinical, and document contexts, based on a conceptual-graph model and using XML language. Mendonca [240] also reviewed NLP systems and examined the role that standardized terminologies could play in the integration between a clinical system and literature resources, as well as in the information retrieval process. By helping clinicians to formulate well-structured clinical queries and to include relevant information from individual patient's medical records, they hoped to enhance information retrieval to improve patient care by developing a model that identified relevant information themes and added a framework of evidence-based practice guidelines.

Borlawsky et al. [41] reviewed semantic-processing approaches to NLP for generating integrated data sets from published biomedical literature. They reported using BioMedLEE and a subset of PhenoGo algorithms to extract, with a high degree of precision, encoded concepts and determine relationships among a body of PubMed abstracts of published cancer and genetics literature, with a high degree of precision.

Lacson [190] described the use of mobile phones to enter into their computer in natural language time-stamped, spoken, dietary records collected from adult patients over a period of a few weeks. They classified the food items and the food quantifiers and developed a dietary/nutrient knowledge base with added information from resources on food types, food preparation, food combinations, portion sizes, and with dietary details from the dietary/nutrient resource database of 4,200 individual foods reported in the U.S. Department of Agriculture's Continuing Survey of Food Intakes by Individuals (CSFII). They then developed an algorithm to extract the dietary information from their patients' dietary records and to automatically map selected items to their dietary/nutrient knowledge database. They reported 90 % accuracy in the automatic processing of the spoken dietary records.

Informatics for Integrating Biology & the Bedside (i2b2) was established in 2004 as a Center at the Partners HealthCare System in Boston, with the sponsorship of the NIH National Centers for Biomedical Computing. It was directed by Kohane,

Glaser, and Churchill (https://www.i2b2.org). Murphy [248] described i2b2 as capable of serving a variety of clients by providing an inter-operable framework of software modules, called the i2b2 Hive, to store, query, and retrieve very large groups of de-identified patient data, including a natural language processing (NLP) program. The i2b2 Hive used applications in units, called cells, which were managed by the i2b2 Workbench. The i2b2 Hive was an open-source software platform for managing medical-record data for purposes of research. The i2b2 had an architecture that was based upon loosely coupled, document-style Web services for researchers to use for their own data, with adequate safeguards to protect the confidentiality of patient data that was stored in a relational database that was able to fuse with other i2b2 compliant repositories. It thereby provided a very large, integrated, data-repository for studies of very large patient groups. The i2b2 Workbench consisted of a collection of users' "plug-ins" that was contained within a loosely coupled visual framework, in which the independent plug-ins from various user teams of developers could fit together. The plug-ins provided the manner in which users interfaced with the other cells of the Hive. When a cell was developed, a plug-in could then be used to support its operations [59]. McCormick and associates [227] at Columbia University in New York reported that in response to an i2b2 team's challenge for using textual data in patients' discharge summaries for testing automated classifiers for the status of smokers (as a current smoker, non-smoker, past smoker, or status unknown), they investigated the effect of semantic features extracted from clinical notes for classifying a patient's smoking status and compared the performance of supervised classifiers to rule-based symbolic classifiers. They compared the performance of a symbolic rule-based classifier, which relied on semantic features (generated by MedLEE), a supervised classifier that relied on semantic features, and a supervised classifier that relied only on lexical features. They concluded that classifiers with semantic features were superior to purely lexical approaches; and that the automated classification of a patient's smoking status was technically feasible and was clinically useful.

Himes and associates [156] at Harvard Medical School and Partners HealthCare System, reported using the i2b2 natural language processing (NLP) program to extract both coded data and unstructured textual notes from more than 12,000 electronic patient records for research studies on patients with bronchial asthma. They found that the data extracted by this means was suitable for such research studies of large patient populations. Yang and associates [339] used the i2b2 NLP programs to extract textual information from clinical discharge summaries and to automatically identify the status of patients with a diagnosis of obesity and 15 related co-morbidities. They assembled a knowledge base with lexical, terminological, and semantic features to profile these diseases and their associated symptoms and treatments. They applied a data mining approach to the discharge summaries of 507 patients, which combined knowledge-based lookup and rule-based methods. They reported 97 % accuracy in predictions of disease status, which was comparable to that of humans. Ware and colleagues [325] also used the i2b2 NLP programs to focus on extracting diagnoses of obesity and 16 related diagnoses from textual discharge summary reports. They reported better than 90 % agreement with clinical experts as the comparative "gold standard."

Kementsietsidis and associates [180] at the IBM Watson Research Center developed an algorithm to help when querying clinical records to identify patients with a defined set of medical conditions, called a "conditions profile," that was required for a patient to have in order to be eligible to participate in a clinical trial or a research study. They described the usual selection process which was to first query the database and identify an initial pool of candidate patients whose medical conditions matched the conditions profile and then to manually review the medical records of each of these candidates. They would then identify the most promising patients for the study. Since that first step could be complicated and very time-consuming in a very large patient database if one used simple keyword searches for a large number of selection criteria in a conditions profile, they developed an algorithm that identified compatibilities and incompatibilities between the conditions in the profile. Through a series of computational steps the program created a new conditions profile and returned to the researcher a smaller list of patients who satisfied the revised conditions profile. This new list of patients could then be manually reviewed for those suited for the study.

Meystre and Haug [241, 243] at the University of Utah described their development of a NLP system to automatically analyze patients' longitudinal electronic patient records (EPRs) and to ease for clinicians the formation of a patient's medical-problem list. They developed from the patients' problem-oriented medical records in their Intermountain Health Care program a problem list of about 60,000 concepts. Using this as a knowledge base, their Medical Problem Model identified and extracted from the narrative text in an active patient's EMR, a list of the potential medical problems. Then a Medical Document Model used a problem-list management application to form a problem list that could be useful for the physician. In the Intermountain Health Care program that used their HELP program, the objective was to use this NLP system to automate the development of problem lists and to automatically update and maintain them for the longitudinal care of both ambulatory and hospital patients. Meystre [242] also reported installing and evaluating an i2b2 Hive for airway diseases including bronchial asthma and reported that it was possible to query the structured data in patients' electronic records with the i2b2 Workbench for about half of the desired clinical data elements. Since smoking status was typically mentioned only in clinical notes, they used their natural language processing (NLP) program in the i2b2 NLP cell. They found the automated extraction of patients' smoking status had a mean sensitivity of 0.79 and a mean specificity of 0.90.

Childs [58] described using ClinREAD, a rule-based natural language processing (NLP) system, developed by Lockheed Martin, to participate in the i2b2 Obesity Challenge program to build software that could query and retrieve data from patients' clinical discharge summaries and make judgments as to whether the patients had, or did not have, obesity and any of 15 comorbidities (including asthma, coronary artery disease, diabetes, and others). They developed an algorithm with a comprehensive set of rules that defined word-patterns to be searched for in the text as literal text-strings (called 'features'), that were grouped to form word lists that were then matched in the text for the presence of any of the specified disease comorbidities. Fusaro and associates [117] at Harvard Medical School reported transferring electronic medical records from more than 8,000 patients into an i2b2 database using Web services. Gainer [122, 344] and associates from Partners Healthcare System, Massachusetts General Hospital, Brigham and Women's Hospital, and the University of Utah described their methods for using i2b2 to help researchers query and analyze both coded and textual clinical data that were contained in electronic patient records. Using data from the records of patients with rheumatoid arthritis, the collaborating investigators were required to develop new concepts and methods to query and analyze the data, to add new vocabulary items and intermediate data-processing steps, and to do some custom programming.

Wynden [336, 337] and associates at the University of California, San Francisco (UCSF), described their Integrated Data Repository (IDR) project that contained various collections of clinical, biomedical, economic, administrative, and public health data. Since standard data warehouse design was usually difficult for researchers who needed access to a wide variety of data resources, they developed a translational infrastructure they called OntoMapper that translated terminologies into formal data-encoding standards without altering the underlying source data, OntoMapper also provided syntactic and semantic interoperability for the grid-computing environments on the i2b2 platform, and they thereby facilitated sharing data from different resources. Sim [306] and associates from UCSF and several other medical institutions employed translational informatics and reported their collaboration in the Human Studies Database (HSDB) Project to develop semantic and data-sharing technologies to federate descriptions of human studies. Their priorities for sharing human-studies data included (1) research characterization of populations such as by outcome variables, (2) registration of studies into the database ClinicalTrials.gov, and (3) facilitating translational research collaborations. They used UCSF's OntoMapper to standardize data elements from the i2b2 data model. They shared data using the National Cancer Institute's caGrid technologies.

Zhang and associates [345] at Case Western Reserve and University of Michigan developed a query interface for clinical research they called Visual Aggregator and Explorer (VISAGE) that incorporated three interrelated components: Query Builder with ontology-driven terminology support; Query Manager that stored and labeled queries for reuse and sharing; and Query Explorer for comparative analyses of query results.

Together these components helped with efficient query construction, query sharing, and data exploration. They reported that in their experience VISAGE was more efficient for query construction than the i2b2 Web client. Logan and associates [216] at Oregon Health and Portland State Universities reviewed the use of graphical-user interfaces to query a variety of multi-database systems, with some using SQL or XML languages and others having been designed with an entity-attribute-value (EAV) schema. They reported using Web Ontology Language (OWL) to query, select, and extract desired fields of data from these multiple data sources; and then to re-classify, re-modify, and re-use the data for their specific needs.

3.5   Summary and Commentary

Levy [197] observed that in the 1950s computers had introduced the information age. Yet in the 1950s patients' medical records were still paper-based and were stored in stacks of charts on shelves in a medical record room. In the early 1960s the development of computers began to allow patient care data to be entered into a computer by using punched paper cards. Data were stored and accessed sequentially in computer flat files that had little structured relationships, and they were aggregated in file-management systems. In the late 1960s structured computer databases began to evolve with associated database management systems, and hospital information systems (HISs) began to be developed using large mainframe computers with random-access disc storage to provide integrated databases that serviced all clinical departments. It was soon found that although a single, large, mainframe computer could readily integrate patient data into a single database, it could not adequately support the information processing requirements for all of the clinical specialty and ancillary services in a large medical center.

In the 1970s the advent of minicomputers permitted many hospital services to have their subsystems' databases directly linked to a central mainframe computer that integrated all patients' data into the patients' clinical records that were stored in the mainframe computer's database [18, 19]. Some patient data were manually encoded before being entered into the database to facilitate billing for payments of claims and for the retrieval of data for management and clinical research purposes. In the 1970s distributed database systems began to be developed, and in the following decades the development of increasingly large and enhanced medical databases was phenomenal.

In the 1980s a diffusion of minicomputers and microcomputers were incorporated into a variety of medical applications. Microcomputer-based systems that had evolved independently for specialized clinical and ancillary services usually became subsystems of larger medical information systems with an integrating central database management system. Storage technology improved, storage devices became cheaper and larger. Registries grew in size to become databases. Databases became data warehouses and a great variety of secondary clinical databases evolved. It was not until the 1980s, when microcomputers became internalized into the popular culture of the United States, that computers became commonly accepted working tools. Van Brunt [320] observed that despite the increasing use of computer technology, there were not yet any noteworthy effects of computers on a physician's mode of practice.

The conversion of natural language English words into a language understandable by a computer was an essential functional and technical requirement since computer applications in all medical specialties and for all health care providers needed to be able to communicate with computers in order to enter, store, retrieve, and manipulate patient data. Accordingly, NLP needed to be developed for retrieving and understanding unstructured data from patients' medical histories and physical examination data, from nursing notes, from operative notes describing surgery, pathology, and other procedures, from diagnostic interpretations of x-rays and electrocardiograms, and from all clinical laboratory test re diagnostic and therapeutic procedures ordered for and received by a patient. English words were entered by typewriter-like keyboard, either encoded or in natural language and later by spoken words.

In the 1990s international communications used computers and local-area networks, and the use of the Internet and the World Wide Web became commonplace. As patient care data expanded in both volume and complexity, frequent innovations in informatics technology provided more efficient computer-based, clinical-information systems in hospitals and in medical offices. Lincoln [203] reviewed the important contributions of computing to medical care and to medical research and observed that there still existed the challenge to formulate appropriate computer logics to properly relate descriptions of disease, rules for medical practice, and general guidelines for health care delivery.

In the 2000s distributed information systems allowed physicians to enter orders and retrieve test results using clinical workstations connected to client-server computers in local-area-networks that linked multiple medical center databases. Hartzband [143] noted that nothing had changed clinical practice more fundamentally than did the Internet, since it provided easily retrieved information by physicians for clinical decision support and by patients in search of self-diagnoses and better understanding of their diseases and of their prescribed therapy. The Internet and the Web not only changed profoundly personal communication between the doctor and the patient but also made possible the global exchange of clinical data and medical knowledge between multiple information sources. In the 2010s federal support greatly increased the use of computer-based electronic patient records (EPRs). Global wireless communications with cloud storage for translational networks evolved that linked data warehouses in collaborating medical centers in the nation; and mobile e-health care for the individual patient.

Through these six decades, the complexity of computer applications greatly increased. More commercial software packages came to market, and software costs became a greater proportion of total computing costs. The development of efficient computer-stored databases was essential for many medical computing applications. Users found it more economical to obtain commercial application programs ("apps") that were packaged to perform specific, commonly needed functions than to develop such programs directly themselves. Specialized commercial application programs included databases, word processing programs, and spreadsheets for tabular processing of numerical data. It became less necessary for the users of such software to know how to program a computer themselves. Information communication systems grew to service large medical centers with all of their inpatient and outpatient clinical departments that included internal medicine, surgery, pediatrics, obstetrics, gynecology, pathology, clinical laboratory, radiology, and others. The great variety of medical applications required a complex, computer-based, information system that communicated data to and from all of the various clinical subsystems.

Since the early 1900s physicians have followed the teachings of the famed clinician, William Osler, to study and learn from their patients and from the medical records of their patients, in order to improve their knowledge of diseases. The process of physician-patient interaction still follows the basic system described at the beginning of this chapter. Technology, however, has added significant new capabilities to aid in decision making and to acquire new knowledge.

References

1. Adams LB. Three surveillance and query languages. MD Comput. 1986;3:11–9.
2. Addison CH, Blackwell PW, Smith WE. GYPSY: general information processing system remote terminal users guide. Norman: University of Oklahom; 1969.
3. Anderson JG, Schweer HM. Physician communication networks and the adoption and utilization of computer applications in medicine. In: Anderson JG, Jay SJ, editors. Use and impact of computers in clinical medicine. New York: Springer; 1987. p. 185–99.
4. Anderson JG, Jay SJ. Computers and clinical judgment: the role of physician networks. Soc Sci Med. 1985;20:969–79.
5. Anderson JG, Jay SJ, Perry J, Anderson MM. Diffusion of computer applications among physicians. In: Salamon R, Protti D, Moehr J, editors. Proc int symp med informatics and education. Victoria: University of Victoria; 1989. p. 339–2.
6. Anderson JG, Jay SJ, Anderson MM, Schweer HM. Why do doctors use computers? Proc AAMSI. 1988;109–13.
7. Anderson JG, Jay SJ, Hackman EM. The role of physician networks in the diffusion of clinical applications of computers. Int J Biomed Comput. 1983;14:195–202.
8. Anderson JG, Jay SJ, Anderson M, Hunt TJ. Evaluating the potential effectiveness of using computerized information systems to prevent adverse drug events. Proc AMIA. 1997;228–32.
9. Anderson RJ, Young WW. Microcomputers as a management tool for hospital pharmacy directors. Proc SCAMC. 1984;231–3.
10. ASTM. Standard specifications for transferring clinical laboratory data messages between independent computer systems. E-1238-88. Philadelphia: American Society for Testing Materials; 1988.
11. ASTM. Standard specifications for transferring clinical observations between independent computer systems. E-1238-88. Philadelphia: American Society for Testing Materials; 1989.
12. Baker RL. An adaptable interactive system for medical and research data management. Methods Inf Med. 1974;13:209.
13. Bakken S, Hyun S, Friedman C, Johnson S. A comparison of semantic categories of the ISO reference terminology models for nursing and the MedLEE natural language processing system. Stud Health Technol Inform. 2003;107:472–6.
14. Bakken S, Hyun S, Friedman C, Johnson S. A comparison of semantic categories of the ISO reference terminology models for nursing and the MedLEE natural language processing system. Proc MEDINFO. 2004;472–6.
15. Ball M. Review of hospital information system approaches. Proc AAMSI. 1982;267–9.
16. Ball M. Medical information systems in the USA, 1980. In: Gremy F, Degoulet P, Barber B, Salamon R, editors. Proc med informatics Europe 1981. New York: Springer; 1981. p. 22–32.
17. Ball M, Snelbecker GE. How physicians in the U.S. perceive computers in their practice. Proc MEDINFO. 1983;1169–72.
18. Ball MJ, Hammon GL. Overview of computer applications in a variety of health care areas. CRC Crit Rev Bioeng. 1975;2:183–203.
19. Ball MJ, Hammon GL. Maybe a network of mini-computers can fill your data systems needs. Hosp Financ Manage. 1975;29:48–51.
20. Barnett GO. Computers in patient care. N Engl J Med. 1968;279:1321–7.

21. Barnett GO, Castleman PA. A time-sharing computer system for patient-care activities. Comput Biomed Res. 1967;1:41–51.
22. Barnett GO, Baruch JJ. Hospital computer project. Memorandum Eight. 1st ed. Boston: Massachusetts General Hospital; 1965.
23. Barnett GO. In: Collen MF, editor. Massachusetts general hospital computer system. New York: Wiley; 1974.
24. Barnett GO. The modular hospital information system. In: Stacy RW, Waxman BD, editors. Computers in biomedical research, vol. IV. New York: Academic; 1974. p. 243–5.
25. Barnett GO. The use of computers in clinical data management: the ten commandments. American Medical Association symposium on computers in medicine. AMA: Washington, DC;1970.
26. Barnett GO, Greenes RA. High level programming languages. Comput Biomed Res. 1970;3:488–94.
27. Barnett GO, Greenes RA, Grossman JH. Computer processing of medical text information. Methods Inf Med. 1969;8:177–82.
28. Barrows Jr RC, Busuioc M, Friedman C. Limited parsing of notational text visit notes: ad-hoc vs. NLP approaches. Proc AMIA. 2000;51–5.
29. Benson T. Principles of health interoperability HL7 and SNOMED. London: Springer; 2010.
30. Best WR. The potential role of computers in medical practice. JAMA. 1962;182:994–1000.
31. Bishop CW. A name is not enough. MD Comput. 1989;6:200–6.
32. Blois MS. Medical records and clinical data bases. What is the difference? Proc AMIA. 1982;86–9.
33. Blois MS. The physician's information environment. Proc SCAMC. 1984;86–8.
34. Blois MS. Medical records and clinical databases: what is the difference? MD Comput. 1983;1:24–8.
35. Blois MS, Tuttle MS, Sherertz DD. RECONSIDER: a program for generating differential diagnoses. Proc SCAMC. 1981;263–8.
36. Blum BI. A history of computers. In: Blum B, editor. Clinical information systems. New York: Springer; 1986. p. 1–32.
37. Blum BI. Design methods for clinical systems. Proc SCAMC. 1986;309–15.
38. Blum BI. A data model for patient management. Proc MEDINFO. 1983;83:748–51.
39. Blum BI. Clinical information systems. New York: Springer; 1986.
40. Blum BI. Information systems for patient care. New York: Springer; 1984.
41. Borlawsky TB, Li J, Shagina L, Crowson MG, Liu Y, Friedman C, et al. Evaluation of an ontology-anchored natural language-based approach for asserting multi-scale biomolecular networks for systems medicine. Proc AMIA TBI. 2010;6–10.
42. Broering NC, Potter J, Mistry P. Linking bibliographic and infomation databases: an IAIMS prototype. Proc AAMSI. 1987;169–73.
43. Broering NC, Bagdoyan H, Hylton J, Strickler J. Biosynthesis: integrating multiple databases into a virtual database. Proc SCAMC. 1989;360–4.
44. Brown B, Harbort B, Kaplan B, Maxwell J. Guidelines for managing the implementation of automated medical systems. Proc SCAMC. 1981;935–41.
45. Bryan M. The year of the data base. Personal Comput. 1988;12:100–9.
46. Buck CR, Reese GR, Lindberg DA. A general technique for computer processing of coded patient diagnoses. Missouri Med. 1966;63:276. 9 passim.
47. Caceres CA. Large versus small, single versus multiple computers. Comput Biomed Res. 1970;3:445–52.
48. Campbell KE, Cohn SP, Chute CG, Rennels G, Shortliffe EH. Galapagos: computer-based support for evolution of a convergent medical terminology. Proc AMIA. 1996;26–7.
49. Campbell KE, Cohn SP, Chute CG, Shortliffe EH, Rennels G. Scalable methodologies for distributed development of logic-based convergent medical terminology. Methods Inf Med. 1998;37:426–39.
50. Campion TR, Weinberg ST, Lorenzi NM, Waitman LR. Evaluation of computerized free text sign-out notes: baseline understanding and recommendations. Appl Clin Inform. 2010;1:304–17.

51. Cao H, Chiang MF, Cimino JJ, Friedman C, Hripcsak G. Automatic summarization of patient discharge summaries to create problem lists using medical language processing. Proc MEDINFO. 2004;1540.
52. Chamberlin DD, Boyce RF. SEQUEL: a structured English query language. Proc of the 1974 ACM SIGFIDET (now SIGMOD) workshop on data description, access and control 1974;249–64.
53. CHCT. Assessment: IOM study of the medical record. Newsletter of the Council on Health Care Technology. IOM-NAS; September 1989:2.
54. Chen ES, Hripcsak G, Friedman C. Disseminating natural language processed clinical narratives. Proc AMIA Annu Symp. 2006;126–30.
55. Chen ES, Hripcsak G, Xu H, Markatou M, Friedman C. Automated acquisition of disease-drug knowledge from biomedical and clinical documents: an initial study. JAMIA. 2008;15:87–98.
56. Childs BW. Future of information system technology. USHealthcare. 1989;6:8–9.
57. Childs BW. Bedside terminals: status and the future. Healthc Comput Commun. 1988;5:12–4.
58. Childs LC, Enelow R, Simonsen L, Heintzelman NH, Kowalski KM, Taylor RJ. Description of a rule-based system for the i2b2 challenge in natural language processing for clinical data. JAMIA. 2009;16:571–5.
59. Chueh HC, Murphy S. The i2b2 hive and clinical research chat. Informatics for integrating biology and the bedside. National Centers for Biomedical Computing. Washington, DC: National Institutes of Health; 2006. p. 1–58.
60. Chute CC, Crowson DL, Bluntrock JD, Crowson DL. Medical information retrieval and WWW browsers at Mayo. Proc AMIA. 1995;68–73.
61. Chute CG, Elkin PL, Sheretz DD, Tuttle MS. Desiderata for a clinical terminology server. Proc AMIA. 1999;42–6.
62. Chute CG. The Copernican era of healthcare terminology: a re-centering of health information systems. Proc AMIA. 1998;68–73.
63. Cimino JJ, Socratous SA, Grewal R. The informatics superhighway: prototyping on the World Wide Web. Proc AMIA. 1995;111–6.
64. Cimino JJ. From data to knowledge through concept-oriented terminologies experience with the medical entities dictionary. JAMIA. 2000;7:288–97.
65. Cimino JJ. Desiderata for controlled medical vocabularies in the twenty-first century. Methods Inf Med. 1998;37:394.
66. Cimino JJ, Barnett GO. Automated translation between medical terminologies using semantic definitions. MD Comput. 1990;7:104–9.
67. Cimino JJ, Clayton PD, Hripcsak G, Johnson SB. Knowledge-based approaches to the maintenance of a large controlled medical terminology. JAMIA. 1994;1:35–50.
68. Cimino JJ, Aguirre A, Johnson SB, Peng P. Generic queries for meeting clinical information needs. Bull Med Libr Assoc. 1993;81:195.
69. Cimino ZQ. Mapping medical vocabularies to the unified medical language system. Proc AMIA. 1996;105–9.
70. Codd EF. A relational model of data for large shared data banks. Commun ACM. 1970;13:377–87.
71. Codd EF, Codd SB, Salley CT. Providing OLAP (On-Line Analytical Processing) to user-analysts: an IT mandate. San Jose, CA: EF Codd and Associates; 1993.
72. Collen M. Hospital computer systems: reasons for failures and factors making for success. In: Public Health in Europe, editor. 1. Health planning and organization of medical care. Copenhagen: Regional Office for Europe, World Health Organization; 1972.
73. Collen MF. General requirements of a medical information (MIS). Comput Biomed Res. 1970;3:393–406.
74. Collen MF. Medical information system (MIS) diffusion in the USA: a historical review. Proc MEDINFO. 1989;1:3–7.
75. Collen MF, Davis LS, Van Brunt EE, Terdiman JF. Functional goals and problems in large-scale patient record management and automated screening. In: Siler W, Lindberg DAB, edi-

tors. Computers in life science research. FASEB monographs. Vol. 2. New York: Springer; 1974. p. 159–64.

76. Connolly TM, Begg CE. Database management systems: a practical approach to design. New York: Addison-Wesley; 1999.

77. Cote RA. The SNOP-SNOMED concept: evolution towards a common medical nomenclature and classification. Pathologist. 1977;31:383–9.

78. Cousins SB, Silverstein JC, Frisse ME. Query networks for medical information retrieval-assigning probabilistic relationships. Proc SCAMC. 1990;800–4.

79. Cooney JP. Uniform hospital discharge data: minimum data set. DHEW Pub No 80-1157, 1980.

80. Crosby EL, Cooney JP. Common data set for hospital management. DHEW Pub No. (HSM 72-306). Washington, DC: U.S. Govt Printing Office; 1972.

81. Curtice RM, Glaser JP. The difference between interfaced and integrated systems. J Med Syst. 1989;13:55–8.

82. Das AK, Musen MA. A comparison of the temporal expressiveness of three database query methods. Proc AMIA. 1995;19:331–7.

83. Davis LS. A system approach to medical information. Methods Inf Med. 1973;12:1–6.

84. Davis LS. Problems facing large health information systems. Proc ACM. 1973;1–2.

85. Demuth AI. Automated ICD-9-CM coding: an inevitable trend to expert systems. Healthc Comput Commun. 1985;2:62.

86. Densen PM, Group AHW. Guidelines for producing uniform data for health care plans. Washington, DC: DHEW Publication No.(HSM); 1972. p. 73–3005.

87. Dick RS, Steen EB, Detmer DE. The computer-based patient record: an essential technology for health care. Washington, DC: National Academy Press; 1991.

88. Dolin DH, Mattison JE, Cohn S, et al. Kaiser Permanente's convergent medical terminology. Proc MEDINFO. 2004;346–50.

89. Dolin RH, Spackman K, Abilla A, Correia C, Goldberg B, Konicek D, et al. The SNOMED RT procedure model. Proc AMIA. 2001;139–43.

90. Doszkocs TE. CITE NLM: natural-language searching in an online catalog. Inf Technol Libr. 1983;2:365–80.

91. Dozier JA, Hammond WE, Stead WW. Creating a link between medical and analytical databases. Proc SCAMC. 1985;478–82.

92. Eden M. Storage and retrieval of the results of clinical research. Proc IRE Trans Med Electron. 1960;265–8.

93. Enlander D. Computer data processing of medical diagnoses in pathology. Am J Clin Pathol. 1975;63:538–44.

94. Farrington JF. CPT-4: a computerized system of terminology and coding. In: Emlet H, editor. Challenges and prospects for advanced medical systems. Miami: Symposia Specialists; 1978. p. 147–50.

95. Feinstein AR. Unsolved scientific problems in the nosology of clinical medicine. Arch Intern Med. 1988;148:2269–74.

96. Fineberg HV. Effects of clinical evaluation on the diffusion of medical technology. In: Mosteller F, editor. Assessing medical technologies. Washington, DC: National Academy Press; 1985. p. 176–210.

97. Fischetti L, Schloeffel P, Blair JS, Henderson ML. Standards. In: Lehmann HP, Abbott P, Roderer N, editors. Aspects of electronic health record systems. New York: Springer; 2006. p. 252–82.

98. Flagle CD. On the requirements for information systems in hospitals. Proceedings of the conference on ADP in hospitals, Elsinore. 1966.

99. Flagle CD. Communication and control in comprehensive patient care and health planning. Ann NY Acad Sci. 1969;161:714–29.

100. Flagle CD. Technological development in the health services. Proc IEEE. 1969;57:1847–52.

101. Forman BH, Cimino JJ, Johnson SB, Sengupta S, Sideli RV, Clayton PD. Applying a controlled medical terminology to a distributed, production clinical information system. Proc AMIA. 1995;19:421–5.

102. Frawley WJ, Piatetsky-Shapiro G, Matheus CJ. Knowledge discovery in databases: an overview. AI Mag. 1992;13:57.
103. Friedman BA, Martin JB. The physician as a locus of authority, responsibility, and operational control of medical systems. J Med Syst. 1988;12:389–96.
104. Friedman C, Johnson SB. Medical text processing: past achievements, future directions. In: Ball MJ, Collen MF, editors. Aspects of the computer-based patient record. New York: Springer; 1992. p. 212–28.
105. Friedman C. A broad-coverage natural language processing system. Proc AMIA. 2000;270.
106. Friedman C. Towards a comprehensive medical language processing system: methods and issues. Proc AMIA. 1997;595.
107. Friedman C, Hripcsak G. Evaluating natural language processors in the clinical domain. Method Inform Med. 1998;37:334–49.
108. Friedman C, Hripcsak G, Shablinsky I. An evaluation of natural language processing methodologies. Proc AMIA. 1998;855–9.
109. Friedman C, Shagina L, Lussier Y, Hripcsak G. Automated encoding of clinical documents based on natural language processing. J Am Med Inform Assoc. 2004;11:392–402.
110. Friedman C, Johnson SB, Forman B, Starren J. Architectural requirements for a multipurpose natural language processor in the clinical environment. Proc AMIA. 1995;19:347–51.
111. Friedman C, Alderson PO, Austin JHM, Cimino JJ, Johnson SB. A general natural-language text processor for clinical radiology. J Am Med Inform Assoc. 1994;1:161–74.
112. Friedman C, Shagina L, Socratous S, Zeng X. A web-based version of MedLEE: a medical language extract and encoding system. Proc AMIA. 1996;938.
113. Friedman RB. Computers. In: Eden HS, Eden M, editors. Micro-computers in patient care. Park Ridge: Noyes Medical Publications; 1981. p. 90–5.
114. Friedman RB, Gustafson DH. Computers in clinical medicine, a critical review. Comput Biomed Res. 1977;10:199–204.
115. Frisse ME. Digital libraries & information retrieval. Proc AMIA. 1996;320.
116. Frisse ME, Cousins SB. Query by browsing: an alternative hypertext information retrieval method. Proc SCAMC. 1989;388–91.
117. Fusaro VA, Kos PJ, Tector M. Electronic medical record analysis using cloud computing. Proc AMIA CRI. 2010;90.
118. Gabrieli ER. Standardization of medical informatics (special issue). J Clin Comput. 1985;14:62–104.
119. Gabrieli ER. Interface problems between medicine and computers. Proc SCAMC. 1984;93.
120. Gabrieli ER. Computerizing text from office records. MD Comput. 1987;4:44–9.
121. Gabrieli ER. A new electronic medical nomenclature. J Med Syst. 1989;13:355–73.
122. Gainer V, Goryachev S, Zeng Q, et al. Using derived concepts from electronic medical record systems for discovery research in informatics integrating biology and the bedside (i2b2). Proc AMIA TBI. 2010;91.
123. Galbraith JK. New industrial state. Boston: Houghton Mifflin; 1967.
124. Gantner GE. SNOMED: the systematized nomenclature of medicine as an ideal standardized language for computer applications in medical care. Proc SCAMC. 1980;2:1224.
125. Giannakopoulos S, Hammer J. Requirements for the small office practice. Proc SCAMC. 1980;3:1778–81.
126. Giebink GA, Hurst LL. Computer projects in health care. Ann Arbor: Health Administration Press; 1975.
127. Glaser JP, Gatewood LC, Anderson JC. Achieving health information system fit. Proc MEDINFO. 1983;61–4.
128. Goldstein L. MEDUS/A: a high-level database management system. Proc SCAMC. 1980;3:1653.
129. Gordon BL. Linguistics for medical records. In: Driggs MF, editor. Problem-directed and medical information systems. New York: Intercontinental Medical Book Corp; 1973. p. 5–13.
130. Gordon BL. Regularization and stylization of medical records. JAMA. 1970;212:1502–7.
131. Gordon BL. Biomedical language and format for manual and computer applications. Methods Inf Med. 1968;7:5.

132. Gordon BL. Standard medical terminology. JAMA. 1965;191:311–3.
133. Graepel PH, Henson DE, Pratt AW. Comments on the use of the Systematized Nomenclature of Pathology. Methods Inf Med. 1975;14:72.
134. Graepel PH. Manual and automatic indexing of the medical record: categorized nomenclature (SNOP) versus classification (ICD). Inform Health Soc Care. 1976;1:77–86.
135. Grams RR, Jin ZM. The natural language processing of medical databases. J Med Syst. 1989;13:79–87.
136. Grams S, Dvorak RM, Pryor TA, Childs BW. Panel: trends in health care information systems. Proc SCAMC. 1984;8:139–42.
137. Greenes RA. Medical computing in the 1980s: operating systems and programming language issues. J Med Syst. 1983;7:295–9.
138. Greer AL. The state of the art versus the state of the science: the diffusion of new medical technologies into practice. Int J Technol Assess Health Care. 1988;4:5–26.
139. Haas RE, Fleishl G. Medical time sharing on a small business computer. Proc San Diego Biomed Symp. 1972;11:359–62.
140. Hammond WE. GEMISCH. A minicomputer information support system. Proc IEEE. 1973;61:1575–83.
141. Hammond WE, Straube MJ, Blunden PB, Stead WW. Query: the language of databases. Proc SCAMC. 1989;13:419–23.
142. Hanmer JC. Diffusion of medical technologies: comparison with ADP systems in medical environment. Proc SCAMC. 1980;3:1731–6.
143. Hartzband P, Groopman J. Untangling the web: patients, doctors, and the Internet. N Engl J Med. 2010;362:1063–6.
144. Haug PJ, Gardner RM, Tate KE, Evans RS, East TD, Kuperman G, et al. Decision support in medicine: examples from the HELP system. Comput Biomed Res. 1994;27:396–418.
145. Haug PJ, Warner HR, Clayton PD, Schmidt CD, Pearl JE, Farney RJ, et al. A decision-driven system to collect the patient history. Comput Biomed Res. 1987;20:193–207.
146. Hendrix GG, Sacerdoti ED. Natural-language processing: the field in perspective. Byte. 1981;6:304–52.
147. Henkind SJ, Benis AM, Teichholz LE. Quantification as a means to increase the utility of nomenclature-classification systems. Proc MEDINFO. 1986;858–61.
148. Henley RR, Wiederhold G. An analysis of automated ambulatory medical record systems. San Francisco: Office of Medical Information Systems, University of California, San Francisco Medical Center; 1975.
149. Hersh WR, Donohue LC, SAPHIRE International: a tool for cross-language information retrieval. Proc AMIA. 1998; 673–7.
150. Hersh W. Information retrieval at the millenium. Proc AMIA. 1998;38.
151. Hersh WR, Greenes RA., SAPHIRE – an information retrieval system featuring concept matching, automatic indexing, probabalistic retrieval, and hierarchical relationships. Comput Biomed Res. 1990;23:410–25.
152. Hersh WR, Hickam DH. Information retrieval in medicine: the SAPHIRE experience. JASIS. 1995;46:743–7.
153. Hersh WR, Leone TJ. The SAPHIRE server: a new algorithm and implementation. Proc AMIA. 1995:858–63.
154. Hersh WR, Pattison-Gordon E, Evans DA, Greenes RA. Adaptation of meta-1 for SAPHIRE, a general purpose information retrieval system. Proc SCAMC. 1990;156–60.
155. Hersh WR, Brown KE, Donohoe LC, Campbell EM, Horacek AE. CliniWeb: managing clinical information on the World Wide Web. JAMIA. 1996;3:273–80.
156. Himes BE, Kohane IS, Ramoni MF, Weiss ST. Characterization of patients who suffer asthma exacerbations using data extracted from electronic medical records. Proc AMIA Annu Symp. 2008;308.
157. Hodgdon JD. ADP management problems and implementation strategies relating to user resistance to change. Proc SCAMC. 1979;843.
158. Hoffman T. The 6th annual medical hardware and software buyers guide. MD Comput. 1989;6:334–77.

159. Hogan WR, Wagner MM. Free-text fields change the meaning of coded data. Proc AMIA. 1996;517.
160. Hogarth MA, Gertz M, Gorin FA. Terminology query language: a server interface for concept-oriented terminology systems. Proc AMIA. 2000;349.
161. Hripcsak G, Allen B, Cimino JJ, Lee R. Access to data: comparing AccessMed with query by review. J Am Med Inform Assoc. 1996;3:288–99.
162. Hripcsak G, Friedman C, Alderson PO, DuMouchel W, Johnson SB, Clayton PD. Unlocking clinical data from narrative reports: a study of natural language processing. Ann Intern Med. 1995;122:681–8.
163. Hucko GM, Hagamen WD. An interactive patient record system and its transfer from a mainframe to microcomputers. Proc SCAMC. 1978;509.
164. Humphreys BL. De facto, de rigueur, and even useful: standards for the published literature and their relationship to medical informatics. Proc SCAMC. 1990;2.
165. Humphreys BL, Lindberg D, D. Building the unified medical language system. Proc SCAMC. 1989;475–80.
166. Hutchinson DR. The office of technology assessment health data study: a preliminary report. Health Serv Res. 1978;13:103.
167. Jacobs H. A natural language information retrieval system. Methods Inf Med. 1968;7:8–16.
168. Jenkin MA. Design concepts for successful computerized information systems. Proceedings of the AAMI 9th annual meeting. New Orleans;1974.
169. Jenkin MA, Cheezum L, Essick V, Gilson K, Jean BB, Mockler N, et al. Clinical patient management and the integrated health information system. Med Instrum. 1977;12:217–21.
170. Johnson KB, Rosenbloom ST. Computer-based documentation: past, present, and future. In: Lehmann HP, Roderer N, Abbott P, editors. Aspects of electronic health record systems. New York: Springer; 2006. p. 308–28.
171. Johnson SB. Conceptual graph grammar: a simple formalism for sublanguage. Methods Inf Med. 1998;37:345–52.
172. Johnson SB, Friedman C. Integrating data from natural language processing into a clinical information system. Proc AMIA. 1996;537–41.
173. Johnston Jr H, Higgins SB, Harris TR, Lacy W. The effect of a CLINFO management and analysis on clinical research. Proc MEDCOMP. 1982;517–8.
174. Kaplan B. The medical computing "lag": perceptions of barriers to the application of computers to medicine. Int J Technol Assess Health Care. 1987;3:123–36.
175. Kaplan B. The computer as Rorschach: implications for management and user acceptance. Proc SCAMC. 1983;664–7.
176. Kaplan BM. Computers in medicine, 1950–1980: the relationship between history and policy. Dissertation abstracts international part A: humanities and social science; 1984. p. 44.
177. Karpinski RH, Bleich HL. MISAR: a miniature information storage and retrieval system. Comput Biomed Res. 1971;4:655–60.
178. Kastner V, Pratt AW. Resourcing. Comput Progr Biomed. 1976;5:189–205.
179. Katz B. Clinical research system. MD Comput. 1986;3:53–5. 61.
180. Kementsietsidis A, Lim L, Wang M. Profile-based retrieval of records in medical databases. Proc AMIA Annu Symp. 2009;312.
181. Kent A. Computers and biomedical information storage and retrieval. JAMA. 1966;196:927–32.
182. King C, Strong RM, Goldstein L. MEDUS/A: distributing database management for research and patient data. Proc SCAMC. 1988;818–26.
183. King C, Strong RM, Manire L. Comparing data management systems in clinical research: 1983 Survey. Proc SCAMC. 1983;715–9.
184. Kingsland LC. RDBS: research data base system for microcomputers; coding techniques and file structures. Proc AAMSI Conf. 1982;85–9.
185. Kling R. Social analyses of computing: theoretical perspectives in recent empirical research. ACM Comput Surv (CSUR). 1980;12:61–110.
186. Korein J. The computerized medical record: the variable-field-length format system and its applications. Inf Process Med Rec. 1970;259–91.

187. Korein J, Goodgold AL, Randt CT. Computer processing of medical data by variable-field-length format. JAMA. 1966;196:950–6.
188. Korein J, Tick LJ, Woodbury MA, Cady LD, Goodgold AL, Randt CT. Computer processing of medical data by variable-field-length format. JAMA. 1963;186:132–8.
189. Kwon IW, Vogler TK, Kim JH. Computer utilization in health care. Proc AAMSI. 1983;538–42.
190. Lacson R, Long W. Natural language processing of spoken diet records (SDRs). Proc AMIA Annu Symp. 2006;454–8.
191. Lamson BG, Russell WS, Fullmore J, Nix WE. The first decade of effort: progress toward a hospital information system at the UCLA Hospital, Los Angeles, California. Methods Inf Med. 1970;9:73–80.
192. Lamson BG. Computer assisted data processing in laboratory medicine. In: Stacy RW, Waxman BD, editors. Computers in biomedical research, vol. II. New York: Academic Press; 1965. p. 353–76.
193. Layard MW, McShane DJ. Applications of MEDLOG, a microcomputer-based system for time-oriented clinical data. Proc SCAMC. 1983;731–4.
194. Ledley RS, Lusted LB. The use of electronic computers in medical data processing: aids in diagnosis, current information retrieval, and medical record keeping. IRE Transactions on Med Electronics. 1960;ME-7:31–47.
195. Ledley RS. Report on the use of computers in biology and medicine. Washington, DC: National Academies; 1960.
196. Levy AH. Information retrieval. In: Ball MJ, Collen MF, editors. Aspects of the computer-based patient record. New York: Springer; 1992. p. 146–52.
197. Levy AH. Recent developments in microcomputers in medicine. Proc AAMSI. 1984;341–5.
198. Levy AH, Baskin AB. Clinical computing-1977. J Med Syst. 1977;1:361–74.
199. Levy AH, Shires DB, Wolf H. Is informatics a basic medical science. Proc MEDINFO. 1977;979.
200. Levy C, Rogers E. Clinician-oriented access to data-COAD: a natural language interface to a VA DHCP Database. Proc AMIA. 1995;933.
201. Lilienfeld AM. Ambulatory medical care records: uniform minimum basic data set. Washington, DC: U.S. Govt Printing Office; 1974.
202. Lincoln TL, Groner GF, Quinn JJ, Lukes RJ. The analysis of functional studies in acute lymphocytic leukemia using CLINFO-A small computer information and analysis system for clinical investigators. Informatics for Health and Social Care. 1976;1:95–103.
203. Lincoln T. An historical perspective on clinical laboratory systems. In: Blum BI, Duncan KA, editors. A history of medical informatics. New York: Addison-Wesley; 1990. p. 267–77.
204. Lindberg D. The impact of automated information systems applied to health problems. In: Holland WW et al., editors. Oxford text of public health, Investigative Methods in Public Health. 3rd ed. New York: Oxford University Press; 1985. p. 55–76.
205. Lindberg D. Computer networks within health care. In: Peterson H, Isaksson A, editors. Communication networks in health care. Amsterdam: North Holland; 1982. p. 109–20.
206. Lindberg D. The growth of medical information systems in the United States. Lexington: Lexington Books Lexington; 1979.
207. Lindberg D. The status of medical information systems technology. In: Shannon R, editor. Hospital information systems. Amsterdam: North-Holland; 1979. p. 19–29.
208. Lindberg D. Impact of public policy on the development, adoption, and diffusion of medical information systems technology. Washington, DC: U.S. Govt. Print. Off; 1978.
209. Lindberg D. The computer and medical care. South Med J. 1972;65:1032.
210. Lindberg D. Computer failures and successes. South Med Bull. 1969;57:18–21.
211. Lindberg D. CONSIDER: a computer program for medical instruction. NY State J Med. 1969;69:54.
212. Lindberg D. The computer and medical care. Springfield: CC Thomas; 1968.
213. Lindberg DAB. Diffusion of medical information systems technology in the United States. J Med Syst. 1982;6:219–28.

214. Lindberg DAB. The development and diffusion of a medical technology: medical information systems. In: Sanders CA, et al., editors. Medical technology and the health care system: a study of the diffusion of equipment-embodied technology. Washington, DC: National Academy of Sciences; 1979. p. 201–39.
215. Linton PH, Willcutt HC. Psychological aspects of computer use. MD Comput. 1985;2:64–7.
216. Logan JR, Britell S, Delcambre LML, Kapoor V, Buckmaster JG. Representing multi-database study schemas for reusability. Proc AMIA TBI. 2010;21.
217. Logan RA, Brenner DJ. Innovative physicians and medical information systems. Proc AAMSI. 1987;197–201.
218. Lupovitch A, Memminger 3rd J, Corr RM. Manual and computerized cumulative reporting systems for the clinical microbiology laboratory. Am J Clin Pathol. 1979;72:841–7.
219. Lussier Y, Borlawsky T, Rappaport D, Liu Y, Friedman C. PHENOGO: assigning phenotypic context to gene ontology annotations with natural language processing. Pac Symp Biocomput. 2006;64.
220. Lyman M, Sager N, Freidman C, Chi E. Computer-structured narrative in ambulatory care: its use in longitudinal review of clinical data. Proc SCAMC. 1985;82–6.
221. Mabry JC, Thompson HK, Hopwood MD, Baker WR. A prototype data management and analysis system (CLINFO): system description and user experience. Proc MEDINFO. 1977;77:71–5.
222. Markus ML. Power, politics, and MIS implementation. Commun ACM. 1983;26:430–44.
223. Mathur S, Dinakarpandian D. Automated ontological gene annotation for computing disease similarity. Proc AMIA TBI. 2010;12.
224. Mays E, Weida R, Dionne R, Laker M, White B, Liang C, et al. Scalable and expressive medical terminologies. Proc AMIA. 1996;259.
225. McCarn DB, Moriarty DG. Computers in medicine. Hospitals. 1971;45:37–9.
226. McCormick BH, Chang SK, Boroved RT. Technological trends in clinical information systems. Proc MEDINFO. 1977;43–8.
227. McCormick PJ, Elhadad N, Stetson PD. Use of semantic features to classify patient smoking status. Proc AMIA Annu Symp. 2008;450.
228. McCray AT. The nature of lexical knowledge. Methods Inf Med. 1998;37:353–60.
229. McCray AT, Sponsler JL, Brylawski B, Browne AC. The role of lexical knowledge in biomedical text understanding. Proc SCAMC. 1987;103–7.
230. McCray AT, Bodenreider O, Malley JD, Browne AC. Evaluating UMLS strings for natural language processing. Proc AMIA. 2001;448.
231. McDonald CJ. Standards for the electronic transfer of clinical data: progress, promises, and the conductor's wand. Proc SCAMC. 1990;9–14.
232. McDonald CJ, Hui SL. The analysis of humongous databases: problems and promises. Stat Med. 1991;10:511–8.
233. McDonald CJ. Medical information systems of the future. MD Comput. 1989;6:82–7.
234. McDonald CJ, Hripcsak G. Data exchange standards for computer-based patient records. In: Ball M, Collen MF, editors. Aspects of the computer-based patient record. New York: Springer; 1992. p. 157–64.
235. McDonald CJ, Tierney WM, Overhage JM, et al. The Regenstrief medical record system: 20 years of experience in hospitals, clinics, and neighborhood health centers. MD Comput. 1992;9:206–16.
236. McDonald C, Blevins L, Glazener T, Haas J, Lemmon L, Meeks-Johnson J. Data base management, feedback control, and the Regenstrief medical record. J Med Syst. 1983;7:111–25.
237. McDonald CJ. Standards for the transmission of diagnostic results from laboratory computers to office practice computers: an initiative. Proc SCAMC. 1983;123.
238. McDonald CJ. Protocol-based computer reminders, the quality of care and the non-perfectability of man. N Engl J Med. 1976;295:1351–5.
239. Melski JW, Geer DE, Bleich HL. Medical information storage and retrieval using preprocessed variables. Comput Biomed Res. 1978;11:613–21.
240. Mendonca EA, Cimino JJ, Johnson SB. Accessing heterogeneous sources of evidence to answer clinical questions. J Biomed Inform. 2001;34:85–98.

241. Meystre SM, Haug PJ. Comparing natural language processing tools to extract medical problems from narrative text. Proc AMIA Annu Symp. 2005;525.
242. Meystre SM, Deshmukh VG, Mitchell J. A clinical use case to evaluate the i2b2 hive: predicting asthma exacerbations. Proc AMIA Annu Symp. 2009;442.
243. Meystre S, Haug PJ. Medical problem and document model for natural language understanding. Proc AMIA Annu Symp. 2003;4559.
244. Miller MC, Levkoff AH, Wong YM, Michel Y. Normal newborn nursery information system. Proc AAMSI. 1983;154–62.
245. Miller PB, Strong RM. Clinical care and research using MEDUS/A, a medically oriented data base management system. Proc SCAMC. 1978;288.
246. Moore FJ. Information technologies and health care: 1. Medical care as a system. Arch Intern Med. 1970;125:157.
247. Morgan MM, Beaman PD, Shusman DJ, Hupp JA, Zielstorff RD, Barnett GO. Medical query language. Proc SCAMC. 1981;322–5.
248. Murphy SN, Mendis M, Hackett K, et al. Architecture of the open-source clinical research chart from informatics for integrating biology and the bedside. Proc AMIA. 2007;548–52.
249. Munoz F, Hersh W. MCM generator: a Java-based tool for generating medical metadata. Proc AMIA. 1998;648.
250. Murnaghan JH. Uniform basic data sets for health statistical systems. Int J Epidemiol. 1978;7:263–9.
251. Murphy G, Waters K. The patient record as a primary component of medical computing. Proc SCAMC. 1979;525.
252. Murphy SN, Morgan MM, Barnett GO, Chueh HC. Optimizing healthcare research data warehouse design through past COSTAR query analysis. Proc AMIA. 1999;892.
253. Myers J, Gelblat M, Enterline HT. Automatic encoding of pathology data: computer-readable surgical pathology data as a by-product of typed pathology reports. Arch Pathol. 1970;89:73.
254. Naisbitt J. Megatrends. New York: Warner Books; 1982.
255. Nelson S, Hoffman S, Kanekal H, Varma A. Making the most of RECONSIDER: an evaluation of input strategies. Proc SCAMC. 1983;852.
256. Nielson J, Wilcox A. Linking structured text to medical knowledge. Proc MEDINFO. 2004;1777.
257. Nigrin DJ, Kohane IS. Scaling a data retrieval and mining application to the enterprise-wide level. Proc AMIA. 1999;901–5.
258. NIH-DIR. General clinical research centers: a research resources directory. 7th ed. Bethesda: Division of Research Services, NIH; 1988.
259. Niland JC, Rouse L. Clinical research needs. In: Lehmann HP, Roderer N, Abbott P, editors. Aspects of electronic health record systems. New York: Springer; 2006. p. 31–46.
260. Nunnery AW. A medical information storage and statistical system (MICRO-MISSY). Proc SCAMC. 1984;383.
261. Obermeier KK. Natural-language processing. Byte. 1987;12:225–32.
262. O'Connor MJ, Tu SW, Musen MA. Representation of temporal indeterminacy in clinical databases. Proc AMIA. 2000;615–9.
263. Okubo RS, Russell WS, Dimsdale B, Lamson BG. Natural language storage and retrieval of medical diagnostic information: experience at the UCLA Hospital and Clinics over a 10-year period. Comput Programs Biomed. 1975;5:105–30.
264. Oliver DE, Shortliffe EH. Collaborative model development for vocabulary and guidelines. Proc AMIA. 1996;826.
265. Oliver DE, Barnes MR, Barnett GO, Chueh HC, Cimino JJ, Clayton PD, et al. InterMed: an Internet-based medical collaboratory. Proc AMIA. 1995;1023.
266. Olson NE, Sherertz DD, Erlbaum MS, Lipow SS, Suarez-Munist O, Fuller LF, et al. Explaining your terminology to a computer. Proc AMIA. 1995;957.
267. OTA. Policy implications of medical information systems. Washington, DC:Office of Technology Assessment; 1977. p. 58–63.
268. Ozbolt JG, Russo M, Stultz MP. Validity and reliability of standard terms and codes for patient care data. Proc AMIA. 1995;37.

269. Pendse N. Online analytical processing. Wikipedia. 2008.
270. Porter D, Safran C. On-line searches of a hospital data base for clinical research and patient care. Proc SCAMC. 1984;277.
271. Powsner SM, Barwick KW, Morrow JS, Riely CA, Miller PL. Coding semantic relationships for medical bibliographic retrieval: a preliminary study. Proc SCAMC. 1987;108.
272. Prather JC, Lobach DF, Hales JW, Hage ML, Fehrs SJ, Hammond WE. Converting a legacy system database into relational format to enhance query efficiency. Proc AMIA. 1995;372–6.
273. Pratt AW. Medicine and linguistics. Proc MEDINFO. 1974;5–11.
274. Pratt AW. Automatic processing of pathology data. Leaflet published by National Institutes of Health. Bethesda: NIH; 1971.
275. Pratt AW. Representation of medical language data utilizing the systemized nomenclature of pathology. In: Enlander D, editor. Computers in laboratory medicine. New York: Academic; 1975. p. 42–53.
276. Pratt AW. Medicine, computers, and linguistics. In: Brown J, Dickson JFB, editors. Biomedical engineering. New York: Academic; 1973. p. 97–140.
277. Pratt AW, Pacak M. Automatic processing of medical English. Preprint No. 11, classification IR 3,4, reprinted by US HEW, NIH; 1969.
278. Pratt AW, Pacak M. Identification and transformation of terminal morphemes in medical English. Methods Inf Med. 1969;8:84–90.
279. Price SL, Hersh WR, Olson DD, Embi PJ. SmartQuery: context-sensitive links to medical knowledge sources from the electronic patient record. Proc AMIA. 2002;627–31.
280. Pryor DB, Stead WW, Hammond WE, Califf RM, Rosati RA. Features of TMR for a successful clinical and research database. Proc SCAMC. 1982;79–83.
281. Ranum DL. Knowledge-based understanding of radiology text. Comput Methods Programs Biomed. 1989;30:209–15.
282. Robinson RE. Acquisition and analysis of narrative medical record data. Comp Biomed Res. 1970;3:495–509.
283. Robinson RE. Surgical pathology information processing system. In: Coulson W, editor. Surgical pathology. Philadelphia: JB Lippincott; 1978. p. 1–20.
284. Robinson RE. Pathology subsystem. In: Collen M, editor. Hospital computer systems. New York: Wiley; 1974. p. 194–205.
285. Rockart JF. On the implementation of information systems. In: Abernathy WJ, Sheldon A, Prahalad CK, editors. The management of health care. Cambridge, MA: Ballinger; 1974. p. 175–86.
286. Roper WL. From the health care financing administration. JAMA. 1988;259:3530.
287. Rothrock JJ. ASTM: the standards make the pieces fit. Proc AAMSI. 1989;327–35.
288. Rutt TE. Work of IEEE P1157 medical data interchange committee. Int J Clin Monit Comput. 1989;6:45–57.
289. Safran C, Porter D. New uses of a large clinical data base. In: Blum BI, editor. Implement health care systems. New York: Springer; 1989. p. 123–32.
290. Safran C, Porter D, Rury CD, Herrmann FR, Lightfoot J, Underhill LH, et al. ClinQuery: searching a large clinical database. MD Comput. 1989;7:144–53.
291. Safran C, Porter D, Lightfoot J, Rury CD, Underhill LH, Bleich HL, et al. ClinQuery: a system for online searching of data in a teaching hospital. Ann Intern Med. 1989;111:751–6.
292. Sager N, Chi EC, Tick LJ, Lyman M. Relational database design for computer-analyzed medical narrative. Proc SCAMC. 1982;797–804.
293. Sager N, Tick L, Story G, Hirschman L. A codasyl-type schema for natural language medical records. Proc SCAMC. 1980;2:1027.
294. Sager N, Friedman C, Chi E, Macleod C, Chen S, Johnson S. The analysis and processing of clinical narrative. Proc MEDINFO. 1986;86:1101–5.
295. Sager N, Bross I, Story G, Bastedo P, Marsh E, Shedd D. Automatic encoding of clinical narrative. Comput Biol Med. 1982;12:43–56.

296. Sager N, Kosaka M. A database of literature organized by relations. Proc SCAMC. 1983;692–5.
297. Sager N, Hirschman L, Lyman M. Computerized language processing for multiple use of narrative discharge summaries. Proc SCAMC. 1978;330.
298. Sager N, Nhã nN, Lyman M, Tick LJ. Medical language processing with SGML display. Proc AMIA. 1996;547.
299. Sager N, Lyman M, Bucknall C, Nhan N, Tick LJ. Natural language processing and the representation of clinical data. J Am Med Inform Assoc. 1994;1:142–60.
300. Schoch NA, Sewell W. The many faces of natural language searching. Proc AMIA. 1995;914.
301. Seol Y, Johnson SB, Cimino JJ. Conceptual guidance in information retrieval. Proc AMIA. 2001;1026.
302. Shanas E. Long-term health care minimum data set. Washington, DC: US Department of Health and Human Services, Public Health Service, Office of Health Research, Statistics, and Technology, National Center for Health Statistics; 1980.
303. Shapiro AR. The SCAMP system for patient and practice management. J Med Syst. 1983;7:127–36.
304. Shortliffe EH. Medical computing: another basic science? Proc SCAMC. 1980;1:490.
305. Shusman DJ, Morgan MM, Zielstorff R, Barnett GO. The medical query language. Proc SCAMC. 1983;742–5.
306. Sim I, Carini S, Tu S, Wynden R, et al. Federating human studies design data using the ontology of clinical research. Proc AMIA CRI. 2010;51–5.
307. Simborg DW. An emerging standard for health communications: the HL7 standard. Healthc Comput Commun. 1987;4:58–60.
308. Smith MB, Burke KE, Torgerson JS, Stollerman JE, Kern DC, Hardy WL, et al. Logical and efficient conversation between patients and the telephone linked computer system. Proc SCAMC. 1988;463.
309. Spackman KA. Rates of change in a large clinical terminology: three years experience with SNOMED Clinical Terms. Proc AMIA Annu Symp. 2005;714.
310. Spackman KA, Hersh WR. Recognizing noun phrases in medical discharge summaries: an evaluation of two natural language parsers. Proc AMIA. 1996;155.
311. Spencer WA, Vallbona C. Application of computers in clinical practice. JAMA. 1965;191:917–21.
312. Starr P. The social transformation of american medicine. New York: Basic Books; 1982.
313. Stearns MQ, Price C, Spackman KA, Wang AY. SNOMED clinical terms: overview of the development process and project status. Proc AMIA. 2001;662.
314. Story G, Hirschman L. Data base design for natural language medical data. J Med Syst. 1982;6:77–88.
315. Summerfield AB, Empey S. Computer-based information systems for medicine: a survey and brief discussion of current projects. Santa Monica: System Development Corporation; 1965.
316. Tatch D. Automatic encoding of medical diagnoses. 6th IBM Medical Symposium. Poughkeepsie, NY: IBM; 1964.
317. Terdiman J. Ambulatory care computer systems in office practice: a tutorial. Proc AMIA. 1982;195–201.
318. Thompson Jr HK. Acquisition and reporting of medical history data. Proc 10th IBM Med Symp. 1977;117–24.
319. Tuttle MS, Campbell KE, Olson NE, Nelson SJ, Suarez-Munist O, Erlbaum MS, et al. Concept, code, term and word: preserving the distinctions. Proc AMIA. 1995;956.
320. Van Brunt E. Computer applications in medical care-some problems of the 1970's: a clinical perspective. Proc SCAMC. 1980;1:454.
321. Van Brunt E, Collen M. Hospital computer systems. In: Collen MF, editor. Hospital computer systems. New York: Wiley; 1974. p. 114–47.
322. Van Brunt E. Factors which limit or constrain the development of medical data processing. Informatics for Health and Social Care. 1976;1:293–9.

323. Wang X, Chused A, Elhadad N, Friedman C, Markatou M. Automated knowledge acquisition from clinical narrative reports. Proc AMIA Annu Symp. 2008;783.
324. Ward RE, MacWilliam CH, Ye E, Russman AN, Richards RR, Huber M. Development and multi-institutional implementation of coding and transmission standards for health outcomes data. Proc AMIA. 1996;438.
325. Ware H, Mullett CJ, Jagannathan V. Natural language processing framework to assess clinical conditions. J Am Med Inform Assoc. 2009;16:585–9.
326. Warner HR, Guo D, Mason D, et al. Enroute towards a computer based patient record: the ACIS project. Proc AMIA. 1995;152–6.
327. Watson BL. Liability for failure to acquire or use computers in medicine. Proc SCAMC. 1981;879–83.
328. Webster S, Morgan M, Barnett GO. Medical query language: improved access to MUMPS databases. Proc SCAMC. 1987;306.
329. Wells AH. The conversion of SNOP to the computer languages of medicine. Pathologists. 1971;25:371–8.
330. Weyl S, Fries J, Wiederhold G, Germano F. A modular self-describing clinical databank system. Comput Biomed Res. 1975;8:279–93.
331. Whitehead SF, Streeter M. CLINFO – a successful technology transfer. Proc SCAMC. 1984;557.
332. Whiting-O'Keefe Q, Strong PC, Simborg DW. An automated system for coding data from summary time oriented record (STOR). Proc SCAMC. 1983;735–7.
333. Willems JS. The relationship between the diffusion of medical technology and the organization and economics of health care delivery. In: Medical technology. DHEW Pub No 79-3254. 1979. p. 92–104.
334. Williams GZ, Williams RL. Clinical laboratory subsystem. In: Collen M, editor. Hospital computer systems. New York: Wiley; 1974. p. 148–93.
335. Wood M. Uniform ambulatory medical care minimum data set. Report of the National Committee on Vital and Health Statistics. DHSS No. (PHS) 81-1161. Washington, DC: U.S. Govt Print Office; 1981.
336. Wynden R. Providing a high security environment for the integrated data repository lead institution. Proc AMIA TBI. 2010;123.
337. Wynden R, Weiner MG, Sim I, Gabriel D, Casale M, Carini S, et al. Ontology mapping and data discovery for the translational investigator. Proc AMIA TBI. 2010;66.
338. Xu H, Friedman C. Facilitating research in pathology using natural language processing. Proc AMIA. 2003;107.
339. Yang H, Spasic I, Keane JA, Nenadic G. A text mining approach to the prediction of disease status from clinical discharge summaries. J Am Med Inform Assoc. 2009;16:596–600.
340. Yianilos PN, Harbort Jr RA, Buss SR, Tuttle Jr EP. The application of a pattern matching algorithm to searching medical record text. Proc SCAMC. 1978;308.
341. Zacks MP, Hersh WR. Developing search strategies for detecting high quality reviews in a hypertext test collection. Proc SCAMC. 1998;663–7.
342. Zeng Q, Cimino JJ. Mapping medical vocabularies to the unified medical language system. Proc AMIA. 1996;105–9.
343. Zeng Q, Cimino JJ. Evaluation of a system to identify relevant patient information and its impact on clinical information retrieval. Proc AMIA. 1999;642.
344. Zeng Q, Gainer V, Goryachev S. Using derived concepts from electronic medical records for discovery reseach in informatics for integrating biology and bedside. Proc AMIA Annu Symp. 2010.
345. Zhang G, Siegler T, Saxman P, Sandberg N, Mueller R, Johnson N, et al. VISAGE: a query interface for clinical research. Proc AMIA TBI. 2010;76.
346. Zhou L, Tao Y, Cimino JJ, Chen ES, Liu H, Lussier YA, et al. Terminology model discovery using natural language processing and visualization techniques. J Biomed Inform. 2006;39:626–36.

Chapter 4
Medical Databases and Patient Record Systems

Morris F. Collen, Warner V. Slack, and Howard L. Bleich

Abstract As computer-based electronic patients' records replaced paper-based charts, hospital medical records departments gave way to computer centers that stored data on magnetic disks. As computer storage became cheaper and database designs became more efficient, medical databases grew in size and variety. Federated databases could store large volumes of aggregated data in multiple partitions, or as functionally oriented databases that were logically interconnected. Directly accessible from clinical applications, they allowed users to simultaneously access and query data for patient care, clinical research, and financial reimbursement. Extended central databases collected and managed data from different databases. Known as data warehouses, they could service ever-increasing volumes of data collected from ever-changing medical technologies. Larger warehouses developed partitions and data marts for subsets of data to serve users with specific needs. The need to store and query large collections of data led to the development of online analytical processing (OLAP), distributed database systems, distributed database management systems, and translational data processing between multiple data warehouses. With more powerful computers in the 1990s, physicians began to enter data directly into the patient's electronic health record using the keyboard, mouse, and clinical workstation. Dedicated computers became database servers to store and integrate multiple databases. In the 2000s electronic health records became more common; in the 2010s federal funding produced more widespread diffusion of electronic health records, and advances in informatics resulted in more efficient data management of expanding, multi-media, patient care databases.

Sections of this chapter are reproduced from author Collen's earlier work *Computer Medical Databases*, Springer (2012).

Author Collen was deceased at the time of publication. Bleich and Slack edited this chapter on his behalf after his death.

M.F. Collen (deceased)

W.V. Slack, M.D. (✉) • H.L. Bleich, M.D.
Harvard Medical School, Division of Clinical Informatics, Department of Medicine,
Beth Israel Deaconess Medical Center, Brookline, MA, USA
e-mail: wslack@bidmc.harvard.edu; bleich@bidmc.harvard.edu

© Springer-Verlag London 2015   207
M.F. Collen, M.J. Ball (eds.), *The History of Medical Informatics
in the United States*, Health Informatics, DOI 10.1007/978-1-4471-6732-7_4

Keywords Electronic patient records • Medical databases • Data warehouses • Federated databases • Distributed systems • Electronic health records • Database management • Clinical data • Genomic data • Translational data processing

Physicians have always followed the teachings of the famed clinician, Sir William Osler, to study and learn from patients and from their medical records, in order to improve their knowledge of diseases. Physicians continue to learn by taking a history of the patient's medical problems, performing a physical examination, and recording their findings in the medical record. To confirm a preliminary diagnosis and to rule-out other possible diagnoses, physicians order tests and procedures that may involve the clinical laboratory, the department of radiology, and other clinical support services. After reviewing the information received from these services, physicians refine their diagnoses and prescribe treatment. For an unusual or complex medical problem, physicians can refer the patient to appropriate clinical specialists. In addition, they can review reports of appropriate therapies by consulting the medical literature.

In the past, the patients' paper-based files were called patients' charts, and the charts were aggregated and stored by medical record librarians within a medical records department or chart room. With the advent of electronic computers, some medical facilities began to store patient's data, not on paper, but rather electronically. Computer scientists called such a collection of computer-stored patients' records a medical database. Health care providers called it a computer-stored patient record (CPR), an electronic patient record (EPR), an electronic health record (EHR), or an electronic medical record (EMR). The most important component of a medical information system is the electronic medical record that contains the data associated with the care of a patient. In addition to the electronic medical record, the medical information system of a hospital or a medical practice contains administrative data needed for clinic scheduling, medical record tracking, insurance coverage, and the like.

In the 1950s with the early development of computers, users began to bring work to a central mainframe computer to be batch-processed. The data were collected, entered, and merged into computer files that were stored on magnetic tape, and a file-management system was designed to enter, store, and retrieve the data. In the 1960s time-shared mainframe computers, that communicated by telephone lines or coaxial cable to remote data-entry terminals and printers, enabled users to process their data concurrently. Time-shared computers provided a more acceptable turnaround time for data services. Initially stored on magnetic tape, data soon moved to random-access, magnetic drums and then discs that were better suited for query and retrieval. High costs for computer storage and slow retrieval times limited what could be done, however.

In the 1970s with the emergence of lower cost, magnetic random-access disc storage, subsystem databases could be more readily merged into larger databases. As the number of databases increased, there was a need for an integrating database management system. The retrieval of subsets of selected data from various databases required both re-organization of the stored data, and an index to the locations of the various data subsets. Attempts were made to design more efficient databases to make them independent of their applications and subsystems, so that a well-designed database could process almost any type of data. Terdiman [317] credited the development of microcomputer technology in the 1970s with many of the subsequent advances in database management.

In the 1980s microcomputers and minicomputers were increasingly used for small databases, often called registries. As storage technology became more efficient and larger, and cheaper storage devices became available, computer-based registries expanded their storage capacity for larger amounts of data, and were then generally referred to as databases. When huge storage capacity became available at relatively low cost, very large collections of data became known as data warehouses. Helvey [175] reported that almost 100 medical online databases on a variety of subjects were distributed by a variety of information producers, vendors, and carriers. The year of 1988 was called the year of the database by Bryan [60], who reported that more than 20 new or improved database management systems became available in that year. In 1989 the total number of computer-stored databases in the world was estimated to be about five million. Most of these databases were small, but some were considered huge, as was the 1990 U.S. census – a million-million bytes, or a terabyte, of data [140]. In 2014, as this is being written, a terabyte of data can easily fit within a laptop computer.

Computer-stored medical databases were considered by Coltri [94] to be one of the most important developments in medical computer software engineering, and to be the equivalent of the heart and the brain of a medical information system (MIS). *Databases* were defined by Wiederhold [360, 363] as collections of related data so organized that usable data could be extracted. Databases were defined by Frawley et al. [140] as logically integrated collections of data in one or more computer files, organized to facilitate the efficient storage, change, query, and retrieval of information. With the advent of medical informatics, the most important computer-stored database needed to support the practice of medicine became the electronic patient record (EPR).

4.1 Medical Database Requirements and Structural Designs

The development of efficient computer-stored medical databases was essential for providing usable medical computing applications. Clinical repositories was a phrase proposed by Johnson [189] as more accurately representing a shared resource of patient data that were collected for the purpose of supporting clinical care. Johnson advised that a large-scale, clinical repository required a data model to define its functional requirements and to produce a formal description, a conceptual schema of all the data generated in the enterprise and how it was related, and a database structural design to define its technical requirements.

Davis [107] recommended that, as a minimum, the major goals of a medical database should be to maintain readily accessible the relevant data for each patient served, and to provide a resource for the systematic retrieval of relevant data from patients' records for any desired primary, secondary, clinical research purpose.

Blum [38] advised that medical databases should be designed so that they could: (1) be used for high volume activities; (2) be non-redundant with each element stored in the database only once; (3) ensure consistency of information; (4) be flexible to allow for change; (5) when storing active patient records, the clinical database needed to store not only the patients' data, but also other associated transactional data, such as when, where, how, and by whom the patients' data were collected.

The requirements and structural designs of a medical database specified that it be compatible with the objectives of the medical enterprise of which it was a part. Since a medical care database usually operated within a larger medical information system (MIS), whether the medical database served as the primary electronic patient record (EPR), or served as a secondary medical database such as a clinical research database with its data derived from the EPRs, both had some similar basic functional requirements.

Technical requirements and structural designs for medical databases were described by Wiederhold [351–363] at Stanford University. Wiederhold, who made important contributions to the development of medical databases, emphasized that the effectiveness of a database depended on its relevance to its organizational purposes, and that a database management system was needed to control, enter, store, process, and retrieve the data. He advised that when using very large databases, it was helpful to apply automated methods for the acquisition and retrieval of textual data.

Data modeling designs to provide the conceptual schema that represented the information in clinical databases were considered by Johnson [189] to be as important for large medical databases as was their structural designs. Johnson defined the conceptual schema for a database as a representation of all of the data types required to manage the data process, whether using a hierarchical, a relational, or an object-oriented structural database design, or whether using a combination of database structural designs. Johnson advised that the structural design of a database needed to provide rapid retrieval of data for individual users, and that it had to adapt to changing information needs of growth and new technology. He also emphasized that the primary purpose of the database structural design was to implement the conceptual schema. To properly build a database, Johnson further advised that it was necessary to develop a model of the database that defined its functional requirements, its technical requirements, and its structural design. The database model needed to provide a formal description – a conceptual schema – of the data to be generated and how the data were related. Thus, the users of the database needed to fully define its functional requirements as to what they wanted the database and its database-management system to do.

Since a medical database usually operated within a database-management system, Johnson [189] advised that the medical database needed to be compatible with the information system of the enterprise of which it was a part. It also needed to be operationally and structurally independent of applications programs even though it contained data produced by these programs.

Coltri [94] noted that although a single structural database model could initially allow for simpler coordination, operation, and reporting, as databases enlarged and became more complex with many functional relationships, and as their components required frequent changes in data content, the ability to design a single, large database that could provide efficient querying became increasingly difficult. Furthermore, as databases grew larger they often developed problems caused by redundant data.

Hierarchical databases were considered by Coltri [94] to be the simplest and the earliest structural design used for medical databases. For a hierarchical database the connections between files, or between fields within files, needed to be defined at the start of the database. The data were organized in what was usually described as a parent-child relationship; where each "parent" could have many "children", but each "child" had only one "parent". Hierarchical data subclasses with inheritance of attributes could also appear in other database designs, such as in relational and object-oriented databases.

Coltri considered as the best known early example of a hierarchically structured, medical database, the one developed in the 1960s by Neil Pappalardo working in the laboratory of Dr. Octo Barnett and associates [21, 24, 165, 195]. Their Massachusetts General Hospital Utility Multi-Programming System (MUMPS) was designed for building and managing dynamic hierarchical databases with interactive computing applications and online transactional processing. MUMPS provided a good structure for medical databases with all their complexity, since its hierarchical structure enabled a more complex design than did a relational table with rows and columns. In the 1980s Meditech, the Department of Defense, and the Veterans Hospitals began installing their MUMPS-based medical information systems; and in the 2000s Epic was also MUMPS-based.

Karpinski [195] described an information storage and retrieval system (MISAR), which would find widespread use in the research analyses of important clinical problems, such as cerebral vascular accidents, berylliosis, and psoriasis. Another early example of a hierarchically structured medical database was that developed in the 1960s by Davis [107, 108, 110, 111], Terdiman [317], Collen, and associates at Kaiser Permanente in Oakland, California, to store electronic medical records (EMRs) for about one million patients. The design of each patient's record included 12 levels of storage that allowed direct access by the patient's unique medical record number to each of the patient's computer-defined office visits, which were subdivided into medically meaningful parts (as "tree branches"), such as laboratory data, medical diagnoses, and clinical services. The database was designed to store all data received.

Relational databases and their management systems were developed in the 1960s for large, shared databases by Codd [77–79] while at the IBM Research Center in San Jose. Codd required that all data in a relational database be in the form of two-dimensional tables with uniquely labeled rows and columns. Every data element was logically accessible through the use of the names of its table and its column. Data transformations resulted from following defined logical rules. In a relational database the data were organized into files or tables of fixed-length records; each record was an ordered list of values, with one value for each field. The information about each field's name and potential values was maintained in a separate metadatabase. The relational database model, because of its simplicity and power, soon became dominant in use, and in the 1970s Structured Query Language (SQL) was developed by Chamberlin and Boyce at IBM to construct, manage, and query relational databases [330]. SQL soon became the standard language used for the programming of relational databases. In 1979 a commercial relational database named ORACLE became available from the ORACLE Corporation. In the 1980s Ashton-Tate developed dBASE for microcomputers [99]. Johnson [190] described an extension of SQL for data warehouses that enabled analysts to designate groups of rows that could be manipulated and aggregated into large groups of data, and then be analyzed in a variety of ways to solve a number of analytic problems. Miller [244] at the University of Pittsburgh described the use of a commercial relational database-management system, called System 1022, that provided its own programming language (1022 DPL), and that permitted clinical data from large groups of patients to be entered, stored, queried, and analyzed for clinical studies. Friedman [143] and associates at Columbia University noted that the typical relational design for a clinical database could seriously impair query performance because a patient's data was typically scattered over many different tables. To circumvent this problem, a query language needed to be added.

Marrs [222] and Kahn at Washington University, St. Louis, described a distributed relational database-management system across multiple sites comprising a single enterprise, when they extended their clinical database for Barnes Hospital to include data from Jewish Hospital in BJC HealthCare – a merger of Barnes-Jewish, Inc. and Christian Health Services – that included 15 hospitals and other health care facilities. After considering alternative approaches, they chose to add the data from Jewish Hospital to their database. They then mapped the data from other facilities into their database and adjusted for differences in syntax and semantics in patient identifiers, medication formulary codes, diagnosis codes, and other information in their patients' records.

Multi-dimensional relational databases were developed as relational databases grew in size and developed multiple dimensions. Relational database structures were considered to be multi-dimensional when they contained multiple attributes, such as time periods, locations, product codes, and other attributes that could be defined in advance and aggregated in hierarchies. Some commercial search-and-query programs, such as Online Analytic Processing (OLAP), were designed for very large relational databases. These generally stored data in a relational structured design, and they used aggregations of data built from a fact-table according to specified dimensions. The combinations of all possible aggregations in the database were expected to be able to provide answers to every query of the stored data that could be anticipated [79].

Connolly [99] described a way of visualizing a multi-dimensional database by beginning with a flat, two-dimensional table of data, adding another dimension to form a three-dimensional cube, or hypercube, and then adding cubes of data within cubes of data, with each side of each cube being called a "dimension."

Pendse [268] described in some detail the history of Online Analytic Processing, and credited the publication in 1962 by Iverson of A Programming Language (APL) as the first mathematically defined, multi-dimensional language for processing multi-dimensional variables. Multi-dimensional analyses then became the basis for several versions of Online Analytic Processing that were developed in the 1970s and 1980s by IBM and others. In 1999 the Analyst module was available from Cognos, a company subsequently acquired by IBM. By the year 2000 new Online Analytic Processing derivatives were in use by IBM, Microsoft, Oracle, and others.

Object-oriented databases were developed in the 1970s at the Xerox Palo Alto Research Center (PARC), and used the programming language Smalltalk [277]. Whereas traditional database programs separately represented the data and procedures for manipulation of the data, in an object-oriented system the objects encapsulated both of these. Object-oriented databases were designed to attempt to bring the database programming and the applications programming closer together. They treat the database as a modular collection of components called objects. Objects were members of an entity that belonged to types or classes of data with their own data and programming codes. Objects incorporated not only data but also descriptions of their behavior and of their relationships to other objects. Objects used concepts such as entities, attributes, and relationships. Objects had an independent existence. Attributes were properties that described aspects of objects; and relationships described the association between objects. Objects were sufficiently modular and independent that they could be copied into other programs. An object-oriented database could serve a network of workstations in which one or more computers were designated as object-servers that would supply applications programs with objects as needed to minimize workstation and server communications.

By the late 1980s some database applications were programmed in object-oriented languages that treated the database as a modular collection of component items [112]. Connolly [99] described some relational variances for an object-oriented database in order to use Structured Query Language (SQL). Barsalou and Wiederhold [27] described their PENGUIN project that applied a three-layered architecture to an object-oriented database that defined the object-based data as a layer of data on top of a relational database-management system, with a hypertext interface between the object-oriented database and the relational database that provided conceptual integration without physical integration. Their workstations were Apple personal computers. They used Apple's HyperCard program for their Macintosh computer that defined and manipulated "stacks" of data corresponding to a relational-database structure, with one field for each attribute, written in the Macintosh HyperTalk language that allowed querying visual images that moved through a hypertext document.

Entity-attribute-value (EAV) databases were designed and developed to help manage the highly heterogeneous data within medical databases, where over several years of medical care a single patient could accumulate thousands of relevant descriptive parameters, some of which might need to be readily accessible from a large clinical database that contained multiple relational tables. Dinu and Nadkarni [119], Nadkarni [257–261], and Brandt et al. [57] described the entity-attribute-value database as an alternative to conventional relational database modeling where diverse types of data from different medical domains were generated by different groups of users. The term entity-attribute-value database was generally applied when a substantial proportion of the data was modeled as an entity-attribute-value even though some tables could be traditional relational tables. Conceptually, an entity-attribute-value design used a database table with three columns: (1) *Entity*, that contained data such as patient identification, with a time-stamp of the date-and-time of the beginning and end of each clinical event; (2) *Attribute*, that identified the event, such a laboratory test, or showed a pointer to a separate attribute table; and (3) *Value*, that contained the value of the attribute (such as the result of a laboratory test). A metadatabase was usually added to help provide definitions of terms, keys to related tables, and logical connections for data presentation, as well as interactive validation, data extraction, and for ad hoc query.

Chen and associates [72] evaluated the performance of an entity-attribute-value design and concluded that the advantage was in supporting generic browsing among many tables of data, as when following changes in a clinical parameter over many periods of time. The entity-attribute-value database also helped to provide schema stability as knowledge evolved and the metadata needed to change. However, attribute-centered queries were somewhat less efficient because of the large number of data tables with many more rows than when using conventional relational databases. Tuck et al. [323] described ways to map object-oriented software systems to relational databases by using entity-attribute-value databases.

Some early medical users of variations of the entity-attribute-value database model were: McDonald et al. [227, 228, 229, 232, 233] in the Regenstrief Medical Record (RMR); Warner [336, 338, 339] and Pryor [271] in the HELP system; Stead [307, 308, 309], Hammond [172] and Pryor [270] in Duke's TMR system; and Friedman [143] and Hripcsak [183] at Columbia University. The entity-attribute-value database model underlies the architecture of Informatics for Integrating Biology and the Bedside, or i2b2. The rapidly increasing volume of computer-based information stimulated the development of larger storage devices and more efficient database-management systems. To some investigators it became apparent that the complex requirements of patient-record databases required combined hierarchical, relational, and object-oriented structural approaches.

Federated databases developed that could store large volumes of aggregated data either in multiple partitions or as functional-oriented databases that were logically interconnected. They were directly accessible to-and-from multiple applications, and they allowed many users to simultaneously access and query data in the various databases [94]. The name data warehouses was applied to large, extended, central databases that collected and managed data from several different databases. They could service the ever-increasing volume of clinical data collected from ever-changing medical technologies. As data warehouses further enlarged, they often developed partitions and data-marts for specialized sub-sets of data in order to better serve users with different functional needs [99]. Data warehouses that could satisfy the needs of different users and to efficiently query large collections of data led to the development of online analytical processing (OLAP) and to translational data processing between data warehouses.

Distributed database management systems that involved the management of data, dispersed in two or more databases located in different computers required some means of communication for the distribution and exchange of data. Distributed database management systems in large organizations were designed as either clusters of computers tightly coupled to a central large mainframe computer, or loosely-coupled in a distributed database system [216].

Translational databases evolved in the late 1990s with more advanced designs of database management systems to: (1) optimize the translation, transformation, linkage, exchange, and integration of the increasingly voluminous medical information that was becoming accessible from many large databases in multiple institutions, by using wide-area-networks, the Internet and the World Wide Web; (2) provide access to high-performance, super-computing resources; (3) facilitate the concurrent query, analyses, and applications of large amounts of data by multi-disciplinary teams; (4) encourage knowledge discovery and data mining, and support the transfer of new evidence-based knowledge into patient care; and, (5) to advance the use of biomedical computational methods. Since most data warehouses were developed from their own legacy data-encoding standards, some reorganization and modification of source data were often required to permit data from different data warehouses to be merged into a single database schema. In this way translational database software evolved.

4.2 Classification of Medical Databases

Lindberg [213] noted that practitioners of medicine needed the help of computers to store and retrieve facts needed to care for their patients; to place these facts in the spectrum of similar observations on other patients in the same hospital or region; and to keep abreast of the ever growing mass of new medical knowledge.

Medical databases can be classified in accordance with their objectives, which can be to serve as patients' electronic records in support of clinical care, as specialized databases to support medical research, as databases designed to support financial claims, or for other objectives. Medical databases collect, integrate, and store data from various sources. They are usually considered to be primary databases if the data were initially collected and used for the direct purposes of the user, and to be secondary databases when data derived from primary databases are stored separately and used for other objectives [156].

Medical research databases may be primary databases when the clinical data were collected to support clinical research, such as for genetics or for clinical trials. But most research databases are secondary, in that they contain selected, de-identified clinical data extracted from primary medical databases used for clinical care. In contrast, in primary patient care databases, the medical record of each patient needs to contain all of the information collected for all of the medical problems of that individual patient. In a secondary research database, it is usually necessary to extract and transfer the selected data from the primary patient-record database into the secondary research database; and all patient data transferred from a primary patient-record database has additional special legal requirements for assuring the data validity, data security, and strict privacy and confidentiality of each patient's data. Garfolo [150] emphasized the importance of the need to de-identify patient data when a clinical database is also used for research.

Claims databases are maintained to account for the payments of financial claims for provided medical services. Among the largest of these are the databases for the Medicare and the Medicaid Programs created by the Social Security Amendment of 1965. The Medicare Program has been funded entirely by the Federal Government and is administered by the Federal Medicare Agency within the Department of Health and Human Services. It provides partial coverage for medical care to virtually all individuals aged 65 years and older. The Medicaid Program comprises a group of 54 programs supported by state and federal funds, and it provides coverage for medical care for economically disadvantaged and disabled persons. It is administered by the states with Federal oversight. In 1972 the Medicaid Management Information System (MMIS) was created to provide fiscal and management control, with defined minimum standards that each state had to meet. When a claims database is used for medical research, the conclusions may be limited to the selected population. In addition, the medical accuracy of diagnoses used for reimbursement has been questioned. Medical record databases of clinical care are generally considered to have more accurate data since they are primarily used for direct patient care, and clinicians need objective quantitative information to weigh the risks versus the benefits of each drug ordered [70].

4.2.1   Clinical Databases

Primary patients' medical databases that store computer-based, electronic patient records (EPRs) are also commonly referred to as electronic health records (EHRs) or as electronic medical records (EMRs). They are the data repositories used by physicians, nurses, medical technologists, administrators, and other health care providers to enter, store, and retrieve patients' data while providing patient care. The National Library of Medicine once defined an electronic patient record (EPR) as a computer-based system for input, storage, display, retrieval, and printing of information contained in a patient's medical record [252].

Clinical databases include a variety of primary and secondary databases that are used by physicians to help them make decisions about diagnosis and treatment. The utility of clinical databases resides in their capacity to store and retrieve huge amounts of information from many patients and from other sources. Michalski [243] described clinical databases as constructed to collect data and to learn more about the phenomena that produced the data. He divided techniques for using clinical databases into: (1) descriptive analyses to extract summaries of important features, such as grouping patients with similar syndromes and identifying important characteristics of each syndrome; and (2) predictive analyses to derive classification rules, such as developing rules that predict the course of a disease.

Primary clinical databases usually include the patients' medical records (PMRs), as well as any separate repositories of data collected in medical offices, outpatient clinics, and hospitals. Patient record databases may contain data collected over long periods of time, sometimes for a patient's life-time. They are accessed by a variety of users for different patient-care purposes, to satisfy legal requirements and assist with administrative issues, such as reimbursement. They must maintain the security, privacy, and confidentiality of the data.

Dick [116] and Steen reviewed the essential technologies needed for a patient-record database, and they believed that in the 1990s no medical database available could serve as a suitable model for computer-based patient records. Camp [64] described some of the complexities of primary clinical databases: (1) at the time patient care information was being obtained, it was not always known what data might be needed in the future, so this tended to enlarge a database with some data that would never be used; (2) the database had to store information that could be differently structured and formatted, and that was often unstandardized; (3) it needed to allow exploring complex data relationships in (frequently) a minimal access time, yet not unduly interfere with the productivity of busy health care providers who were not computer programmers; and (4) primary clinical databases tended to lack patients' data for events that occurred between recorded visits to their health care providers.

Connolly [99] noted that since most clinical data were time-stamped data, it was necessary that data transactions be recorded and retrieved in their correct time sequence. Graves [163] added that another requirement for a medical database was to provide a natural language processing (NLP) program that had the capability to query textual information, such as were obtained by patient interviews and that could include expressed feelings and experiential information. The availability of online access to clinical databases greatly facilitated the search and retrieval of information needed by physicians for clinical decision making. The factors that influenced the rate of diffusion of medical databases and other computer applications in medical practice were studied by Anderson [2] and Jay at Purdue and Indiana Universities who concluded that physicians had the major role in the diffusion of clinical databases.

Specialized clinical databases can be disease specific, such as for genetic diseases or cancers; or be organ specific such as for heart or kidney disease. Or they can be device specific such as for chest x-rays; procedure specific such as for coronary artery bypass surgery, clinical specialty specific such as for pediatric disorders; therapy specific such as for anti-viral drugs, or population-specific such as for a geriatric or a racial group. Safran [284] observed that a clinical database could be used to look up data on an individual patient, to find data on patients with similarities to the patient being cared for; to find data about patients who share one or more attributes; or to analyze data patterns for trends or relationships. Fries [144] noted that some of the most important clinical problems were chronic, such as arthritis, cancer, and heart disease; and a study of the management of these disorders could benefit from specialized chronic diseases databases.

Large medical centers often have many specialized clinical databases for various inpatient and outpatient clinical services in addition to databases for clinical support systems for the clinical laboratory, radiology, pharmacy, and others [7]. As a result, they usually need a distributed database-management system to link them. Each clinical subsystem's database needs extract-transfer-load (ETL) programs to move data to-and-from its subsystem database and the central, integrated, clinical database. Secondary clinical records include data abstracted from the primary patient record. Clinicians have long been encouraged to study their patients' records, to abstract data of interest from these primary patients' records, and to store such data in secondary databases such as in registries for use by investigators for clinical, epidemiological, or health services research [34].

Metadatabases are developed to: (1) store metadata that describe the primary data contained in a database; (2) provide a data dictionary with definitions of terms, and a list of coded data in the database with their codes; (3) serve as a thesaurus to recognize different terms that have similar meanings; and (4) provide a lexicon of standard, accepted, defined, and correctly spelled terms. A metadatabase needs to contain associated relevant information to aid in the storage and retrieval of data; by providing linkages to other data items and files; by providing keys to related tables; by providing logical connections for data presentation, interactive validation, and data extraction; by permitting ad hoc query; and by providing users with interfaces for any metadata additions or corrections. A data dictionary is usually initiated as a part of a metadatabase by selecting commonly used terms from a standard medical dictionary and from related medical literature. It needs to permit the addition of new terms – new data items – such as for new procedures. As lexicons became the basis for automated natural-language processing, they usually included syntactical information, such as whether the word was a noun, verb, or other, as well as semantic information, such as the meaning in the language of medicine [225]. It was soon obvious that medical text processing required a comprehensive data dictionary, a lexicon of standard, accepted, defined, and correctly spelled terms; and that such a dictionary had to list all data items stored in the computer database, with their definitions, and with any associated information and codes required for their storage and retrieval, as well as linkages to other data items and files.

For a primary patient record database, its metadatabase needed to provide any special instructions for conducting clinical procedures; needed to describe all processes and procedures such as clinical laboratory tests; and needed to specify the normal and the "alert" boundary limits for each clinical test and procedure. Warner [337] emphasized that the purpose of a metadatabase was to minimize the chance of ambiguity in data representation between the point of data entry and the point at which the data were used. Anderson [3] credited the Veterans Administration (VA) with publishing the first data dictionary as a part of the VA's computer-based medical records. Hammond [169, 171, 172] and Stead described in some detail the metadatabase developed for Duke University's TMR (The Medical Record). Their metadatabase included patients' identification data, and it defined and coded all clinical variables including patients' medical problems, diagnostic studies, and therapies. They used their metadatabase as a dictionary to define the codes for their computer-based, clinical laboratory system that was linked to their TMR system. The metadatabase contained patients' demographic and examination data, clinical reports and messages, and professional fees and accounting data. An alphabetically arranged thesaurus provided definitions of synonyms. Codes and their text equivalents were defined in the metadatabase. The user could enter a code directly or type text and let the program find the code. Their dictionary permitted modification and updating of specific functions, and it allowed for differences between various specialties and clinics. Major sections of the dictionary were devoted to system specifications, medical problems, laboratory studies, providers' names, supplies, and therapies; demographic data, subjective, and physical examination data; and places of encounter, professional fees, accounting, messages, and report control.

As an example of the type and format of information contained in the dictionary, the medical problem section included the problem name, any corresponding standard coding scheme, and a flag to identify the problem as temporary or permanent. An alphabetically arranged section permitted synonym definitions. A cross-reference section listed possible causes and manifestations of the given problem; gave subjective and physical parameters to be followed for that problem; recommended studies and therapies for that problem; and identified items to be displayed in a flow sheet specific to that problem.

Ostrowski [265] employed The Medical Record in a group practice in Los Angeles and found the data dictionary to be an important part of the database-management software. In addition to a data dictionary, a thesaurus of accepted synonyms was required. Although it was possible in a metadatabase to search and retrieve computer-stored text by matching desired words, it was easier to search and retrieve by numbers and letters.

4.2.2   Genetics Databases

Genetics is the study of heredity. Genetics databases are used to plot a family pedigree, to manage clinical care, and to provide decision support for the diagnosis and treatment of genetic diseases [241]. Modern genetics can be traced to Mendel, whose plant breeding experiments in the mid-1800s produced the underlying basis of genetics [29]. Watson [343] and Crick described the structure of deoxyribonucleic acid (DNA), and this radically changed the study of genetics and initiated new generations of genetic databases and genomic databases. Each cell in the human body contains 46 chromosome – strands of DNA composed of 23 chromosome pairs. One chromosome of each pair is inherited from each parent. DNA is composed of four nucleic acids: guanine (G), cytosine (C), adenine (A), and thymine (T) that are formed into base pairs. Guanine (G) always pairs with cytosine (C), while adenine (A) always pairs with thymine (T). These base pairs of nucleic acids are linked into chains that are wound in a spiral called a double helix. A specific group of base pairs is called a gene, and each gene is found in a specific location on a chromosome. Chromosomes carry 50,000–100,000 genes, which produce the proteins that carry out specific functions in human development and cellular activity. DNA contains instructions for making all of the proteins that our bodies need. The map of the proteins in the human body is called the proteome. A mutation is a genetic disorder that results from a cell division in which there is a change from the normal sequence of base pairs in a gene. If the mutation occurs in only one gene – if the other gene remains intact and the protein(s) which that gene encodes can still be made – then the individual may be a carrier and not show the disease; but if both paired genes are defective the person usually displays the genetic disease [346].

Genetic linkage databases must be able to satisfy the complex hierarchical structures of patients' demographic and genetic data and deal with the pedigrees, the kindred or family trees that are used in genetic research. Genetic linkage refers to the tendency of genes to be inherited together as a result of their proximity on the same chromosome. Such linkage can be quantified by measuring recombination frequencies from family studies. A computer can help genetic researchers determine the linkage of genes within a chromosome.

Genetic linkage databases began to be reported in 1959 when McKusick, at the Johns Hopkins University described a genealogical database with census and vital statistics data for 18,000 Old Order Amish who were living in Lancaster County, Pennsylvania, and in Holmes County, Ohio [90]. McKusick's goal was to collect data on all Amish in the area, who then numbered about 50,000. He gathered a complete census by family units, recording for every individual their date of birth (and death) and date of marriage. He then assembled a total genealogy by tracing ancestors as completely and as far back as possible. In the case of this relatively closed population, to which almost no new members had been added since its founding, the genealogy aimed for completeness. Between the 1700s when the Amish began to arrive in America and 1986, the total genealogy consisted of at about ten generations. Output of the program included the printed pedigree up to 12 generations, the cumulative percentage completeness of the pedigree for each generation, the cumulative consanguinity in each generation, the common ancestors together with their contribution to the total consanguinity, and if desired, the sex-linked coefficient of consanguinity. Medical data, blood group, sociological and other data were stored with the unique identification number of each individual [236, 239]. McKusick [235] described the problems involved in studying genetic linkage in man as involving the identification of genetic loci that are on the same chromosome, and the determination of how far apart these loci are.

It was usually easy to determine if a trait was determined by a gene on the X chromosome as opposed to a gene on an autosomal chromosome. In 1962 McKusick [237, 238] published a catalog of traits in man linked to the X chromosome. He periodically revised this catalog, and in 1966 published his classic book on the *Mendelian Inheritance in Man*, which aimed to be a comprehensive gene encyclopedia. In 1987 the Online Mendelian Inheritance in Man (OMIM) also became available by online computer retrieval; and the 1988 edition of OMIM listed over 2,000 genetic disorders.

Murphy [256] and associates at Johns Hopkins University used a computer to estimate genetic linkage. Using data from large human pedigrees of gene linkage problems, they devised a computer program to calculate the probability that two genes on the same chromosome would part company during hereditary transmission. Their program determined the genotypic possibilities for each person in the pedigree, calculated the probability of obtaining the pedigree for various crossover values, and expressed the results as a logarithm of the ratio of this probability to that for a specified crossover value. From these calculations, they could determine confidence limits for their estimates [255].

Chung [74] at the University of Wisconsin, reported on the early use of a library of programs called SEGRAN, which employed IBM 650 and Control Data Corporation model CDC 1604 computers to study human pedigrees in a variety of diseases. They also studied the genetic effects on children of the ABO blood groups of their parents where incompatibility was found to cause a 12 % loss of incompatible children. They developed physical maps that could specify actual distances between landmarks along the chromosomes [51].

In 1975, the department of medical genetics at the Indiana University School of Medicine designed and implemented a Medical Genetics Acquisition and Data Transfer System (MEGADATS). They collected human pedigree data and laboratory test results on appropriate individuals, performed retrievals from the database within or across several pedigrees, and maintained confidentiality of the patient data. The system was designed to store and retrieve information collected on approximately 15,000 families seen over 14 years. In 1978 the database included 525,000 individuals. Retrievable information included family pedigrees, genotyping, and physical and laboratory diagnostic information. The linkage of family members was achieved by a set of pointers to other family records [194]. In 1983 the MEGADATS database continued to store data on the 525,000 individuals in the 15,000 families. It was used to study Huntington's disease, a hereditary disorder of the central nervous system which can cause rapid, jerky, involuntary movements. A Huntington's chorea project was initiated with the aim of searching for the basic defect, for improving methods of diagnosis, and for developing more effective methods of treatment and prevention [153]. Gersting [154] also described in some detail a revised version, MEGADATS-4, as a relational database-management system that required little or no programming to carry out a variety of genetics applications, and that included patient's files related by family-member fields to manage pedigrees.

Skolnick and associates [304] at the Church of Jesus Christ of Latter-day Saints (LDS) operated an extensive program, initiated in 1906, for collecting and storing genealogical records of the membership of the Mormon Church Skolnick's project began as an extraction of data from these records for the construction of family genealogies, which would ultimately be linked with medical data to investigate genetic factors in various diseases. In 1973, the system began to use video terminals for data entry, using as many as six terminal operators to enter coded data on individuals and families. A team of researchers at the University of Utah began to use these records to develop a database linked to medical records to investigate the genetic transmission of several diseases. In 1974, they introduced a system of automatic record linkage that by 1978 resulted in the computerized genealogy of 170,000

Utah families, with data for 1.2 million persons stored in a dedicated database on a Data General Eclipse minicomputer [28].

In 1978 they published the initial results of their first effort to use the LDS records to study demography. These large sibships led to pedigrees of 2,000–5,000 individuals over six or seven generations for Mormon pioneers [303]. In 1980 these investigators described their general database system, the Genealogical Information System (GENISYS), as using a high-level query language that allowed researchers to access data without the need for prior training. It provided the ability to analyze selected data sets, to add new data to existing files, and to accommodate familial relationships present in genetic data [118]. In 1980 they also reported a new basis for constructing high-level, genetic-linkage maps by detecting DNA sequence polymorphisms as polymorphic marker loci linking groups with similar restriction fragment length polymorphisms (RFLPs), and then using pedigree analysis to establish high-level linkage relationships that could be useful in developing models for human inheritance [54].

In 1988 the LDS group reported developing a relational database for their Utah population called the Human Genetics Database Management System (HGDBMS) that facilitated data collection and retrieval for human genetics research. In addition to the representation of pedigree data, it also included programs for the management of clinical parameters, blood samples, and genotype processing. It was used for genetic and epidemiologic studies, and was designed to be extended and customized to fit the needs of different genetic applications by adding relations, attributes, forms, and reports. Since their genetic analyses, such as gene mapping, linkage studies, and segregation analysis, were designed around studies of pedigrees, the representation of genealogical data was a major issue for the development of the genetics database management system. The system design had to incorporate the ability to link individuals and families together to form genealogical records. Seuchter [291] wrote that a genotype processing unit contained information about the genotyping of the extracted DNA. The genotype knowledge unit contained genotypic information gathered during the different studies.

The management of human genetic data involves a large number of different data structures including pedigrees, clinical data, genotypic data, and laboratory information, all received from a variety of sources and at different times. To analyze pedigree structures linked to family trees, Prokosch [269] developed a rule-based expert system for the Utah Population that performed the preliminary analysis of pedigree data. For a simple pedigree, this could lead to the final result, but when the program detected a complexity, for example, consanguinity, it would automatically trigger further analysis with the appropriate procedure. Galland [149] and colleague described in some detail a gene mapping expert system (GMES) that they added to help in locating genes on one of the 23 pairs of chromosomes. They used an expert system shell called frames plus objects (FROBS) that allowed a mixed approach using objects-and-rules capabilities and algorithms that provided an interface to further programming.

Mitchell and associates [251] at the University of Missouri, Columbia, described their Clinical Genetics Data-Management System (MEDGEN). They further reported the development of their Genetics Office Automation System (GOAS) for the Medical Genetics Unit of the University of Missouri that was implemented on an IBM PC/XT personal computer. GOAS included primary databases for the records of their patients. In addition, it had secondary reference databases that contained diagnostic and family data that were linked by a six-digit patient number to the primary databases, using a form that was completed from GOAS databases and sent to the Missouri Genetics Disease Program [106].

Buyse [63] described Birth Defects Information System (BDIS), an online, computer-based, information retrieval and decision-support system that contained data from over 1,000 types of birth defects. Also, the Missouri Information Retrieval Facility provided summaries of current clinical information on a broad range of birth defects. Its Diagnostic Assist Facility provided interactive decision support for complex and multi-system birth defects and genetic disorders. By comparing signs and symptoms from a patient's record with those of the more than 600 conditions in the knowledge base, the program could suggest potential diagnoses and provide information on what was needed to confirm a diagnosis. Finally, Yu [368] at Columbia University in New York described a database of genetic diseases and family histories for 22,292 patients collected from electronic medical discharge summaries using a natural language processing system.

The Genetic Sequence Data Bank (GenBank) was chartered to provide a computer database of all known DNA and RNA sequences and related biological and bibliographic information. GenBank was founded in 1982 under a contract by the National Institute of General Medical Sciences (NIGMS) with IntelliGenetics, Inc. of Mountain View, California, and co-sponsored by the National Library of Medicine (NLM) and by the Department of Energy. In the mid-1980s it was managed at Stanford University. By 1989 GenBank contained data on 30 million nucleotides, the building blocks of DNA and RNA, in 26,000 different entries in biological material and organisms ranging from viruses to humans. Cross-referencing was established with the Human Gene Mapping Library, allowing users of GenBank to identify and compare newly sequenced human genes with those mapped previously [315]. The Human Gene Map was to fix each gene to a particular region of one of the 23 pairs of human chromosomes, and to define the complete set of sequences of adenine, thymine, cytosine, and guanine that make up a human being. By 1989, less than 2 % of the estimated 100,000 human genes had been mapped [242].

The goal of the human genome project was to provide new approaches to the treatment of the more than 3,000 inherited genetic diseases, many of which were already mapped to specific chromosomes. The project was authorized with the hope that it would link existing databases and help disseminate crucial information to researchers around the world. Collins [93] reviewed how changes in chromosomes and mutations can help identify disease-causing genes, and how mutations in specific genes can cause disease. He wrote that most of the genes that cause genetic disorders were identified by functional cloning, which required biochemical or structural information about the defect underlying the disease, and he listed recent targets of positional cloning in the human genome. In 1992, management of GenBank was transferred to the National Center for Biological Information, which now maintains on the World Wide Web the Human Gene Map that charts the locations of genes in the 23 pairs of human chromosomes.

Human genome databases began to be developed in many academic centers to study the association of genes with diseases, and to find commonality between seemingly dissimilar clinical disorders. This research was aimed at a better understanding of the etiology of disease, and at the development of more effective drugs and treatments. A collaborative genome center database was reported by Miller [245] and associates at Yale University School of Medicine that had Internet collaboration with the Albert Einstein College of Medicine. Graves [164] and associates at the Baylor College of Medicine described their genome database for the Baylor Human Genome Center. Evans [129, 130] and associates at Creighton University applied data mining algorithms to family history data to automatically create hereditary disease patterns. They noted that in most hereditary syndromes, to find a correspondence between genetic mutations within a gene (genotype) and a patient's clinical history (phenotype) was challenging. To define possible genotype and phenotype correlations, they used data mining technology whereby the clinical cancer histories of gene-mutation-positive patients were used to help define valid patterns for a specific DNA intragenic mutation. For each hereditary disease, such as hereditary colon cancer or breast cancer, a set of rules that contained clinical data were evaluated by clinical experts as relevant, valid, and likely to classify a patient as positive or negative for having the cancer. They applied their algorithm to patients with family histories suggestive of hereditary colon cancer and found the conclusions of their computer recognizer and those of clinical experts to be in close agreement. They developed rules for data mining algorithms derived from breast cancer patients known to have the BRCA1 or BRCA2 genes, and found that "true" patterns for a specific DNA intragenic mutation could be distinguished from "false" patterns with a high degree of reliability. They also reported using data mining algorithms to characterize DNA mutations by patients' clinical features.

Weiland [346] at Kaiser Permanente (KP) Northwest Region described the KP Human Genome Project that was initiated to study the clinical impact of genetic information, and to develop guidelines as to who should be screened and who should receive genetic counseling. When completed, this Human Genome Project was expected to identify about 4,000 genetic disorders, and to assist clinicians in the diagnosis and management of genetic diseases. Weiland found that physicians without genetics training were ill equipped to interpret complex genetic tests or to provide genetic counseling. In 2005, a Research Program for Genes, Environment, and Health (RPGEH), affiliated with the University of California in San Francisco, was launched by Kaiser Permanente's Northern California Division of Research to study genetic and environmental factors that influence common, important diseases. This research established registries for cancer, diabetes, asthma, autoimmune disease, osteoporosis, obesity, and other diseases. Based on a membership of more than three million Kaiser Health Plan members in Northern California, the clinical, genetic, and other information from more than 500,000 consenting members were collected from their electronic medical records, from samples of their saliva or blood and from their self-reported health surveys (www.rpgeh.kaiser.org).

Mathur [223] and associates at the University of Missouri-Kansas City described the Disease Ontology they used for automated annotation of genetic records to measure disease similarity. Corvin [102] and associates described the Genome-Wide Association Studies (GWAS) that had published nearly 400 articles that identified common genetic variants that predispose to a variety of common human diseases.

The human genome, the full set of chromosomes that account for inheritable traits, is estimated to have about ten million single nucleotide polymorphisms (SNPs) that constitute about 0.1 % of the genome. Cooper et al. [101] noted the availability of newer gene-chip technology that can identify and measure a half-million SNPs, and that can be used to support studies to identify SNPs and corresponding genes that are associated with disease. In addition, Cooper reported a genome-wide database (GWAS) study of Alzheimer's disease that contains 312,318 SNP measurements on 1,411 patients. Denny [114] and associates at Vanderbilt University, used genetic data in their longitudinal electronic medical records (EMRs) for phenome-wide association scans (PheWAS), and used the International Classification of Diseases version 9 (ICD-9) codes found in patients' records to approximate the clinical disease phenome. They then developed a code translation table to automatically define 776 different disease populations. They genotyped 6,005 patients in their DNA databank at five single nucleotide polymorphisms (SNPs) for previously reported disease-SNP associations for Crohn's disease, multiple sclerosis, and other diseases. Their phenome-wide association scans generated case and control populations as well as disease-SNPs associations. They demonstrated that it was possible to couple genome-wide and phenome-wide association scans to discover gene-disease associations in patients with genetic diseases [114].

4.3   Internet Medical Databases

Internet medical databases were used by Anderson [6] and associates at the University of California-Fresno Medical Center to provide medical information for their clinical decision-support system by adding online access to the National Library of Medicine's MEDLINE and other databases. They modified the CONSIDER program developed by Lindberg [213] and the RECONSIDER program developed by Blois [33] to use for differential diagnoses, and they added provisions for time-series analysis, electrocardiogram signal-analysis, radiology digital-image analysis, and an images database. Chaney [71] and associates at Baylor College in Houston, reported developing an Integrated Academic Information Management System (IAIMS) supported by the National Library of Medicine (NLM) that used hypertext in a Virtual Network employing UNIX software and SUN workstations.

In the 1990s Internet medical databases began to be used by some medical information systems for Web-based, electronic patient records (EPRs). On the other hand, McDonald et al. [226] wrote that provisions to maintain adequate confidentiality of data were not yet available via the Internet. In 1994 Willard [364] and associates at the University of Minnesota deployed a Web-based, clinical information system claimed to be less expensive to develop and operate than client-server systems used previously. Their system provided services to physicians and to patient-care areas with connections to their hospital communications network. They reported a significant savings in physicians' time and a substantial reduction in interpretive errors. Cimino [75] and associates at the Columbia-Presbyterian Medical Center in New York, developed a clinical workstation for their hospital surgery service that used the Web client-server architecture. They used a Netscape server, Navigator clients, Macintosh computers, and Internet protocols on their local-area network. Their files were in Hypertext Markup Language (HTML) format, and used Uniform Resource Locators (URLs) to point to additional sources on the Internet. They built a clinical information browser, and they considered Netscape's standard security features to be adequate.

In the 1990s the Internet quickly and reliably delivered text, email, music, and images by employing a variety of digital communication technologies. By 1995 about 13,000 Web sites allowed public access. A User's Network (USENET) was available for discussion groups that focused on medical subjects, and mailing list services commonly called listserv provided hundreds of medicine-related mailing lists covering all specialties in medicine. The National Institutes of Health could be accessed at http://www.nih.gov, and databases of the National Library of Medicine could be accessed at http://www.nlm.nih.gov. In addition, many medical centers allowed public access to medical services through Web servers [157].

In 1998 the Web transmitted about five million emails each minute. It also began to be used by some physicians for consultations and education [53]. In 1999 private corporations and colleges sponsored the evolving Internet-2, and the Federal government supported the Next-Generation Internet using fiber-optic digital networks to develop the infrastructure for faster transmission of text, voice, and video. The Web had already established a global consumer market place of virtual stores that sold a variety of products and services, and it was becoming an important provider of health information to both patients and clinicians [350]. In 1991 Berners-Lee, the founder of the World Wide Web, established a Web Virtual Library with hypertext links to transmit textual, graphic, and video information. The Web Library became associated with the National Institutes of Health (NIH) and its National Library of Medicine (NLM), with a group of international academic institutions, and with government and commercial providers. A user could connect to the NLM Web server, to the Web Virtual Library of Medicine and Biosciences, and to many other databases [234].

Buhle [61] and associates at the University of Pennsylvania School of Medicine, founded OncoLink, an electronic library of audio, graphic, images, and video about cancer – all disseminated via the Web. In 1994 it was estimated to have 20 million users. Hypertext links led users to other sources. OncoLink employed Gopher services, developed at the University of Minnesota, to provide hierarchical menus of information. It used the public domain Web browser, Mosaic, and HTTPs, an encrypted version of the HyperText Transport Protocol, to communicate text files and graphics over the World Wide Web. OncoLink software was implemented on DEC 3000 AXP Model 800 computers.

Hersh et al. [178] described CliniWeb, a searchable database of clinical information accessible on the Web that provided a database of clinically-oriented, Universal Resource Locators (URLs) indexed with the Medical Subject Headings or MeSH terms, the controlled vocabulary used by the National Library of Medicine to index the biomedical literature. CliniWeb served as a test bed for research in defining the optimal methods to build and evaluate a clinically oriented Web resource. Hersh also observed that the National Library of Medicine, the Centers for Disease Control and Prevention, the Food and Drug Administration, the National Cancer Institute, and other health-related government agencies all used the Web to disseminate information free of charge.

Lowe [219] and associates at the University of Pittsburgh, reviewed the evolution of the Internet and of the Web, and described them as rapidly evolving from a resource used primarily by the research community, to a global information network offering a wide range of services. They described the Web as a network-based, distributed hypertext system, with links to component objects or nodes (such as text, sound, images and video) embedded in a document or in a set of documents. The nodes could be linked to associated nodes to form a database, and the user could navigate from one node to another based on the user's needs rather than on fixed data linkages defined in more usual information-retrieval systems. They described their WebReport system that used a Web-based database to store clinical images with their associated textual reports for diagnostic procedures, including gastrointestinal endoscopy, radiology, and surgical pathology. Their WebReport used the HyperText Markup Language to provide physicians in their offices with ready access to radiographic images and associated reports [220]. The history of the Internet and of the World Wide Web and their contributions to medical informatics has been described by Shortliffe [295], Glowniak [157], Hafner [166], and Shortliffe [295, 296]. Shortliffe considered the ARPANET, which led to the Internet, to be one of the most compelling examples of how government investments led to innovations with broad economic and social effects.

4.4 Medical Database Management Systems

Database managementsystems were designed to capture and process data stored in a computer in a way that permitted their ready retrieval [17]. For a medical information system the database management system needed to store and retrieve patients' data in a way that supported a computer-based patient record. A database management system could either interface with files that were physically independent but had logical relationships and could be organized and reorganized in accordance with the needs of the different applications; or store the files in one site so that they were actually physically integrated in a collated patient record. Blum [39] emphasized that the usefulness of a clinical information system depended on its database management system.

Walters [332] considered the main contribution of database management science was to distinguish between what information should be stored in a system from how it should be stored. Wiederhold [360] defined a database management system as the hardware and software that controlled, stored, processed, and retrieved the data in the database. A database management system was defined by Blum [39, 40, 44] as software consisting of a collection of procedures and programs with the requirements for: (1) entering, storing, retrieving, organizing, updating, and manipulating the data within its database; (2) managing the utilization and maintenance of the database; (3) including a metadatabase to define application-specific views of the database; (4) entering each data element only once, even though the same data might be stored in other subsystems; (5) retrieving, transferring, and communicating needed data in a usable format, and having the ability to create inverted files indexed by key terms; (6) maintaining the integrity, security, and the required level of confidentiality of the data; and (7) fulfilling all management, legal, accounting, and economic requirements. A metadatabase was usually added to provide definitions of terms, keys to related tables, logical connections for data presentation, interactive validation, and data extraction, as well as for ad-hoc query. Database managementsystems soon replaced the earlier file-based systems that often stored the same data in many files where retrieval and coordination could be more difficult.

After a review of medical record database structures used in the 1990s, Stead et al. [309] reported that the major problem for a patient-record database management system was the [36] difficulty of mapping complex logical structures into a physical media. They concluded that patient-record databases were more complicated than were databases used for other purposes, that no existing database structural design was adequate for developing, as an example, a common national patient-record database, and that some combination of database designs would be needed.

Database management systems were required when the computer processing of large amounts of data and their storage in a manner to permit their ready retrieval, was no longer a trivial problem. Some early examples of the development of medical database management systems were: the Massachusetts General Hospital Utility Multi-programming System (MUMPS), Duke University's Generalized Medical Information System (GEMISCH), Kaiser Permanente's MFCS, and the Veterans Administration's File Manager. The evolution, design, implementation, and management of computer-stored databases have been described by: Blum [37, 39, 42], Collen [83–86, 89, 96], Connolly [99], Coltri [94], Duke [124], and Campbell-Kelly [67].

Distributed database management systems involved managing physically dispersed data in two or more databases located in different computers, and used some means of communication to exchange of data. Distributed database management systems in large medical centers were designed either as clusters of computers tightly coupled to a central large mainframe computer, or were loosely-coupled in a distributed database system [217]. Distributed medical database systems evolved in the 1970s with the introduction of lower cost minicomputers and more efficient communication networks that brought computers closer to the users. In a distributed database system with a cluster of specialized subsystem databases, each subsystem collected and stored the data locally generated. A communications network then provided linkages not only for data entry and retrieval from an integrated central database, but also for other subsystem databases as needed. In a large medical center, if each clinical service developed its own database to satisfy its own specific functional and technical requirements, an integrating database management system was needed to provide generalized data retrieval. This arrangement allowed physicians to use clinical workstations connected to client-server minicomputers connected in a local area network (LAN) that linked the entire hospital. Patient data could be generated and used at the local sites, collected from all of the distributed databases, and integrated into a central, computer-based patient record [83]. Since the computers were often made by different manufacturers and used different software platforms, to construct and maintain the interfaces needed to interchange data could be difficult and expensive. This stimulated the evolution of specialized communications computers and networks for the distribution of data. Small computers were linked together, often connected to a central mainframe computer from which data could be downloaded. Wess [349] noted that the design and implementation of a distributed database system was more complex than that of a simple networked, data communications system.

In the 1970s, a variety of forms of networks for distributed database systems began to appear, either linked together or connected to a central mainframe computer from which data could be communicated to-and-from the distributed smaller computers. Blois [32, 35] advocated the use of a communications processor that would perform code conversion and provide a high-speed communicating link to each distributed computer. In 1971 Blois initiated a distributed database system for the medical facilities at the University of California, San Francisco (UCSF) Hospital. He used a separate, dedicated, communications minicomputer to connect computers from different vendors, and he established a local-area network (LAN) for medical data communications. Blois separated data communications from data processing. After developing modular subsystems that could stand alone, he linked them in a communications network using specific data communications standards adopted at the onset. His distributed database management system required a reliable, high-bandwidth, communications computer to perform communications code conversion, and a high-speed link to each subsystem.

Wasserman [340, 342] while associated with Blois, proposed that a distributed database system should be capable of functioning at all levels of data acquisition, data manipulation, data retrieval, and data communications for a variety of applications, and he advocated for distributed medical databases to support an interactive information system with clinical work-stations. A distributed database management system was then needed to manage physically dispersed data in multiple databases located in different computers, and to provide some means of communications for the exchange of data.

Walters [333], at the University of California, Davis, linked microcomputers with their databases to a remote, large host computer using MUMPS-based software. Zeichner [369] at Mitre Corporation and Tolchin [319] at Johns Hopkins University described their distributed database spread over a variety of different, independent minicomputers. They used microcomputer-based, interface units between each network minicomputer processor and a communications bus. Data exchange used protocols between network units, so each new or modified application or device could interact with the communications bus. In 1980 the Johns Hopkins group used a fiber-optic, local area network to integrate several subsystems built by three different manufacturers, each with a different operating system. They used microprocessor-based, network-integrating units to perform the conversions of communications codes needed to exchange data [41, 321]. Tolchin [320] at the Johns Hopkins University and Simborg [298] at the University of California in San Francisco (UCSF) reduced the problem of interfacing multiple incompatible computers when they implemented at the UCSF medical center a fiber-optic, local area network that integrated four different minicomputers. A fifth host computer was interfaced to the network to provide a monitoring service for performance analysis. In 1985 they expanded their distributed clinical-information systems, all linked by Ethernet technology that supported 10-megabit-per-second data rates [322].

Hammond and associates [171] at Duke University reported implementing an Ethernet local area network for three types of computers connecting their clinical laboratory system to their central "The Medical Record" (TMR) database. Steinbach [312] described an early hospital communication system that used a DEC VAX minicomputer and MUMPS software to combine voice and data communications using a combination of cabling and bundled telephone lines connected to modems. Kuzmak [205] described their use of a central, clinical results database to contain reports from the clinical laboratory, radiology, and surgical pathology. A local area network permitted reports to be viewed from any terminal, personal computer, or clinical workstation in the hospital.

4.5   Patient Data Security, Privacy, and Confidentiality

Data security involves the protection of data against theft, unauthorized access, and unintentional access. Data protection for any computer-based medical information system (MIS) means protecting the privacy, confidentiality, security, and integrity of each patient's medical data against unauthorized access, intentional or not, for reading, copying, altering, or destroying. In addition, data security requires that the information system itself be protected from theft, vandalism, fire, flood and other destructive forces. Blum [45, 47] defined data protection in a medical information system as involving data safety and data security; where data safety includes protection against destruction, manipulation, or falsification of data, as well as theft of recording media. Primarily concerned with physical media, data safety protects against the loss of data, the introduction of invalid data, and the deliberate misuse of data. Maintenance of data confidentiality has long been a tradition between patient and physician; communications between them have been considered privileged.

Computer-based medical record systems have the same requirements for maintaining the confidentiality of patient data as do paper-based medical record systems. In comparison with paper records, computer-based systems provide advantages and disadvantages. Simon [301] emphasized that computer databases have to be given the highest protection from abuse, yet one needs to be careful that crude methods of protection do not deprive society of needed information. In the 1980s precautions were implemented for protecting the data of patients with a diagnosis of drug abuse, or with positive tests for the acquired immunodeficiency syndrome (AIDS) [347]. These issues had to be re-addressed as technology moved the patient record from pieces of paper collected in folders and stored in file cabinets at the doctor's office to electronic health records stored in a large, central facility.

Privacy is viewed as the individual patient's right to control personal information. Confidentiality is defined as the obligation of the health professional and the hospital to safeguard the privacy of information in the medical record, whether stored on paper or in a computer [168, 280]. Springer [306] in a review of state law relating to computer-based medical records listed the following threats to information privacy in a time-sharing medical information system: (1) accidental infiltration by computer malfunction, user errors, or software errors; (2) deliberate infiltration by wire-tapping or hacking, electromagnetic pickup, examination of carbon copy papers, entrance of files by browsing, or legitimate access to a part of a system to ask unauthorized questions; (3) masquerading as a legitimate user after having obtained proper identification through wire-tapping or other means; (4) "between-lines" entry, as when a legitimate user was inactive but still held an open communication channel; or (5) "piggyback" entry by selective interception of communication between user and computer and the substitution of a modified message.

Springer also defined as distinct from security and confidentiality, data reliability in that most state laws and the Joint Commission on Accreditation of Hospitals (JCAH) required medical record data contributed by physicians, nurses, and other health care professionals to be signed. This requirement was the basis for introducing acceptable electronic signatures for computer-stored transactions. In the 1980s, rubber stamp signatures and computer printed signatures began to appear on printouts [276].

It was always the hospital's responsibility for its inpatients and the physician's responsibility for office patients, to safeguard medical records against loss, tampering, or use by unauthorized persons. By the late 1960s a concern of many was how to control access to computer files and how to safeguard the entry and retrieval of data from public and private computer databases [104, 141, 179, 354]. McNamara [242], in the law division of the American Medical Association, asked how, when a patient consented to have data entered into an electronic record, could confidentiality be protected when the data were sent to a computer 1,000 miles away? Levinson [207] pointed out that paper-based records provided incomplete protection in that patients' charts were often left unattended. Anyone wearing a white coat or carrying a stethoscope could often obtain a patient's chart without providing adequate identification. Perhaps computer-based records, hidden behind user names and passwords, provided better protection. On the other hand, once breached, a computer offered the temptation of data theft on a massive scale.

In 1970, IBM published a 36-page manual on data security in a computer environment, and in that same year, the state of California passed a law stating that any attempt to obtain by deceit personal data from computerized files is a misdemeanor. The National Academy of Sciences initiated a study, led by Westin [355] at Columbia University, which reviewed problems associated with the maintenance of privacy of patients' records kept in large, computer-stored databases. This study reported on the status of the Kaiser Permanente system as an example of an early advanced user of computers for clinical medicine. The study concluded that data within the patients' computer records were subject to the same regulations governing their privacy and confidentiality as data in the hospital record room; that unauthorized disclosures from medical records had not played a prominent role in increasing the concern about privacy; and that the medical community had received little criticism connected to unauthorized disclosure.

Ware [335] chaired an Advisory Committee on Automated Personal Data Systems, appointed by Casper Weinberger, then the Secretary of the Department of Health, Education, and Welfare, which recommended a Code of Fair Information Practice. This code advocated safeguards for automated personal data systems, namely: (1) the existence of a record-keeping system that contained personal data must not be kept secret; (2) an individual must have access to personal information and how it is used; (3) an individual's information collected for one purpose must not be used for any other without that individual's prior consent; (4) an individual must be able to correct or amend personal information that is incorrect; and (5) any organization creating or using records of identifiable personal data must ensure the reliability of the data for their intended use and must take precautions to prevent misuse. This committee also advised against using the Social Security number as a standard universal personal identifier, and recommended that its use be limited to federal programs that had a specific federal legislative mandate to use it.

In 1977 a Privacy Protection Study Commission, created by the Privacy Act of 1974, submitted a report that also recommended that the use of the Social Security number and other labels by private organizations be monitored. They advised that the federal government should not consider taking any action that would foster the development of a standard, universal label for individuals, or that would develop a central population register, until such time as significant steps had been taken to implement safeguards and policies regarding permissible uses and disclosures of records [215]. Ware [334, 335] summarized the recommendations of this Privacy Protection Study Commission's report: (1) the patient's right to see and copy his medical record; (2) the patient's right to have errors in his record corrected or amended; (3) performance standards be kept for record-keeping systems in order to protect and control access to records; (4) enforcement of an expected level of confidentiality for medical records; (5) control of disclosures to third parties so that only information necessary to the purpose of the request is disclosed and a requirement that disclosures made without an individual's authorization must be reported to the individual; (6) a requirement that individually signed authorization for release of information must be specific in all details; and (7) a requirement that the release of information pursuant to an authorization must be noted in the record from which the disclosure is made.

In 1977 the American Medical Association (AMA) issued guidelines on procedures for the management of computer-based patient records, and for procedures to control access to the databases [173]. Jelovsek [185] chaired a committee on standards for the Society of Computer Medicine, and published guidelines for user access to computer-based medical records. Westin [352, 353] extended his earlier study under the auspices of the National Bureau of Standards, and Westin [351] reported that experience under the Federal Privacy Act of 1974, where federal health care and health insurance activities are involved, showed that clear rules of confidentiality had worked well.

Blum [47] described the security of the Johns Hopkins Oncology Center Clinical Information System. Through software control, each terminal provided access to only those data required to perform the functions for which that terminal was designed. For example, the terminal in use at an inpatient nursing station allowed access to information only about patients in that unit. Terminals in the admissions office could display the current census and scheduled admissions, but not clinical data. Access to clinical data was controlled by passwords, but access to nonclinical processes was not.

Thus measures were developed to protect confidentiality for patient computer-based records that usually included some means of controlled access. Authorized users obtained access to specified subsets of data by entering an assigned password, or by using a machine-readable identification card with which each user selected an alphanumeric code that thereafter served as a password. Groups of users, identified by their user identification codes, would be able to access, read, or enter data into specified clinical files. Every transaction with a patient's record was logged with the user's identification code.

Cryptography could be used for databases that required a higher level of protection. It transformed messages into forms that rendered them unintelligible to unauthorized persons. Feistel [132] explained that cryptography could be achieved by ciphers or by codes. A cipher assigned substitute symbols to some given set of alphabet characters. With a cipher one could encode any message. A code was intrinsically semantic in character and could convey only meanings thought of in advance and provided for in a secret list such as a code book. Cryptography used a code to transform (or encrypt) the original text into a cryptogram, which could then be decrypted by a person who knew the code and could convert it back to the original text. A computer encryption program would usually read the file into memory, byte by byte, encrypt it, and write it back to disk in exactly the same place, so that the rewritten encrypted file overwrote and erased the original file. Software encryption algorithms became available in the 1980s, and they were used to encrypt data transmitted over a network, since security problems increased with network accessibility.

For the strictest privacy, such as that sometimes required for psychiatric records, data isolation was usually maintained by storage in a locked file accessible only to authorized psychiatrists and psychologists [283]. Curran [105] described the protection measures established by a multistate psychiatric information system developed by Laska: Each terminal had access only to its own files, a password was required to identify the user, the computer recorded every transaction, and guards were posted 24 h a day to prevent unauthorized persons from entering the computer room. It was concluded that adequate legal and administrative protection could provide the confidentiality and privacy required of an electronic medical record in the mental health field [247]. A special problem of maintaining patient confidentiality arose when researchers found large databases to be especially useful for collecting data on large numbers of people. They soon recognized that it was necessary to place restrictions on the research use of medical databases to protect the identity of the patients and to preserve the confidentiality of the data without interfering unduly with the enhancement of analytic power inherent in computer technology [247]. Lindberg [212] wrote that in the 1970s the increased number of collaborative studies using networked medical computer systems created a problem for protecting patient confidentiality, and he cited Laska's multistate psychiatric information system as a model of good data protection. In the 1980s the increasing mobility of patients across state lines and the emergence of multistate health care providers resulted in a need for uniform regulations in all states governing the use and disclosure of health care information. In recognition of this problem, the Uniform Health-Care Information Act was drafted in 1985, and was recommended for enactment in all states [62]. By the end of the 1980s the usual forms of data protection included frequent changes of assigned passwords that authorized access to patient data from certain terminals. It was thought that the highest risk to security at that time was from unauthorized access via telephone lines that could connect into computer networks.

The Standards for Privacy of Individually Identifiable Health Information (Privacy Rule) for the first time established a set of national standards for the protection of certain health information. The U.S. Department of Health and Human Services (HHS) issued the Privacy Rule to implement the requirement of the Health Insurance Portability and Accountability Act (HIPAA). Public Law 104–191, enacted on August 21, 1996, required the Secretary of Health and Human Services (HHS) to publicize standards for the electronic exchange, privacy, and security of health information. HIPAA required the Secretary to issue privacy regulations governing individually identifiable health information if Congress did not enact privacy legislation within 3 years of its passage. When Congress did not act, the Department of Health and Human Services developed a proposed Privacy Rule that was released for public comment on November 3, 1999. The Department received 52,000 comments. The final regulation of the Privacy Rule was published December 28, 2000. In March 2002, the Department proposed and released for public comment modifications to the Privacy Rule. This release generated 11,000 comments. The final modifications were published on August 14, 2002. A text combining the final regulation and the modifications can be found at 45 CFR Part 160 and Part 164, Subparts A and E. The Privacy Rule standards address the use and disclosure of individuals' health information called protected health information by organizations subject to the Privacy Rule, called covered entities, as well as standards to help individuals understand and control how their health information is used.

Within HHS, the Office for Civil Rights (OCR) is responsible for the implementation and enforcement of the Privacy Rule, voluntary compliance activities, and civil monetary penalties. A major goal of the Privacy Rule is to assure that health information is properly protected while allowing the flow of health information needed to provide high quality health care. The Privacy Rule strikes a balance between access to information needed to care for the patient and the protection of the patient's privacy. The healthcare marketplace is diverse, and the Privacy Rule is designed to be flexible enough to cover the variety of uses and disclosures that need to be addressed.

Data security involves the protection of data from unauthorized alteration and from accidental or intentional disclosure to unauthorized persons. Data security is dependent on adequate system security such as protection from illegal access to computer rooms or to the databases, illicit use of data communications by hackers, or illegal modification of programs. A serious threat to data security is tampering by an authorized employee or by someone who illegally obtained a valid password from an associate.

As shared files and remote access became more common, security became more complex. In the 1980s, with the proliferation of personal computers, the security of computer-stored medical data was threatened by access via telephone lines [58]. Access from personal computers in the home or office had to be controlled with a level of security comparable to that which obtained within the medical center. Some systems installed call-back procedures for remote users: (1) the user had to dial from a predetermined authorized telephone number; (2) the computer answered the call and queried the user for a password and telephone number; (3) the computer then terminated the call; (4) if the user's password and telephone number as typed matched an entry in an authorization table the computer called back and requested log in [367]. Determined outsiders could sometimes break in by patching into an authorized telephone line and taking over the call after the authorized user hung up and before the computer logged out [246].

Medical facilities that were a part of a communications network were especially vulnerable to intentional or accidental altering or destroying of data. For example, a group of teenagers who intended no harm used a home telephone and a computer terminal to access a computer in the Department of Radiology at New York's Sloan Kettering Cancer Center [197].

Computer viruses are uninvited programs that can copy themselves into other programs and destroy data or perform other activities. Some viruses are programmed like a time bomb that can check the date, perform a task such as print a message, and then execute destructive code. Worms are self-contained, independent, self-propagating programs that enter operating systems and networks but do not destroy data. Both viruses and worms were difficult to detect; once detected, they can require a great deal of time for skilled programmers to eliminate. As an early example, on November 2, 1988, the Internet, which on that date connected about 180,000 corporate, university, military, and medical research computers in the United States, was invaded by an unsolicited worm that attached itself to every operating-system program that it entered, and soon shut down the network. A graduate student in computer science at a computer terminal in Cornell University had entered his worm program of coded instructions through an electronic mail program that was linked to the Internet. Every computer in the Internet that received the message entered that message into its operating system, which was then instructed to set up files that repeatedly replicated the worm program until the replications overloaded the storage capacity of the computer and shut it down. An estimated 6,000 of the 60,000 computers in the Internet were infected. The invading worm did not erase data or programs [9]. However, also in November 1988 a newspaper reported that a virus in the computers of an East Coast hospital caused the destruction of 40 % of its medical records [177]. Juni [192] described how the Department of Nuclear Medicine at the William Beaumont Hospital in Royal Oak, Michigan, discovered that their Macintosh II personal computer began to show occasional random malfunctions, such as nonexistent names in their patient directory. It turned out that 70 % of the programs for their database had been altered. Their system harbored two separate computer viruses, and floppy disks used by the staff for word processing contained at least one of these viruses.

Data integrity means assuring the completeness and accuracy of data, and protecting against invalidation – another important requirement for a computer-based patient record. In the traditional patient care setting, the paper-based medical record required the highest standards of data integrity; it was the definitive document and the final source of information about a patient's past care. If the paper-based patient record was transferred or copied, the original document was handled with great care to preserve its original format and content, and to avoid accidental destruction or alteration in case the record had to be reviewed for reasons of medical or legal challenge. When data, such as medical orders, were transcribed from a written format to a computer, the risk of error was introduced. Accordingly, it was generally recommended that physicians and nurses enter patient care data directly into the computer without clerical intermediaries [280]. In a computer-based system there was also the possibility that a computer software or hardware malfunction could result in accidental deletion or alteration of data, an issue usually addressed by maintaining adequate backup files. When it was especially critical to minimize errors and to maximize reliability, such as for NASA space launches, three independent computer systems operated concurrently to process all real-time critical data.

The practice of medicine usually uses a sequential decision-making process dependent on time-sequenced data transactions for frequently changing medical problems. As a patient's condition changes, data collected on consecutive examinations may differ. An acute illness often produces dynamic, changing information with a high rate of data collection. The patient's record has been traditionally oriented by time, by data source, and by medical problem. The record has to document when each procedure was done. In some cases, it has to show when a test was ordered, when the specimen was collected, when the specimen arrived in the laboratory, when the test was completed and the result entered into the computer, when the physician displayed the result, and when the physician took action if any was needed. In addition, the record has to keep track of the identity of each person who participated in the process, and of each medical problem that led to the test being done.

In the case of treatment, the patient's record has to document the status of each continually changing medical problem, and it has to document each of the physician's orders that pertained to that problem. The medical record has to permit reconstruction of what happened in the past, and of exactly what information was available at that time [89, 92, 329].

For professional audits and medico-legal problems, a patient's computer-based record often underwent many reviews over time. When a past treatment or patient's outcome was questioned, the medical record had to be reassembled, restored, and re-constructed in the same format, in the same transaction-time sequence, and with the same content as when it was used by the health care professionals at the time when the patient's care under question had been given. With the increasing complexity of distributed databases, avoiding accidental alterations of data, and ensuring absolute fidelity of the processing, merging, and transmitting of patient data became increasingly difficult. In such a case, data integrity meant that the data in the patient's computer-stored record always had to be in total and absolute agreement with the data entered by every user at every instant. This was an acutely sensitive requirement for direct patient care because overlapping or simultaneous entry of considerable amounts of data for one patient could occur within a few seconds, such as from automated laboratory analyzers and from intensive care monitoring systems.

The use of patients' records for administrative reviews of utilization of resources and of the quality of patient care could compromise the confidentiality of patients' data, a problem that could be accentuated by the speed and power of the computer [212]. Separate from the ability to monitor the quality of patient care, it is important to monitor the quality of the data processing. In a study of a large database of vital records, Schwartz and associates [289] found significant error rates in the spelling of patients' names. They also found the same patient identification (ID) number assigned to more than one patient. If one patient is assigned two or more ID numbers, there is no problem provided that all numbers point to the same record.

Error detection and correction methods are advocated, including error checks based on repeat entry (such as was routinely done to verify keypunched data). Validity checks, such as rejection of entries that lie outside a predetermined range, are also important, as are redundancy checks such as check digits – numbers computed from the values of a numeric identifier and appended to it. If a patient's identification number includes a check digit, the computer can compute a check sum; if the check sum differs from the one included with the patient's number, the computer can signal an error.

Physical security of the computer and its databases against accidental destruction of data was recognized from the beginning as being important. In addition, it was evident to physicians that striving for 100 % reliability – a non-existent, non-attainable goal – was important. Collen [89] pointed out that an information system with a relatively high reliability of 98 % would still have an average downtime (that is, being inoperable) of 1 h in every 50 h, or be down 1 day in every 2 months. Such lack of reliability is unacceptable in the setting of acute patient care.

Measures taken to promote reliability usually involved either fail-safe or fail-soft systems. Fail-safe systems had uninterruptible power supplies to ensure against unanticipated power failures, continually maintained redundant devices for the backup of essential computer equipment (such as would be needed for a database computer), and duplicate computer terminals and other critical equipment. Fail-soft systems used alternative backup modes to collect transaction data during a system or component failure, and then updated the master database when the operation was restored. In addition, as advocated by Davis [107], a strong preventive maintenance program reduced failure. Uninterruptible power supplies were employed in the late 1960s. By the 1980s, for local area networks (LANs) where multiple computers could store data in temporary databases before forwarding them to a central database, uninterruptible power supplies became essential for the protection of the communications network. Fireproof safes and offsite storage for archival and backup magnetic tapes and disks were increasingly used to prevent accidental loss of essential data. In the 1980s when personal computer hard disk storage was at first notorious for breakdown, frequent backup procedures were a necessity. Barnett [22] described the duplicate hardware measures taken in the early 1970s for the Massachusetts General Hospital's computer system to ensure reliability. They used redundant systems in a hierarchical fashion; if one computer was inoperative, its modules could be shifted to another. Activities of the highest priority would continue, while those of lower priority, such as programming development, were temporarily halted.

4.6   Development of Paper-Based Patients Records

Physicians have followed the teachings of the famed clinician, Sir William Osler, to study and learn from their patients and from their medical records, in order to improve their knowledge of diseases. Physicians continue this learning process by taking a history of the patient's medical problems, performing a physical examination, and then recording the history and physical findings in the patient's medical record. To confirm a preliminary diagnosis and to rule-out other possible diagnoses, physicians refer the patients for selected tests and procedures that usually involve the clinical laboratory, radiology, and other clinical-support services. After reviewing the information received from these services, physicians usually arrive at a more certain diagnosis, and then prescribe appropriate treatment. For an unusual or a complex medical problem, physicians can refer the patient to a specialist, and they can review evidence-based reports of appropriate therapies by consulting relevant medical literature and bibliographic databases.

It was always a problem for busy physicians to adequately document and maintain their patients' records. In the 1950s before the advent of computers, the traditional hand-written, paper-based patient record was a collated series of documented encounters between the patient and the health professional that had been collected serially over time. The patients' records in a solo practitioner's office for a relatively small number of patients could consist of paper cards with the identification and business data handwritten or typed, and with handwritten notes about medical problems, diagnostic tests, and treatments to remind the practitioner at the time of subsequent visits. In a small group practice, records were usually written on plain sheets of paper, stored chronologically in a folder or envelope, and filed in cabinets alphabetically by the patient's last name.

In a large group practice, or in a hospital, each patient would be assigned a unique medical record number, and all information for that patient would be stored in one or more folders filed under that record number in a common medical record department. If a patient was scheduled to see two or more physicians on the same day, one physician often needed the chart beyond the time that a subsequent appointment began. In contrast to data in a computer, the paper chart could not be in more than one place at a time.

When the number of physicians in a group increased and the storage area outgrew the space allocated for filing cabinets, the cabinets were replaced by a medical records department with racks of shelves on which the patients' records were stacked in the alphabetical order of the patients' last names, or in the numerical order of their medical record numbers. In large medical centers some clinical specialties stored their specialty records separately. Psychiatrists and psychologists almost always stored their records in separate, locked cabinets to provide an additional measure of privacy and security. Clinical laboratory test results were usually kept in the laboratory for a limited time, and the final test reports were permanently stored in the patients' records. Original x-ray images were typically stored in the radiology departments, and copies of the radiologist's interpretations were filed in the patients' records. Electrocardiograms (ECGs) were usually stored in their original graphic form in the electrocardiography department, with a copy and its interpretation for the patient's chart. Relevant postal mail correspondence, textual reports from pathology, consultations, surgical notes, and other procedures were also filed in patients' medical records.

Patients' records were also used to support claims for reimbursement for services provided. Health care insurers usually required case summaries with standardized codes to represent diagnoses and procedures.

If a patient was hospitalized, inpatient care was documented in the patient's chart. Upon discharge, a hospital discharge summary was prepared by the attending physician. These paper documents were collated in a manually stored file that constituted the outpatient record. When a patient returned for a clinic visit, the physician could retrieve the outpatient chart and review data from prior visits together with any new reports received in the interim, such as laboratory test results, x-ray reports, or hospital discharge summaries. After seeing the patient, the physician could modify or add a diagnosis, change the treatment, and record the events of the current visit. Thus the outpatient record was a physician's primary means of documenting the continuity of care. For patients with chronic problems and recurring episodes of illness over many years, the record could become voluminous, which could make retrieval of specific data from prior visits increasingly difficult.

As an information source, paper-based hospital records were inefficient. When several physicians were attending the same patient, only one of them at a time could use the paper-based record. After discharge from the hospital, at the time of a follow-up visit to the outpatient department, the paper-based medical record had to be sent to the outpatient clinic. Urgently ill patients arriving in the emergency room often waited for their medical records to arrive. When the desired information was located, physicians' notes were sometimes illegible. Some patients had separate medical records in several hospitals and physicians' offices, which then required the patient's authorization for any part of their record to be transferred.

After years of inactivity, old paper-based records were sometimes destroyed or transferred to microfiche. Children's records were generally required by law to be retained until 1 year after a child's 21st birthday. Tufo [324] studied five large medical facilities where hospitals and clinics used conventional paper-based patient records and reported that 5–10 % of patients were seen in the clinics without an available record, 5–20 % of hospital records were incomplete. Of the missing information, 75 % consisted of laboratory test results and x-ray reports, and 25 % consisted of lost, incomplete, or illegible textual data from patients' previous visits.

4.7   Development of the Electronic Patient Record (EPR)

Computer-stored databases were the origins of modern electronic patient records (EPRs). A computer-stored database that serves as an electronic patient record is an essential component of every computer-based outpatient information system, of every hospital information system, and of every comprehensive medical information system. For many reasons electronic medical records became an early objective of people who worked in medical informatics. To locate and retrieve bulky, paper-based charts was often burdensome and time-consuming. Often, the paper-based chart was unavailable to a physician in a group practice when colleagues also needed it. Early forecasts that electronic patient records would become widespread [254] proved optimistic. Some investigators thought that the absence of electronic patient records was the main problem limiting the diffusion of medical information systems [206].

In the 1950s physicians began to work with information scientists to develop a more efficient computer-based hospital record. Patient identification data, length of hospital stay, and codes representing attending physicians, diagnoses, and procedures were keypunched onto cards for tabulating and sorting by machine [14, 55]. Although this approach produced some improvement over manual processing of data, a great number of punched cards were necessary and storage space for the cards was required. Also, to keypunch, verify, sort, and tabulate the data was tedious.

In the 1960s medical record departments used keypunched cards to index medical records. The Joint Commission on Accreditation of Hospitals mandated indices of diseases, surgical operations, and physicians. Medical record librarians coded the data and recorded the codes on work sheets that were then sent to a data processing center where the coded data were punched into machine-readable cards. Periodically the cards were batch processed to tabulate the data. The process was simple and affordable even for small hospitals. By the mid-1960s reports appeared describing the use of electronic digital computers in medical records departments. Ausman [12] and associates at Roswell Park Memorial Institute in Buffalo, New York, reported on their computer-based medical record system which had been under development for several years. Hospital admission data, patient's history information, physical examination data, and nurses' notes were manually recorded on forms and then keypunched into cards that were read into an IBM 360 computer. The system also used portable punch cards for many fixed-format data entry applications, including requisitions for procedures, laboratory test results, and vital signs (temperature, pulse and respiration). A book of portable punch cards was contained in a specially designed hand-held holder, and the user, guided by a plastic overlay, entered data by punching holes with a stylus. A card reader then tabulated the data. Ausman [12] was enthusiastic about this method of data entry, for it did away with the need for keypunch operators. He suggested its use would be limited only by the ingenuity of the user.

In 1969 the National Center for Health Servicers Research and Development [262] reported that computer-based medical record projects were being conducted by: Ausman at Health Research, Inc. in Buffalo, New York; Robinson at Bowman Gray School of Medicine; Schenthal at Tulane University; and Weed at the Cleveland Metropolitan General Hospital. In the 1970s some pathologists and medical record transcriptionists were using word processing programs, either by magnetic tape coupled to an IBM Selectric typewriter (MTST), or by a display terminal with keyboard data entry directly into a computer [290]. Some early examples of electronic patient records in hospital information systems were those developed at the Texas Institute of Research and Rehabilitation, University of Missouri-Columbia, University of Vermont, and El Camino Hospital in Sunnyvale, California. Some early electronic patient records for office and hospital practice were developed at the Latter Day Saints Hospital, Massachusetts General Hospital, Kaiser Permanente, and Johns Hopkins Hospital.

In the 1980s a hospital information system provided the medical records department with record-tracking and location for paper-based medical charts. Computer-based records did not need this application, but some hospitals had hybrid record systems that retained some paper-based records. An automated record-tracking system at the Lutheran Hospital of Southern California, with an annual experience of 23,000 hospitalized and 200,000 ambulatory patients, provided specific information about the location, movement, and use of each patient's record [297]. In 1980 at Parkland Memorial Hospital in Dallas, Texas, with 40,000 admissions and 215,000 outpatient visits in 1980, an automated chart-location system to check charts in-and-out improved the ability to manage a large volume of charts that had a high activity rate [250]. Parkland Hospital's system also tracked deficiencies in the completion of paper-based charts by the medical staff, a common problem for medical librarians.

At the University of California in San Francisco (UCSF), Simborg and associates [299] reported that their medical records department system became operational as an integrated module in their hospital information system, and that it provided medical record location tracking, control of incomplete medical records, medical transcription for discharge summaries, operative notes and correspondence, and management statistics – all entered by typing with a word processing module. The processing of narrative textual data contained in patients' records was a major technical problem. For a patient who had a long stay in the hospital due to a serious disease with complications, the amount of text in the patient's record could be voluminous, and would include the admission history and physical examination, followed by many progress notes, consultation and laboratory reports, and perhaps surgery and other special procedure reports.

Functional requirements for patients' hospital electronic records were generally similar to those for patients' records in a clinic, though many hospitals had specialized services that added to the complexity of their medical records. Clinicians needed to review relevant data collected during the present and past hospitalizations, as well as data collected in prior clinic visits, in order to assess the current status of the patient. Davis [107] proposed that as a minimum, the two major goals of the electronic patient record should be to: (1) maintain and readily provide relevant clinical and administrative data for each patient; and (2) provide a resource for the systematic retrieval of medical data across large numbers of electronic patient records for administrative and clinical studies. The electronic patient record had to document each patient's care by collecting and storing administrative and clinical data. It had to contain all data collected: (1) from the patient (identifying data and medical history); (2) from physicians' examination findings, diagnoses, orders, treatments, consultations, and progress reports); (3) from the nurses (nursing procedures, medications administered, and nursing progress notes), from aides and medical attendants (height, weight, temperature, and vital signs); and (4) from clinical support services (laboratory, pharmacy, radiology, electrocardiography, pathology), for every episode of illness during the periods for which the patient received care [108, 111, 329]. Fries [145] considered the ideal patient's record to have the following characteristics: once data was recorded, a user should be able to readily refer to it again; an authorized user should be able to find out why specific services were provided; and data should be displayed such that each individual observation was seen in the context of related observations.

In a large medical group practice or in an academic center, the electronic patient record had to process, integrate, and communicate each patient's data in a timely way as needed by all authorized users. The number of medical consultants and technical specialists in a large medical center required the electronic patient record to readily integrate, retrieve, and communicate patient care data wherever collected and whenever requested. When several physicians were involved in the care of the patient, the electronic patient record had to be accessible to every physician taking care of the patient at any hour of the day or night. The capability for many physicians to simultaneously query a patient's electronic patient record at any time was a benefit that had no counterpart in the paper-based patient record.

The electronic patient record had to have the flexibility to retrieve and arrange the relevant patient data in a variety of readable and usable formats, such as by time, by source, or by medical problem (that is, to be problem oriented). Physicians often want data presented in reverse chronological order, so the most recent data is presented first. Psychiatrists and psychologists wanted their patients' data to be sequestered and locked to preserve its privacy and confidentiality. Some specialists, such as ophthalmologists, wanted their data kept separately.

From a review of 17 computer-based outpatient information systems), Rodnick [278] and associates concluded that the most important service that an electronic patient record could provide was an up-to-date patient profile that included the patient's social information, prescribed medicines, a medical problem list; any patient care flow-sheets, tables, and graphical displays that showed the course of the patient's health and therapy status. The electronic record should also have query capabilities to permit searches of the patient's record to help determine any needed additional data, tests, or procedures. Zimmerman [370] asked, in a questionnaire of 21 physicians, which components of a patient record they looked at in more than 10 % of instances when they used the record. Ninety percent specified laboratory test results; 81 % looked at the patient's history for prior diseases and treatments; 76 % looked at allergies; 71 % looked at vital signs and x-ray reports; 67 % looked at hospitalizations, prior operations, and at the patients' discharge summaries; 57 % looked at patients' problem lists; and 24 % specified injuries. Zimmerman listed the major functions of a patient's encounter form to be to record data collected during an outpatient visit that included: provider identification, patient identification, sources of payment for care, and visit date, as well as the patient's medical complaints, diagnoses, diagnostic procedures, treatments, and disposition. Zimmerman concluded that structured, electronic patient' records could help office practitioners obtain needed information in patient care.

Stead [311] emphasized that the electronic patient record should support the decision making processes involved in patient care, and improve the quality of clinical decision making. (1) The electronic patient record should provide alerts and reminders to physicians and nurses to call attention to important or newly available test results and clinical findings. (2) For every patient, the electronic record needed to be able to communicate and provide linkages for exchange of data with other affiliated patient care facilities. (3) It should facilitate access to and linkages with the relevant medical literature and outside factual and knowledge databases in order to support clinical decision making. (4) It needed to permit access to abstracts of specified data items for an individual patient or for a specified group of patients; and it had to be able to generate secondary records for patient registries for medical research and education. Electronic patient records also had to store data that described the sequence of activities used to provide patient care services, data that could be used for health services evaluation. (5) The electronic record also had to help with the surveillance, monitoring, auditing, and assessment of a physician's and of a hospital's activities. It had to facilitate utilization review and support quality assurance programs with clinical alerts and reminders. (6) The electronic record had to maintain the integrity and restorability of the record for the required legal time (that is, for up to 21 years for some pediatric records), and it had to provide extra protection for patients with socially sensitive diagnoses and for famous persons, whose records could attract inappropriate attention. (7) The electronic record had to accommodate continual addition as needed throughout the lifetime of the patient. (8) And the electronic record had to accept new types of data resulting from innovations in patient care. Gabrieli [146] extended this last requirement beyond the individual patient to permit multi-generational record linkage, so that the clinical records for a patient's parents, children, and siblings could be linked.

Although patients' records vary widely in size, format, and content, they have been the primary means of recording health care processes and services that were provided to the patient, and the data contained in a patient's record have usually provided the basic and legal representation of the care received. Therefore it is essential that whether it is paper-based or electronic-based, the patient's record is able to collect, store, process, retrieve, transfer and communicate the needed data accurately, reliably, and efficiently. The composite of all component records during the life of a patient makes up the patient's continuing, longitudinal, lifetime medical record, and as advocated by Stead [307] it should be an accurate and complete medical database built by collecting health and medical care information over the patient's lifetime.

Technical requirements and structural designs for an electronic patient record need to satisfy the functional requirements specified by users. Gordon [159, 160] proposed that a [111] standardized format should become an integral part of the patient record, thus offering some ease in data entry and information retrieval. When computer technical specialists first designed the structure of the earliest computer-based patient records, they generally mechanized the approach of the medical record librarian, who took a paper folder for each patient, placed into it a set of individual pages and thereby established the patient's file. These files were then stored in cabinets or on racks in the medical records department. The file consisted of structured sheets beginning with the cover page, and followed by administrative data, physicians' notes, nurses' notes, laboratory test results, pharmacy data, x-ray reports, and other documents such as operative notes and hospital discharge summaries. The paper-based patient's file was readily increased in size by the addition of more sheets. In the early computer-based systems, just as in a manual paper-based record system, each patient's record was treated as a separate file. The computer-stored electronic patient record was the aggregate of an individual patient's data; it served in place of the patient's chart.

Electronic patient records were initially stored as fixed-field, fixed-length computer files as a carryover from business data processing. As in the manual paper-based chart, each type of data was entered into a specifically defined field (location) in the computer's magnetic storage device, and each field of data (such as the patient's identification data) was programmed to store a predetermined amount of data. To save storage space, data were coded, and they were entered from pre-coded forms. Time elapsed between the initial recording of a patient's data on a paper form and its subsequent entry into a computer. Furthermore, when data for an outpatient visit were collected on encounter forms, that is, when the physician did not interact with the computer, there was no opportunity for clinical decision support or for the receipt of clinical alerts or reminders.

Soon more flexible variable-field, variable-length records were developed that could accept textual data, whether coded or not. Whenever new data needed to be entered into an existing electronic patient record at Kaiser Permanente in Oakland, Davis [108, 111] transferred the patient's entire electronic patient record to the computer memory, opened the specific fields that were to receive new data, and once the new data had been entered, he returned the entire integrated record back to the database. As an alternative, Barnett [23] at Massachusetts General Hospital stored sequentially the strings of newly entered data, and linked these time-stamped strings by pointers to the patient's identifying data. In this way, a logically integrated patient record could be presented to the health professional even though the individual items of the patient's data might be distributed throughout various parts of one or more databases.

As the volume and variety of data in patients' files grew, and as data elements arrived from many sources, each stamped with time and date, it became increasingly difficult to find and retrieve specific items or sets of data that were stored in a large electronic database. In the traditional paper-based medical record, a time-source-orientation was usually maintained for data and documents; to perpetuate this familiar approach and to facilitate the storage and retrieval of specific data in patients' records, database designs in the 1960s usually linked the individual patient's data in a hierarchical, tree-structured, mode [186]. In the late 1970s relational and object-oriented databases began to be used.

Hospital inpatient medical records are more complex than outpatient records. The medical record system for a large hospital that used integrated inpatient and outpatient records was the most difficult to design and implement. The patient's medical record in a hospital was often so complex, and was used in such a variety of ways that substantial differences arose in the approaches taken by different developers of computer-based medical records.

The increasing interest in computer-based patient records was recognized by Ball [18] who classified hospital information systems into those with and those without electronic patients' records. Level (I) record systems primarily offered data-collection and message-switching. They transmitted orders, captured charges, prepared a bed census, and sometimes reported laboratory test results. However, because they did not maintain an electronic patient record file, they could not meet the requirements for a total information system. Level (II) record systems maintained a complete computerized patient record during the patient's hospital stay and handled clinical information as well as requisitions for procedures. Shannon [292, 293] and Ball further divided Level (II) systems with a patient record into subclasses A, B, and C systems, according to their comprehensiveness.

The patient's medical record in a hospital is the repository in which information about the patient is collected and stored while the patient is hospitalized. The medical records department is responsible for arranging with physicians for the completion of their patients' records with their discharge diagnoses and abstracted summaries. Paper-based medical charts were often stored in multiple record rooms; for example, inpatient records were commonly stored separately from outpatient records.

It was the responsibility of the medical records department to keep track of the medical records; for paper-based medical records this task was sometimes difficult. Prior to computer-based hospital information systems, medical record librarians were responsible for the storage, integrity, and security of the paper-based medical charts; for tracking records as they moved through the hospital; and for making the records available to all authorized users in a timely way. They maintained a master index of diagnoses and provided periodic statistical reports. The medical records department often arranged for medical transcriptionists who transcribed physicians' dictated narrative textual reports (such as for surgery, pathology, and radiology), that were then filed in the patients' records. In a hospital with paper-based records, all the documents collected while a patient was in the hospital were almost always collated in chronological order, on a clipboard or in a loose leaf notebook, and usually beginning with the nurses' graphical charts of the patient's vital signs (temperature, pulse, and respiratory rates). Most physicians manually wrote the patient's medical history, physical findings, diagnostic impressions, and progress notes on paper forms, which were collated in chronological order in one section of the paper-based medical record. Laboratory test results, x-ray reports, surgical operative reports, and nurses' notes were also clipped in the chart. These charts were kept in racks at the nursing stations near the patient's bedside, so they would be readily available for physicians and nurses when they visited their patients. Shortly after discharge, the documents were bound together in a paper folder that was stored on shelves in the hospital's medical records department. Folders were filed sequentially, either alphabetically by the patient's last name, or numerically by the patients' medical record number.

Most computer-based patient records were organized in a time-oriented sequence; that is, the data were filed chronologically, and were presented in order of the date and time of day the data were collected. A source-oriented record was one collated by the department of origin; for example, surgical notes, ophthalmologic notes, and clinical laboratory tests were each grouped by department. Source-oriented data were usually filed in a time-oriented sequence within departmental records; for example, all laboratory results were grouped together and then sequenced within the laboratory file by date and time.

In the 1970s, with the advent of lower cost minicomputers, large medical groups and clinics began to acquire dedicated minicomputers for their outpatient practices [155]. In the 1970s and 1980s with the introduction of personal computers, outpatient information systems became more affordable for the individual doctor's office and the implementation and diffusion of computers was facilitated by the publication of a number of books to guide physicians on how to select an electronic patient record to meet the needs of their practices. Some early published books included: *Computers in Medicine: A Primer for the Practicing Physician*, by Krasnoff (Charles C. Thomas, 1967); *Computers for the Physician's Office*, by Zimmerman and Rector (Research Studies Press, 1978); *Computers for Medical Office and Patient Management*, edited by Day and Brandejs (Van Nostrand Reinhold Company, 1982); *Computerizing Your Medical Office*, by Sellars (Medical Economics Books, 1983); *Using Computers in the Practice of Medicine: Professional and Clinical Guidelines for Managing Your Practice and Improving Patient Care*, by Solomon (Prentice-Hall, Inc., 1984); *Information Systems for Patient Care*, edited by Blum (Springer-Verlag, 1984); and *The Physician's Computer Workbook*, by Tuttle (Burgess Communications, 1985).

In 1985 Jelovsek published *Doctor's Office Computer Prep Kit* (Springer-Verlag) that contained guidelines for developing detailed functional requirements for an outpatient information system using a series of questions to be answered by the office manager, the insurance forms manager, the billing manager, the medical records manager, the patient accounts and receivables manager, and the receptionist. In 1987 Oberst and Long wrote *Computers in Private Practice Management* (Springer-Verlag). Symbolic of the popularity of the subject in the later 1980s, Mayo and Ball published, in the *Disease-a-Month* series, *How to Select a Computerized Medical Office Practice System* (1988; Year Book Publishers).

In the 1970s, with the advent of lower-cost minicomputers, an increased effort was made to have a computer-based office information system. Henley [176] and associates reported developments in more than 200 sites in the United States. Of these, 175 were developing patient record systems, and 17 had operational outpatient medical records at sites that they visited.

The information systems they reviewed, and the primary persons whom they interviewed at each site were, in the chronological order of their visits: (1) Fries at Stanford University Medical Center, Stanford, California; (2) Leavitt at Insurance Technology Corporation in Berkeley, California, a workmen's compensation insurance company that used the system in the San Francisco Bay Area to monitor the care of about 1,200 patients a year with industrial injuries; (3) Thompson in the Department of Health Services in Los Angeles County, California, that operated a large county-wide system with terminals at 48 different sites, providing primarily patient identification data, clinic registration and appointment scheduling (since 1968), with a limited amount of clinical information, for about 550,000 patient visits a year; (4) Thompson at the East Los Angeles Child and Youth Clinic, California, a Los Angeles County-supported clinic that collected patient data on forms, coded the data (done by a medical technician), and entered the data by keypunch, off-line and batch processed, to provide a supplement to the paper-based medical record for about 10,000 patients; (5) Laska at Rockland State Hospital, Orangeburg, New York; (6) Brunjes at Yale University School of Medicine in New Haven, Connecticut; (7) Barnett at the Harvard Community Plan in Cambridge, Massachusetts; (8) Fakan at Medical Data Systems Corporation in Olmsted Falls, Ohio; (9) Schneeweiss at the Medical University of South Carolina in Charleston; (10) Penick in Appalachia II Health District, Greenville, South Carolina; (11) Hammond at Duke University Medical Center, Durham, North Carolina; (12) McDonald at the Indiana University Medical Center, Indianapolis; (13) Robbins at the Cardiovascular Clinic, Oklahoma City; (14) Vallbona and Evans at Baylor College of Medicine, Houston, Texas; (15) Garratt at the Indian Health Service in Tucson, Arizona; (16) Craemer at the U.S. Naval Air Station Dispensary in Brunswick, Maine; and (17) Lyman and Tick at Bellevue Hospital, New York University Medical Center.

These institutions comprised five clinics (hospital-based or neighborhood), four university medical centers, four health maintenance organizations (HMOs), a solo general practice, a county health department, and a specialty group practice. Eleven of the sites provided primary patient care. Eight of the 17 sites were sponsored by local, state, or federal government; six were private, nonprofit corporations; three were organized as private, for-profit corporations. The authors considered seven of these sites to be academic institutions. Seven sites were supported largely by federal grants, two by institutional funds, and the remainder by user charges.

Henley [176] further reported that all sites stored in their electronic records the patients' chief medical complaints or symptoms, and that more than half of them coded the patients' problems. Two sites – Yale and the Indian Health Service – implemented a problem-oriented electronic medical record. The patient's history of present-illness was entered at 12 sites, and the past history, at least to some degree, was entered at most sites. A limited amount of physical examination data were collected and stored in coded form at 14 sites. Progress notes were stored primarily by sites able to process free text. Current medications were stored at 14 sites, and past medications were stored at 10. Psychiatric data were stored at ten sites. Follow-up data were stored at the majority of sites, routine laboratory tests at eight sites, x-ray studies at seven sites, electrocardiograms at six sites, and medications at five sites. All the systems provided patient identification data and search capabilities. Computer-generated encounter reports with progress notes and data from prior visits were provided at 15 sites; 15 provided patient profiles summarizing the medical status; 11 permitted online inquiries into the database; 11 included some type of problem list; 8 provided computer-generated flow sheets with tabular presentation of visit and laboratory data; and 2 sites used the computer to produce histograms. Graphical data, x-ray images, electrocardiographic tracings, and referral letters were excluded.

The Harvard Community Health Plan (HCHP) and the Brunswick Naval Air Station dispensed with the traditional paper-based record completely at the patient-physician encounter. The greatest reliance on computer availability of the record existed at the Naval Air Station in Brunswick, where the medical record was kept entirely on the computer and was not posted until the patient registered for an appointment. Summaries were printed in preparation for appointments at Bellevue, Indian Health Service, and at the Harvard Community Health Plan. According to Henley [176], Harvard Community Health Plan's COSTAR was a relatively comprehensive electronic record with much of the data in coded form; it was the first civilian system to dispense with the traditional paper-based record.

Henley [176] also reported that for the 17 sites visited in 1974 and 1975, total operating costs ranged widely from $1 to $50 per-patient year and from $0.50 to $22 per-patient office visit. As examples, the operational cost of COSTAR at the Harvard Community Health Plan was reported to be $15 per-patient per year and $3 per office visit. Duke University's TMR system was reported to have a total operational cost of $22 per patient year and $10 per patient visit. Regenstrief's RMR system had a total operational cost of $101 per patient year and $22 per office visit [176]. In 1977 McDonald et al. [233] estimated the cost of the RMR system of their computer-based patient record at $2.02 per patient office visit. In 1979 an evaluation of the Johns Hopkins outpatient Minirecord and appointment system estimated the cost to be $0.63 per patient visit [202, 203].

Fourteen sites reported better patient care as manifested by earlier identification of high-risk patients (for example, those with hypertension). In addition, sites reported increased access to care because of fewer missed appointments, and increased availability of paper records at the time of the patient's visit. Reduction of costs was claimed by 12 sites. All but one site agreed that the computer-based record was more available, and most agreed that it provided more timely data for administrative decisions. Most agreed that one of the major contributions of the computer-based medical record system was to provide for a more complete, up-to-date, medical record, and that it facilitated peer review and was better at meeting requirements for quality review. Henley concluded that the successful implementation and operation of an outpatient information system depended on health care providers, in most cases physicians. Since the physician was usually the initial point of data capture, the physicians' acceptance and cooperation was essential for success.

Henley [176] reported that eight sites used large, commercial, time-sharing computers (six were manufactured by IBM); nine sites used minicomputers (seven were manufactured by Digital Equipment Corporation); six used distributed shared systems; and three used small dedicated systems. All were aimed at medical support functions. None of the minicomputer systems had been established before 1970. A variety of programming languages was represented: four sites used MUMPS, three used PL/1, three used assembly language, two used COBOL, two used FORTRAN, and the remainder used other languages. Most of the sites provided online operations; only four were primarily dedicated to batch-processing. Three of the 17 sites initially had some inpatient services; the others were developed specifically for outpatient functions.

For data entry, none of the 17 sites used menu selection from a terminal display as was then being used by some hospital information systems. Most sites used full-page paper encounter forms, some of which were medical problem specific, with pre-labeled check boxes. Codes that corresponded to the checked boxes were then entered into the computer. At some sites the users wrote numerical values that could be entered into the computer. Many sites used interactive display terminals. Five used mark-sense forms and a mark-sense reader that automatically assigned codes by reading the location of the mark on the form. Eleven sites allowed free text to be written on the forms, and five permitted dictation that was then entered from interactive keyboard terminals. Some sites employed clerks to code diagnoses and to abstract data from the encounter forms. Three of the 17 sites had the capacity for the health care providers to enter data directly into the computer using the display terminal.

Storage requirements for a single outpatient visit varied from 100 to 1,500 bytes and for all visits for one patient requirements ranged from 500 to 100,000 bytes, depending on the number of visits, complexity of care, redundancy of data, and degree of data compression. The number of online terminals used varied from 1 to 6 Henley [176] also reported that the reliability of the computers was not a major concern – an important difference between an outpatient information system with its relatively low rate of data entry, and a hospital information system with its 24-h high-density rate of information processing. In 1975 none of the 17 outpatient information systems visited had begun to use computer networks or distributed databases; each practice stored its data in its own database. Most database designs used at these sites were hierarchical; beginning with the patient's identification data, followed by medical problems and diagnoses, treatments provided, and follow-up care. Some used a relational database with a tabular design that laid out parallel files, with each medical record identified by the patient's identification number. Clearly evident was a lack of coordination and uniformity that would allow for transfer of data between sites. Nor could the separate databases be combined to support collaborative research.

Even though there were ample demonstrations of substantial development at these 17 sites, there was little evidence of technology transfer to other locations. Henley [176] explained this lack of diffusion as mostly due to differences between innovation and prototype development versus adoption and diffusion. Henley stated that it took more courage, foresight, imagination, capital investment, and willingness to take risks at the stage of adoption and diffusion than it did at the stage of innovation and prototype development. In addition, a major marketing effort would be needed to promote widespread acceptance.

The protection of patient data privacy, though at the time limited, was generally considered adequate at the sites visited. A few sites reported access violations or attempts to gain unauthorized access. Rockland State Hospital prohibited data for its psychiatric patients from being shared among institutions, although the normal legal access to data at the individual sites was maintained.

Kuhn and Wiederhold [204], from Stanford University also reviewed the state of development in the 1970s of approximately 175 computer-based, ambulatory medical record systems in the United States, including COSTAR, the COmputer STored Ambulatory Record developed at the Massachusetts General Hospital for use by the Harvard Community Health Plan; Duke University's The Medical Record (TMR); and the Regenstrief Institute's Regenstrief Medical Record (RMR). They reported that most were still in a state of development and evaluation, limited in medical scope, and primarily providing administrative services such as patient registration, billing, and appointment scheduling. Future links to the laboratories and pharmacy were anticipated. The authors concluded that successful implementation and operation was critically dependent on the training of the health care providers who used the system; on the presence of strong leadership – usually a physician turned computer specialist; and on effective administrative and financial services provided by the system.

In 1981 another group led by Kuhn [202, 203] and Wiederhold revisited these sites and found that: (1) the user interface needed better methods for collecting and displaying data; (2) the predominant hardware was the minicomputer; (3) there appeared to have been little innovation in software development since 1975; and (4) health care providers did not readily accept and were not motivated to fully use the systems. Still, most of the developers were involved in transferring parts or all of their systems to new sites as the technical constraints on transfer diminished.

Distributed data processing began to appear in the early 1980s using minicomputers connected by local area networks (LANs). Microcomputers were also linked with minicomputers, with all computers supported by a shared central database for the computer-stored electronic patient records, and this advanced the diffusion of outpatient information systems into larger medical group practices [349]. By the mid-1980s reports claimed that an array of personal computers inter-connected by a LAN could provide the basis for an efficient and cost-effective outpatient information system [128], and that battery-powered personal computers could serve as portable data transfer devices to an office computer [11]. Personal computers began to be used for communications between practitioners and patients. Also, a physician's office computer could dial a patient's telephone and leave a reminder about an upcoming appointment [113]. Microcomputer-based clinical workstations connected to a central communications computer in a local area network began to be used in larger clinics for clinical alerts and reminders [231].

By the mid-1980s commercial vendors were marketing the Massachusetts General Hospital's COmputer-STored Ambulatory Record (COSTAR), Regenstrief's Medical Record (RMR), and Duke University's The Medical Record (TMR) systems. By the end of the 1980s, Tang [316] observed that the demands on the electronic patient record as a repository of patient information had increased dramatically for several reasons: (1) the increased number of patients' encounters since people were living longer and received more care for both acute and chronic medical problems; (2) the dramatic increase in the number and use of diagnostic procedures, with many procedure results being recorded on different media (such as film, video, digital images, graphs and charts); and (3) at many outpatient clinics, patients were being seen by many different health care providers. Finally, some early adopters needed to reduce the amount of space required to store medical records.

Initial adoption of an electronic patient record required the transfer of data residing in the paper-based record into the database of the computer. On the other hand, the transfer of an entire old record was rarely necessary and could be costly, so selective abstraction was usually employed. The line between over- and under-extraction of data was ill defined [151]; judgment calls do not come cheap. When considering the inclusion of all old data with the thought that some later retrospective search might require it, Spencer [305] advised against this approach. In contrast, Lindberg [213] discouraged attempts to abbreviate the electronic patient record since different portions of the same record could be relevant for different future purposes.

Stead [311] noted that in the 1980s Duke's *The Medical Record* (TMR) was the only record of physician-patient encounters in the outpatient information system for the nephrology clinic of the Durham Veterans Administration Medical Center. Stead referred to TMR as a *chartless* record rather than as a paperless record, and he noted that after 15 years of false starts, computer-based patients' records were becoming a reality.

Clinicians needed to determine whether computerized records should supplement or replace the paper chart. Since most medical facilities in the 1980s maintained a hybrid (paper-based and computer-based) patients' record system, McDonald [229] noted that as long as the entire medical record could not be fully obtained from the computer, the continued use of paper and the double entry of some information would be required. He forecasted a continuing decline in the cost for information systems that would eventually favor electronic storage of the entire record. Jelovsek [187] also observed that electronic storage of medical records lagged behind computer applications in banking and manufacturing, since financial benefits were less apparent for patient records. Also, because third-party payers did not then reimburse for electronic medical records, financial support for most development was limited to government or private foundation grants.

The relatively slow diffusion of outpatient information systems led Van Brunt [328] to suggest more limited functions, such as an essential medical data file or stable events summary – a limited set of medical and demographic data that were considered clinically important and immutable. Typical elements included dates of hospitalization and associated final diagnoses, known drug sensitivity, dates and names of surgical or major investigative procedures, and names of drugs that had been prescribed to treat important or chronic diseases.

In 1988 a survey of members of the American Association of Medical Systems and Informatics (AAMSI) that requested their assessment of computer-based medical records, indicated that appropriate hardware and software were already available. The remaining deficiencies in the electronic patient record systems at that time included interfaces that were not user friendly; were unable to accept unstructured input; were more difficult with data entry than by handwriting; were lacking voice input; and were failing to address the intellectual needs of users. Lack of physician acceptance was the major reason for lack of use. Medical record keeping is highly individualized, whereas automated records require a uniformity and consistency that some physicians find unacceptable [209]. By the end of the 1980s a satisfactory electronic patient record that could process outpatient data for continuing patient care was not yet available to physicians. At that time electronic patients' records, instead of being paperless, often produced more paper than before; disposable computer printouts were used by physicians as temporary records backed up by the computer-based record. Clearly, potential benefits of the electronic record had yet to be realized.

And yet, after four decades of unsuccessful attempts to develop a generally acceptable computer-based electronic patient record, the Institute of Medicine (IOM) of the National Academy of Sciences recognized this need as a high-priority. In 1989, the IOM established a *Patient Record Project* with three subcommittees to define the functional requirements for a computer-based patient record, to determine that record's technical specifications, and to develop a national strategy for that record's diffusion. The result was the publication of *The Computer-Based Patient Record* [116], and of *Aspects of the Computer-Based Patient Record* [16]. By the end of the 1980s Stead [309] suggested that the increasing volume and complexity of patient data stored in electronic patient records required a combination of hierarchical, relational, and object-oriented designs. In the 1980s, users generally agreed that an ideal patient record – one that could provide some combination of a time-oriented, source-oriented, and problem-oriented record, one that could satisfy the functional requirements of its users – had yet to be designed. It was apparent that to convert a paper-based medical record into a computer-based electronic record could be difficult, since the paper-based chart was usually a collection of irregularly entered, unstandardized textual data, mostly handwritten and sometimes illegible, and often replete with diagnostic impressions and verbose descriptions [345]. Gordon [159, 160] addressed the problems of the variable organization, format, and vocabulary in paper based medical records, and proposed a standardized format, not only to facilitate manual information retrieval, but also to prepare for electronic entry, processing, storage, and retrieval. Stead [308] and Hammond also concluded that problem-oriented, time-oriented, encounter-oriented data, with graphical displays of subjective and physical findings, and with test results, clinical diagnoses, and records of therapies, must be able to be mixed and matched upon demand; their name for a medical record that could satisfy these requirements was a demand-oriented medical record.

During the 1990s, with the advent of more powerful computers and more user friendly software, physicians began to use keyboard terminals and clinical workstations to enter data directly into electronic patient records. In the 2000s, encouraged by federal financial support, electronic patient records became more common. In addition, advances in informatics technology led to more efficient data management of expanding databases, and to the inclusion of multi-media data [94].

In the 1990s it was hoped that the computer-based electronic patient record would provide round-the-clock access to a patient's data from more than one location simultaneously; improve the legibility and organization of data; improve the accuracy and comprehensiveness of the record; improve the speed of data retrieval; preserve the confidentiality of the data; discourage redundant testing, suggest lower cost diagnostic and therapeutic alternatives, and thereby improve the efficiency and reduce the cost of providing care; provide clinical decision support; facilitate the monitoring of quality of care; provide aggregate data needed for health services research; facilitate claims and financial reimbursement; and produce a wide variety of administrative reports.

In the 1990s commercial proposals for providing outpatient information systems became commonplace, and in the 2000s the federal government encouraged physicians to have an outpatient information system with a computer based patient record.

Physicians who used computer-based medical records wanted them to allow displays in time-oriented, source-oriented, and problem-oriented representations of the data. Depending on the comprehensiveness of the data items stored in the various files, properly designed retrieval programs could generate the various displays and printed reports requested.

Portable electronic patients' medical records were initiated in the late 1970s with the advent of smart cards, which were similar in size to plastic credit cards but contained one or more microprocessor, integrated-circuit, silicon chips for data storage and processing. These cards could store enough data for essential information from a patient's record [172]. But concerns about confidentiality of portable data, lack of standards for data transfer from one care provider to another, and cost deterred use [218]. By the mid-1980s lower-cost laser optical cards were being tried. The optical card could store a lot of data. Both encoded and read with a laser, the data were then manipulated with software as with any other computer storage device. In 1985 a subsidiary of Blue Cross-Blue Shield in Maryland offered a laser optical card that could be carried in a wallet. The card could hold up to 800 pages of medical information. The portable card reader-writer was connected to an IBM personal computer [230].

The optical write-once read-many (times) (WORM) card used by Vallbona and his colleagues for a patient-carried medical record in a community clinic could store 1.76 megabytes of digitized information – about 700 pages of text. Their Health Passport contained identification data, medical problems, medications, laboratory and x-ray results, and some medical history items. They reported that patients carried their cards when they visited the clinic, and that the optical card reader-writer functioned well. Once written onto the card, information could not be removed; Vallbona considered the card an ideal mechanism for recording clinical information [327].

4.8 Diffusion of Electronic Health Records

In the 2000s, the federal government's financial support for the development, implementation, and diffusion of computer-based electronic patient records markedly increased. The record of a healthcare provider's services to a patient had been called the paper-based patient record or patient's chart, but now it began to be called the computer-based electronic patient record (EPR), or the electronic medical record (EMR), or the clinical electronic patient record (CEMR) when used primarily for patient care. Garrett [152], in the Office of the National Coordinator for Health Information Technology (ONC) recognized that the term electronic medical record (EMR) was used mainly by physicians for the record of a patient's sick care in a hospital or clinic, so federal agencies began to use the term electronic health record (EHR) to include both health care and sick care.

In April 2004, a presidential Executive Order created the position of National Coordinator for Health Information Technology, organizationally located within the Office of the Secretary for the U.S. Department of Health and Human Services (HHS) [201]. The mission of the Office of the National Coordinator for Information Technology (ONC) was to promote development of a nationwide Health Information Technology infrastructure that allowed for electronic use and exchange of information, and to ensure secure and protected patient health information; to improve health care quality and reduce health care costs; to improve coordination of care and information among hospitals, laboratories, physicians and health care providers; to improve public health care activities and facilitate health and clinical research; to promote early detection, prevention and management of chronic diseases; to promote a more effective marketplace and reduce health disparities; to provide leadership in the development, recognition, and implementation of standards and the certification of health information technology products; to provide policy coordination and strategic planning for health information technology adoption and health information exchange, and to establish governance for the Nationwide Health Information Network. In 2009 Kolodner was appointed Chief of the Office of the National Coordinator for Health Information Technology [96, 115, 133].

In 2009 the United States Congress passed the American Recovery and Reinvestment Act (ARRA) that directed about $20 billion in new funds to the healthcare industry, including about $2 billion for health information technology [56]. In 2010 only 1 % of hospitals in the United States were reported to have an operational medical information system (MIS) with patients' electronic health records (EHRs) [179]. The Federal government announced it would subsidize qualifying physicians who purchased an electronic health record (EHR) system that met Federal certification requirements, and who demonstrated compliance with the Federal definitions for "meaningful use" [167, 366].

In 2010 President Obama signed into law the Patient Protection and Affordable Care Act (PPACA) to provide affordable health insurance to most Americans, to improve access to primary care, and to lower its costs [120]. In addition, the president signed the Healthcare Reconciliation Bill which introduced changes in the PPACA to reflect agreements between the House and the Senate [142]. In 2010 Blumenthal, Chief of the Office of the National Coordinator for Health Information Technology (ONC), established an Electronic Health Record Certification Program to ensure that physicians adopted electronic health records that could satisfy the specified requirements for meaningful use and thus entitle them to the federal subsidy.

An electronic health record had to be able to store and retrieve an individual patient's information collected over time. The information had to include the patient's demographics, medical history, current medications, doctor's notes, and important administrative information. Issues concerning electronic health records included data exchange, privacy, security, and patient's consent. Meaningful use was defined by increasingly complex stages comprising sets of requirements and qualifications established in order for an institution to be eligible for Federal funding based on the adoption and use of an electronic health record in accordance with the provisions established by the Healthcare Information Technology for Economic and Clinical Health (HITECH) Act [174].

The HITECH Act established one set of awards that provided $386 million to 40 States and qualified State-Designated Entities to build the capacity for exchanging health information across the health care system, both within and between states through the State Health Information Exchange Cooperative Agreement Program; and another set of awards that provided $375 million to create 32 Regional Extension Centers (RECs) to support the efforts of health professionals, starting with primary care providers, to become meaningful users of electronic health records. Together these programs were to help modernize the use of health information, and improve the quality and efficiency of health care for all Americans [48].

The HITECH legislation provided direct financial subsidies to physicians for adopting and demonstrating qualified meaningful use of certified information technology in amounts of up to $44,000 to physicians who were not hospital-based and who participated in the Medicare electronic health record incentive program, or up to $63,750 if they were participating in the Medicaid electronic health record incentive program [294]. The final rules for meaningful use Stage 1 were released in July 2010. Participants in the program needed to satisfy the criteria by using certified technology to improve the quality, safety, and efficiency of health care, and reduce health disparities; engage patients and families; improve care coordination for population and public health; maintain privacy and security of patient health information; and be able to capture and share patients' electronic data, and use uniform standards for clinical procedures and summary reports [48–50]. Advancing to Stage 2 in 2014 required further integration within increasingly complex subsystems that required adequate database management systems, and that required vendors to have better data standards to support interoperability for data exchange within and between electronic health record systems. Further stages of requirements for meaningful use were expected to be released later, including defined requirements for recording patients' outcomes.

In 2011, commercial vendors of electronic health records reported that MEDITECH had 1,212 installations, Cerner 606; McKesson Provider Technologies 573, Epic Systems 413, and Siemens Healthcare 397. By the middle of 2011, the Centers for Medicare and Medicaid Services (CMS) reported that 77,000 health care providers were registered in the CMS program; and CMS had paid $400 million in meaningful use incentives to physicians and hospitals [253]. By 2012 electronic health systems were in widespread use. CMS reported that more than 40 % (132,000) of the primary health care providers, and more than 3,300 hospitals in the United States had enrolled in the program, and that CMS had paid out more than $5 billion in meaningful use incentives to more than 93,000 physicians [221]. The majority of physicians who responded to a survey reported satisfaction with their electronic records. Vendors used by the largest percentage of respondents were Epic with 22 %, Allscripts with 10 %, and Cerner with 9 % [97]. In 2012, the chief of the Office of the National Coordinator for Health Information Technology, Mostaashari, reported that the Certified Health IT Product List (CHPL) contained more than 500 certified products. The 2011 and 2014 lists are posted on the web [73].

4.9 Evaluation of Patient Record Systems

To evaluate a patient record system, whether it be for a physician's office, a hospital, or both, and whether paper-based or electronic, requires an assessment of the effects on medical outcomes, patients' satisfaction with the care provided, physician's satisfaction with the use of the system, and the system's effects on health care costs.

Flagle [139] at Johns Hopkins University proposed that an evaluation of an information system should include three groups of criteria: (1) From a societal point of view, the most important criteria were economic. What were the values or utilities that the information system provided and what were its costs? This led to cost-effectiveness analyses that compared the costs of alternative means for performing a specified process. (2) Flagle called his second set of criteria cybernetic, in that they measured how well the information system functioned in observation, analysis, communication, control, and planning. (3) Flagle's third set of criteria related to human factors. How compatible was the information system with the perceptions, capabilities, and motivations of its users?

Flagle [138] further described four measures for evaluating the effects, contributions, and costs of a technology to a health service: (1) component technical performance measures such as response time and cost-per-procedure; (2) subsystem technical performance measures such as capacity and lifecycle cost; (3) service process measures such as patients' acceptance and patients' admission cost to the health service; and (4) patients' outcomes and end results, such as disability and per capita cost. Flagle [137] also described the process of *technology assessment* as a method of problem formulation that forces the examination of a technology beyond its immediate intended effects, by a comprehensive definition of the technology and its competitors; by identification of levels within society of interest from individuals to organizations; by assessment of its impact on the parties of interest; and by forecasting the outcomes of various policy systems that encourage or discourage its development. Flagle [136] proposed an evaluation matrix with three dimensions: policy/societal, managerial/institutional, and operational/clinical, which combined considerations of the patients with those of health care professionals and policy makers. Later Flagle [135] outlined a comprehensive evaluation methodology that included: designing the evaluation study; measuring changes in structure, process, and outcome; and measuring costs and benefits. Flagle [134] considered technology assessment as a process in which the independent variable is *system structure* as modified by technological changes; and the dependent variables are *system processes* such as volume of service, accuracy of data, timeliness of information flow, health outcomes, and social and economic impact on society, since the system model needed to be set in the social, political, and economic context in which it interacted.

Klarman [200] proposed that the process of evaluating information technology was primarily that of an economic assessment as to: did it reduce costs, and by how much? Even when the computer helped in the diagnostic process, the basic test was still cost reduction. With respect to services that were rendered in the past, does the new system save money, or does it expand services for the same amount of money? Although economists emphasized measurements of direct costs and direct benefits, some did not include indirect benefits, such as postponement of disability and death, or less tangible benefits, such as improved quality of care and quality of life.

Goldman [158] at the University of Missouri, Columbia, emphasized the need to evaluate information systems, since the information gained provided feedback that the designer needed to direct future evolution. He recommended that a proper system evaluation include: (1) An experimental design that measured the effects of the new system compared to a control environment in which the innovation had not been implemented. (2) A data-collection and analysis plan for assessing the effects, using statistical tests of significance made with a quantitative measure of confidence, as well as judgmental assessments of importance that relied on human experience and that were made with a qualitative measure of confidence. Statistical significance alone is insufficient; thoughtful judgment is still required. To rephrase, as has been said, "To be a difference a difference has to make a difference." (3) Definition of the basic work units, such as the patient's medical record in an information system. (4) Definition of the system components, including not only functional components, such as a nursing unit, but for each component there should be assessed its costs for labor, material, equipment, and overhead. Goldman also advocated that attention be focused on personnel performance and attitude, micro-costs, information audit, and benefits. Few evaluations satisfied Goldman's recommendations.

Barnett [21, 22] offered a different approach by asking if management would pay to support the computer system from non-government funds over a prolonged period of time, and if other institutions successfully implemented a similar system.

Collen [81] proposed a matrix to serve as a guide for measuring the extent to which an electronic patient record system achieved its specified requirements and objectives. This required that consideration be given to the objectives of four groups of stakeholders: (1) patients, which included measuring the system's effects on patients' health outcomes, and the length and costs of the care process; (2) health professionals, as to the ease of entering orders and receiving test results, and the extent of the support for clinical decision-making; (3) administrators, as to the system's effects on operating costs, and its support of managerial decisions; and (4) policy makers, as to the system's effects on overall costs and outcomes of patient care.

Weinstein [348] described the differences between cost-effectiveness and cost-benefit analyses. The purpose of cost-effectiveness analysis is to assess the efficiency with which resources were applied to achieve specified desired benefits; for example, what was the cost of procedure "A" versus procedure "B" to make a particular diagnosis? In the health care context, cost-effectiveness analysis typically assumes that the objective is to achieve a desired health benefit, given the level of expenditure or the health care budget. In cost-benefit analysis the goal is to develop a single measure of net value for each program or procedure being evaluated, and this requires that health benefits be assigned monetary values so they can be compared with the cost of resources expended. King [198] noted that system benefits took the forms of: (1) cost savings, cost reductions, or cost avoidance; (2) improved operational performance, lower error rates, increased speed for performing certain tasks, increased capacity and volume of information processing and storage; and (3) such intangibles as improved quality of information, improved decision making, and enhanced morale.

Lindberg [210, 211, 214] proposed five approaches to evaluating the worth of an electronic patient record: (1) The marketplace outcome, as to what was preferred and would prevail in the marketplace, since more valuable systems would compete successfully against less valuable offerings. Lindberg observed that in the 1970s, the marketplace had selected predominantly business office applications; for clinically-oriented applications the market place had concluded that their worth was slim or as yet undiscovered. (2) He described as an operations research approach the development of a study design with an explicit set of variables to be examined, and with an analytic methodology based on statistically valid procedures. (3) He advocated cost and economic analyses such as were described above. (4) He advocated a technology assessment approach which included studies of the social, ethical, and legal effects of the information system, such as its effects on data privacy. (5) Lindberg wanted to evaluate the scientific impact, or the extent to which an information system could influence or advance other fields of medicine, and serve as the technical infrastructure for scientifically advanced concepts in medicine. He cited, as an example, the effect of expert systems in clinical decision making, which he pointed out could not emerge from evaluations such as a cost-benefit analysis. He emphasized the difficulty in quantifying this type of benefit when he stated that there was reason to expect the benefit from an electronic patient records would be a summation of small gains, plus the very large potential gain in the additional desirable activities that such a system would permit, such as in the support of clinical decision making. Lindberg advised that a meaningful cost-benefit evaluation for a major electronic health record system would take a minimum of 5 years, and might well require 10 years.

Prior to the advent of electronic patient record systems, virtually no studies were done to evaluate paper-based patients' records. The traditional paper-based patient records contained a collated series of documents that described encounters between the patients and their health professionals over a period of time. Prior to the advent of computers, when solo practitioners saw patients in their offices, the case records were usually hand written or transcribed on sheets of paper that were stored chronologically in paper folders or envelopes. For physicians in a group practice, where one patient might see several specialists, all patient care information was generally collated in an integrated paper-based medical record. Each patient would be assigned a unique medical record number; and all charts would be collected and filed in the sequential order of their medical record numbers in a common medical record room. A common problem in a group practice occurred when a patient needed to see more than one physician on the same day. The patient's paper-based chart was often still needed in the first doctor's office and therefore unavailable to the physicians being seen subsequently.

An early evaluation of a comprehensive electronic patient record system was reported in 1962 by Roach [275] at Systems Development Corporation in Santa Monica, California. The system was deployed in a 400-bed hospital using 40 computer terminals at an estimated cost of $500,000–1,000,000 to buy, plus $125,000–250,000 per year to operate, with anticipated savings of $240,000 per year from a 23 % reduction in nursing staff.

In 1964 the total cost for the electronic patient record system developed for the diabetes clinic of the University Hospitals of Cleveland, Ohio, was reported to be approximately $2 per patient visit [208]. According to Barnett, the cost in 1965 for the Computer-Stored Ambulatory Record (COSTAR) system at the Harvard Community Health Plan (HCHP), including its hardware and its support personnel, was approximately $1.50 per patient visit, and the cost for the computer to process the medical data, including the input of data and computer generation of reports and medical statistics, was reported to be 60 cents per patient visit [165].

On the other hand, few evaluations of electronic patient record systems provided data on the costs and effectiveness of patient care or on clinical functions. Most reports that appeared in the first few decades analyzed the effectiveness and costs for implementing the business and administrative functions [16]. By the end of the 1960s there had occurred sufficient development of electronic patient information systems in medical facilities that questions arose as to how to accurately evaluate their costs and effectiveness. Interest in this evaluation process was spurred by the report of Jydstrup [193] that the average cost in hospitals for information handling was 22–25 % of a hospital's total operating cost.

In a 1974 survey of 17 ambulatory care centers, Rogers [279] found that physicians in outpatient clinics who were randomly assigned to see patients while they used an electronic patient record ordered significantly more clinical laboratory tests than they did when they saw patients without the system (12.2 tests ordered per patient with the electronic record, compared to 8.1 without it). Nevertheless, the physicians thought the additional tests appropriate, given the chronicity and severity of illness in the patient population studied. When office-visit scheduling conflicts occurred, and physicians assigned to see patients with the electronic record system actually saw control patients and vice versa, the investigators found no carry-over, that is, no system effect on control patients.

Vickery [331] reported the use of an electronic patient record system by physician assistants who treated ambulatory patients using specified algorithms or protocols. Some used computer-generated encounter forms interactively with visual display terminals for the input of data, whereas others used computer-generated paper encounter forms with data recorded on the forms as in the manual system. A total of 609 patients' records were audited for errors of omission or commission of data items. The researchers estimated the skill of the physician assistants by comparing the encounter forms produced by them with those produced by their supervising physicians. Whether physician assistants used the manual system or the computer-supported system, the frequency of their errors and their estimated skill was not significantly different. An audit that compared data recorded in the manual charts with those prescribed by the clinical algorithms found a mean of one error of data omission per chart, whereas no errors occurred when computer-generated forms programmed to follow the specified algorithm were used. It was concluded that a significant portion of the omissions represented failure to record data that had in fact been collected.

In a later study Kuhn [203, 204] noted that the analysis of a specific site had to consider all resources required, including the costs of installation, transition, technical support, and training of personnel. The acceptance of the patient care providers (doctors, nurses, technologists, and administrators) appeared to be best when they were involved in the system design, when they participated in the decision to install the system, and when they received adequate training in its use. From an analysis of 58 responses to a questionnaire, it was concluded that a computer-based patient record system was viewed as affording distinct benefits to its users, and that it was preferred to the prior paper-based record system.

Kuhn [203] revisited Duke's TMR, Regenstrief 's RMR, Harvard Community Health Plan's COSTAR, as well as the Arthritis Research Information Office Network (ARION) in Wichita, Kansas, an administrative and clinical outpatient information system developed by a private-practice physician to collect data for the Arthritis, Rheumatism, and Aging Medical Information System (ARAMIS) project at Stanford University, and for the Family Practice medical information system in Bailey, Colorado, which provided administrative services to a family practice clinic. They reported that only one-third of all systems they had identified had achieved full operational status. In most cases, the systems were limited in medical scope or were providing primarily administrative services, such as patient registration, billing, and appointment scheduling. Several of the promising systems visited in 1975, particularly COSTAR, were undergoing transfer from a prototype demonstration in the research setting to the commercial market.

The Office of Technology Assessment [266] cited a study done by Bolt, Beranek, and Newman for the National Center for Health Services Research (NCHSR) that analyzed a clinic operated by 11 physicians in Nashua, New Hampshire. That study concluded that between $87,000 and $142,000 in data processing and personnel salaries could be offset by a computer-based outpatient information system, and that such a group practice could benefit from a capital investment for electronic health records of between $275,000 and $460,000.

Some evaluations of the problem-oriented medical record soon followed Weed's publications. Tufo [325] and associates at the Given Health Care Center of the University of Vermont College of Medicine reported that the problem-oriented medical record permitted their practitioners to double the ratio of patients to physicians, to decrease the rate of hospitalizations, and to decrease the use of ambulatory medical care. In an evaluation of the problem-oriented medical record in the medical services of Fort Sam Houston in Texas, Stuart [314] and associates reported that the great majority of physicians thought the problem-oriented medical record was an improvement over the traditional record for both clinic and hospital patients, and that it provided a clearer picture of a patient's health problems. They also felt that it made the record more understandable; that it helped the physicians to provide better care and to manage patients' care more efficiently; and that it improved physicians' teaching rounds.

On the other hand, after 5 months of use, Stuart [313] reported that there had not yet been enough time for physicians to learn to use the problem-oriented medical record with high consistency and proper attention to all its elements. A comparison of a paper-based problem-oriented medical record to a paper-based traditional source and time-oriented record in the clinics of the medical department of the Beach Army Hospital at Fort Worth, Texas, found no significant difference between the two groups in the number of problems identified, objective data documented, or completeness of follow-up. When the computer-based problem-oriented medical record was used, time needed for data entry and retrieval was reduced as compared to the paper-based problem-oriented medical record.

Rubin [282] observed that although Weed's problem-oriented record was useful to track and audit problems that were listed, an incidental or unexpected abnormality not reflected in the problem list, such as a nurse recording an elevated blood pressure measurement, might easily be overlooked.

Salmon [285] noted that the problem-oriented medical record generally allowed one problem to be considered at a time during a long period of the patient's care. When a patient had many problems, he advocated a graphical timeline in which the patient's visits were plotted along the horizontal axis, and each problem identified at that visit was plotted as a vertical bar. With such a plot, the temporal profile of problems that arose and that were resolved could be appreciated graphically.

An issue often reported with Weed's problem-oriented medical record was the need to train physicians to enter data with links to specific problems. Feinstein [131] considered it difficult to accommodate to Weed's problem-oriented medical record due to the frequent need to rearrange data. In addition, he observed that data entry was faster in a time-oriented record. Others thought that the problem-oriented medical record placed too much emphasis on the patient's chart.

Richart [272, 273] conducted a 4-year study that compared the electronic patient information system in the Kaiser Foundation Hospital in San Francisco with the manual systems in the Kaiser Foundation Hospitals in Oakland and Walnut Creek. The evaluation plan included comparisons before and after system installation, for a short-term test of the electronic system's ability to increase message legibility; increase speed of data dissemination; control information flow; handle volume; improve reliability and accuracy of data; and increase cost-effectiveness while decreasing unnecessary use and duplication. Annual comparisons were conducted. The first round of data collection occurred in April and May of 1969. Observations were organized in terms of patient care and communications activities, thus providing four groups of basic measurements: (1) activities that involved patient care and communication; (2) activities that involved patient care but no communication; (3) activities that involved no patient care but that did involve communication; and (4) activities that involved neither patient care nor communication. Baseline studies showed that all three hospitals were initially similar in that their total costs for communication, whether for patient care or not, represented 35–39 % of total operating cost [273]. After installation of the electronic patient records system, nursing functions in patient care (communication with patients) were found to be adversely affected by computer-terminal introduction, whereas patient care-communications were made more efficient. Richart [272] also observed that the electronic patient record shortened the time needed to evaluate hospital activities to a number of days, as compared to the weeks or months necessary in the manual mode.

Collen [91] reported a cost analysis of the Kaiser Permanente pilot electronic patient record system. Total annual system cost was $1.2 million, of which 40 % was spent for staff services, 40 % for equipment, and 20 % for database storage to provide electronic medical records for both inpatients and outpatients. Unit costs were about $2.50 per patient for each of 50,000 multiphasic screening examinations; $0.06 per test for 50,000 clinical laboratory tests; $0.05 per prescription for 15,000 pharmacy prescriptions; $1.00 per admission for 10,000 hospital admissions; $0.17 per-visit for 90,000 doctor's office visits; $1.35 per electrocardiogram for 40,000 procedures; and $0.03 per retrieval for each of 5,000 requests per terminal for information from a patient record.

Bond [52] provided an early cost evaluation of an electronic patient record system by analyzing the costs in three hospitals operated by the Third Order of St. Francis in Peoria, Illinois, that shared an online system. Bond reported improvements in admissions procedures – significantly less time to admit patients, and significantly improved staff utilization. The probability of erroneous information being introduced into the care process was reduced by more than 20 % in those areas served by the electronic patient record. On nursing stations the flow of orders improved by 36–44 %; in the clinical laboratories order flow improved by 21–34 %; and in the radiology department patient processing time was reduced by 25–27 %.

Simborg [300] and associates at Johns Hopkins Hospital reported on the early effects of their electronic patient record on patient care in one acute medical unit consisting of 31 beds, as compared to a similar, manual, paper-based patient record in a unit that served as the control. They found a significant reduction in error rates in carrying out physician orders in the experimental unit that used the electronic patient record as compared to the manual, paper-based, control unit. With the new system, they reported a transcription error rate of 1.7 % for the 856 orders examined, and six communication errors caused orders to be carried out incorrectly. In contrast, with the manual record the transcription error rate was 7.3 % for the 857 orders examined, and 38 communication errors caused orders to be carried out incorrectly. They also found that nurses spent 40 % of their time in direct patient contact after implementation of the electronic patient record compared to 23 % with the paper-based record. With respect to indirect care (*administrative time*) nurses spent 32 % of their time in this way after implementation of the electronic patient record compared to 45 % before. In the control unit, nurses spent 38–41 % of their time on indirect care. The authors concluded that the costs of the electronic patient record system were effectively offset by improved effectiveness of the staff.

Schmitz [288] reported a cost analysis of the Medelco electronic patient record system installed at the Deaconess Hospital in St. Louis, Missouri. The direct expense attributed to the system for 1970 and 1971 was $223,021, or $1.37 per patient day during the first complete fiscal year of operation. Offsetting this expense was an increase in revenue from recovery of previously lost charges of about $2.18 per patient day. It was concluded that the system had been economically beneficial to the hospital.

Vallbona [326] reported that when research and development costs were excluded, the electronic patient record at the 81-bed Texas Institute for Research and Rehabilitation cost $14.47 per patient day. He estimated that if the electronic patient record system were to operate at its capacity of 200 hospital beds, cost per patient day would decline to $4.20.

A comprehensive evaluation of an early electronic patient record system was that of the Technicon system installed in the El Camino Hospital in Mountain View, California. Gall [148] estimated that most of the potential savings for their electronic patient record system was in labor, mostly in nursing services that Gall categorized as those that were developed as planned, those that required an explicit effort called the *benefits-realization process*, and those described as *spin-off benefits* made possible by the system but were not integral to it. He considered the benefits-realization process to be a unique endeavor, separate and distinct from implementation, but of equal or greater importance. Benefits realization undertakes to aggregate small labor savings, spread over many employees and three daily shifts, into partial or full-time equivalents that become candidates for staff reduction. Gall further suggested that possible revenue sources included lost charges and late-charge write-offs, cash-flow improvements, and volume changes in ancillary service orders or in patient care throughput. Hodge [181] in considering the lost-charges benefit for the El Camino Hospital agreed that an automated charge-collection system in an electronic patient record could reduce or eliminate charges lost in manual information processing. On the other hand, he noted that services provided by El Camino Hospital were for the most part reimbursed on the basis of cost or through some form of prospective reimbursement. For such hospitals, failure to capture individual charges would have little impact on the hospital's revenue.

In El Camino Hospital's admitting department, Norwood [263] reported that the Technicon system had enabled a labor reduction of five full-time equivalents. When a patient was transferred from one bed to another, or was discharged or expired, the system made the necessary record changes and notified the affected departments. A 1973 survey of staff physicians at El Camino Hospital reported that about 90 % of their orders were entered directly into the system by obstetricians and gynecologists, about 80 % were entered by surgeons, but only 30 % were entered by internists. On average, 70 % of all physicians' orders were entered directly by the physicians into the computer system. Half of all physicians surveyed responded that they were in favor of retaining the system [344]. Cook [100] reported that if one asked any nurse at the El Camino Hospital what she thought of the Technicon system, one would receive a positive response. Gall [147] reported after 3 years of online operation, the system had accomplished wide-spread user acceptance from both physicians and nurses, and that by December 1973, the system was considered to be cost effective compared to the prior manual system.

El Camino also compared their experience with that of six nearby hospitals, similar in size that also provided short-term, acute-care services. Gall [147] found a significant decrease of 3.5 nursing hours per admission at El Camino as compared to the other hospitals. The savings in cost for nursing personnel totaled $54,000 per month. Other labor savings in support areas consisted of labor reduction in the business office and in medical records yielding an additional $3,400 per month, for a total monthly labor savings of $68,100. The major ancillary services in the El Camino Hospital affected by the Technicon system (laboratory, radiology, pharmacy, central services, and admissions) showed a cost reduction and cost containment of 1 h per admission, or the equivalent of $10,000 per month. Gall concluded that the total cost savings that could be attributed to the Technicon system at the El Camino Hospital by the end of 1973 averaged $86,600 per month.

Anderson [8] reported that the use of personal order sets by physicians at the Methodist Hospital of Indiana, which had installed the Technicon Hospital Information System in 1987, resulted in faster order entry and results reporting, a significant decrease in error rate for entering orders, decreased nursing paperwork, and greater use of the direct order entry mode by physicians.

A study by the Office of Technology Assessment (OTA) of the United States Congress also concluded that the El Camino Hospital realized substantial cost savings in labor from its installation of the Technicon system. OTA reported estimated savings attributed to the computer system ranged from $72,000 to $189,000 per month, whereas the fixed operational cost of the system was $89,800 per month. Net benefits, after payment for the costs of the system, were estimated to range between $30,000 and $50,000 per month or $3–5 per patient day. Labor savings, particularly in nursing, accounted for about 95 % of the Technicon system's total cost savings. Savings in materials made up much of the other 5 %. As a comparison, the OTA reported that the operating costs for an electronic patient information system for a hospital ranged from $4 to $9 a day, and represented from 4 % to 7 % of the total hospital operating budget [266].

In 1979 the Battelle Columbus Laboratories, under a contract from the National Center for Health Services Research and Development, completed a 7-year evaluation of the El Camino Hospital's Technicon system [25], which generally affirmed the reported findings by Gall [147]. The Battelle group first reported on some non-economic benefits, such as a significant reduction in pharmacy errors, improvement in the accuracy and completeness of the paper medical records, an overall decrease in variance in medical orders and reporting results, and improved communications at all levels of the hospital. There was a decrease in turnaround time for tests and procedures in the clinical laboratory, radiology, and electrocardiography; patients were admitted faster because physicians' orders were entered sooner; laboratory test results were more available to physicians during evening rounds; treatments and medications were begun earlier and modifications to treatment plans initiated sooner; elective surgery admissions were processed faster and patient satisfaction was increased by the reduction in the time consumed in being admitted to the hospital. The cumulative effects of these benefits contributed to shorter hospital stays.

Coffey [80] summarized for the National Center for Health Servicers Research and Development the results and findings of the Battelle evaluation as follows: (1) the Technicon Hospital Information System improved the efficiency of nursing care, and through staff attrition and care for a greater number of patients, reduced nursing costs per patient by 5 %. (2) The average length of stay at El Camino was shortened by 4.7 %. (3) The overall effect of the system on total hospital expenses could not be estimated conclusively; however, (4) the total hospital cost per patient day, including the cost of the Technicon system, rose 3.2 % during the operation of the system, a statistically significant increase. This increase was explained in part by the reduction in average length of stay. Monthly overall expenses rose 7.8 % from the pre-system period, a change largely explained by the greater flow of patients through the El Camino Hospital. Although nurses strongly favored the Technicon system, the community physicians who admitted their patients to the El Camino Hospital required several years to accept the system and use the light-pen terminals to enter their orders directly. At the end of the initial 4-year study, 61 % of physician users voted to retain and extend the system, a number that increased to 80 % several years later [211]. Despite all the favorable results reported from the several independent evaluations of the Lockheed-Technicon system at the El Camino Hospital, some still considered the economic models used to be controversial.

Emlet [127] and associates at Analytic Services in Falls Church, Virginia, developed a detailed cost-benefit method for the evaluation of the Department of Defense *Tri-Service Medical Information System* (TRIMIS). In addition to an assessment of the economics, they defined 11 areas of effectiveness to consider in measuring to what extent TRIMIS achieved the defined objectives of the Department of Defense. These areas included quality, availability, accessibility, and acceptability of health care; appropriateness of utilization; recruitment, retention, and training of personnel; absenteeism of personnel; performance of personnel; response to changing needs; organizational image; and contributions to society. For each of these areas, they identified specific measures and indicators for the evaluations to be performed, pre-and post-implementation, and to be collected on site at the various installations in army, navy, and air force hospitals [126]. For example, indicators of accessibility of care included barriers to access and attitudes of patients as well as measures of access that could be influenced by TRIMIS, including waiting times for appointments and for admissions [69]. The evaluation of a multihospital system such as TRIMIS encompassed not only how well the system met the objectives of the individual hospitals, but also how well TRIMIS met the overall objectives of the Department of Defense for all facilities that used it [68]. In the end, however, Analytic Services completed no evaluations; they lost the evaluation contract to Arthur D. Little, Inc.

Grann [162] evaluated the attitudes of clinic personnel before and after the implementation of TRIMIS for outpatient appointments in 12 clinics at the Walter Reed Army Medical Center. At first, physician users of the computer-based appointment system viewed it with disfavor, but attitudes became more favorable after they had used it for several months. Grann suggested that new-user training of computer systems would be more effective if it attempted to inculcate realistic perceptions of, and positive attitudes toward the system. Mishelevich [248, 249] analyzed the costs of the Parkland Online Information System at the Parkland Memorial Hospital in Dallas, and reported that in 1979 costs were $5.81 per inpatient day, $3.64 per emergency room visit, and $3.05 per outpatient visit. Mischelevich also analyzed radiology procedures and reported a savings in time for processing requisitions and reports and a decrease in volume due to the elimination of duplicate procedures.

Kennedy [196] and associates summarized some of the findings of the prior decade. They reported that among specialty groups, obstetricians, gynecologists, urologists, surgeons, and radiologists were most favorably disposed to an electronic patient record, whereas internists and general practitioners were the least receptive. As a whole, physicians were less favorable than nurses to electronic patient records.

Kennedy concluded that the use of electronic patient records could enable hospitals: (1) to reduce errors in the administration of medications and the performance of laboratory tests; (2) to decrease the time and costs of transmitting medical orders. (3) To reduce duplicative and unnecessary procedures; (4) to reduce clerical activities; (5) to eliminate misplaced reports; (6) to decrease time and costs of reporting test results; and (7) to expedite the completion of the patient's medical record.

Kennedy [196] added that in addition to its other uses, the electronic patient record was being used increasingly for clinical decision-making. Kennedy also confirmed that the overall effect of an electronic patient record on a hospital's expenses was not to increase per-patient costs significantly, even though a decreased length of stay would cause the cost-per-patient day to go up.

Schlager [287] provided comparative costs for an outpatient information system in a two-office, three-physician family practice, with an average workload of 30 patients per day. The reported costs to update and maintain a patient's record was $1.32 for the computer-based system, compared to $2.56 for similar activities with a manual, paper-based system.

Drazen [122] at Arthur D. Little concluded from a study of methodologies used in the 1970s to measure the cost effectiveness of electronic patient records, that one of the most common reasons for implementing an electronic patient record was to increase staff productivity by reducing paper work. Drazen [123] found that labor savings (notably in nursing time) in a hospital was the largest cost reduction identified or predicted, and she described techniques used to estimate the amount of these savings: (1) Task analysis, which identified individual activities affected by the electronic patient record. (2) Job-content analysis, which focused on differences in time spent when the same job was performed in different ways. (3) Work sampling which documented staff time allocated to information handling in different service units. (4) Trend analysis, which monitored changes in productivity of personnel after implementing an electronic patient record.

Drazen emphasized that turning time savings into labor-force reductions required a deliberate effort to reorganize services and thereby to improve work-methods, redistribute job titles, and redefine job roles among various labor categories. Without active benefits realization, activity displacement might result in increased idle time rather than payroll savings. Drazen also observed that a hospital typically incurred a large initial capital cost and then realized economic benefits only incrementally and in later years. She defined the cost effects of an electronic patient record as changes that could be expressed in dollars. From a review of published evaluations in the 1970s, she reported that two basic techniques had been used to analyze the cost effects of an electronic patient record. In one method, before and after costs were compared. In the other method, cost effects were predicted before the system was implemented based on baseline data concerning hospital operations, knowledge of potential system effects, and the experience of other users. Drazen observed that predictive methods were useful for decision makers who were considering installation of an electronic patient record, but only the retrospective study of actual experience could provide data that could be used to develop or validate predictive models.

Drazen required a careful accounting of costs, including expenditures for services and equipment obtained from a vendor, and expenditures for in-house personnel required to install, maintain, and use the system. When system costs were being compared with labor savings, she proposed that the costs of a *benefits-realization effort* to bring about the necessary operational changes be included as well.

Drazen [123] concluded that cost savings were rarely the only motivation for implementing an electronic patient record since improved information handling resulted in benefits that were difficult to measure in economic terms. Furthermore, she pointed out that the evaluation of revenue implications of an electronic patient record was complex and had to consider reimbursement patterns; while more complete capture of lost charges never reduced revenue, it often had no effect, as when a patient's hospitalization was reimbursed by case-mix.

Whiting-O'Keefe and associates [357] studied the effectiveness of their Summary Time-Oriented Record (STOR) flow sheets as a sole clinical information source and reported that 59 % of the physicians in their rheumatic diseases clinic did not request the full medical record [356]. They also studied the effect on the accuracy of physicians' prognostic capabilities by using their computer-based time-oriented flow sheets to supplement a traditional paper-based medical record. In two medical clinics of the University of California at San Francisco, more than 1,100 patients were randomized into two groups. In one group, the physician received the medical record and the computer-based time-oriented flow sheets, whereas in the control group only the medical record was provided. After the patients left the clinic, physicians made predictions about events in the patient's future clinical course recorded on a form as probabilities. In 617 visits in the arthritis clinic, the authors reported that clinicians were better able to predict their patients' future symptom changes and laboratory test results when computer-based time-oriented flow sheets were added to the medical record than when they were not.

In a second study, the use of only computer-based time-oriented flow sheets (without the medical record) did not decrease in the physician's predictive abilities. In addition, in 74 % of 514 visits in the rheumatic diseases clinic, clinicians did not exercise their option of calling for the full medical record. The authors concluded that the improved flow of information from the computer-based time-oriented flow sheets could improve the clinical decision-making process.

Tierney and associates [318] at the Regenstrief Institute reported a 13 % reduction in the number of outpatient diagnostic tests ordered when physicians, about to order selected tests, were shown previous results from these same tests.

The relatively slow early diffusion of outpatient information systems and computer-based patient records Van Brunt [328] to suggest simpler, more limited functions, such an essential medical data file to be composed of a limited set of medical and demographic data that were considered clinically important and immutable. Typical elements would include dates of hospitalization and associated final diagnoses, drug sensitivities, dates and names of surgical or major investigative procedures, and names of drugs that had been prescribed to treat important diseases for more than a transient period.

In her work for Arthur D. Little with the Department of Defense's TRIMIS program, Drazen [121] employed a *formative* type of evaluation, which she called *implementation monitoring*; that was designed to track information about the system's operation, use, and benefits from the time the site was being prepared for system installation through the time that a stable operation was achieved. This provided an early warning of where hospital operations and computer systems would have to be changed if the expected benefits were to be gained. This process involved four steps: (1) selecting aspects of performance and benefits to be monitored, which included identifying items critical to the system's success; (2) specifying how to measure each aspect in discrete, unambiguous units; (3) specifying a schedule for the monitoring process; and (4) specifying performance criteria and determining the kind of performance expected at specified times in the implementation schedule.

Through the second half of the 1980s, Arthur D. Little, Inc. conducted for the Department of Defense a comprehensive evaluation of TRIMIS. The approach they took in performing the economic analysis of TRIMIS involved comparing its incremental lifecycle costs and benefits with the costs and benefits of manual systems operations, while considering only the costs and benefits attributed to the computer system. The cost-benefit analysis encompassed the expected lifetime of the information system, and examined the associated costs and benefits from the date of installation to the end of the system's life expectancy of 8 years. They grouped the identified benefits from TRIMIS into six major categories: increased availability of health professionals, increased availability of other hospital staff members, increased service capacity, savings of materials, improved health status of patients, and increased effective time of active duty military personnel. The methodology was focused on those benefits expected to contribute substantial, measurable, dollar-valued benefits. The costs associated with the purchase, installation, operation, and maintenance of TRIMIS were organized into costs for hardware, software, communications, and other expenses, including those for site preparation, training, personnel, supplies, and overhead. A computer-based cost-benefit analysis model was developed in which all cost items were inflated for future years using a Department of Defense inflation index; and benefits and costs in future years were discounted to present value using a 10 % discounted rate as mandated by Department of Defense regulations [286].

From a 1980 survey Ball [19, 20] reported that six vendors who sold *Level II* hospital information systems had a cost range for hardware and software of $4.00–7.50 per patient day. A *Level II* system was defined by Ball as a large, comprehensive hospital information system with an electronic patient record system to capture and maintain the entire patient record. In addition, it had a database that could be queried for patient medications and other data. Ball found that for simpler *Level I* systems, of which 18 vendors had sold more than 500 as of the spring of 1980, their cost range was $1.50–2.75 per patient day.

The Office of Technology Assessment [267] of the United States Congress expanded the evaluation of technology to measure not only intended and expected effects, but also to assess effects and costs of intangible and unintended consequences. Assessing the positive and negative effects of *unintended consequences* that result from implementation of an electronic patient record system required the collection of post-implementation data to measure unanticipated events. The collection of such data added complexity and expense, since data about unplanned effects were usually unavailable. This would require *sensitivity analysis* with varying estimates and assumptions to substitute for missing data to estimate the potential range of costs of the unintended effects [87].

Blum [46] proposed that an electronic patient record could also produce such measurable benefits as surveillance of diagnosis, therapy, and laboratory results to identify potential incompatibilities; management of information overload by producing reminders when tests were overdue or changes in therapy were suggested; and decision-making support and protocol-directed management by using patient care plans.

Wilson [365] and McDonald at the Wishard Memorial Hospital in Indianapolis reported their experience with almost 2,000 adult patients seen in their emergency room. Twenty-five percent of the patients also had been seen in their medical clinics and had prior computer-stored records of their medical problems. Internists who had received a printed summary of the patients' computer-stored records in addition to other information, ordered an average of 2.7 tests compared to 3.2 tests ordered by physicians who did not receive the computer-stored summary. No difference was found in the rate of ordering tests by emergency-room surgeons who received the computer-record summaries.

Jacobs [184] analyzed the costs of training personnel to use an electronic medical record at the 450-bed St. Vincent Hospital in Portland, Oregon. All new users were required to take a 3-h class, whereas experienced users took a 1- or 2-h class. Although the hospital had planned for a 1-year training program, implementation took 5-years in which 4,356 individuals were instructed in the use of the system, generating 8,670 h of training and resulting in $106,500 in direct training costs. Jacobs concluded that this represented a 500 % increase over the original statement by the vendor for implementation, and an excess of 100 % over the original hospital estimate for training costs.

To evaluate users' satisfaction with an electronic medical record generally involved surveys. Counte [103] and associates at Rush-Presbyterian-St. Lukes Medical Center in Chicago conducted a survey of employees in clerical positions using the admission, discharge, and transfer (ADT) system in the hospital. The admission, discharge, and transfer system linked 13 hospital departments and 40 hospital wards. From a total of 305 employees trained to use the hospital information system, 68 were randomly selected to participate in the study. Surveys were taken 1 month prior to implementation, 6 months after implementation, and again 1 year after implementation. Counte reported that results of the analyses suggested that, over the 1-year period, employee attitudes toward the system became less favorable, although levels of job satisfaction increased. They also found that employees' attitudes toward computers in general were predictive as a measure of adaptation to the computer system [199].

Zoltan-Ford [372] surveyed several professional groups and found that pharmacists had the best attitudes toward and experiences with computers, as also did certified public accountants. Physicians tended to be the most moderate in their opinions – neither overly positive nor overly negative. More than lawyers, physicians believed that computer benefits outweighed costs.

Alexander [1] surveyed 42 clinicians in a psychiatric facility who entered data into a computer-based drug-ordering system that provided guidelines for prescribing and compared them to 31 similar clinicians who were also required to enter their drug orders into the system, but who received no such feedback. Alexander found that in contrast to physicians who did not receive the feedback, those who received it ordered significantly fewer drugs in exception to guidelines. Clinicians in both groups retained their generally favorable attitudes toward the guidelines and drug review. However, clinicians who were not exposed to the guidelines became more negative toward computers, while clinicians who experienced the review system did not. Alexander concluded that tangible feedback was important to maintain clinical support for an electronic medical record.

Bleich [31] and associates at Harvard Medical School's affiliate, Beth Israel Hospital in Boston, reported widespread acceptance by both physicians and staff of their hospital-wide, clinical computing system. They concluded that the key to widespread acceptance and enthusiastic use is an electronic medical record that requires neither user manuals nor training time, and that provides major help to doctors, nurses, and other clinicians in the care of their patients.

Although it was commonly reported that an electronic medical record decreased errors in patient care, Lloyd [216] reported on a study of errors in recording diagnoses by physicians on the discharge of patients from a hospital. An automated patient discharge abstract system, called the Patient Treatment File (PTF), was used by the Veterans Administration (VA). In this study, patient records for calendar 1982 were reviewed for concordance between the abstract produced by the Patient Treatment File and the manual medical record. Physicians were judged responsible for correctly stating summary diagnoses appropriate for: the patient's hospital stay, for specifying the primary diagnosis, and for listing all procedures performed. Medical record personnel were responsible for the complete analysis of each medical record and the accurate selection of codes. Of 1,829 medical records examined, they reported that 82 % were discordant with the Patient Treatment File in at least one field. Of these, 62.1 % were considered to be physicians' errors (missed procedures or diagnoses, inappropriate primary diagnoses, or inactive diagnoses called active); 34.5 % were considered to be medical record personnel's coding errors (incorrect decision about what to code or use of incorrect code); and 3.4 % were data entry errors in dates or in clinical data.

Bailey [13] surveyed 39 items including terminal response time, ease of use, and form of output, and scored each item on a seven step Likert scale from extremely satisfied to extremely dissatisfied. Bailey found that all users (those involved with direct patient care, those who worked in medical records, and those who worked in accounting) were most satisfied with accuracy, ease of use, response time, need for the system, and confidence with the system. Dissatisfaction was expressed with systems integration, timeliness of reports, user training, inability to correct errors, and data security.

Anderson [4] and associates at the Methodist Hospital of Indiana surveyed physicians about their use of electronic medical records. Physicians who joined the medical staff took 5 h of training in use of the electronic medical record in their clinical practice. Physicians with prior education in computing entered and retrieved orders more frequently than did those without such experience, but prior computer education had little effect on rates of retrieval of patient lists and laboratory results. Anderson et al. [5] further found that physicians' perceptions of the potential effects of computer-based systems on medical practice significantly affected the frequency with which they used these systems in practice, and this effect was similar for both attending and resident physicians.

In 1987 a survey of 3,000 health care executives was conducted by Zinn and DiGiulo. The authors categorized benefits of electronic medical records as *quantitative*, with tangible results, measurable in dollars; and as *qualitative*, which, while important, were intangible, and more difficult to measure. Zinn [371] found that responses to the survey indicated that 43 % of the benefits achieved in their institution were quantitative, whereas 57 % were qualitative. Zinn [371] also reported that benefits actually achieved were timely capture of information (84 %), decreased lost charges (81 %), improved access to information (79 %), standardization of procedures (70 %), improved cash flow (69 %), improved staff productivity (63 %), better staff-patient relations (61 %), increased revenue (60 %), reduced length of stay (58 %), improved organizational communications (56 %), reduced labor and material costs (50 %), and improved quality of care (46 %). Some subsystems that were reported as not being implemented at that time because of lack of expected quantitative benefits were bedside computer terminals (75 %), nursing management (38 %), radiology (36 %), laboratory (30 %), order entry (23 %), pharmacy (20 %), comprehensive electronic medical records (19 %), and medical records (10 %). The reasons given for not achieving desired benefits were: lack of system functionality which implied that the system did not do what was wanted (28 %); lack of effective methods to achieve benefits (26 %); lack of administrative commitment (20 %); and institutional unwillingness to change (19 %).

By 1989 significant cost benefits were being realized by a variety of commercially installed electronic patient information systems. As reported by Johnson [188] who cited the resultant savings at: El Camino Hospital to be $2 million per year, Sacred Heart Hospital to be $1,021 million per year, Waukesha to be $3.8 million in 3 years, Medical Center of Central Georgia projected to be $13 million in 7 years, Presbyterian Albuquerque to be $336,000 per year, University of Missouri – pay-back in 2 years, and Ochsner Clinic – pay-back in 2 years. The assessment of an electronic patient information system was found to be difficult and complex due to its many tangible and intangible costs and benefits. From the 1960s to the 1980s, methods evolved from early tabulations of direct costs to later attempts to assess, in addition, intangible benefits. Gradually, through the years, evaluations were increasingly reported as positive; computer systems became more comprehensive, and users became more experienced.

In the early 1980s it was evident that microprocessors would have a major influence on the office practice of medicine. Eden [125] predicted that microcomputers would have a decentralizing effect on medical practice since primary care physicians might be more willing to work in isolated areas if they had computer-based access to consultative and bibliographic services. In 1982 as a follow-up report that had been reviewed by Henley's group in 1974, Kuhn [203] concluded that, in a general assessment of an automated, ambulatory medical record system, flexibility, modularity, programming language, computer and software support, and ease of modification were all important. The analysis of a specific site needed to consider the resources required, installation time and costs, technical support, training of personnel, and costs for startup, transition, and routine operation. Schlager [287] provided comparative costs for an outpatient information system in a two-office, three-physician family practice, with an average workload of 30 patients per-day; and reported that a patient record could be updated and maintained for $1.32 for the computer-based system, compared to $2.56 for similar activities associated with maintaining a manual, paper-based record system.

Gorman [161] described evaluation of electronic health records based on the degree to which the system fulfilled its purposes as specified by the users in their functional requirements. Fernandopulle [133] reported the experience in a not-for-profit health care system in southern New Jersey; and cited as benefits of the new electronic health record to be: the ready access to patients' records; the prescribing of medication refills that required only a fraction of the time previously required; communication with consultants and colleagues made easier; and summaries of patient care compiled more easily. Cited as challenges were periods of slow response time; down-time; unnecessary clinical alerts and warnings; inability to maintain accurate medication lists for patients cared for by multiple physicians; and an increase in time required for physicians to document in comparison with their paper charting. Another issue was difficulty in correcting dysfunctional software.

On evaluating their electronic health records, some physicians reported difficulties in qualifying for the Centers for Medicare and Medicaid Services (CMS) incentive payments because of inability to fulfill mandated requirements for *meaningful use*, particularly the requirement for inter-operability of patient data with other systems. Issues included the lack of standards for the exchange of data between systems sold by different vendors and the absence of universal patient identification numbers. Beyond this, concerns arose about data security and privacy should patients' data to be stored in the "cloud."

Some physicians complained about frequent modifications, additions, or enhancements to their electronic health record system. Physicians also complained that it was difficult to modify an item to satisfy a desired routine; or to modify an automatic alert that was not appropriate for their practice; or to satisfy some meaningful use requirement by the specified date. Also many changes were introduced without adequate training of the users.

The common difficulty in achieving interoperability and data exchange between systems from different vendors was generally attributed to a lack of incentives for vendors to standardize on data transfer between competitive systems. In addition, some vendors had concerns related to maintaining privacy if confidential data were sent elsewhere. Some vendors struggled to maintain compatibility between the many distinct applications and subsystems within their own systems; to maintain an additional compatibility would not be easy or inexpensive, particularly in an economically competitive marketplace [302].

Since many physicians faced difficulties in adopting an electronic health records, the Office of the National Coordinator for Health Information Technology (ONC) funded 60 Health Information Technology Regional Extension Centers (RECs) to assist healthcare practitioners to adopt and meaningfully use their electronic health records [224]. The Rand Corporation prepared a *Guide to Reducing Unintended Consequences of Electronic Records* that described how unintended consequences could occur at any time during and after an electronic health records was implemented, and how that could result from complex interactions between technology and the surrounding work environment. To avoid some adverse unintended consequences, they recommended: (1) actively involving clinicians and staff in the reassessment of the quality of technology solutions; (2) continually monitoring for problems and for errors, and addressing any issues as quickly as possible; (3) reviewing skipped or rejected alerts; (4) requiring departmental review and sign-off on orders created outside the usual parameters; (5) providing an environment that protects staff involved in data entry from undue distractions when using the technology; and (6) monitoring free text entry that could disable the ability to provide decision support [191].

DesRoches [115] and associates in Boston medical centers reviewed data collected by a national survey of electronic health records among acute care hospitals, as to whether their implementation was associated with better performance on standard process-of-care measures, lower mortality and readmission rates, shorter lengths-of-stay, and lower inpatient costs. They found a lack of relationships, and suggested that if electronic health records were to play an important role in promoting effective and efficient care, they needed to be used in a way that would better drive the health care system toward these goals. Romano [281] studied electronic health records employing a clinical decision support system (CDSS), and reported no consistent improvement in the quality of outpatient care. Bitton [30] and associates in Boston medical centers observed that the notion of health information technology (HIT) improving patient care was not new; and that the encouragement of vendors by Federal policy makers in the 2010s to make quality measures more automated in electronic health records was laudable but insufficient, and that physicians and hospitals needed to demand that vendors generate timely, comprehensive data on quality and cost of care for all their patients.

Some health insurers complained that providers' requests for reimbursement of claims when using electronic health records were greater than before, and that the use of electronic health records increased the costs of medical care. Physicians responded that some items needed for proper reimbursement and previously missed, owing to manual coding of handwritten reports, were now more readily identified in computer-based electronic health records.

4.10 Summary and Commentary

Medical databases rapidly grew in size and variety as computer storage became cheaper and database designs became more efficient. Federated databases developed that could store large volumes of aggregated data in multiple partitions, or as functionally oriented databases that were logically interconnected. They were directly accessible to-and-from multiple applications, and allowed many users to simultaneously access and query data [94]. Data warehouses was the term applied to large, extended, central databases that collected and managed data from several different databases; they were capable of servicing the ever-increasing volume of data collected from the ever-changing medical technologies. As data warehouses further enlarged they often developed partitions and data-marts for specialized subsets of data to better serve users with different functional needs [99]. Data warehouses that satisfied the needs of different users to efficiently store and query large collections of data led to the development of online analytical processing (OLAP), and of distributed database systems, distributed database management systems, and of translational data processing between multiple data warehouses.

As computer-based electronic patients' records (EPRs) replaced paper-based charts, the hospital medical records department gave way to a computer center that stored data on magnetic disks. With more powerful computers in the 1990s, physicians began to enter data directly into the patient's electronic health record using the keyboard, mouse, and clinical workstation. Dedicated computers became database servers to store and integrate multiple databases. In the 2000s electronic health records became more common; in the 2010s federal funding produced more widespread diffusion of electronic health records, and advances in informatics resulted in more efficient data management of expanding, multi-media, patient care databases.

References

1. Alexander MJ, Siegel C. Opinions and feelings: the validity of attitudes toward computers. Proc SCAMC. 1984; 540–2.
2. Anderson J, Jay S. The diffusion of computer applications in medicine: network locations and innovation adoption. Proc SCAMC 1984; 549–52.
3. Anderson J. Personal communications to M. Collen. 1986.
4. Anderson JG, Jay SJ, Schweer HM, Anderson MM. Teaching physicians to use a computer-based information system. Proc AAMSI. 1987a; 207–12.
5. Anderson JG, Jay SJ, Anderson MM, Schweer HM. What do physicians think about computers? Proc AAMSI. 1987b; 213–7.
6. Anderson JG, Jay SJ, Anderson M, Hunt TJ. Evaluating the potential effectiveness of using computerized information systems to prevent adverse drug events. Proc AMIA. 1997;9:228–32.
7. Anderson RJ, Young WW. Microcomputers as a management tool for hospital pharmacy directors. Proc SCAMC. 1984; 231–3.
8. Anderson JG, Jay SJ, Perry J, Anderson MM. Diffusion of computer applications among physicians. In: Salamon R, Protti D, Moehr J, editors. Proceedings international symposium on medical informatics and education. Victoria: University of Victoria; 1989. p. 339–42.
9. AP (Associated Press). Felony indictment in computer virus case. San Francisco Chronicle July 17, 1989; A4(col 1).

10. Ash SR, Mertz SL, Ulrich DK. The computerized notation system: a portable, self-contained system for entry of physicians' and nurses' notes. J Clin Eng. 1983;8:147–56.
11. Ash SR, Ulrich DK, Laxton DE. The total recall program: a relational office database interfacable with briefcase computers. Proc SCAMC. 1984; 429–32.
12. Ausman RK. Automated storage and retrieval of patient data. Am J Surg. 1967;114:159–66.
13. Bailey JE. A tested model for measuring and analyzing hospital computer users' attitudes. Proc AAMSI. 1987; 202–6.
14. Baird HW, Garfunkel JM. Electronic data processing of medical records. N Engl J Med. 1965;272:1211–5.
15. Ball MJ, Jacobs SE. Hospital information systems as we enter the decade of the 80's. Proc SCAMC. 1980;1:646–50.
16. Ball M, Magnier EA, Raney WO. Thinking of automating your business system? Hosp Financ Manage. 1970;24:12–5.
17. Ball MJ, Collen MF. Aspects of the computer-based patient record. New York: Springer; 1992.
18. Ball MJ. Computers: prescription for hospital ills. Datamation. 1975;21:50–1.
19. Ball MJ, Jacobs SE. Information systems: the status of level 1. Hospitals. 1980a;54:179–86.
20. Ball MJ, Jacobs SE. Hospital information systems as we enter the decade of the 80s. Proc SCAMC. 1980b:646–50.
21. Barnett G. Medical information systems at the Massachusetts General Hospital. Proc International Conference in Health Technology Systems. ORSA Health Applications Section. 1974a; 286–95.
22. Barnett GO. Massachusetts General Hospital computer system. In: Collen MF, editor. Hospital computer systems. New York: Wiley; 1974.
23. Barnett GO, Greenes RA. High level programming languages. Comput Biomed Res. 1970;3:488–94.
24. Barnett GO, Greenes RA, Grossman JH. Computer processing of medical text information. Methods Inf Med. 1969;8:177–82.
25. Barret JP, Hersch PL, Cashwell RJ. Evaluation of the impact of the Technicon medical information system at El Camino Hospital. Part II. Columbus: Battelle Columbus Labs; 1979.
26. Barrett JP, Hersch PL, Caswell RJ. Evaluation of the impact of the implementation of the Technicon Medical Information System at El Camino Hospital. Part II: economic trend analysis. Final report 1972; 27.
27. Barsalou T, Wiederhold G. A cooperative hypertext interface to relational databases. Proc SCAMC. 1989; 383–7.
28. Bean LL, May DL, Skolnick M. The Mormon historical demography project. Hist Methods: J. 1978;11:45–53.
29. Beaty TH, Khoury MJ. Interface of genetics and epidemiology. Epidemiol Rev. 2000;22:120–5.
30. Bitton A, Flier LA, Jha AK. Health information technology in the era of care delivery reform: to what end? JAMA. 2012;307:2593–4.
31. Bleich HL, Beckley RF, Horowitz GL, Jackson JD, Moody ES, Franklin C, et al. Clinical computing in a teaching hospital. N Engl J Med. 1985;312:756–64.
32. Blois MS, Henley RR. Strategies in the planning of hospital information systems. Tech Report #1. San Francisco: Office of Med Inform Systems, University of California.
33. Blois MS, Tuttle MS, Sherertz DD. RECONSIDER: a program for generating differential diagnoses. Proc SCAMC. 1981; 263–8.
34. Blois MS. Information and medicine: the nature of medical descriptions. Berkeley: University of California Press; 1984.
35. Blois MS, Wasserman AI. The integration of hospital information subsystems. San Francisco: Office of Medical Information Systems, University of California, San Francisco Medical Center. 1974.
36. Blum BI, Duncan K. A history of medical informatics. New York: Addison Wesley; 1990.
37. Blum BI. Information systems at the Johns Hopkins Hospital. Johns Hopkins APL Tech Rev Dig. 1983;4:104–7.
38. Blum B. Design methodology. Proc SCAMC. 1989; 277–95.

39. Blum BI. A history of computers. In: Blum B, editor. Clinical information systems. New York: Springer; 1986. p. 1–32.
40. Blum BI. Design methods for clinical systems. Proc SCAMC. 1986b; 309–15.
41. Blum BI, Tolchin SG. The impact of technology on hospital information systems. Hawaii Int Conf Syst Sci. 1981; Jan 9, 1989; 14.
42. Blum BI. TEDIUM and the software process. Cambridge, MA: MIT Press; 1990.
43. Blum BI, Johns CJ, McColligan EE, Steinwachs DM. Low cost ambulatory medical information system. J Clin Eng. 1979;4:372–7.
44. Blum BI. Clinical information systems. New York: Springer; 1986.
45. Blum BI, Lenhard RE. Privacy and security in an oncology information system. Proc SCAMC 1978; 500–8.
46. Blum RL. Displaying clinical data from a time-oriented database. Comput Biol Med. 1981;11:197–210.
47. Blum RL, Wiederhold G. Inferring knowledge from clinical data banks: utilizing techniques from artificial intelligence. Proc SCAMC. 1978; 303–7.
48. Blumenthal D. Advancing health information exchange: a message from the Office of the National Coordinator (ONC), Health and Human Services (HHS). 2010.
49. Blumenthal D. Meaningful progress toward electronic health information exchange. A message from ONC, HHS. 2009.
50. Blumenthal D, Tavenner M. The meaningful use of a regulation for electronic health records. N Engl J Med. 2010;363:501–4.
51. Bokuski M. Correlating gene linkage maps with physical maps of chromosomes. Natl Libr Med News. 1989; 6.
52. Bond EJ. Hospital information system effectiveness. In: Bekey GA, Schwartz MD, editors. Hospital information systems. New York: Marcel Dekker; 1972. p. 131–48.
53. Borowitz SM, Wyatt JC. The origin, content, and workload of e-mail consultations. JAMA. 1998;280:1321–4.
54. Botstein D, White RL, Skolnick M, Davis RW. Construction of a genetic linkage map in man using restriction fragment length polymorphisms. Am J Hum Genet. 1980;32:314.
55. Bradley F, Vermillion CO, Anderson W. Medical records on punch cards. II. Mod Hosp. 1954;82:83–4. passim.
56. Brailer DJ, Blumenthal D. Guiding the health information technology agenda. Health Aff. 2010;29:586–95.
57. Brandt CA, Morse R, Matthews K, Sun K, Deshpande AM, Gadagkar R, et al. Metadata-driven creation of data marts from an EAV-modeled clinical research database. Int J Med Inform. 2002;65:225–41.
58. Brannigan VM. Remote telephone access: the critical issue in patient privacy. Proc SCAMC. 1984; 575–8.
59. Brook RH, Harris TR, Lewis CE. Sizing up primary care needs. Patient Care. 1977 (July 15); 70–111.
60. Bryan M. The year of the data base. Personal Comput. 1988; Jan; 100–9.
61. Buhle Jr E, Goldwein JW, Benjamin I. OncoLink: a multimedia oncology information resource on the Internet. Proc AMIA. 1994; 103–7.
62. Burnett KK, Battle H, Cant GD. Uniform Health-Care Information Act. Chicago: National Conference of Commissioners on Uniform State Laws; 1985.
63. Buyse ML. Computer-based information retrieval and decision support for birth defects and genetic disorders. Pediatrics. 1984;74:557–8.
64. Camp HN, Ridley ML, Walker HK. THERESA: a computerized medical consultant based on the patient record. Proc MEDINFO. 1983; 612–4.
65. Campbell KE, Cohn SP, Chute CG, Shortliffe EH, Rennels G. Scalable methodologies for distributed development of logic-based convergent medical terminology. Methods Inf Med. 1998;37:426–39.
66. Campbell-Kelly M, Aspray W, Ensmenger N, Yost JR. Computer: a history of the information machine. Boulder: Westview Press; 2009.
67. Campbell-Kelly M. Origin of computing. Sci Am. 2009;301:62–9.

68. Carlisle RG. A concept and methodology for evaluating automated information systems for multi-facility health care systems. Proc SCAMC. 1979; 334–8.
69. Carlisle RG. Measures and indicators of health care system effectiveness and economy. In: Emlet H, editor. Challenges and prospects for advanced medical systems. Miami: Symposia Specialists, Inc; 1978. p. 191–7.
70. Carson JL, Ray WA, Strom BL. Medical databases. In: Strom BL, editor. Pharmacoepidemiology. New York: Wiley; 2000. p. 307–24.
71. Chaney RJ, Shipman FM, Gorry GA. Using hypertext to facilitate information sharing in biomedical research groups. Proc SCAMC. 1989; 350–4.
72. Chen RS, Nadkarni P, Marenco L, Levin F, Erdos J, Miller PL. Exploring performance issues for a clinical database organized using an entity-attribute-value representation. JAMIA. 2000;7:475–87.
73. CHPL. Certified Health IT Product list. 2015. Office of the National Coordinator: healthit.gov.
74. Chung CS. Genetic analysis of human family and population data with use of digital computers. Proc of 3rd IBM Medical Symposium Endicott: International Business Machines. 1961; 53–69
75. Cimino JJ, Socratous SA, Grewal R. The informatics superhighway: prototyping on the World Wide Web. Proc SCAMC. 1995; 111–5
76. Clayton PD, Urie PM, Marshall HW, Warner HR. A computerized system for the cardiovascular laboratory. IEEE Proceedings of Conference on Computers in Cardiology, Bethesda, Maryland 1974; 97.
77. Codd EF. Further normalizations of the data base relational model. In: Rustin R, editor. Data base systems. Englewood Cliffs: Prentice-Hall; 1972. p. 33–64.
78. Codd EF. A relational model of data for large shared data banks. Commun ACM. 1970;13:377–87.
79. Codd EF, Codd SB, Salley CT. Providing OLAP (on-line analytical processing) to user-analysts: an IT mandate. San Jose, CA: Codd and Associates. 1993; 32.
80. Coffey RM. How a medical information system affects hospital costs: the El Camino hospital experience. NCHS&R, DHEW Pub No. (PHS) 80–3265; 1980.
81. Collen M. A guide matrix for technological system evaluation. J Med Syst. 1978;2:249–54.
82. Collen M. Problems with presentation of computer data. In: Anderson J, editor. Information processing of medical records. Amsterdam: North-Holland; 1970. p. 407–11.
83. Collen MF. A history of medical informatics in the United States, 1950 to 1990. Indianapolis: American Medical Informatics Association; 1995.
84. Collen MF. The origins of informatics. JAMIA. 1994;1:91–107.
85. Collen MF. Clinical research databases – a historical review. J Med Syst. 1990;14:323–44.
86. Collen MF. Origins of medical informatics. West J Med. 1986;145:778–85.
87. Collen MF. The cost-effectiveness of health checkups – an illustrative study. West J Med. 1984;141:786–92.
88. Collen MF. Foreword. Proc AMIA. 1982.
89. Collen MF. General requirements of a medical information (MIS). Comput Biomed Res. 1970;3:393–406.
90. Collen MF. Medical bibliographic databases. In: Collen MF, editor. Computer medical databases. London: Springer; 2012.
91. Collen MF. Automated multiphasic health testing. In: Collen MF, editor. Multiphasic health testing services. New York: Wiley; 1974. p. 274–94.
92. Collen MF, Van Brunt EE, Davis LS. Problems of computerization of large computer medical record systems. Inform Health Soc Care. 1976;1:47–53.
93. Collins FS. Identification of disease genes: recent successes. Hosp Pract (Off Ed). 1991;26:93–8.
94. Coltri A. Databases in health care. In: Lehmann HP, editor. Aspects of electronic health record systems. New York: Springer; 2006. p. 225–51.
95. Commission for Privacy Protection. Personal privacy in an information society: the report of the Privacy Protection Study Commission. Washington, DC: The Commission; 1977.

96. Conn J. Commonwealth Fund names Dr. David Blumenthal as next president. Modern Healthcare.com. 2012a.

97. Conn J. No single winner in doc's EHR rankings. Modern Healthcare.com. 2012b.

98. Connelly D. The deployment of a World Wide Web (W3) based medical information system. Proc AMIA. 1995; 771–7.

99. Connolly TM, Begg CE. Database management systems: a practical approach to design. New York: Addison-Wesley; 1999.

100. Cook M. Introduction of a user-oriented THIS into a community hospital setting-nursing. Proc MEDINFO. 1974; 303–4.

101. Cooper GF, Hennings-Yeomans P, Visweswaran S, Barmada M. An efficient Bayesian method for predicting clinical outcomes from genome-wide data. Proc AMIA Annu Symp. 2010; 127–31.

102. Corvin A, Craddock N, Sullivan PF. Genome-wide association studies: a primer. Psychol Med. 2010;40:1063–77.

103. Countie MA, Kjerulff KH, Salloway JC, Campbell BC. Implementing computerization in hospitals: a case study of the behavioral and attitudinal impacts of a medical information system. In: Anderson J, Jay SJ, editors. Use and impacts of computers in clinical medicine. New York: Springer; 1987. p. 224–37.

104. Curran WJ, Stearns B, Kaplan H. Privacy, confidentiality and other legal considerations in the establishment of a centralized health-data system. N Engl J Med. 1969;281:241.

105. Curran WJ, Kaplan H, Laska EM, Bank R. Protection of privacy and confidentiality: unique law protects patient records in a multistate psychiatric information system. Science. 1973;182:797–802.

106. Cutts JW, Mitchell JA. Microcomputer-based genetics offer database system. Proc AAMSI. 1985; 487–91.

107. Davis LS. Data processing facilities. In: Collen M, editor. Hospital computer systems. New York: Wiley; 1974. p. 32–51.

108. Davis LS. Prototype for future computer medical records. Comput Biomed Res. 1970;3:539–54.

109. Davis LS, Terdiman J. The medical data base. In: Collen MF, editor. Hospital computer systems. New York: Wiley; 1974. p. 52–79.

110. Davis LS. A system approach to medical information. Methods Inf Med. 1973;12:1–6.

111. Davis LS, Collen MF, Rubin L, Van Brunt EE. Computer-stored medical record. Comput Biomed Res. 1968;1:452–69.

112. Dawson J. A family of models. Byte. 1989;14:277–86.

113. DeBrota D. Man/microcomputer telephone communication. MD Comput. 1986;3:24.

114. Denny JC, Ritchie MD, Basford MA, Pulley JM, Bastarache L, Brown-Gentry K, et al. PheWAS: demonstrating the feasibility of a phenome-wide scan to discover gene-disease associations. Bioinformatics. 2010;26:1205–10.

115. DesRoches CM, Campbell EG, Vogeli C, Zheng J, Rao SR, Shields AE, et al. Electronic health records†™ limited successes suggest more targeted uses. Health Aff. 2010;29:639–46.

116. Dick RS, Steen EB, Detmer DE. The computer-based patient record: an essential technology for health care. Washington, DC: National Academy Press; 1991.

117. DiGiulio LW, Zinn TK. Actualizing system benefits – part V. Comput Healthc. 1988;9:30–2.

118. Dintleman SM, Maness AT, Skolnick M, Bean LL. In: Dyke B, Morrill WT, editors. GENISYS: a genealogical information system. New York: Academic; 1980. p. 94–114.

119. Dinu V, Nadkarni P. Guidelines for the effective use of entity-attribute-value modeling for biomedical databases. Int J Med Inform. 2007;76:769–79.

120. Doherty RB. The certitudes and uncertainties of health care reform. Ann Intern Med. 2010;152:679–82.

121. Drazen EL, Seidel FJ. Implementation monitoring: a critical step towards realizing benefits from hospital information systems. Proc SCAMC. 1984; 148–51.

122. Drazen EL, Metzger J. Methods for evaluating automated hospital information systems. Proc SCAMC. 1980;1:673–8.

123. Drazen EL, Metzger J. Methods for evaluating costs of automated hospital information systems. NCHRS research summary series. DHHS Pub No. (PHS) 81–3283.
124. Duke JR, Bowers GH. Scope and sites of electronic health records systems. In: Lehmann HP, Roderer N, Abbott P, editors. Aspects of electronic health record systems. New York: Springer; 2006. p. 89–114.
125. Eden HS, Eden M. Changes: the technology's effect on the health care system. In: Eden HS, Eden M, editors. Microcomputers in patient care. Park Ridge: Noyes Medical Publications; 1981. p. 47.
126. Emlet HE. Methodology for evaluation of medical information systems. In: Emlet H, editor. Challenges and prospects for advanced medical systems. Miami: Symposia Specialists; 1978. p. 183–90.
127. Emlet HE, Carlisle RG. Measures and indicators for evaluation of innovations to the health care system. Falls Church: Analytic Services; 1977.
128. Epstein MH, Epstein LH, Emerson RG. A low cost micro-computer based local area network for medical office and medical center automation. Proc SCAMC. 1984; 793–5.
129. Evans S, Lemon SJ, Deters CA, Fusaro RM, Lynch HT. Automated detection of hereditary syndromes using data mining. Comput Biomed Res. 1997;30:337–48.
130. Evans S, Lemon SJ, Deters C, Fusaro RM, Durham C, Snyder C, et al. Using data mining to characterize DNA mutations by patient clinical features. Proc AMIA. 1997b; 253–7.
131. Feinstein AR. The problem with the "problem-oriented medical record". Ann Intern Med. 1973;78:752–62.
132. Feistel H. Cryptography and computer privacy. Sci Am. 1973;228:15–23.
133. Fernandopulle R, Patel N. How the electronic health record did not measure up to the demands of our medical home practice. Health Aff. 2010;29:622–8.
134. Flagle CD. Methodological problems in technology assessment of medical informatics. Proc AAMSI. 1985; 414–8.
135. Flagle CD. Evaluation of healthcare. Proc MEDINFO. 1983; 46–9.
136. Flagle CD. Information requirements for evaluation and planning of innovative health services. Proc MEDINFO. 1980; 615–9.
137. Flagle CD. An overview of evaluation methods. In: Goldman J, editor. Health care technology evaluation. Lecture notes in medical informatics. New York: Springer; 1979. p. 33–42.
138. Flagle CD. Evaluation and control of technology in health services. Conference on Technology and Health Care Systems in the 1980's. DHEW Pub (HSM) 73-3016. 1972; 213–24.
139. Flagle CD. Evaluation techniques for medical information systems. Comput Biomed Res. 1970;3:407–14.
140. Frawley WJ, Piatetsky-Shapiro G, Matheus CJ. Knowledge discovery in databases: an overview. AI Mag. 1992;13:57.
141. Freed RN. Legal aspects of computer use in medicine. In: Medical progress and the law. Durham: Duke University School of Law. 1967; 674–706.
142. Frieden J. Obama signs Healthcare Reconciliation Bill. MePage Today, March 30, 2010.
143. Friedman C, Hripcsak G, Johnson SB, Cimino JJ, Clayton PD. A generalized relational schema for an integrated clinical patient database. Proc SCAMC. 1990; 335–9.
144. Fries JF. The chronic disease data bank: first principles to future directions. J Med Philos. 1984;9:161–80.
145. Fries JF. Alternatives in medical record formats. Med Care. 1974;12:871–81.
146. Gabrieli ER. Interface problems between medicine and computers. Proc SCAMC. 1984; 93–5
147. Gall J. Computerized hospital information system cost-effectiveness: a case study. In: van Egmond J, de Vries Robbe PF, Levy AH, eds. Amsterdam: North Holland. 1976; 281–93
148. Gall J. Cost-benefit analysis: total hospital informatics. In: Koza RC, editor. Health information systems evaluation. Boulder: Colorado Associated University Press; 1974. p. 299–327.
149. Galland J, Skolnick MH. A gene mapping expert system. Comput Biomed Res. 1990;23:297–309.
150. Garfolo B, Keltner L. A computerized disease register. Proc MEDINFO. 1983; 909–12.

151. Garrett L, Stead WW, Hammond WE. Conversion of manual to total computerized medical records. J Med Syst. 1983;7:301–5.
152. Garrett P, Seidman J. EMR vs EHR – what is the difference? HealthITBuzz, January 2011.
153. Gersting J, Conneally P, Beidelman K. Huntington's disease research Roster support with a microcomputer database management system. Proc SCAMC. 1983; 746–9.
154. Gersting JM. Rapid prototyping of database systems in human genetics data collection. J Med Syst. 1987;11:177–89.
155. Giannakopoulos S, Hammer J. Requirements for the small office practice. Proc SCAMC. 1980; 1778–81.
156. Glichlich RE, Dreyer NA. Registries for evaluating patient outcomes: a user's guide AHRQ Pub. # 7-EHC001-1. Rockville: Agency for Healthcare Research and Quality; 2007. p. 1–233.
157. Glowniak JV. Medical resources on the Internet. Ann Intern Med. 1995;123:123–31.
158. Goldman J. Evaluation of technological innovations in health. In: Koza RC, editor. Health information system evaluation. Boulder: Colorado Associated University Press; 1974. p. 45–61.
159. Gordon BL. Terminology and content of the medical record. Comput Biomed Res. 1970;3:436–44.
160. Gordon BL. Regularization and stylization of medical records. JAMA. 1970;212:1502–7.
161. Gorman PN. Evaluation of electronic health record systems. In: Lehmann HP, Abbott P, Roderer N, editors. Aspects of electronic health record systems. New York: Springer; 2006. p. 401–15.
162. Grann RP. Attitudes and effective use of computers among hospital personnel. Proc SCAMC. 1984; 543–7.
163. Graves J. Design of a database to support intervention modeling in nursing. Proc MEDINFO. 1986;240:242.
164. Graves M, Bergeman ER, Lawrence CB. A graph conceptual model for developing human genome center databases. Comput Biol Med. 1996;26:183–97.
165. Grossman JH, Barnett GO, Koepsell TD, Nesson HR, Dorsey JL, Phillips RR. An automated medical record system. JAMA. 1973;224:1616–21.
166. Hafner K, Lyon M. Where wizards stay up late: the origins of the Internet. New York: Simon & Schuster; 1996.
167. Halamka JD. Making the most of federal health information technology regulations. Health Aff. 2010;29:596–600.
168. Hammon GL, Drake MV. Hospital data processing presents unique security needs. Hospitals. 1976;50:103–5.
169. Hammond W, Stead W, Straube M, Kelly M, Winfree R. An interface between a hospital information system and a computerized medical record. Proc SCAMC. 1980;3:1537–40.
170. Hammond WE, Straube MJ, Blunden PB, Stead WW. Query: the language of databases. Proc SCAMC. 1989;13:419–23.
171. Hammond WE, Stead WW, Straube MJ. Planned networking for medical information systems. Proc SCAMC. 1985; 727–31.
172. Hammond WE, Stead WW, Feagin SJ, Brantley BA, Straube MJ. Data base management system for ambulatory care. Proc SCAMC. 1977; 173–87.
173. Harris DK, Polli GJ. Confidentiality of computerized patient information. Am Med Assoc (Resolution 38, A-77). Comput Med (Special report). 1977;1–6.
174. Health Information Technology for Economic and Clinical Health (HITECH) Act. American Recovery and Reinvestment Act of 2009 (ARRA) Pub. L. No. 111-5. 2009.
175. Helvey W, Brdlik M, Peterkin K. Online medical databases – 1985: status and prognosis. Healthc Comput Commun. 1985;2:28.
176. Henley RR, Wiederhold G. An analysis of automated ambulatory medical record systems. San Francisco: Office of Medical Information Systems, University of California, San Francisco Medical Center; 1975.
177. Herger W. New law can fight computer viruses. USA Today. 1988.
178. Hersh WR, Brown KE, Donohoe LC, Campbell EM, Horacek AE. Clini web: managing clinical information on the World Wide Web. JAMIA. 1996;3:273–80.

179. HIMSS Analytics. Essentials of the U.S Hospital IT Market. Chicago: Health Information Management and Systems Society; 2011.
180. Hinman EJ. The patient-carried personal health record. In: Hinman EJ, editor. Advanced medical systems: the 3rd century. Miami: Symposia Specialists; 1977. p. 55–62.
181. Hodge MH. Medical information systems: a resource for hospitals. Germantown: Aspen Publishers, Inc; 1977.
182. Hoffman LJ. Computers and privacy: a survey. ACM Comput Surv (CSUR). 1969;1:85–103.
183. Hripcsak G, Allen B, Cimino JJ, Lee R. Access to data: comparing AccessMed with query by review. JAMIA. 1996;3:288–99.
184. Jacobs P. Training for an MIS implementation: what does it really cost? Proc SCAMC. 1984; 156–9.
185. Jelovsek F, Smith R, Blackmon L, Hammond W. Computerized nursery discharge summary. Methods Inf Med. 1977;16:199–204.
186. Jelovsek FR. Doctor's office computer prep kit. New York: Springer; 1985.
187. Jelovsek FR. The medical record: session overview. Proc SCAMC. 1983; 99–100.
188. Johnson RL. Economic benefits of hospital system automation. US Healthc. 1989;6:38–40. concl.
189. Johnson SB. Generic data modeling for clinical repositories. JAMIA. 1996;3:328–39.
190. Johnson SB, Chatziantoniou D. Extended SQL for manipulating clinical warehouse data. Proc AMIA. 1999; 819–23.
191. Jones SS, Koppel R, Ridgely MS, Palen TE, Wu S, Harrison MI. Guide to reducing unintended consequences of electronic health records. Rockville: Agency for Healthcare Research and Quality; 2011.
192. Juni JE, Ponto R. Computer-virus infection of a medical diagnosis computer. N Engl J Med. 1989;320:811–2.
193. Jydstrup RA, Gross MJ. Cost of information handling in hospitals. Health Serv Res. 1966;1:235.
194. Kang K, Merritt A, Conneally P, Gersting J, Rigo T. A medical genetics data base management system. Proc SCAMC. 1978; 524–9.
195. Karpinski RH, Bleich HL. MISAR: a miniature information storage and retrieval system. Comput Biomed Res. 1971;4:655–60.
196. Kennedy OG, Colligon SJ, Protte DJ. Impact of medical information systems on health care in the U.S.A. Proc MEDINFO. 1980; 1058–62.
197. Khosrowpour M. Managing computer fraud/crime in healthcare organizations. Healthc Comput Commun. 1987;4:59–62. 64.
198. King JL, Schrems EL. Cost-benefit analysis in information systems development and operation. ACM ACM Comput Surv(CSUR). 1978;10:19–34.
199. Kjerulff KH, Counte MA. Measuring attitudes toward computers: two approaches. Proc SCAMC. 1984; 529–35.
200. Klarman HE. Application of cost-benefit analysis to health systems technology. In: Collen M, ed. Technology and health care systems in the 1980s. DHEW Pub (HSM) 73-3016. 1973; 225–50.
201. Kolodner RM, Cohn SP, Friedman CP. Health information technology: strategic initiatives, real progress. Health Aff. 2008;27:w391–5.
202. Kuhn IM, Wiederhold G, Rodnick JE. Automated medical record systems in the U.S. In: Blum BI, editor. Information systems for patient care. New York: Springer; 1984. p. 199–271.
203. Kuhn IM, Wiederhold G, Rodnick JE, Ransey-Klee D, Benett S, Beck DD. Automated ambulatory record systems in the US. NTIS Publication (1982, August). 1982; 178–89.
204. Kuhn IM, Wiederhold G. The evolution of ambulatory medical record systems in the US. Proc SCAMC. 1981; 80–5.
205. Kuzmak PM, Arseniev M, Tolchin SG, Bergan E. Proposal for interfacing MUMPS to an open systems interconnection network architecture. Proc MEDINFO. 1986; 853–7.

206. Lamson BG. A panel session. Computers in medicine: problems and perspectives. Proc AFIPS Conf. 1971; 195.
207. Levinson D. Information, computers, and clinical practice. JAMA. 1983;249:607–9.
208. Levy RP, Cammarn MR, Smith MJ. Computer handling of ambulatory clinic records. JAMA. 1964;190:1033–7.
209. Liggett B. Why computerized medical records systems are not widely used. Comput Med Record News. 1968;1:1–7.
210. Lindberg D. The impact of automated information systems applied to health problems. In: Holland WW, editor. Oxford Oxfordshire: Oxford University Press. 1985; 55–76.
211. Lindberg D. The growth of medical information systems in the United States. Lexington: Lexington Books; 1979.
212. Lindberg D. Special aspects of medical computer records with respect to data privacy. In: Williams B, ed. Proc 2nd Illinois Conf Med Inform Syst. 1975; 35–8.
213. Lindberg D. The computer and medical care. Springfield: CC Thomas; 1968.
214. Lindberg DAB. The development and diffusion of a medical technology: medical information systems. In: Sanders CA et al., editors. Medical technology and the health care system: a study of the diffusion of equipment-embodied technology. Washington, DC: National Academy of Sciences;1979;201–39.
215. Linowes DF. Personal privacy in an information society: the report of the Privacy Protection Study Commission. Washington, DC: US Govt Print Office; 1977. 052-003-00395-3.
216. Lloyd SS, Rissing JP. Physician and coding errors in patient records. JAMA. 1985;254:1330–6.
217. London JW. A computer solution to clinical and research computing needs. Proc SCAMC. 1985; 722–6.
218. Long JM. On providing an automated health record for individuals. Proc MEDINFO. 1986; 805–9.
219. Lowe HJ, Lomax EC, Polonkey SE. The World Wide Web: a review of an emerging internet-based technology for the distribution of biomedical information. JAMIA. 1996;3:1–14.
220. Lowe HJ, Antipov I, Walker WK, Polonkey SE, Naus GJ. WebReport: a World Wide Web based clinical multimedia reporting system. Proc AMIA. 1996b; 314.
221. Manos D. CMS pays out more than $5B in incentives. HealthcareIT News. 2012.
222. Marrs KA, Kahn MG. Extending a clinical repository to include multiple sites. Proc AMIA. 1995; 387–91.
223. Mathur S, Dinakarpandian D. Automated ontological gene annotation for computing disease similarity. Proc AMIA TBI. 2010; 12.
224. Maxson E, Jain S, Kendall M, Mostashari F, Blumenthal D. The regional extension center program: helping physicians meaningfully use health information technology. Ann Intern Med. 2010;153:666–70.
225. McCray AT. The nature of lexical knowledge. Methods Inf Med. 1998;37:353–60.
226. McDonald CJ, Overhage JM, Dexter PR, Blevins L, Meeks-Johnson J, Suico JG, et al. Canopy computing: using the Web in clinical practice. JAMA. 1998;280:1325–9.
227. McDonald C, Blevins L, Glazener T, Haas J, Lemmon L, Meeks-Johnson J. Data base management, feedback control, and the Regenstrief medical record. J Med Syst. 1983;7:111–25.
228. McDonald CJ, Hammond WE. Standard formats for electronic transfer of clinical data. Ann Intern Med. 1989;110:333–5.
229. McDonald CJ, Tierney WM. Computer-stored medical records: their future role in medical practice. JAMA. 1988;259:3433–40.
230. McDonald CJ, Tierney WM. The Medical Gopher: a microcomputer system to help find, organize and decide about patient data. West J Med. 1986;145:823.
231. McDonald CJ, Blevins L, Glazener TT, Lemmon L, Martin D, Valenza M. CARE: a real world medical knowledge base. COMPCON. 1984; 187–91.
232. McDonald CJ, Murray R, Jeris D, Bhargava B, Seeger J, Blevins L. A computer-based record and clinical monitoring system for ambulatory care. Am J Public Health. 1977;67:240–5.

233. McDonald CJ, Wilson G, Blevins L, Seeger J, Chamness D, Smith D, et al. The Regenstrief medical record system. Proceedings of the Annual Symposium on Computer Application in Medical Care 1977b; 168.

234. McKinney WP, Wagner JM, Bunton G, Kirk LM. A guide to Mosaic and the World Wide Web for physicians. MD Comput: Comput Med Pract. 1994;12:109–14. 141.

235. McKusick VA. Some computer applications to problems in human genetics. Methods Inf Med. 1964;4:183–9.

236. McKusick VA, Talbot SA. Analysis of genetic linkage in man with assistance of digital computer. Proc 1st IBM Medical Symp. Poughkeepsie, NY: IBM. 1959; 217–27.

237. McKusick VA. Forty years of medical genetics. JAMA. 1989;261:3155–8.

238. McKusick VA. Mendelian inheritance in man: catalogs of autosomal dominant, autosomal recessive, and X-linked phenotypes. Baltimore: Johns Hopkins University Press; 1988.

239. McKusick VA. Computers in research in human genetics. J Chronic Dis. 1966;19:427–41.

240. McNamara JJ. Legal aspects of computerized medical records. JAMA. 1968;205:153–4.

241. Meaney FJ. Databases for genetic services. J Med Syst. 1987;11:227–32.

242. Merz B. 700 genes mapped at world workshop. JAMA. 1989;262:175.

243. Michalski RS, Baskin AB, Spackman KA. A logic-based approach to conceptual data base analysis. Inform Health Soc Care. 1983;8:187–95.

244. Miller MC, Levkoff AH, Wong YM, Michel Y. Normal newborn nursery information system. Proc AAMSI. 1983; 154–62.

245. Miller PL, Nadkarni PM, Kidd KK, Cheung K, Ward DC, Banks A, et al. Internet-based support for bioscience research: a collaborative genome center for human chromosome 12. JAMIA. 1995;2:351–64.

246. Miller RA, Schaffner KF, Meisel A. Ethical and legal issues related to the use of computer programs in clinical medicine. Ann Intern Med. 1985;102:529–36.

247. Miller RF. Computers and privacy: what price analytic power? Proc ACM. 1971; 706–16.

248. Mishelevich DJ, Gipe WG, Roberts JR, et al. Cost-benefit analysis in a computer-based hospital information system. Proc SCAMC. 1979:339–49.

249. Mishelevich DJ, MacGregor WD, Gipe WG, Granfill LD. Distribution of data processing costs for a hospital information system on a cost-per-incident-of-service basis. Proc SCAMC. 1980:658–64.

250. Mishelevich DJ, Kesinger G, Jasper M, Inga P, Robinson AL, Gaige W, et al. Medical record control and the computer. Top Health Rec Manage. 1981;2:47–55.

251. Mitchell JA, Loughman WD, Epstein CJ. GENFILES: a computerized medical genetics information network. II. MEDGEN: the clinical genetics system. Am J Med Genet. 1980;7:251–66.

252. Moorman P, Schuemie M, van der Lei J. An inventory of publications on electronic medical records revisited. Methods Inf Med. 2009;48:454–8.

253. Mosquera M. $400 M in EHR incentives delivered. Government Heathcareitnews. 2011.

254. Mount SA. Annual administrative reviews: medical records. Hospitals. 1965;39:125.

255. Murphy EA, Sherwin RW. Estimation of genetic linkage: an outline. Methods Inf Med. 1966;5:45–54.

256. Murphy EA, Schulze J. A program for estimation of genetic linkage in man. Proceedings of 3rd IBM Medical Symposium." International Business Machines, New York. 1961.

257. Nadkarni PM, Cheung K. SQLGEN: a framework for rapid client-server database application development. Comput Biomed Res. 1995;28:479–99.

258. Nadkarni PM, Marenco L. Easing the transition between attribute-value databases and conventional databases for scientific data. Proc AMIA. 2001; 483–7.

259. Nadkarni PM, Brandt CM, Marenco L. WebEAV: automatic metadata-driven generation of web interfaces to entity-attribute-value databases. JAMIA. 2000;7:343–56.

260. Nadkarni PM, Marenco L, Chen R, Skoufos E, Shepherd G, Miller P. Organization of heterogeneous scientific data using the EAV/CR representation. JAMIA. 1999;6:478–93.

261. Nadkarni PM, Brandt C, Frawley S, Sayward FG, Einbinder R, Zelterman D, et al. Managing attribute – value clinical trials data using the ACT/DB client-server database system. JAMIA. 1998;5:139–51.

262. NCHSR&D. Summary report on hospital information systems. Springfield: National Center for Health Services and Health Care Technology Programs; 1969.

263. Norwood D. Introduction of user-oriented THIS into a community hospital setting: introduction and system description. Proc MEDINFO. 1974; 295–8.

264. ONC. The Office of the National Coordinator for Health Information Technology. HealthIT. hhs.gov.ONC 2012.

265. Ostrowski M, Bernes MR. The TMR data dictionary: a management tool for data base design. Proc SCAMC. 1984; 829–32.

266. OTA. Policy implications of medical information systems. Washington, DC: Office of Technology Assessment; 1977. p. 58–63.

267. OTA. The implications of cost-effectiveness analysis of medical technology. Washington, DC: Office of Technology Assessment; 1980.

268. Pendse N. Online analytical processing. Wikipedia. 2008; 2008.

269. Prokosch HU, Seuchter SA, Thompson EA, Skolnick MH. Applying expert system techniques to human genetics. Comput Biomed Res. 1989;22:234–47.

270. Pryor DB, Stead WW, Hammond WE, Califf RM, Rosati RA. Features of TMR for a successful clinical and research database. Proc SCAMC. 1982; 79–84.

271. Pryor TA, Gardner RM, Clayton PD, Warner HR. The HELP system. J Med Syst. 1983;7:87–102.

272. Richart RH. Evaluation of a hospital computer system. In: Collen MF, editor. Hospital computer systems. New York: Wiley; 1974. p. 341–417.

273. Richart RH. Evaluation of a medical data system. Comput Biomed Res. 1970;3:415–25.

274. Rind DM, Davis R, Safran C. Designing studies of computer-based alerts and reminders. MD Comput. 1995;12:122.

275. Roach CJ. Patient data processing – the key to hospital automation. Am J Med Electron. 1962;1:51.

276. Roach J, Lee S, Wilcke J, Ehrich M. An expert system for information on pharmacology and drug interactions. Comput Biol Med. 1985;15:11–23.

277. Robson D. Object-oriented software systems. 1981.

278. Rodnick JE, Wiederhold G. A review of automated ambulatory medical record systems in the United States: charting services that are of benefit to the physician. Proc.MEDINFO. 1977; 957–61.

279. Rogers JL, Haring OM, Phifer JF. Carry-over of medical information system influence to control patients. Eval Health Prof. 1984;7:43–51.

280. Romano CA. Privacy, confidentiality, and security of computerized systems: the nursing responsibility. Comput Nurs. 1987;5:99.

281. Romano MJ, Stafford RS. Electronic health records and clinical decision support systems: impact on national ambulatory care quality. Arch Intern Med. 2011;171:897–903.

282. Rubin AD, Risley JF. The PROPHET system: an experiment in providing a computer resource to scientists. Proc MEDINFO. 1977; 77–81.

283. Sadock RT, Saunders SA. A security system for a computerized medical record. Proc SCAMC. 1984; 854–7

284. Safran C, Chute CG. Exploration and exploitation of clinical databases. Int J Biomed Comput. 1995;39:151–6.

285. Salmon P, Rappaport A, Bainbridge M, Hayes G, Williams J. Taking the problem oriented medical record forward. Proc AMIA. 1996; 463–7.

286. Schauffler HH, Koran RE. A methodology for estimating costs and benefits of medical information systems. Proc SCAMC. 1984; 152–5.

287. Schlager DD. A comprehensive patient care system for the family practice. J Med Syst. 1983;7:137–45.

288. Schmitz HH. An evaluation of the immediate financial impact of the hospital information system at Deaconess Hospital. In: Koza RC, editor. Health information systems evaluation. Boulder: Colorado Associated University Press; 1974. p. 265–82.

289. Schwartz SR, Stinson C, Berlant J. Computers in psychiatry. MD Comput. 1985;2:42–50.

290. Seidel K, Peeples J. The evaluation and implementation of an automated medical transcription. In: Anonymous Chicago: American Hospital Association, Center for Hospital Management Engineering. 1977; 67–90.
291. Seuchter SA, Skolnick MH. HGDBMS: a human genetics database management system. Comput Biomed Res. 1988;21:478–87.
292. Shannon JA. Federal support of biomedical sciences: development and academic impact. J Med Educ. 1976;51:1–98.
293. Shannon RH, Ball MJ. Patient-oriented classification of medical data-aid to systems-analysis and design. Biosci Commun. 1976;2:282–92.
294. Shea S, Hripcsak G. Accelerating the use of electronic health records in physician practices. N Engl J Med. 2010;362:192–5.
295. Shortliffe EH. Networking health: learning from others, taking the lead. Health Aff (Millwood). 2000;19:9–22.
296. Shortliffe EH. The next generation Internet and health care: a civics lesson for the informatics community. Proc AMIA. 1998; 8–14.
297. Siemon JH, Kuratomi RM. Automated record tracking as a component of a management information system. In: Topics in health record management. Germantown: Aspen Systems; 1982. p. 54–65.
298. Simborg DW. Local area networks: why? what? what if? MD Comput. 1984;1:10–20.
299. Simborg DW, Shearer M, Daniels L, Moss J. A medical records department system: a vital node in a hospital information system. Proc SCAMC. 1981; 830.
300. Simborg DW, Macdonald LK, Liebman JS, Musco P. Ward information-management system: an evaluation. Comput Biomed Res. 1972;5:484–97.
301. Simon HA. What computers mean for man and society. Science. 1977;195:1186–91.
302. Sittig DF, Campbell E, Guappone K, Dykstra R, Ash JS. Recommendations for monitoring and evaluation of in-patient computer-based provider order entry systems: results of a Delphi survey. Proc AMIA Annu Symp. 2007; 671–5.
303. Skolnick M. The Utah genealogical database: a resource for genetic epidemiology. Banbury Rep. 1980;4:285–97.
304. Skolnick M, Bean L, May D, Arbon V. Mormon demographic history I. Nuptiality and fertility of once-married couples. Popul Stud. 1978;32:5–19.
305. Spencer WA. An opinion survey of computer applications in 149 hospitals in the USA, Europe and Japan. Inform Health Soc Care. 1976;1:215–34.
306. Springer EW. Automated medical records and the law. Germantown: Aspen Publishers; 1971.
307. Stead WW. A quarter-century of computer-based medical records. MD Comput. 1989;6:74–81.
308. Stead WW, Hammond WE. Computer-based medical records: the centerpiece of TMR. MD Comput. 1988;5:48–62.
309. Stead WW, Wiederhold G, Gardner RM. Database systems for computer-based patient records. In: Ball MJ, Collen MF, editors. Aspects of the computer-based patient record. New York: Springer; 1992. p. 83–98.
310. Stead WW, Hammond WE. Demand-oriented medical records: toward a physician work station. Proc SCAMC. 1987; 275–80.
311. Stead WW, Hammond WE, Straube MJ. A chartless record: is it adequate? J Med Syst. 1983;7:103–9.
312. Steinbach GL, Busch JF. Combining voice and data communication in a hospital environment. Proc SCAMC. 1985; 712–7.
313. Stuart RB, Bair JH. The effect of the problem-oriented medical record on comprehensiveness of care as reflected in the clinical record. Houston: Fort Sam, Health Care Studies Division, Academy of Health Sciences; 1972. p. 1–13.
314. Stuart RB, Rahm AE, Bair JH. Army physicians' attitudes toward the problem-oriented medical record. Houston: Fort Sam, Health Care Studies Division, Brook Army Medical Center; 1972. p. 1–15.
315. Swyers JP. Genetic data base service. Research Resources Reporter. 1989 (Dec); 13–4.

316. Tang PC. Futurescope, the advent of electronic medical records. Decisions Imaging Econ. 1989;2:4–10.
317. Terdiman J. Ambulatory care computer systems in office practice: a tutorial. Proc AMIA. 1982; 195–201.
318. Tierney WM, McDonald CJ, Martin DK, Hui SL. Computerized display of past test results: effect on outpatient testing. Ann Intern Med. 1987;107:569–74.
319. Tolchin SG, Blum BI, Butterfield MA. A systems analysis methodology for a decentralized health care information system. Proc SCAMC. 1980; 1479–84.
320. Tolchin SG, Stewart RL, Kahn SA, Bergan ES, Gafke GP, Simborg DW, et al. A prototype generalized network technology for hospitals. J Med Syst. 1982;6:359–75.
321. Tolchin SG, Stewart RL, Kahn SA, Bergan ES, Gafke GP, Simborg DW, et al. Implementation of a prototype generalized network technology for hospitals. Proc SCAMC. 1981; 942–8.
322. Tolchin SG, Arseniev M, Barta WL, Kuzmak PM, Bergan E, Nordquist R, et al. Integrating heterogeneous systems using local network technologies and remote procedure call protocols. Proc SCAMC. 1985; 748–9.
323. Tuck D, O'Connell R, Gershkovich P, Cowan J. An approach to object-relational mapping in bioscience domains. Proc AMIA. 2002; 820–4.
324. Tufo HM, Speidel JJ. Problems with medical records. Med Care. 1971;9:509–17.
325. Tufo HM, Bouchard RE, Rubin AS, Twitchell JC, VanBuren HC, Weed LB, et al. Problem-oriented approach to practice: I. Economic impact. JAMA. 1977;238:414–7.
326. Vallbona C, Spencer WA. Texas Institute for Research and Rehabilitation Hospital Computer System (Houston). In: Collen MF, editor. Hospital computer systems. New York: Wiley; 1974. p. 662–700.
327. Vallbona C, Brohn J, Albin J. Pilot test and preliminary evaluation of an optical card medical record system. Proc MEDINFO. 1989; 809–12.
328. Van Brunt E. Selected observations on ambulatory care: office practice. Proc AMIA. 1982; 202–5.
329. Van Brunt E, Davis LS, Terdiman JF, Singer S, Besag E, Collen MF. Current status of a medical information system. Methods Inf Med. 1970;9:149–60.
330. VanName ML, Catchings B. SQL-a database language sequel to Dbase. Byte. 1989;14:175.
331. Vickery DM. Computer support of paramedical personnel: the question of quality control. Proc MEDINFO. 1974; 281–7.
332. Walters RF. File structures for database management systems. MD Comput. 1987;5:30–41.
333. Walters RF. Microprocessors as intelligent front-end devices for medical information systems. Med Inform (Lond). 1979;44:139–50.
334. Ware WH. Old practices in a new age endanger information privacy. Hosp JAHA. 1977;51:133–9.
335. Ware WH. Records, computers and the rights of citizens. Report of the Secretary's Advisory Committee on Automated Personal Data. Washington, DC: US Govt Print Office; 1973.
336. Warner H, Morgan J, Pryor T, Clark S, Miller W. HELP-a self-improving system for medical decision-making. Proc MEDINFO. 1974; 989–93.
337. Warner HR. Data sources. In: Computer-assisted decision making. New York: Academic; 1979. p. 6–101.
338. Warner HR. History of medical informatics at Utah. In: Blum BI, Duncan KA, editors. A history of medical informatics. New York: Addison-Wesley; 1990. p. 357–69.
339. Warner HR. Computer-based patient monitoring. In: Stacy RW, Waxman B, editors. Computers in biomedical research, vol. III. New York: Academic; 1972. p. 239–51.
340. Wasserman AI. Minicomputers may maximize data processing. Hosp JAHA. 1977;51:119–28.
341. Wasserman AI, Stinson SK. A specification method for interactive medical information systems. Proc SCAMC. 1980;3:1471–8.
342. Wasserman AI, Pircher PA, Shewmake DT, Kersten ML. Developing interactive information systems with the user software methodology. IEEE Trans Softw Eng. SE-12(2):326–45.
343. Watson JD, Crick FHC. Molecular structure of nucleic acids. Nature. 1953;171:737–8.

344. Watson RJ. Medical staff response to a medical information system with direct physician-computer interface. Proc MEDINFO. 1974;74:299–302.
345. Waxman BD. Biomedical computing 1965. Ann NY Acad Sci. 1966;128:723–30.
346. Weiland AJ. The challenges of genetic advances. Healthplan. 2000;41:24–30.
347. Weinstein M. Securing and safeguarding paperless records. Am Coll Phys Obs. 1988 (July/August); 17.
348. Weinstein M. Economic evaluation of medical procedures and technologies: progress, problems and prospects. In: Wagner J, ed. Medical technology. DHEW Pub No (PHS) 79-3254. NCHSR Research Proc Series. 1979; 52–68.
349. Wess Jr BP. Distributed computer networks in support of complex group practices. Proc SCAMC. 1978; 469–77.
350. Westberg EE, Miller RA. The basis for using the internet to support the information needs of primary care. JAMIA. 1999;6:6–25.
351. Westin AF. New developments and problems in health care confidentiality. Proc SCAMC. 1979; 380–1.
352. Westin AF. A policy analysis of citizen rights: issues in health data systems. National Bureau of Standards Special Pub 467. Washington, DC: US Govt Print Office; 1977.
353. Westin AF. Computers, health records, and citizen rights. National Bureau of Standards Monograph 157. Washington, DC: US Govt Print Office; 1976.
354. Westin AF. Legal safeguards to insure privacy in a computer society. Commun ACM. 1967;10:533–7.
355. Westin AF, Baker MA. Databanks in a free society: computers, record keeping and privacy. New York: Quadrangel Books; 1972.
356. Whiting-O'Keefe QE, Simborg DW, Epstein WV. A controlled experiment to evaluate the use of a time-oriented summary medical record. Med Care. 1980;18:842–52.
357. Whiting-O'Keefe QE, Simborg DW, Epstein WV, Warger A. A computerized summary medical record system can provide more information than the standard medical record. JAMA. 1985;254:1185–92.
358. Wiederhold G. Databases, a tutorial. Proc AAMSI. 1984; 423–30.
359. Wiederhold G. Modeling databases. Inf Sci. 1983;29:115–26.
360. Wiederhold G. Databases for ambulatory care. Proc AMIA. 1982; 79–85.
361. Wiederhold G. Summary of visit to the Research Center, Rockland Psychiatric Center, Orangeburg, NY, on January 9, 1974. CDR-4 HRA Contract. 1975.
362. Wiederhold G, Walker MG, Blum RL. Acquisition of medical knowledge from medical records. Proc Benutzer-gruppenseminar Med Syst. 1987; 213–4.
363. Wiederhold G. Database technology in health care. J Med Syst. 1981;5:175–96.
364. Willard KE, Hallgren JH, Sielaff B, Connelly D. The deployment of a World Wide Web (W3) based medical information system. Proc AMIA. 1995;771–5.
365. Wilson GA, McDonald CJ, McCabe GP. The effect of immediate access to a computerized medical record on physician test ordering: a controlled clinical trial in the emergency room. Am J Public Health. 1982;72:698–702.
366. Wilson JF. Making electronic health records meaningful. Ann Intern Med. 2009;151:293–6.
367. Winters S, Hurt S, Turney SZ. Levels of security in a critical care hospital data system. Proc SCAMC. 1984; 517–23.
368. Yu H, Hripcsak G. A large scale, cross-disease family health history data set. Proc AMIA. 2000; 1162.
369. Zeichner ML, Brusil PJ, Tolchin SG. Distributed processing architecture for a hospital information system. Proc SCAMC. 1979; 859–65.
370. Zimmerman J. Towards generalized automated ambulatory care record systems. Proc MEDINFO. 1977;77:473–7.
371. Zinn TK, DiGiulio LW. Actualizing system benefits – part II. Comput Healthc. 1988;9:38–40.
372. Zoltan-Ford E. Professional persons' attitudes toward computers: comparative analyses and some suggestions. Proc SCAMC. 1984; 536–9.

Chapter 5
Outpatient Information Systems (OISs) for Ambulatory Care

Morris F. Collen, Warner V. Slack, and Howard L. Bleich

Abstract Of the relatively few outpatient information systems (OISs) operational in the United States in the 1960s, most were in ambulatory clinics that shared time on mainframe computers with affiliated hospitals. In the 1970s some larger physician practices launched standalone OISs on minicomputers. With the advent of microcomputers in the 1980s, OISs began to diffuse rapidly, some as federally funded pilots. By the end of the 1980s, about 80 % of physicians had some type of computer in their offices, primarily for administrative and business functions; computer-based patient records and other OIS clinical applications were still infrequently used. When admitting a patient to the hospital, few physicians could transfer data from their OIS to the hospital information system. For the most part, lack of standardization made the interchange of data difficult or impossible. However, three OISs achieved notable success in the 1970s and 1980s. Each was developed in an academic environment and led by a committed physician; each developed a "chartless" record, continuously updated and stored in the computer; two of the three had linkages to large affiliated hospitals. Yet they were the exception. Few evaluations of OISs were convincing as to their benefits. Low physician adoption of OISs suggested computer-based records were not considered more efficient for office practice than paper-based records. Expectations for the 1990s were that OISs would change to support electronic claims reporting and quality of care monitoring. In the 2010s, federal funding became available for physicians who purchased electronic health record systems complying with "Meaningful Use."

Keywords Outpatient information systems • Clinical applications • Physician adoption • Computer-based patient records • Administrative applications • Electronic health records • Interoperability • Success factors

---

Author Collen was deceased at the time of publication. Slack and Bleich edited this chapter on his behalf after his death.

M.F. Collen (deceased)

W.V. Slack, M.D. (✉) • H.L. Bleich, M.D.
Harvard Medical School, Division of Clinical Informatics, Department of Medicine, Beth Israel Deaconess Medical Center, Brookline, MA, USA
e-mail: wslack@bidmc.harvard.edu; bleich@bidmc.harvard.edu

© Springer-Verlag London 2015
M.F. Collen, M.J. Ball (eds.), *The History of Medical Informatics in the United States*, Health Informatics, DOI 10.1007/978-1-4471-6732-7_5

The care of most ambulatory patients is provided in the home as self-care by the patient, with the help of the family and personal caregivers. The professional care for ambulatory outpatients in the United States is usually provided outside of the hospital, in the offices of physicians in solo practice or in groups of health professionals in medical centers, or in clinics of the outpatient departments associated with large hospitals.

5.1   OIS Functional Requirements and Technical Designs

In 1974 Henley and Wiederhold [81] asked users of 17 OISs why they had installed their systems, and they found the main objective for the most part to be to improve the quality of their patients' care. These users expected to accomplish this objective by using their OISs to improve patient care management, to increase patient adherence with physicians' orders, to improve the continuity of care, to permit the implementation of quality-of-care procedures using the patient's record as the source of information, and to facilitate the collection of data for subsequent research. Other important objectives were to: improve patient record availability, to improve cost management by utilization-review, to provide faster and more accurate processing of patients' billings and insurance claims, and to reduce operating costs by increasing the productivity of personnel.

Functional requirements of an OIS for the care of ambulatory patients are generally similar to those of a hospital information system for the care of hospitalized patients. Hospitalized patients, however, are usually sicker and receive more intensive treatment than do ambulatory patients. Although a smaller volume of patient data is generally entered into the patient's record during an office visit than during a hospital stay, the accumulated collection of data from many office visits over a long time period can produce a voluminous patient record. O'Desky and associates [131] recommended that the functional requirements of an OIS include: an integrated electronic database providing patients' medical records and meeting patients' care needs. It should also have provisions to satisfy business, accounting, office administration and management needs; and it should support administrative and clinical decision making. Blum [14] noted that OISs could be less expensive and require fewer sub-systems than hospital information systems, but that both needed to satisfy similar requirements, including: accurate patient identification data; administrative and business requirements, such as billing and third-party claims submissions; comprehensive patient records; patient scheduling and tracking functions; provision for utilization review and quality assurance; natural language word processing for forms and correspondence; protection and security of access to the computing system and information within it; and backup capabilities to protect the data if any component of the system failed. For a large medical group or clinic, the OIS needed to be interfaced to information subsystems operating in the clinical specialty services. It should also be interfaced to computer subsystems in the clinical laboratories, radiology department, and pharmacy; and when possible, the OIS should be interfaced as well as to the information system of an affiliated hospital.

Blum also deemed it important for the OIS to fulfill requirements for decision support and continuing medical education, and when possible, be capable of linking to outside databases, such as to those at the National Library of Medicine, and to affiliated clinical research databases. He summarized the basic functions of the OIS: to support preparation for a patient's visit; to record key patient data for the visit; to update the patient's medical record; and to use the patient's record for medical, administrative, financial, and research applications.

Technical requirements and designs for an OIS are governed by its functional requirements, whether it was to be built as an in-house development or purchased from a commercial vendor, and whether it was to be a part of a larger center's medical information system or to be a physician's standalone system. Blois [12] observed that consideration of the elements underlying the design of the OIS needed to take into account the physicians' personal medical knowledge and experience. And he observed that the hardware, software, and communications technology for an OIS have first to be specified, then either developed or purchased, and finally installed and operated in a manner capable of satisfying the functional requirements of its users.

There are difficulties in achieving these goals, however. When differences in technical designs and data standards for OISs evolve to meet different institutional requirements, problems of interoperability arise between the OISs and hospital information systems of different vendors. Technical requirements and designs of OISs vary from institution to institution. Although patients' records are usually chronologically arranged so all data entries begin with the date and time, followed by the patient's clinical information, structural organization can vary widely; an OIS that works in one medical group may be inoperable in another.

Feinstein [49] suggested the arrangement of medical records being one of catalogs of data with the arrangement of information based on the source, such as the clinician or laboratory, and the chronology of the information. Thus each transaction in a patient's care would be entered into the record with the name of the source or service, the date and time the service was ordered, and the date and time it was performed, all with a description of the service and the results. Such a time-oriented record often used flow charts that organized multiple data items into a graphic or tabular, time-oriented format, such as for temperature, medication records, laboratory test results, and other serially collected information. Early examples of such source and time oriented OISs were those developed by Fries [58, 59], as well as by Wiederhold [188] whose Time-Oriented Database contained clinical information organized chronologically and generally collected in the form of time-oriented flow sheets.

The Problem Oriented Medical Record was developed in the 1960s by Weed [182–185] who listed rules for recording data in the patient's medical record: a numbered list of problems that included every problem in the patient's past and present history and that served as an updated table of contents for the record; a plan for the diagnostic and therapeutic orders for each of the problems, numbered accordingly, with progress notes and procedure reports preceded by the number and title of each problem; and graphs, tables and flow sheets kept on all problems when the data and time relationships are complex.

With Weed's approach, each numbered problem would be associated with progress notes organized in four parts: (S) subjective, (O) objective, (A) assessment, and (P) plan (often referred to as: S-O-A-P notes). Weed advocated that data involving physical findings, vital signs, laboratory test values, and medications could best lead to sound interpretations and decisions if they were organized by problems, with flow sheets to reflect temporal relations. A numbered list of both active and inactive problems would serve as the index to the patient's record and the progress of medical care.

With Weed's computing system, clinicians used structured formats with display terminals for some information entry. However, progress notes, consultation reports, and operative and other special procedure reports were usually dictated to transcriptionists; with the advent of word processing programs, such reports were then entered by the transcriptionists into the computer-based patients' records.

5.2 OIS Administrative Subsystems

Some of the earliest applications of computers in outpatient information systems were for standard business services, such as accounts payable and receivable, general ledger, payroll, inventories, statements for patient billing, and preparation of third-party insurance claims for reimbursement. In the early 1970s Bolt, Beranek, and Newman developed for physicians' offices a standalone, minicomputer-based Ambulatory Care Center Support System to provide accounts receivable and billings to patients and third-party payers; this was reported to be successful in labor savings and improvements in cash flow [30].

Administrative and office management subsystems for OISs were developed in the late 1970s, and included administrative help with utilization of services, personnel staffing and scheduling, and patient registration and appointment scheduling [51]. Jelovsek and associates [85] affirmed that early medical accounting practices were generally thought to be similar to the accounting practices in other businesses, so most computer applications in early physicians' offices were derived from financial systems that had been written by accountants. On the other hand, they noted that two OISs, Barnett's COSTAR and the Duke Medical Center's The Medical Record (TMR) developed by Hammond and associates, were designed primarily to accommodate the computer-based patient record, with financial programs being added subsequently. This approach was important. It is easier to add business applications to a computer-based patient record, than to add a computer-based patient record to an administrative office system.

By the early 1980s, some OISs, such as Duke's TMR, also produced a variety of management reports including daily logs of patients' visits, laboratory work sheets of ordered tests and pending and final test results, lists of patients with problems in need of attention, and lists of patients who failed to keep appointments. Such OISs also produced periodic reports of clinic activity, such as lists of diagnoses reported, tests ordered, treatments given, and other measures of utilization of resources; and they also provided periodic comparative utilization reports to support administrative planning [86].

By the mid-1980s OIS administrative systems included word processing programs for management reports and correspondence, as well as programs for tracking medical records [50]. The installation of OIS administrative systems enabled a more efficient tracking of records than with paper-based medical records, which could be difficult to locate. At the Lahey Clinic in Burlington, Massachusetts, where on any day in 1971 about 15,000 records were active, a medical record tracking system was linked to the computer-based master patient index for patient identification. Computer displays were designed to enter each request for a medical record, to monitor the location of the medical record, to record the person requesting the record, and to cancel a record request [28]. A medical record tracking system with similar functions was also developed at the Parkland Outpatient Clinic of the University of Texas Health Science Center in Dallas, where up to 1,000 patients per day were cared for, and where, before installation of the record-tracking system, 30–40 % of the patients were seen without their charts because their charts could not be located. After installation of the record-tracking system in their 78 clinics, chart availability improved dramatically [126].

In the 1980s an increasing number of large pre-payment medical group practices – health maintenance organizations, such as Kaiser Permanente – developed a need for monitoring the utilization of medical services and their costs, in order to better fulfill their goals. With their OISs, they could monitor the practice patterns of their physicians for ordering diagnostic procedures and prescription medications. They could also monitor physicians' rates of patient referrals to clinical specialists and assess the health status of their patients by diagnostic groupings and rates of occurrence of medical problems [32].

Patient appointment scheduling systems for office visits required computer programs for patients' registration, and these systems needed more complex and specialized programs to fit different-sized physician groups and different specialists' needs. The scheduling of appointments for new, return, and re-scheduled visits all required filling appointment times for each health professional by date, time, and length of visit. Accurate identification of each patient was an essential requirement for the scheduling of appointments and procedures.

In 1964 an automated appointment system was initiated in the outpatient department of the Peter Bent Brigham Hospital in Boston. Teletype input-output terminals were connected to a Univac computer. By 1967, for the medical clinics of 60 physicians, almost one-half of all appointments were made on the automated system. The noise from the Teletype printers, however, created an auditory problem [87]. In 1971 the Boston Children's Medical Center was also operating an automated appointment system for outpatient visits. A video terminal in each clinic was used by receptionists for making office appointments in response to requests either by telephone or in person [61].

In 1973 a large central clinic appointment system had been developed and was operational at the Lahey Clinic in Boston (together with their record-tracking system) which provided up to 180,000 office appointments per year [61]. This Clinic's central appointment service was accessed by telephone, and used a pool of 31 video display terminals all located in one large room. The terminals were connected to an IBM 370/145 computer that serviced the entire Lahey Clinic data system. The system stored all physician appointment schedules, recorded all patient appointments, sent out reminder notices to scheduled patients, provided daily appointment lists to clinic receptionists, and reported appointment and utilization statistics to the clinic management [136]. Furthermore, associates at the Lahey Clinic tested the use a self-administered patient history questionnaire to improve the routing of new patients to appropriate specialists in the group. Using a statistical method, the questions to which the patient answered "yes" were assigned a predictive value as to which specialist the patient should be referred. When implemented, they found this scheduling tool more effective than their prior method of scheduling patients in accordance with each patient's request.

In 1974 the Kaiser Permanente medical care program in its Northern California region initiated a computer-based patient appointment system that maintained appointment schedules for each physician, nurse practitioner, and procedure room. It provided a weekly work pattern for each physician and adjusted for designated types and lengths of the appointments. In 1977 a central database with identification data for 1.3 million patients was implemented for the scheduling of office appointments for one Kaiser medical center, with a network of display terminals connected to an IBM computer center [31]. By the mid-1980s this patient appointment, registration, and reporting system had grown to serve Kaiser's health plan membership of almost 2 million people, who made close to 8 million office visits per year to 2,000 physicians in 20 outpatient medical centers [103].

By the mid-1970s the majority of the 17 OIS sites described in the study by Henley and Wiederhold [81] provided patient identification during office visit registration; 14 of 17 collected utilization statistics for planning and budgeting; and 6 had interactive scheduling systems for patient appointments. Complex scheduling algorithms were also available for scheduling on holidays as well as for different specialists, and for mixed appointment and walk-in clinics. This reduced the long waiting times for unscheduled patients who came during peak-load periods. Another example of a flexible clinic appointment system was that employed by Duke's The Medical Record (TMR) system, which supported a multi-specialty group practice. The TMR system included algorithms to simplify the making of an appointment with a given clinic and provider at a given time. The TMR system also provided user-specific modules to permit scheduling for specialized settings. For example, their RENAL program had a module to assist in the scheduling of dialysis patients [72].

In another setting, Blum and associates at the Johns Hopkins clinics used their TEDIUM program, operated with a microcomputer, to give providers and clinics sets of tables to use for their availability schedules.

Roach [135] reviewed ten of the more sophisticated computer-based, patient appointment scheduling systems available in the mid-1980s. Most allowed for variable-length appointment slots, restricted slots for specified appointment types, sequences for controlled overbooking, controlled scheduling (for holiday, post-holiday, and long-range scheduling), block scheduling of multiple patients into a single slot, automatic sequential scheduling of multiple appointments for predictable follow-up situations, listings of patients waiting for open appointments, filling open slots when patients canceled appointments, and reminder notices of forthcoming appointments.

5.3 Patient Identification and Record Linkage

Accurate patient identification is an essential requirement for every health care program and computer-based system. Even though this can be difficult – particularly in years gone by when computer technology limited users to alphanumeric data for names, codes, gender, and birthdates, and the technology could not process textual information – it is necessary to register each patient in the computing system correctly and in sufficient detail such that every subsequent encounter with the information system will be performed with the intended patient of record. Even when the patient's identifying information arrives from different sources, it must be accurate and safe within the patient's electronic registry. All medical information systems and their subsystems must accurately identify each patient and accurately link all records and other relevant information collected for that patient. Accordingly, each OIS that collected specimens from a patient, or generated products from procedures, such as electrocardiogram and pathology reports, had to identify each report or specimen. The OIS had then to link accurately all of the data that resulted from the patient's tests and procedures and store this information in the designated patient's computer-based record [35].

Identification (ID) numbers are generally assigned to patients upon their first outpatient visit or hospital admission. Each ID number is unique; and with the addition of the patient's name, gender, and birthdate these data usually provide the accurate identification of a patient. With well working medical information systems, all data collected on a patient during an outpatient visit or a hospitalization are linked by the patient's ID number; and the same ID number is used on subsequent outpatient visits and hospital admissions. Thus current test and procedure results can be compared to prior results. Subsystems within a medical information system in the hospital or its associated clinics usually use the same patient ID number that had been assigned to the patient on the first visit for care; and the ID number is then recorded on each requisition for clinical services. Although patient visits to outpatient clinics and medical offices not affiliated with the patient's hospital sometimes used the referred patient's hospital ID number, the outpatient clinics often assigned their own accession numbers for their procedures provided to the patient; this could create problems with misidentification.

The first items of patient data usually entered into a patient's electronic medical record are the patient's name, and a numerical code – the medical record number – which is distinct from the patient's ID number, and which uniquely represents the record of the individual patient. It was soon found, however, that there could be a high error rate in computer-stored patient identification data. Names were often misspelled; and similar-sounding, common names could be spelled differently, as for example Johnson, Jonson, or Jensen. Phonetic coding systems, such as the Russell Soundex code, were developed to help users search through such variations of names with similar sounds. A Soundex Code was created using the first letter of the last name and then numbers that were assigned to the remaining letters in the name. It then organized the names into groups that sounded alike but were spelled differently [179].

Additional identification problems were created when people changed their names through marriage, resulting in the filing of their records under their new name in a different alphabetical listing. It was important, therefore, for the computer-based record to maintain a history of name changes. A parent and a child of the same gender could also have the same name, and in that case an important identifying difference for their records would be their birthdates. Furthermore, different people could have the same birthdate and the same birthplace. Thus, accurate patient identification usually required the patient's full name, the patient's gender, the patient's birthdate, and a unique medical record number assigned to the patient and that served as the basic linkage, together with the patient's ID number, for all the patient's data during his or her lifetime of care within the health care delivery system. To increase the reliability of identification, the systems sometimes included additional identifying items, such as the person's birthplace, the mother's maiden surname, and the mother's birthplace [195]. Gabrieli [60] proposed four general criteria for collecting and providing patient identification: specific data for positive determination of the individual; readily available data for authorized inquiry; data confidentiality preserved with data unavailable without positive authorization; a comprehensive database to include every member of the health care community; and a universal database coordinated with military files, school records, and hospital records.

As early as 1965, Moore [127] at the Los Angeles County General Hospital initiated an identification file for one million patients by using a punched-card system. His patient identification database included the patient's medical record number, name, birthdate, birthplace, mother's maiden surname, gender, and ethnic group. Moore's approach also employed a Soundex code for surnames to accommodate different surname spellings. There soon evolved a variety of patient identification numbering codes. The most common was the Social Security Number, which had been authorized in 1961 as a United States Citizen's identifier for federal agencies resulting from an executive order issued in 1943. In 1961, the Internal Revenue Service (and most states soon thereafter) began to use this identification method for taxpayer identification. Soon the Department of Defense, the Veterans Administration, the Indian Health Service, banks, credit bureaus, stock and bond brokers, retail stores, utilities, insurance companies, motor vehicle departments, and employers found use for this personal number [156].

The Social Security Number would become the key linkage for most computer-based databases in both the public and private sectors. As a result, most medical care programs would not use the number for patients' medical record numbers because its use could permit a federal agency or a private business organization to invade inappropriately the privacy of a person's medical record. Furthermore, the number was not always uniquely assigned. Duplicate Social Security Numbers have been issued [104].

Once an identification (ID) number was assigned to a patient, that ID number should never be assigned to another person. However, mistakes do happen, and to protect against two patients having the same ID number and thereby to protect the privacy and accuracy of medical information, most health care programs assign their own patient medical record numbers in addition to their patients' ID numbers. After a medical record number had been assigned to a patient, this number would be the first information entered into the computer terminal when a patient's electronic record was to be retrieved. Such an entry then would result in the system displaying the full identification data for the patient. This would enable the registering clerk to verify that the medical record number did in truth represent the person.

To minimize errors, such as wrong or transposed digits in entering medical record numbers, mathematical strategies were developed. Lindberg at the University of Missouri-Columbia [97, 98] added a seventh-place *check digit* to each patient's unique ID number, which he also used to help detect and prevent transcription errors. The check digit was calculated by the computer from the preceding 6 digits of each patient's number using the modulus 11 method; the computer system would accept data only if the patient's ID number, including the check digit was correct.

Other efforts to decrease errors in patient identification used algorithms to provide the system user with a probability estimate of a match between the information provided by the patient and the records contained in the patient's file [1]. A master patient record index was typically used by hospital medical record departments to locate a patient's medical record and to determine whether a new medical record number should be assigned to a patient admitted to the system, or whether there were prior admissions, for example, that the patient had neglected to mention. With the advent of electronic medical information systems, the development of increasing numbers of patient identification systems would improve the efficiency and accuracy of linking patient's data for multiple visits to a single patient's medical record. Stewart [161] proposed such a computer-based system to provide a convenient means of linking all patient-related data and thereby decreasing the time required to enter, correct, and update accurate patient identification information.

5.4 Patient's History and Physician's Examination Data

The patient's medical history, as recorded in the patient's record, is the primary documentation of information obtained directly from the patient, or from the patient's family or other knowledgeable persons. The medical history usually includes the description of the patient's current medical problems or chief complaints, with detailed supporting data on the present and past history of these problems. The medical history also includes a review of systems to elicit past and present symptoms of all body systems, from head to toe. The medical history is usually divided into categories that list both body systems (head, chest, abdomen, pelvis, and extremities) and organ systems (brain, heart, lungs, liver, and others), as well as family, social, occupational, and environmental histories.

In their effort to standardize the medical history, Wakefield and Yarnall [177] divided the history into the problem history, which included all the patient's current medical problems; and the database history, which included the rest of the patient's history. (As noted above, Weed based his entire patient record, including the medical history, on the problem-oriented approach.) The problem history would be the more difficult to standardize, and most physicians have continued to evolve their own history-taking style. The database history is more routine and repetitive and more suitable to standardization, programming and automation.

The collection of information by the direct interviewing of a patient is an essential process as the physician begins to formulate the patient's diagnosis. Accordingly, a large proportion of a physician's time during an office visit (particularly with a new patient) is occupied with acquiring a good medical history. For most office patients, an experienced physician asking appropriate probing questions, will know within a few minutes, and with a high probability of being correct, what is medically wrong with the patient; and the rest of the visit will be used to confirm the preliminary diagnosis and to "rule out" other possible conditions. Still, accumulating the history can be time-consuming, and the medical history is often incomplete due to time limitations beyond the physician's control.

Through the years, a variety of methods have been developed to collect reliable information for clinical decision-making and to save time. Some physicians employed nurses, physician assistants, or other allied health professionals to take patients' medical histories; and some used paper-based questionnaires that permitted the patient to self-administer the initial history. Physicians continually sought to develop alternative technologies to interrogate the patient by some method other than by a human interviewer; but the goal of providing an acceptable and effective alternative has proven difficult. Paper-and-pencil self-administered questionnaires have been used extensively in office practice in the effort to save physician's time and to provide data for subsequent entry into the patient's record. They are usually a composite of closed questions in which the patient responds either with a number (for example, when asked for age) or with a choice of alternative responses; for example, "yes" or "no," "true" or "false," "I don't understand," or with a choice of other, multiple responses. If the technology and human factors permit asking branching multilevel questions, then after a first question is answered, second-level questions can be used to obtain more detail; and a third-level and even fourth-level of questions can follow to simulate more closely a human interviewer. Open narrative or free-answer questions for which the patients record their responses in their own words are more subjective and less readily standardized.

In the 1950s, paper-based patients' records were the most common method used by physicians in their offices to enter and store data from their ambulatory patient's history and physical examination; and then to enter data from follow-up visits and to record progress reports. The data were entered mostly in textual form by hand on a paper card or on a paper encounter form; or by dictating the information to a transcriptionist who typed the paper record for the patient's paper chart.

The *Cornell Medical Index-Health Questionnaire* developed by Brodman and associates [24], was among the first to become widely used as a model for self-administered questionnaires. It was a paper-and-pencil questionnaire used in the New York Hospital's general medical clinic; and it consisted of 4, letter-sized, paper sheets on which were printed 195 questions corresponding to those typically asked in an initial comprehensive medical interview. After each question the patient circled "Yes" or "No" [23]. Brodman [22] later reported the use of a computer to process the questionnaires, and to study patients' responses in association with specific diseases.

In 1951 Kaiser Permanente (KP) in Oakland, California, initiated a self-administered health questionnaire – modified from the Cornell Medical Index – within its multiphasic health testing program. This questionnaire contained 95 questions and was incorporated in 1955 into the Oakland and San Francisco multiphasic programs [40]. Then in 1963, the KP automated multiphasic health testing programs began operating with an IBM 1440 computer system. Two hundred common health questions were printed on prepunched IBM cards, one question to a card. The patient responded by taking the card from the top section of a divided letter box and dropping the card into the middle section if the answer was "yes", or into the bottom section if the answer was "no." A card that contained the patient's identification data was placed on top of the pile of "yes" cards and read into a computer by a punched card reading machine [39]. The results of the questionnaire were thereby entered and stored in the patient's electronic record and also printed on a health-checkup summary report.

Patients who answered "yes" to selected complex medical questions were then given a second deck of cards for sorting into "yes" and "no" responses, and this served as a second-level questionnaire [39]. A history question with a large number of possible choices, such as for obtaining the patient's occupation, was presented as a list of 170 common occupations printed on a portable punch card; and with a stylus, the patient punched a hole under the name of the occupation that most closely corresponded to the patient's work. The punched card was then read into the computer with the other questionnaire punch cards [38]. The KP history questions were tested for reliability of the patients' responses when using punched cards; and it was found that it did not matter in what sequence the questions were asked, or whether the questions were presented to patients on paper forms or on punch cards [175]. This approach to an automated self-administered questionnaire was economical since the decks of question cards could be reused many times. Furthermore, the deck of cards needed only to be counted for completeness and did not need to be resorted since the questions could be asked in any order. The card-sorting method of providing an automated self-administered health questionnaire continued to be used in the KP multiphasic testing program until the late 1970s, when it became impossible to replace the worn-out card-punch and card-read equipment that were no longer manufactured. The use of paper forms was then reinstituted for the patients' histories, with the "yes" responses being entered into the computer by clerks using keyboard terminals.

Since these questionnaires were more reliable for what Wakefield and Yarnall [177] called the database history than for the collection of information about patients' medical problems, these self-administered histories were used only for health checkups in the multiphasic and health appraisal programs. In the 1960s, using the Minnesota Multiphasic Personality Inventory (MMPI) as a model, Kaiser Permanente had developed its own Neuromental Questionnaire (NMQ) that consisted of 155 psychological questions to which the patient responded by sorting the prepunched cards into sections of a letter box labeled "true" or "false". These psychological questionnaire responses were used later for epidemiological and clinical studies [55]. Ausman [2] also used portable punch cards for the input of a variety of data including the patient's temperature, pulse, and respiration, as well as the results of clinical laboratory tests.

In 1958 Rockhart and McLean [137] at the Lahey Clinic studied self-administered histories that were mailed to patients. In 1971 they tested their first Automated Medical History Questionnaire. The patients' responses to this paper-and-pencil questionnaire were keypunched and then batch processed by computer, with a printout of questions and answers filed in the patient's chart. The questionnaires were mailed to patients in advance of their clinic visit so the results could be used to aid in the scheduling of patients with appropriate specialists and the printout of responses could be available at the time of the patient's visit [122]. Rockart reported that in general, the patients' acceptance was good; and that physicians' acceptance of the questionnaire was positive. After processing more than 40,000 patient history questionnaires, the authors found increasing physician acceptance with use of the questionnaire [138]. However in 1975 the Lahey Clinic discontinued the regular use of the questionnaire because some physicians found it to be inadequate for their needs [121].

Slack [139, 148], at the University of Wisconsin and later at the Harvard Medical School, is generally credited with the most substantive early contributions to patient-computer dialog. Slack's first patient history program, which he used in early 1965, contained 450 screening questions. Each question had four possible responses: "Yes", "No", "Don't know", and "Don't understand." The questions were presented by a modified version of the method used by Kaiser Permanente in that each question was printed on a punched data-processing card. After the patient had sorted Slack's cards by placing each card into an appropriate slot of a divided tray, the sorted cards were fed into an automatic punched card reader that transmitted the responses to a computer, which then generated a summary printout of the patient's responses.

Slack [148] soon abandoned the use of questionnaire cards; and in 1965, he and his colleagues used a digital computer with a display terminal and teletype printer to obtain patients' medical histories, directly online [151]. He used a LINC (Laboratory Instrument Computer), which he borrowed from a research laboratory at the University of Wisconsin. The patient faced the computer screen, which displayed questions asking the patient to respond by pressing one of four numbered keys on the keyboard corresponding to the same four choices that Slack had used for the card-sort questions. If the patient pressed the "no" key, the computer proceeded to the next question. A "yes" response, such as to a positive symptom, initiated branching to a second-level questionnaire that requested more detail about the frequency, duration, and intensity of the symptom. Subsequent branching was a function of responses to both the current question and to any related prior questions.

Slack also employed open-ended questions, such as "What is your occupation?" for which the patient typed the response using the full keyboard. Slack concluded that the computer, with its branching capability, gave the system great flexibility and permitted more detail and better control in the interview; and branching questions could be as complex as was necessary to obtain the desired detail of response. In his first pilot study of 50 ambulatory patients to elicit a history of allergies, the computer printout was superior to the physician-recorded past histories; but was less detailed when dealing with the present illness of asthma [139]. Slack [150] further reported that with their computer-based history system, they had taken 160 allergy, 128 gynecologic, and 70 general medical histories; and they concluded that automated self-administered histories were particularly useful for the collection of routine health information, though not as good as was the physician for clinical problem histories.

Slack [155] also used branching sequences to provide patient education when the interview indicated the patients' need to learn about their medical problems. He used the "Don't understand" response as an indication to branch to educational sequences to teach the meaning of medical terms. He was initially concerned with how patients would accept the computer, so he concluded each interview with questions designed to ascertain the patient's reaction to the program; and Slack [154] reported that patients were highly favorable to the use of a computer as a medical history-taker. Generally the patient-machine rapport was quickly established, and patients earnestly participated in the medical interview. Attendants reported that gynecology patients routinely indicated a preference for the computer as an asker of questions dealing with subjects of a personal or private nature. Slack [148, 152] later added nutritional and psychological counseling to his interviewing programs. Slack's allergy history questionnaire was translated into Spanish and demonstrated with a LINC in Santiago, Chile [146]. By 1969 Slack reported having conducted approximately 800 computer-based interviews at the University of Wisconsin Hospitals; and he and his colleagues had conducted clinical trials on histories designed for patients with a variety of problems, such as bronchogenic carcinoma, epilepsy, and psychiatric problems, as well as thyroid and gastroenterology disorders [147].

In the 1970s Slack and Slack [153] moved to the Harvard Medical School where he continued his work with computer-based patient histories, now using a DEC PDP-9 computer that was programmed similar to its predecessor LINC. Bloom [13] and others in Slack's group described a program they called Converse, developed as a variant of their original MUMPS-based questionnaire program that provided faster response times for display screens. Converse was a means to work with the computer, for the most part in English, to construct, edit, and operate computer-based interviews, and to analyze responses and generate written summaries.

Converse was based on writing the text for the interview, frame by frame, with the text of each frame to be displayed when the interview was conducted. In addition to choices for the "yes," "no," "don't know," and "don't understand" responses, Slack added a fifth choice, "skip it," to allow a patient the option of not responding to a question. In 1980 Slack's group added an interview for headaches [147]. Slack summarized and published his extensive experience in *A History of Computerized Medical Interviews* [147].

In conjunction with subsequent studies of patient-computer dialogue, Mayne and associates [106, 107] at the Mayo Clinic described an experimental project to obtain automated self-administered patient histories using an IBM 7040 computer with an experimental graphics display terminal that projected photographic images stored on 16-mm color film. The patient responded to displayed questions by using a light pen to touch response areas arranged over the projected image. The computer then printed a summary statement for each patient. Mayne asked approximately 300 questions answerable by "yes" or "no"; using branching secondary questions for "yes" responses to obtain more details about the patient's symptoms. In a study of 154 Mayo Clinic patients, Mayne reported that patients' reactions were favorable and patients' performance was successful and that physicians' reactions were generally favorable. He also reported and that agreement between the automated questionnaire in comparison with the traditional record was 94 % for the patient's chief complaint and 95 % for all symptoms and for past surgery and past illness information. Mayne concluded that given the total set of patients' responses, the performance of the automated medical history for data collection was substantially better than that of physicians.

Also at the Mayo Clinic, Kiely and associates [94] reported their evaluation of the histories obtained from patients who used a visual display terminal with a light-pen selector and a television-tube display developed by Lockheed. They used 600 display screens for a patient-entered general history and a physician-entered set of results of a physical examination and reported that preliminary testing of physician reaction suggested that internists would be willing to use such a system when it was fully developed.

However, in 1969 the Mayo Clinic group concluded that the high cost of the equipment necessary to administer automated questionnaires with individual computer terminals precluded their large-scale use in patient care [109]. Accordingly, from a stored library of questions, they developed a computer generated, pencil-and-paper questionnaire, with patient-identification on each patient's questionnaire. The patient responded to each question by placing a pencil mark in appropriate positions for "yes" or "no." When the forms were passed through an optical mark-sense scanner, the responses were read into the computer, which would then generate an appropriate second-level questionnaire for more detailed information; and the computer could then go on to develop an individual third-level questionnaire.

In a series of evaluations comparing the same history questions given to patients by the mark-sense paper-and-pencil questionnaire and a card-sort method, as pioneered by Collen [42], the Mayo group found that patients preferred the paper-and-pencil format, and concluded that a mark-sense paper-and-pencil questionnaire offered substantial advantages over a card-sort questionnaire. They also reported that their first-level questionnaire showed a correct recording of the chief complaint to be 93.8 %, when compared with the physicians' records; and more than 99 % of all summary sheets contained some useful information when compared to their physician-recorded medical records [105]. However, after a few years of use, the Mayo internists discontinued using the paper-and-pencil mark-sense questionnaire for their patients, whose medical problems were considered too complex. In addition, the paper questionnaires were judged not useful for determining the urgency of a patient's problems. Although the clinicians had been initially enthusiastic, after months of use they concluded that the questionnaires accumulated too many positive but unimportant responses that they then had to pursue, and that the data collected were not sufficiently helpful in making clinical decisions [108].

Kanner [92] at the University of Kentucky College of Medicine had his patients complete a pencil-and-paper questionnaire, following which a secretary entered the positive answers, in medical textual language, into a file in a programmed electric typewriter – the IBM Magnetic Tape/Selectric Typewriter. The secretary was then able to leaf through the file containing the answered questions and whenever a positive response was observed, the machine was directed to advance the memory tape to the correct position. The typewriter then automatically typed out the response; and the responses on the magnetic tape could be transferred to a computer for printout. Kanner [91] later replaced his paper forms with data processing cards on which the patients marked their responses; the cards were then processed by a Hewlett-Packard programmable calculator with a built-in tape cassette and a punched card reader. Strong [164] at the Massachusetts Institute of Technology (MIT) developed an off-line questionnaire device called the Question and Response Kit, which presented question frames printed on a linear plastic tape that also stored the branching logic for the questions. Given the patient's responses, the logic program determined the next frame to be presented. The responses were stored on magnetic tape, and after the questionnaire had been completed by the patient, the magnetic tape on which the responses were stored was read into the computer, which then generated the printout.

Barnett and associates [7] at the Massachusetts General Hospital began to use automated history taking in the late 1960s. Their self-administered questionnaire contained "yes" or "no" questions, multiple-choice questions, and free-text questions. They used a visual display computer terminal for the patient-administered history interview that enabled both the entry of textual responses to open ended questions on a keyboard and the selection of responses to multiple choice questions by touching with a finger, a capacitance sensitive wire overlaying the response to the question [165]. Following the interview, a summary was printed and made available to the physician. After the physician had approved and signed the report, it was placed in the patient's paper-based medical record.

Barnett's group also evaluated their computer-based history. They compared the patients' responses to the computer-based history with the histories recorded by physicians in their standard medical records. They reported that for their automated medical history, patients' attitudes were favorable, but that physicians' attitudes were mixed. The automated histories recorded more items than were found in the physician-recorded medical records, but there was a high degree of agreement between the items in the computer's summary and the physician-recorded summaries [65].

Yarnall and associates [193] reported that in a general medical clinic, an automated screening history was favorably accepted by 96 % of patients; and time saving was claimed by physicians in 77 % of the cases. Although false positive responses were noted, the greatest usefulness of the automated history to physicians was the recording of negative responses, which helped them to focus on real problems.

At the end of the 1960s, a group at MIT and Harvard Medical School's affiliated Beth Israel Hospital surveyed self-administered medical histories and provided a bibliography of 180 references on questionnaires used between 1961 and 1969 [27, 163]. They described the automated questionnaire devices of 27 manufacturers and concluded that there did not yet exist a device that fully satisfied the requirements for automated medical histories [27, 164].

In the early 1970s there was an increase in commercial interest in automated patient histories that would meet the needs at the time for the more than 200 automated multiphasic health testing programs operating in the United States. Among the first of these commercial systems was that developed by Haessler [68], and marketed by Searle Medidata, Inc. Although most history takers used CRT display terminals, Searle's terminal used a carousel projection system with 320 questions, each contained on a quadrant of a 35-mm slide. The top half of the displayed screen was occupied by the question; and from two to five response choices were displayed next to five buttons along the right-hand margin of the screen. The display terminal was connected to a computer, programmed to permit branching to any of the questions depending on the patient's responses. The patient's responses were stored in the computer, which generated the history report when the interview was completed. The advantage with this terminal was that it could project questions and graphics in color; the disadvantage was that only the vendor could change a question by remaking the slide. Also, the system was expensive for its time. After three revisions and experience with 7,000 patients per month, Haessler [69] reported that although most patients felt comfortable with the system, physicians' attitudes were reserved. A trial with the program at Kaiser Permanente had resulted in similar findings, and with time, Searle abandoned this technological approach to automated histories.

With the objective of better integrating the automated medical history into their medical information system, Brunjes [25] at Yale University classified patient's symptoms in a three-dimensional matrix based on body systems and functions, abnormal symptoms, and physical signs together with the source of the information, such as from the patient, physician, or laboratory.

Goldstein [62] at NIH attempted to facilitate the entry of the patient history by physicians by providing them with lists of numbered phrases. The first-level list contained 25 organ systems, and the physician selected the organ system appropriate to the patient's problem. The program then presented a corresponding second-level listing of problems. A third-level list of modifiers to the selected symptoms was then available. The physician chose appropriate phrases from these lists in order to construct the history. The computer program then arranged the phrases to present the final history, which was in a detailed, chronological order.

Waxman [181] did an evaluation of paper-based self-administered questionnaires for new office patients seen by a five-physician group practice in internal medicine in Washington, DC. This approach, in which the responses to the questions were then keyed into a computer terminal, generated a printout of the history, which in turn saved 20–30 min for each new patient workup. In this low-volume situation, the program offset the computer cost by about $12 per history.

Friedman and associates [56] at the University of Wisconsin used the telephone as a low-cost, easy-to-use, and widely available computer terminal. The history questions were recorded on tape; with a minicomputer-controlled stereo tape recorder, the tape could be stopped at any desired location. When a patient telephoned the voice-response unit, the voice-activated unit picked up the call, and the computer started the tape recorder. A spoken message instructed the user to enter the appropriate response via the keypad on the telephone. A "Y" was dialed if the answer was *yes*; an "N" was dialed if the answer was *no*; an "I" was dialed if the patient did not know the answer; an appropriate number was dialed to answer a multiple choice question. The responses were then decoded and used by the computer to make a decision to skip to a new question, to start a pre-recorded verbal message, or to stop the tape.

Buchan [26], in an office practice in Troy, Ohio, used a standard Eastman Super 8-mm movie-film camera with single-frame exposure capability, to photograph individual medical history questions. Fifty feet of color film were mounted in an endless-loop film cartridge and displayed by a projector, in which the projected film could be selectively frozen on a single frame or advanced at 6, 12, 18, or 24 frames per second under software control. The displayed questions were also accompanied by a voice presentation of the questions, such as for foreign-language narration. A microprocessor was programmed to control the variable film frame advances and the audio cassette tape drives. Buchan reported a substantial patient preference for this phototerminal questionnaire presentation over CRT terminal presentation for a small sample of patients and noted that on the basis of cost-per-problem discovery, it compared favorably with other self-administered medical history systems.

Of 17 OISs reviewed by Henley and Wiederhold [81], all clinical sites collected and stored in their computer-based records – by one means or another – some data elements of the patient history, most in coded format supplemented with some text. Only one OIS, the Duke TMR, used a patient-administered history system. In 1970 the Duke group had begun to use a self-administered (by patients) history questionnaire containing 389 questions. The forms were read by an optical scanner on to magnetic tape, from which the data were transmitted to an IBM 360 computer, operating in a batch mode. The system was programmed to store the data and to generate the summary reports for the physicians [167]. In 1971 the Duke group had developed several subspecialty questionnaires, with patients responding to questions displayed on a computer-driven cathode ray tube [101]. By 1972 they had processed almost 3,000 patients' histories; doctors using them reported substantial time savings [100].

By 1973 approximately 7,000 histories had been processed by the Duke approach, which included a number of subspecialty histories [78]. Among these was a psychiatry screening questionnaire for a general medical clinic, used to elicit degrees of anxiety, depression, and alcoholism, and a neurological questionnaire, first used in 1970 [78]. Duke's headache questionnaire contained 173 questions; only about one-third of which were presented to any given patient, depending on the type of headache and the complexity of the patient's problems. Each question presented to the patient was selected by the computer program on the basis of the answers to the preceding questions [160]. The Duke group also evaluated the use of an audio system, with prerecorded questions presented on a magnetic audio cassette tape. The patient would listen to the spoken questions and then respond on a keyboard with "yes," "no," "don't understand," or "repeat." The group concluded that the audio mode of automated history taking was the more effective approach when the patient population was of borderline literacy [76].

Warner [180] used a self-administered questionnaire for patients in his multiphasic screening program in Salt Lake City. Questions were presented to the patients on a terminal displaying a one-digit number preceding each question. The patients used a numerical keyboard to enter the numbers corresponding to the questions to which their answer was "yes." Warner used a list of 320 questions, of which at least 50 had to be answered. Warner's group used a sequential Bayesian approach to direct the course of the computer-based history and to arrive at a list of likely diagnoses based on the patient's responses to the questions. The patient would be presented with a sequence of questions until the Bayesian program indicated that the probability of the patient having a particular diagnosis exceeded 90 %. This diagnosis would then be suggested on the history printout, accompanied with a list of the questions to which the patient had answered "yes."

Williams [190] at the University of Illinois, Urbana, also approached medical history taking by considering the likely diseases, and focusing on those questions necessary to elicit a diagnostic set of symptoms. They observed that the development of such logic occasionally flowed in the reverse direction, an approach they called retrograde mapping.

By the mid-1970s considerable experience had been accumulated regarding self-administered patient questionnaires using a variety of technologies. In 1975 McLean and associates [120] published an extensive bibliography of manual, automated, and computer-processed medical histories that contained 720 citations from the world literature. Also in 1975, Wakefield and Yarnall [177] published an extensive compilation of self-administered medical history questionnaires that included 17 different design approaches and 105 examples. They described 24 paper-and-pencil questionnaires that were put directly into the medical record without processing; 3 questionnaires that were manually processed by some form of manual review; 5 machine-processed questionnaires using an off-line programmed electric typewriter; 18 off-line computer-processed punched cards or mark-sense forms; 4 online computer-processed questionnaires using teletypewriters; 10 computer-based systems using images stored on film strips, carousel slides, or microfiche; 1 audio system for patients to listen to the questions; and 21 cathode ray tube terminal systems for computer-based, interactive branching questionnaires.

The continuing difficulties in obtaining automated patient histories and their associated high costs produced a few evaluations on the comparative cost-effectiveness of the alternative technologies available. The medical history takers were evaluated as to the usefulness of the history questions and the acceptability and costs of the history taker. The reliability or reproducibility of a question was measured by the consistency with which it elicited the same response. Collen and associates [41] studied patients' responses to a set of 204 questions presented on a printed form in comparison with the same questions individually presented on pre-punched cards, so that each patient answered each question twice. They found that patients answered "yes" to the same 7 % of questions by either method; 20 % changed an answer from "yes" to "no" on the second or retest questionnaire, but less than 2 % of questions were changed from "no" to "yes." Neither the method of questioning, nor the order in which the questions were asked, significantly changed the answers. It was evident that, when a patient said "no" to a question, the response was a reliable one; but a "yes" response was more changeable, possibly indicating more uncertainty on the part of the patient and suggesting that "yes" responses needed more detailed secondary branching questions to obtain reliable information.

The validity of answers to history questions was studied by Hershberg and associates [82] using 20 screening, first-level questions from the medical history questionnaire used at the Lahey Clinic. They measured the sensitivity of each question answered "yes" by patients who had the disease associated with the symptom addressed by the question, as well as the specificity of the question for obtaining a "no" response by patients without the disease. Depending on the criteria applied, they found great variability in the validity of the history questions. They concluded that because of their extremely low sensitivity and specificity values, certain questions appeared to have only limited usefulness in screening for disease states. This study confirmed the need for second- and third-level branching of questions to obtain more valid responses from patients.

An extensive evaluation of the cost-effectiveness of automated medical history taking in ten office practices with a variety of practice types and specialties, was conducted by Bolt, Beranek and Newman in their Computer Aids in Physician's Offices Project [17]. After patients completed 1,000 automated histories, which took between 30 and 70 min per history, the group reported that important positive responses were recorded that were not recorded with the conventional, physician-taken histories. Close to half of the physicians were able to save from 5 to 15 min in history taking time by using the automated history. However, the group concluded that physicians would be unwilling to pay for the expensive terminals.

Although in the 1980s a variety of technologies were available in the effort to decrease the costs and improve the effectiveness of automated patient histories, most physicians still used paper-and-pencil questionnaires in their office practice.

Psychiatrists began to automate interviews for their patients in the 1980s. When medical transcriptionists began using computer-based word-processing programs for physician-dictated reports, this permitted direct entry of data into the computer-based patient record. Direct voice input of limited data sets for some subspecialties, such as radiology and orthopedics, was also being tested by the end of 1980s.

Developers of OISs were resigned to the reality that systems for physicians to enter clinical information, such as the results of physical examinations, would likely remain experimental until more powerful clinical workstations would permit free text and voice-recognition input. By the late 1980s, however, advances in clinical workstations offered hope that they might provide a more useful interface for physicians. Barnett's group at the Massachusetts General Hospital used a Hewlett-Packard (IBM-compatible) workstation with a mouse pointer for selecting items from a controlled vocabulary shown on the display, and they used the keyboard for entering narrative text. An interactive, branching, hierarchical representation of terms that represented physical findings allowed the physician to move up or down the vocabulary tree structure, and to construct an appropriate report similar to that found in the traditional written paper record.

Williams [191] at the University of Illinois, Urbana, used an Apple Macintosh to expand on his prior work using the PLATO (Programmed Logic for Automated Teaching Operations) system to display in one window a graphic sketch of the body area being examined, which the user could modify by copying icons onto the anatomic caricature. From another window in the display, the user could select the appropriate terms representing observations or interpretations. The graphic screen and text was stored and could be retrieved, together with findings from previous examinations.

The hospitalized patient's history is usually obtained by the physician interviewing the patient (or a family member when the patient is incapable of providing a history). The results are then entered into the patient's hospital record by the physician. Whereas ambulatory patients can provide much of their medical history by responding to a formatted questionnaire, hospitalized patients are usually in bed when they are interviewed; to have the medical history entered directly into the computer by a patient in bed is generally not feasible.

Some investigators, however, have tested a method for patients' self-administered histories. Weed [183] used self-administered questionnaires with "yes" or "no" cards that were then entered by a keyboard into the computer. Weed also used a display terminal that allowed ten choices for the patient in response to each question, with the patient responding by touching the desired choice displayed on the screen. When the patient's history was completed, a computer printout was produced showing the patient's responses by body systems, in a narrative form. Alternatively, Warner's group at the LDS Hospital used interviewer-administered histories, with the interviewer asking the questions and entering the responses into the computer terminal, as guided by the HELP system, which later guided the physician through a set of possible diagnoses [79].

In the 1950s, physical examination data were recorded manually health practitioners and listed in the patient's paper-based record by body systems, often in an unstandardized format. For a routine physical examination, physicians sometimes used paper-based forms to check "positive" or "negative" to a preprinted list of possible findings. Physicians would then write their related comments as free text in designated areas. The data from completed encounter forms were filed in manila folders or envelopes that were stored in the Medical Records Department. In their day-to-day patient care, physicians accepted the need to complete a variety of paper forms, so the use of paper encounter forms became a familiar data acquisition mode for them. Later, perhaps years later, information on the forms could be entered into the patient's electronic medical record.

Often physicians found paper forms to be inflexible in their organization and limiting in the way they could record unanticipated information. In addition, paper forms precluded direct interaction with the computer for online decision support. Perhaps more important, time elapsed between the recording of the data on paper and entry of those data into the computer where they became available to clinicians in the practice.

Thompson [168] observed that a physician's time was the most expensive cost-per-unit of time in health care, and it was hoped that the computer might help save time in recording the results of physical examinations. Initially the approaches to entering physical findings into the computer were similar to those used for entering the patient's history, except that physical findings were obtained from the health practitioner rather than from the patient. Just as for patients' histories, paper-and-pencil check-off forms were used by some health practitioners to record findings, which could then be entered by clerks into the computer. Some physicians marked their findings on specially designed forms, readable by optical character or mark sense readers. For simple examinations, such as those required for routine employment or school health evaluations, most findings could be checked as "negative" or "positive," and abnormalities could be described further by writing prose for later keyboard entry into the computer. The data were then printed by the computer in the format desired by the practitioner; text was printed just as it had been entered.

Hammond and associates [78] at Duke University implemented in their TMR system a general physical examination program based on a form that allowed the physicians to enter abnormalities by checking appropriate items. Special check sheets were constructed by the different subspecialties to fit their particular needs, and physicians would select the appropriate form for their use. The completed forms were than submitted to a computer for processing and for generating a summary.

Slack and associates [155] at the University of Wisconsin described the use of a LINC computer, with a cathode ray display (CRT) display, a keyboard entry, and a Teletype printer, for the direct entry of the physical examination findings by the physician without any clerical intermediary. The terminal displayed a series of questions for the physician representing the usual findings recorded in such an examination, and presented multiple-choice response options similar to Slack's history questionnaire, where "yes" indicated the presence of an abnormality and "no" indicated its absence. The system also permitted "uncertain" and "not examined". At the end of each major section (for example, head, chest, abdomen, or extremities), the physician was asked to enter relevant findings not included in the program, and these entries then became part of the patient's record. Slack first tested this program on the gynecology service and reported the reaction to the program by participating physicians was one of general approval.

Juergens [90] at the Mayo Clinic reported the use of a television-type video display tube with a light-pen selector for the physician to enter physical examination findings. The physician selected from displayed message elements by pointing the light pen to the appropriate item; with the click of the pen switch, the data were entered into the computer. Physicians could enter free text by using the terminal keyboard. The authors reported, however, that the structured displays were sufficiently comprehensive so that almost no use was made of the keyboard. They tested their approach with findings from examination of the heart and found that when physicians entered their findings with the patient present, it took them almost twice as long as it did when they wrote out their findings in traditional fashion. On the other hand, the authors found the positive acceptance of the new technique by both physicians and patients to be encouraging.

5.5 Examples of Early Office Information Systems (OISs) for General Care

Primary general practice medicine requires a broad domain of medical knowledge. Primary care generalists are usually the first practitioners seen by patients before visiting specialized physicians. Primary care is sometimes considered to require a simpler level of medical technology, because primary care physicians often refer patients to clinical specialists for complex procedures. In reality however, primary care generalists must have a broad domain of medical knowledge, for they encounter a great variety of diseases.

Vallbona [171] emphasized the important potential for computer-based office systems to provide clinical information support for primary care physicians. Computer-based information systems for general primary care in office practice have to satisfy the same functional and technical requirements that apply to other OISs. These include patient identification, registration and scheduling, administrative and business functions, and clinical information. Most primary care is provided in solo or group physician offices. The early OISs described in this section include published descriptions of computer-based systems that were operational prior to the year 2000. These OISs sometimes then expanded into hospitals and joined the hospital information systems to become fully developed medical information systems.

The earliest reported computer-based OIS was described by Schwichtenberg [144] when the Lovelace Foundation undertook, as a project for the United States Air Force Research and Development Command, the development of a method of recording on punch cards the detailed medical information for members of the US Air Force program, *Man in Space*. Schwichtenberg credited Robertson of Asheville, North Carolina, with first using machine-readable, mark-sense punch cards in medical practice. Schwichtenberg used specially printed mark-sense cards to record information collected from medical examinations of Air Force pilots at the Lovelace Clinic. The information included each pilots' medical history and physical findings, and reports from specialty examinations, clinical laboratories, and x-ray examinations. Some history and physical findings were also recorded by the medical examiner on pre-coded data-entry sheets, which were then sent with the mark-sensed cards to an IBM facility for processing and storing in their database. After the Man in Space program was taken over by the National Aeronautics and Space Administration (NASA), this punched-card and patient record system was continued for a time for astronaut candidates.

Schenthal [139] and Sweeney at Tulane Medical School developed an OIS that used a computer to process medical record data for outpatients. They used mark-sense cards to record information, and a mark-sense card reader to submit the information to an IBM 650 computer equipped with magnetic-tape storage. In their pilot study, their OIS contained information from clinic patients stored on magnetic tape. The database consisted of coded diagnoses, physical findings, sigmoidoscopy reports, clinical laboratory test results, and chest x-ray reports as well as medical histories derived from the 195 questions of the Cornell Medical Index. In their first 12 months of operation, their system held the medical records of patients in the Tulane University Cancer Detection Clinic. Schenthal [141] then used the computer to search the stored records of 361 women seen during the prior 12 months for reports of significant cardiac murmurs. He thereby demonstrated the ability of their system to locate rapidly, from a large collection of patients' records, a group of patients meeting a desired combination of requirements. The time required for the investigation of clinical records could thereby be reduced from man-months to machine-minutes.

By 1963 the Tulane group had stored on magnetic tape more than 2,000 active outpatient records in 8 clinical specialties [141]. They used checklists for collecting data from each specialty clinic, and keypunch operators entered English-language text for comments not included in the checklists [194]. The group soon modified their database design from the original fixed-field, fixed-length, records on magnetic tape to variable-field, variable-length records more suited the storage of natural language text. Sweeney also developed a program, GYPSY, for the storage, retrieval, and analysis of data in patients' records. Sweeney was the first Professor of Computer Medicine in the United States, and one of his principal contributions was to introduce physicians to the direct use of computers in ambulatory patient care.

In 1971 the Computer-Stored Ambulatory Record (COSTAR) system was developed by Barnett and associates as the OIS for the Harvard Community Health Plan (HCHP), a comprehensive group-practice medical-care program established in 1969 in Boston. The COSTAR system used the Massachusetts General Hospital Utility Multi-Programming System (MUMPS) language and operating system. Barnett [4] described COSTAR's objectives: provide HCHP with a membership file; improve the availability of patient care information in accessibility, timeliness of retrieval, legibility, and organization; provide automatic retrieval and display of selected information; provide information processing for administrative services as well as for clinical laboratory, x-ray, and electrocardiogram reports; provide the data retrieval and analysis required by HCHP management for operations, budgeting, and planning; support programs in quality assurance; provide reports required by government agencies; and conduct a broad range of research projects [4, 5, 63, 66].

Barnett [4] described the COSTAR computer-based patient record as containing information from each encounter with a patient, including interactions in the health center, emergency ward, and affiliated hospital – as well as information from telephone communications – all captured by completion of structured encounter forms, which were the system's basic data input documents. The COSTAR encounter forms were manually completed by the health professionals at the time of each patient visit. On these forms, physicians recorded their diagnoses, their orders for diagnostic tests and treatments, and their patient's disposition. Different encounter forms were designed for each of the medical specialties, as well as for nursing care and for social services. A form was printed for the patient's first visit; and individualized forms were computer-generated for subsequent visits. These served also as progress notes for each visit. For a routine visit to the health center, the patient's identifying data were recorded on the encounter form by a clerical person before the physician saw the patient.

Administrative data were entered by clerks using remote terminals connected by telephone lines to the computer located in the Laboratory of Computer Science at the Massachusetts General Hospital. Medical information was entered by the patients' physicians on a precoded entry form, with provision for appropriate modifiers and free text. Space was provided for diagnoses and medications that were not among the precoded options. Data on the forms were than coded by record-room personnel using a code directory, and then entered into the computer by the keyboard of a visual display terminal. The code directory was a structured list of problems, medications, and laboratory tests that had been recorded in the COSTAR system during the previous 7 years.

The encounter forms were structured to meet the specific needs of each of the Harvard Community Health Plans' 15 clinical specialties. For example, the pediatric encounter form contained a list of problems and treatments most commonly encountered in pediatrics. Self-encoding checklists reduced the amount of time for physicians to record clinical information and reinforced their use of a common vocabulary. The physician could choose to enter free text and to link each free-text comment to a particular medical problem, and this enabled the selective retrieval of all data about the problem. HCHP physicians could also dictate notes, which were then entered into the computer the following morning. All computer-stored data were available on demand from a computer terminal display, or by computer-generated printouts requested through the HCHP medical records department.

For scheduled patient visits, a pre-specified set of computer-generated records was automatically prepared and distributed to the care area prior to the visit. The basic data-display format was the status report, which was produced for all scheduled visits. The status report was designed to provide an index and summary of the patient's current medical status, and it included any prior hospital discharge data, currently active medications, important previously taken medications, a list of laboratory tests with the date and results of the most recent tests, and any outstanding consultations. A status report was also generated after the entry of new information to the record. This report also included all active diagnoses, and the current medications [66].

After a patient visit and completion of the encounter forms, the computer-generated output was destroyed to avoid the cost of having the medical record room handling and filing the paper chart. A paper medical record was available on each patient, but it contained only archival data, electrocardiograms, diagrams of lesions, communications such as postal letters, the complete text of pathology or radiology reports, and the original medical history questionnaire that had been completed by the patient [4]. The printed-paper encounter forms were clipped to the patient's medical record binder in chronological order to form a computer-generated, paper-based patient's chart. Only the latest patient status report remained in the patient's chart.

Barnett [10] recognized the need for a metadatabase defining all terms that were allowed in patient records. Each element in the directory corresponded to a unique COSTAR code; and each COSTAR code was assigned to a particular division in the directory (diagnoses, laboratory tests, and other data). This directory of terms served as the unifying element that enabled users of COSTAR to identify specific information among the structured database.

Barnett located visual display terminals in all patient care areas to provide access to the full computer-based patient record. Thus, the physicians could review the status report, encounter reports, laboratory data, and patient visits associated with any specific problem, and they could obtain a flow chart of any problem, laboratory test, or medication. Physicians reported the selective recording and retrieval of specific types of data as flow charts to be a valuable supplement to the information available on their status report. Flow charts, specific to individual specialties, were found to be particularly useful for tracking the measurements, immunizations, and developmental milestones of children, and for tracking the prenatal visits of obstetrical patients. The computer's ability to display information in a variety of formats without redundant entry of data was a distinct advantage over the manual system [4].

In the 1970s Barnett's COSTAR system was unique as an operational OIS which had replaced most of the functions of the traditional, paper-based medical record. In 1973 the Harvard Community Health Plan COSTAR system had been operational for 2 years, maintaining the medical records for 20,000 patients who had made 80,000 visits [66]. Teletype terminals that permitted interactive order entry were readily available. Barnett was reluctant to use clerical personnel to enter physician's orders, because he did not want physicians to bypass the clinical decision support capabilities. This decision support included online checking for the completeness, accuracy, and acceptability of an order as well as for providing physicians with pertinent information about specific patients. COSTAR's online, interactive system could check the physician's order against data in the computer for drug-drug and drug-laboratory interactions, as well as for known allergies. Hence Barnett felt it important for the physicians to perform the order entry [6].

In 1975 Barnett reported that the COSTAR system had added a quality assurance program that detected deviations from a set of standards developed by the HCHP physicians and provided immediate feedback to physicians. In 1976 Barnett [4] reported that the HCHP employed a staff of 34 (full-time equivalent) physicians and 23 (full-time equivalent) nurses who handled 550 daily office visits from a membership of 37,500 persons.

The COSTAR system at the time operated on a DEC PDP-15 computer located in the laboratory's computer center connected by leased telephone cable to the HCHP facilities. Twenty display terminals and several printers were located at HCHP for COSTAR's use. The medical information in COSTAR was available 24 h a day, 7 days a week. COSTAR also provided a patient tracking system to monitor the continuity of care. If a physician checked the box on the encounter form that was labeled with "follow-up important," and if there had not been a visit with this physician in a specified time period, the computer automatically generated a medical record printout of the patient's visits since the date on which that physician requested the follow-up visit. This prompted the physician to make a decision about the need for contacting the patient to make an appointment.

By 1978, COSTAR had gone through four revisions in its design at the HCHP, and Barnett [8] described an expanded version called COSTAR 5. This was developed in collaboration with industry and with the support of the Intramural Division of the National Center for Health Services Research. Barnett [9] noted that COSTAR 5 was being implemented at seven different medical sites.

By the early 1980s COSTAR in HCHP had added an accounts receivable and billing module, an expanded patient registration and patient scheduling module, a report-generator module, a medical query language with increased data-retrieval capabilities, and an enhanced medical record module, together with data protection and backup capabilities. COSTAR enabled replacement of the traditional paper-based medical record, with direct entry of patient data from encounter forms, by clerks using CRT display terminals. The availability of the patient record in COSTAR facilitated the preparation of bills, follow-up reminders, and quality-assurance procedures.

Kuhn [96] reported that in December 1980 in the United States, there were 26 operational COSTAR installations and 11 planned installations. At the Laboratory of Computer Science, the cost of COSTAR development was estimated at 2–3 million dollars, and the development and transfer efforts were estimated to have totaled 10 million dollars. Kuhn also commented on the importance of the federal government's support of activities directed toward the transfer and commercialization of COSTAR: the National Center for Health Services Research supported the software design and developmental activities; supported the preparation of technical and user documentation; sponsored the installation of COSTAR as a demonstration site; and awarded a contract to the MITRE Corporation to facilitate the transfer of a COSTAR-5 to a community-based network of five clinics in San Diego County.

Bowie [19] and Fiddleman [52], at the MITRE Corporation, described how COSTAR had also been supported by Digital Equipment Corporation (DEC). In 1978, when DEC decided not to market COSTAR, the National Center chose the

MITRE Corporation as DEC's replacement. Kerlin [93] at the MITRE Corporation noted that COSTAR's early test sites were funded by the federal government and affirmed that the commercial sector did not view COSTAR as a viable product to market. To encourage the transition of COSTAR from a government-financed program to a commercial product, the federal government supported the MITRE Corporation, from October 1979 through February 1983, to debug, test, and document what would be a public domain version of COSTAR.

The number of COSTAR systems grew to 73 in 1982 [93], and the importance of COSTAR was reflected by the inclusion of two full sessions of papers on COSTAR in the1980 Symposium on Computer Applications of Medical Computing (SCAMC). By the end of the 1980s the COSTAR system was widely disseminated in the United States, being used in more than 120 sites. It was available from a number of different vendors, and a magnetic-tape copy of the public-domain programs could be obtained from the COSTAR Users Group [3]. The COSTAR system was one of the most important of Barnett's contributions to medical informatics, and it was one of the first OISs to provide a patient record that was fully computer-based.

The MUMPS programming language, which was used in the development of COSTAR, had general applicability as an operating system and became the basic technological groundwork for large, multi-facility medical information systems, such the Veterans Administration's system. The MUMPS technology also provided the groundwork for commercial vendors, such as Meditech and Epic.

In the 1960s the problem-oriented patient record pioneered by Weed was applied to office and hospital patients' records at the University of Vermont in Burlington. Using as an example of a typical case history – an elderly ambulatory patient with 11 different medical problems – Weed [184] described how to collect the data to form the patient's record, how to complete the medical problem list, how to prepare a diagnosis and treatment plan, how to maintain narrative progress notes and flow sheets, and how to provide a discharge summary. In addition to the use of Weed's system at the Given Health Care Center of the University of Vermont [18, 169, 170], computer-based, problem-oriented patient records were deployed in office practices. Hall [70] described the successful use of such records in a nephrology clinic in a large medical center, and Cross [45] used problem-oriented records in a private physician's office in a small town. Problem-oriented records were also used by nurse practitioners to prepare flow sheets for medical problems [142].

Weed described the problem oriented medical record as the basis for his hospital-based Problem-Oriented Medical Information System (PROMIS). Weed applied his problem-oriented approach to all data in the patient's medical record, including the patient's history, physical examination, progress notes, and record summaries. Weed helped to direct physicians into a more structured approach for collecting and documenting patient care data in the medical record.

In 1963 Collen and associates at Kaiser Permanente were operating automated multiphasic testing systems for ambulatory patients in both the San Francisco and Oakland medical centers [33, 36]. In 1968 a subsidiary computer center containing an IBM 360/50 computer was established in Kaiser Permanente's Department of

Medical Methods Research to develop a prototype medical information system that included clinical laboratory and pharmacy subsystems [37]. Their multiphasic testing system already provided patients' identification data, appointment scheduling, specimen labels, quality control procedures, clinical laboratory test results, and physician's interpretations of electrocardiograms and x-rays. Their system also included clinical decision support, with alert and warning signals for findings of results outside of predetermined limits, advice rules for secondary sequential testing, and "consider" rules for likely diagnoses. All patient data were stored in computer-based patient records as well as in research databases.

The automated multiphasic testing programs in San Francisco and in Oakland each encompassed the information for an average of 150 health checkups per day. For electrocardiograms, pathology, and radiology reports, an IBM magnetic tape/ selectric typewriter was used for processing written or dictated text. With slight modifications in their typing routines, secretaries used these typewriters to store, on analog magnetic tape, the patient's identification information together with the procedures performed, the results of diagnostic tests, and the physicians' reports. These data were transmitted to a magnetic tape receiver located in the central computer facility. By means of a digital data recorder-and-converter, a second tape was created in a digital form acceptable for input to the patient's computer-stored medical record in the IBM 360 computer.

In 1971 all patients' hospital and outpatient diagnoses began to be stored on computer tapes [34]. In the 1980s a regional clinical laboratory was established, and its computer was linked to the Kaiser Permanente regional computer center. In the 1990s Kaiser Permanente contracted with the vendor Epic to develop a medical information system for its nine-million members. By1992, laboratory, pathology, and radiology data – and by 1994 clinical data for outpatient visits – were all being stored in computer databases. By 2000, computer-stored patient data were available for 2.8 million Northern California Kaiser Permanente members [54], and by 2010 the Northern California Kaiser Permanente electronic patient record database contained more than 3 million active patients' records,

In 1969, engineers from the Lincoln Laboratory at MIT, in collaboration with physicians at the Beth Israel Hospital in Boston, and supported by contracts from the federal government, worked on an outpatient information system. The project's objectives were to develop computer-supported, problem-oriented protocols to help non-physician practitioners to provide care for patients who had common medical problems, such as headaches, low-back pains, upper-respiratory infections, and lower-urinary-tract infections. The computer-supported system was discontinued after a few years because it was more expensive than was a manual, paper-based system [61].

In 1969, Hammond and Stead [78] at Duke University began to develop a minicomputer-supported medical information system they called Generalized Medical Information System for Community Health (GEMISCH). The computer-stored records consisted of user-defined, fixed-length sections as well as variable length sections allowing for narrative text. The Duke group's stated objectives were for it to be error free; to be reliable; to have rapid response characteristics; to be operable 24 h a day, 7 days a week; and to have simple and precise input procedures acceptable for clerks, technicians, nurses, and physicians. For their system to be economically feasible, they added basic administrative functions.

In the 1970s with the availability of mass storage devices for minicomputers, the Duke Group recognized that these devices could be used for medical applications requiring large online databases. They planned to use the modularity of minicomputers to enable them to purchase the amount of computing power required, and to increase that power as the need developed. They considered the minicomputer to be especially well suited to the medical environment. Furthermore, a distributed network of minicomputers could provide the extensible framework upon which a responsive and reliable system could be built.

The Duke group's initial developmental effort began in their obstetrics clinic, with the goal of working toward the design and implementation of a generalized online information system utilizing minicomputers. They soon installed a clinical laboratory system designed to allow for the ordering and reporting of laboratory data. Data entry methods included both interactive video terminals and batch-processed mark-sense forms. During its initial development, the GEMISCH system was also used as a basis for the design of automated, self-administered questionnaires to elicit the patients' medical histories [101]. In 1974 GEMISCH applications were operated on a Digital Equipment Corporation (DEC) PDP-11 minicomputer and included a primary care system for their University Health Services Clinic.

By 1974 the system had been used to process more than 15,000 mark-sense patients' histories. Interactive questionnaires were also used, with visual display terminals for recording the histories of patients who had headaches, dizziness, low-back pain, or angina. By 1974 more than 6,000 obstetric patients' records had been processed, and encounter data for more than 1,000 patients per week were being entered into the system [73].

Confidentiality of patient data was assured by "protect" codes [74]. The Duke group also developed an information retrieval language that used basic statement types to enable users to retrieve selected subsets of records, to list specified information retrieved from the records, and to produce summary reports [178]. In 1975 they merged their programs into a higher-level language and an enhanced database management system, which they continued to call GEMISCH.

Wiederhold and associates [189] visited the Duke University Medical Center and described the status of the computing at that time. Their computer-based patient records now included diagnostic and treatment orders, laboratory test results, medications, and follow-up findings. The system was processing close to 30,000 patient visits per year in the internal medicine clinic, with some use of the system as well in the obstetrics clinic. Patients' data were for the most part recorded on paper encounter forms. Written text on the forms was entered into the computer by clerks using display terminal keyboards. Patients' histories and physical examination data were recorded on mark-sense forms for entry into the computer. Patient registration was done online by means of display-terminal and keyboard entry.

In 1975 the computer-stored record was limited to 16,000 characters. It included patient identification data, medical history and physical examination data, medical problems, diagnostic and treatment orders, laboratory test results, medications, and follow-up findings. Selected additional data for research purposes could also be stored. When a patient was seen in the clinic, the traditional paper-based medical record was available, containing the original encounter forms with narrative text from prior visits, supplemented by computer-generated printouts and summary reports from prior encounter forms.

The general development of the Duke system was supported in part by grants from the Robert Wood Johnson Foundation and the National Institutes of Health. By 1977 Duke had an enhanced database management system written in the GEMISCH language, which featured a modular design for the various administrative and clinical applications. Hammond [76] reported that more than 40,000 patients' records were maintained in online files, with about 60,000 annual encounters.

In 1980 the Duke group described their further development and experiences with their computer-based medical record system, which they now called The Medical Record system (TMR), and which was now operational within three settings: the University Health Services Clinic with an active file of 33,000 patients; the Woman's Clinic of the Department of Obstetrics and Gynecology with an active file of 7,000 patients [75]; and the Renal Dialysis Unit of the Durham Veterans Hospital with an active file of approximately 300 patients.

Duke University's TMR now used two PDP-11 minicomputers supported by DEC's RSX-11D and the UNIX operating systems. GEMISCH continued to be the name for the database management system, with a hierarchical data structure and a variable-length text section. GEMISCH records were accessed through an alphanumeric identification number or by the patient's name. TMR contained essential components of a computer-based, electronic patient record, and human interaction with TMR could function at an acceptable level [75].

Hammond [75, 76] considered the Duke data dictionary to be a key to the success of TMR. Their metathesaurus defined and coded all clinical variables. This provided the necessary flexibility to permit editing and to allow for the differences between medical specialties and outpatient clinics. It contained a medical vocabulary together with related information, such as algorithms, decision-making rules, and users' passwords. TMR was dictionary driven, and the TMR programs were modularly constructed. The monitor module controlled the program flow. The demographic module supported the collection of demographic, provider, and insurance data. Another module supported the input and display of patients' history and physical examination findings. The problem module supported the entry, deletion, and modification of patients' clinical problems as well as a problem-oriented chart review. The therapy module supported a formulary of prescribed drugs. The studies module supported the ordering of tests, the entry of test results, and the viewing of results. The flow module supported time-oriented presentations of patient's problems. The encounter module supported the entry of data associated with a patient's visit. The accounting module supported financial processes; and the appointment module supported Duke's multispecialty appointment system.

When a patient arrived for an appointment, a route sheet for the collection of data, a pre-visit medical summary, and results from studies of the previous four visits were printed [75]. The patient then saw the physician, who recorded data, orders, and prescriptions on the route sheet. The patient then met with a clerk, who entered the orders and requisitions, which were then printed out in the appropriate laboratories or clinical departments. The clerk also entered the patient's problems, procedures, and other data pertaining to the visit. The cost of the visit was then calculated and displayed, and a copy of the bill could be given to the patient.

Laboratory results were entered by the laboratory technologists as they became available. The print module then printed all components of the record, including various flow sheets and administrative, financial, and medical reports. TMR thus provided to physicians what Stead called a demand output; it provided physicians with problem-oriented records, time-oriented flow sheets, protocols, decision-support algorithms, and information about possible drug-drug interactions, as requested. By 1980, TMR was interfaced with Duke's hospital information system [75]. By 1981, TMR was used in the nephrology clinic in Durham's Veterans Administration Medical Center. Physicians there could write supplemental notes which were then entered into TMR as text [134].

In the 1980s, TMR became commercially available [96]. In 1981 the California Primary Physicians, a large internal medicine group in Los Angeles, purchased the system and implemented it with a PDP 11/45 computer from Digital Equipment Corporation, and they reported that the financial impact exceeded expectations [166]. Operating costs were reduced in their data processing, transcription, and laboratory departments due to reduction in dictation and forms processing costs and to more efficient procedures for reporting diagnostic information to the physicians.

In 1983 TMR had been implemented in 11 sites [77]. In its use at the Duke medical center, TMR did not replace the paper-based patient record, but it was used to produce the encounter notes and record summaries that kept the paper records current. Stead [159] called TMR a chartless record, not a paperless record; manual or word-processed textual narratives were still needed as a supplement to the electronic record when the physician wanted to describe in detail the reasoning behind a decision. By the late 1980s the TMR system at Duke contained records of more than 200,000 patients. TMR provided linkages to referring physicians; it responded to queries for data elements stored in the TMR database; and it supported inverted files for clinical research. TMR also provided clinical reminders, protocols, and decision rules. Stead and Hammond were an extraordinary physician-engineer team, working together through the 1970s and 1980s to develop a record system to meet the needs of Duke's medical center patients.

In 1971 Vallbona initiated an OIS at the Casa de Amigos Neighborhood Health Clinic in Houston, one of a network of seven neighborhood clinics, all staffed by physicians on the faculty of Baylor's Department of Medicine. The OIS was used to generate a supplement to the traditional paper-based records. Information was abstracted from each patient's paper chart by medical clerks. The information was then coded and entered into Baylor's computing system by punched cards. A diskette was then produced with the summaries of the patients' data, which were then entered into a minicomputer located in the clinic. The OIS provided a patient identification and appointment module; it provided a patient information file, which served as the database for a Health Illness Profile, with a list of each patient's problems, medications, health status of body systems, health risks, and prior hospitalizations; it provided protocols and algorithms to support examinations of patients for their diagnosis and treatment; and it provided a set of home-care plans for patients to follow.

By 1974 the clinic minicomputer contained more than 4,200 Health Illness profiles, which were retrievable on demand [172]. The Health Illness Profile, which was inserted at the front of each patient's paper chart, was considered by the physicians to be the most valuable module in their OIS [174], for it provided a concise summary of the important medical events in a patient's past experience with the clinic [47].

In 1971 Fakan, at the Medical Data Systems Corporation in Olmsted Falls, Ohio, provided an OIS called AUTOMED for close to 100 physicians in 32 different solo and group practices. Health professionals recorded data into paper-based medical records. Clerks then entered the data using keyboard display terminals connected by telephone lines to a UNIVAC computer. The OIS records contained patient identification data, history of present and past illnesses, physical examination data, a medical problem list, medical orders, and treatment plans. A variety of reports were printed in the physicians' offices. In most offices, the traditional paper based record was maintained, even though the computer-based record was readily accessible at any time. The OIS also provided business and accounting functions Henley and Wiederhold [81].

In 1971, Craemer in Brunswick, Maine, introduced an OIS to the U.S. Naval Air Station Dispensary, a primary care clinic serving close to 15,000 active-duty and retired Navy personnel and their dependents, with close to 20,000 office visits a year. Physicians dictated their notes, and the text was entered into the OIS by transcriptionists using display terminal keyboards. Patients' medical problems and diagnoses were then coded, and stored by keyboard entry. Laboratory findings were entered by technologists. Computer services were provided by a commercial vendor located 100 miles away. The medical record available during a patient's visit was a computer-generated abstract that contained a limited amount of medical information. More medical record information could be obtained within a few seconds from an online terminal, when it was needed during the visit Henley and Wiederhold [81].

In 1972 the Arizona Health Plan, a prepaid group practice in Phoenix, Arizona, began to use an OIS for a practice of close to 17,000 patients. Self-funded, this OIS used paper encounter forms for physicians to record data during the office visits. Clerks then entered the data into the computer-stored patient record. Patients' problem lists, medications, and brief medical summaries were retrievable by computer terminals and printouts. The OIS was also used as a means of monitoring clinical performance and utilization practices [61].

In 1972 Haas and Fleishli [67] at the University of Nebraska Medical Center used a time-sharing hospital mainframe IBM computer to provide an OIS for 17 family clinics throughout the city of Omaha. The clinics were run by different agencies, yet all entered data into a single central online database.

In 1973 the Regenstrief Medical Record system was developed by McDonald and associates at the Regenstrief Institute for Health Care and the Indiana University School of Medicine. This OIS was first implemented in the diabetes clinic of Wishard Memorial Hospital in Indianapolis. By 1977 the general medicine clinics, the renal clinic, and two community-based clinics located 3 miles from the central computer site had been added to the OIS. The system included the medical records of 19,000 ambulatory patients with 40,000 visits per year [115]. The Regenstrief Medical Record system used a PDP11/45 computer, which ran under the RSTS/E operating system. The computer programs were written in BASIC-PLUS. The system provided time-sharing services 24-h per-day, 7 days per-week. Patients' records within the medical record file contained data stored in a coded format, with some free-text entry as well. Within a given file, the data fields appeared in the same location in each patient's record [113]. A set of utility programs included commands for storing, editing, sorting, and reporting data, as well as for conducting administrative analyses. Other database files included the clinical laboratory subsystem, the pharmacy subsystem, the patient registry file, the patient appointment file, the physician registry file, the physician schedule file, and a dictionary of terms.

The Regenstrief system was intended to complement rather than replace the paper-based patient record. For each patient served, the system contained a core medical record, which included medical treatments, results of laboratory tests, and reports of x-ray studies and electrocardiograms. By 1982 the medical database contained 60,000 patients' records of variable length, with the data coded or stored as free-text narrative. A metathesaurus provided a dictionary of terms, and defined the kinds of data that could be stored in the medical record files.

At the time of a patient's visit, a three-part patient encounter form was generated for each patient's return visit and made available to the physician. With the first part, the physician was able to identify the patient, to note the active problems from the last visit, and to see the active treatment profile. The second part, a summary report, included historical and treatment information, results from laboratories, radiology reports, electrocardiogram results, and nuclear medicine reports, all in a modified flow-sheet format [118]. With this time-oriented view of the data, the physician could quickly find the most recent data, such as blood pressure or blood sugar, and compare these to previous levels. An asterisk was placed beside each abnormal value. The objective of the patient's summary report was to facilitate data retrieval and help the physician organize the data [115].

At the time of the visit, physicians would record numeric data for later optical-machine reading into the computer. Space was provided for written orders. Within the space for orders, there were suggestions for diagnostic tests that might be needed. The physician would update the patient's problem list by drawing a line through problems that had been resolved and by writing in new problems that had arisen. The physician recorded progress notes in the space beside the problem list. Current prescriptions were listed at the bottom of the encounter form in a medication profile. The physician refilled (by writing "R") or discontinued (by writing "D/C") after each medication listed. New prescriptions were written underneath this list. The patients would then take a carbon copy of this section to the pharmacy as their prescriptions.

The Regenstrief system also provided the physician with a surveillance report for each patient seen, written in a structured English format using the CARE language [118]. This report provided physicians "reminders" about important clinical conditions [115]. The development of these reminders was engineered by physician-authored protocols; each protocol defined the clinical condition that would trigger the reminder [82]. In 1 year, the CARE program generated more than 70,000 reminders for 30,000 patient visits [112]. The CARE program also enabled non-programmers to perform complex queries of the medical records. Thus the three-part encounter form helped physicians with their clinical decisions as well as with their recording and retrieving tasks. McDonald [115] explained that the Regenstrief system used paper-based reports rather than visual displays as the primary means for transmitting information to the physician because this mode of data transfer was inexpensive, portable, and easy to browse. Also, paper reports could be annotated by hand.

Clerks entered physician-recorded information into the Regenstrief system by means of computer terminals. In the clinical laboratories, the information was transferred directly to the Regenstrief system by the laboratory computers. Pharmacy prescription information was collected from both the hospital and outpatient pharmacy systems. Essential information from hospital stays, such as diagnoses, was transferred from hospital case-abstract tapes. Two modules, the database management system and the pharmacy system, could be purchased from the Digital Equipment Corporation [96].

In the early 1980s, the Regenstrief system shared their DEC VAX 11/780 computer with the clinical laboratory and pharmacy systems [117]. By the mid-1980s at the Regenstrief Institute for Health Care, any patient seen by the General Medicine Service, in the emergency room, in the outpatient clinics, or in the hospital wards had been registered with the Regenstrief computer-based medical record system [116]. Then in 1988, the Regenstrief system was linked to the laboratory, radiology, and pharmacy systems within the University of Indiana hospitals and the local Veterans hospital [114]. Thus, Indiana University physicians who rotated their work in those hospitals could use the same programs to find and analyze clinical data for patient care. The query program permitted users, through the CARE program, to generate clinical care reminders across sets of patients in the Regenstrief medical record database. The CARE programs also provided a means for statistical analyses of groups of patients. In 1988 the Regenstrief system contained more than 24 million observations on 250,000 patients. In 1 year patient information was captured for more than 300,000 outpatient visits and for 20,000 hospital admissions.

By the end of the 1990s, the Regenstrief system served a large network of hospitals and clinics [119] and had become a leading OIS model in the United States. Among McDonald's outstanding contributions was his focus on the computer's capabilities for providing in real time, reminders to physicians about problems in need of attention as reflected in the outpatient care database. In addition, he evaluated by controlled clinical trials, the effect of these computer reminders on the quality of care. McDonald's CARE program contributed to the clinical decision support of patient care, just as Warner's HELP program and Duke's TMR supported care for hospitalized patients.

In 1974 the Johns Hopkins Hospital clinics initiated their OIS with a computer-based patient record, called the Minirecord system [15, 88]. The Minirecord system was developed with a grant from the Hopkins Applied Physics Laboratory to produce a prototype demonstration of how medical care could benefit from the use of an information system. The goal was to have a low-cost auxiliary medical record, with rapid retrieval of computer-generated problem and medication lists, developed in parallel with the hospital information system [16].

The Minirecord system was designed to support the needs of Johns Hopkins Hospital's Hamman-Baker Medical Clinic, which provided long-term care for 7,000 chronically ill patients. Access to the Minirecord would be available by online visual display terminals in the medical clinic, in the emergency department, and in selected inpatient units. Once in operation, the Minirecord supplemented the traditional paper-based record. Encounter forms were used for each patient visit. These contained places for the physician to record the patient's chief medical problem, pending and final diagnoses, medications, procedures, progress notes, and schedule of upcoming visits. The information on the encounter forms was then keypunched for entry into the Minirecord.

The Minirecord was merged with the outpatient registration system, which enabled the encounter forms – with pertinent information from previous visits – to be printed prior to each patient's visit, or on demand for unexpected or emergency visits. Once the OIS was deployed, there were Minirecords for 92 % of the patients' charts, with substantial improvement in the availability of information about patients' problems and therapies administered [16, 89].

Following the implementation of the prototype system on the Applied Physics Laboratory's computer, the system was modified to operate on the Johns Hopkins Hospital central computer. Access to the record system was available to physicians in the medical clinic, the emergency department, the primary care walk-in clinic, the orthopedics clinic, the oncology clinic, and selected inpatient units.

In 1981 Johns Hopkins Hospital completed a revised Minirecord, called the Core Record System. The new system complimented the automated ambulatory medical record and was available online at strategically located terminals. Data were also printed as part of the physician's visit record. The Core Record System, which was integrated into the existing hospital administrative systems, provided online patient registration, the processing of charges, a clinic-oriented appointment system, management reports, and a database for retrospective analyses [110].

In the 1970s an international surge of interest in multiphasic testing systems spurred some practitioners to use the technology of their OISs to integrate the resultant data into a computer-based patient record. In 1972 Cordle [44], at the University of North Carolina, described how a clinic made up of a group of general internists in Charlotte had implemented an OIS for their general practice. Their OIS was based on pre-coded encounter forms from which an operator keypunched the data into cards, which were then read into the computer. They also operated an automated multiphasic testing system, with a self-administered patient history and automated test stations that were connected directly to the computer. The computer then provided online reports, available at the conclusion of the patient's visit.

Miller and associates [125] at the University of Missouri-Columbia reported a field demonstration project supported by the Missouri Regional Medical Program, in which a relatively advanced OIS was installed and operated in a private, rural physician's office. By visual display terminals connected by telephone lines to Lindberg's central computer at the University of Missouri, Bass, a solo general practitioner in a distant small town, was able to enter patients' histories from a self-administered patient questionnaire. He could also enter physical examination results, laboratory test results, electrocardiogram interpretations, and x-ray reports. His OIS could then produce printouts of his patients' medical records and conduct statistical analyses of relevance to his practice, using information within electronically stored records.

In 1972, Brunjes at the Yale University School of Medicine began to operate an OIS for 15,000 patients of the Community Health Care Center Plan. Data were collected by physicians who made check marks on office visit encounter forms, supplemented with a small amount of text. The data were subsequently keypunched onto cards that were read into the computer. The OIS record contained patient identification data, present illness, active medical problems, current medications, physical examination data, treatment plans and therapeutic procedures, together with follow-up progress notes from completed encounter forms. The original encounter forms remained in the patients' charts, but searches from the computer-based patient record could be made using the patient's enrollment identification number and information from single or multiple visits Henley and Wiederhold [81].

In 1973 Braunstein and associates at the Medical University of South Carolina in Charleston initiated an OIS at the university-affiliated Family Practice Center. The center trained resident physicians in family practice, in addition to providing general care for 7,000 patients who made 25,000 office visits a year. Medical data were dictated by physicians to medical transcriptionists, who then entered the data into two PDP-15/75 computer systems by display terminal keyboards distributed throughout the center. A relatively comprehensive computer-stored patient record included medical history, physical examination, problem list, physicians' orders, diagnoses, treatments, medications, laboratory findings, x-ray and electrocardiogram reports, and progress notes. At each patient's visit, a paper record of the stored information was organized in a problem-oriented format and printed for use by the patient's physician. The pharmacy was also integrated into the system, so that before they were filled, prescriptions could be screened for drug-drug interactions and a patient's allergies [20, 21].

In 1973, Penick in the Appalachia II Health District of Greenville, South Carolina, in collaboration with Clemson University, developed an OIS for 46,700 mostly indigent patients who made 93,500 visits per year in a four-county area of the South Carolina Department of Public Health. Data were collected in the OIS in six of the clinics. Some clinics used encounter forms, with check marks and provision for text; some clinics used mark-sense forms; and some clinics used direct entry to the computer by display terminal and keyboard, connected through telephone lines to a mainframe computer at Clemson University. Clinicians saw patients with their traditional paper-based record, but at all six sites the computer-stored record was available on a display terminal. It provided data from previous visits, laboratory results, and referrals to other contacts within the public-health system. In addition, patient scheduling was provided by the OIS for 135 clinics in the system [81].

Nelson and associates [130] at Dartmouth Medical School initiated the Primary Care Cooperative Information (COOP) Project, which consisted of a network of 16 small, free standing, primary care practices in Maine, New Hampshire, and Vermont that were working with the medical school faculty. An outpatient encounter form was completed after each patient's visit and mailed to Dartmouth where it was keypunched and entered into a computer. With their information in the computer, each practice received periodic management reports and inter-practice comparisons together with billing services. After 2 years of experience, however, it was concluded that for a network of small medical practices, it would be more cost effective to have a distributed system with microcomputers housed in each practice.

With the advent of lower-cost minicomputers in the 1970s, an increased effort was being made in many locations to develop OISs. Henley and Wiederhold [81] reported the development of OISs in more than 200 sites in the United States; 175 of these were developing electronic medical record systems, 17 of which had operational, state-of-the-art systems. Eleven of the 17 sites provided primary patient care; 7 were largely supported by federal grants, 2 were supported from institutional funds, and the rest were supported primarily by users. The authors considered seven of these sites to be academic institutions [81].

Henley and Wiederhold [81] also completed a review of the accomplishments of these 17 operating, state-of-the-art, computer-based OISs. They reported that all sites stored the patients' chief complaints or symptoms; and all sites provided patient identification data together with search capabilities on the information within the patients' electronic records (11 of the sites had online search capabilities).

Whiting-O'Keefe et al. [186] at the University of California in San Francisco reported on their Summary Time Oriented Record (STOR), designed to replace most of the traditional paper-based chart in their outpatient clinics. STOR contained a computer-generated, tabular, flow-charted summary of the patient's electronic medical record, which included patients' problems, physical examination findings, laboratory test reports, and treatments provided. The physician's written notes, with radiology reports, pathology reports, and discharge diagnoses in free text, were also available to the physician at the time of the patient's visit. STOR retained this information for the seven most recent clinic visits of each patient. On the reverse side of STOR's printed summary form, an encounter form was available for the physician to use to write free-text notes or orders, which would then be entered into the patient's record for subsequent retrieval and use.

In 1983, STOR was interfaced by a local area network to radiology, pathology, clinical laboratories, and to a central transcription service for dictated reports. For the most part, physicians preferred the summaries generated by STOR to the traditional paper-based records [187]. In 1985 STOR was approved for clinic-wide implementation in the University of California ambulatory care clinics [80].

Shapiro [145] reported an enhanced version of the South Carolina ambulatory medical program (SCAMP), which served 180 primary care physicians. SCAMP also used transcriptionist intermediaries and clinical personnel to enter data into the computer. It permitted physicians to create their own reminder rules by filling in blanks in displayed menus or templates. It supported online retrieval and examination of patients' problems and other computer-stored patient data. By means of video display terminals it included the capability of searching natural language text. With displayed menus users could format reports.

Stoneburner [162] listed 73 vendors of OISs in the United States. Friedman and McDonald [57] reported that more than 100 different varieties of personal computers were available for use by physicians. In 1984, Polacsek published his first "Medical Software Buyer's Guide," a collection of 86 predominately microcomputer-supported OISs. His 1985 Guide included over 150 OISs. In 1986 he described 657 OISs; and in 1987, his fourth Buyer's Guide included more than 900. Many of these included software for office management systems, clinical specialty systems, and hospital, laboratory, pharmacy, and radiology systems [132].

Knight and associates [95] at the University of North Carolina at Chapel Hill added a clinical prompting program to their OIS for a general medical group practice in the clinics of the North Carolina Memorial Hospital. This was used primarily to remind physicians when to use preventive-medicine health-promotion procedures. In response to a survey, 65 % of the participating physicians said they liked being reminded, and 97 % said they would include a prompting system in any future private practice.

In the 1970s and 1980s the three OIS systems that received the most recognition in the United States, as best satisfying the functional and technical requirements for clinical office practice, were the COSTAR, TMR, and Regenstrief systems described above. In the 1990s and 2000s, a variety of more advanced electronic health record systems began to be appear, and in the 2010s, with financial support from the Center for Medicare and Medicaid, there would be a rapid diffusion of OISs in the United States.

5.6   Telemedicine and Mobile Health Care

In the 1970s portable medical records began to be carried by patients on smart cards. Similar in size to credit cards, smart cards contained integrated-circuit chips for data processing and memory storage. These cards could store enough data for the essential information from a computer-based patient's record [83]. However, their relatively high initial cost, concerns about protecting confidentiality, and lack of standards for data storage deterred widespread use [102].

By the mid-1980s, the development of lower-cost laser optical cards was being explored. The optical card was not a smart card, but rather a large-capacity storage device. Information in the optical card could be encoded and read with a laser; and the information could be manipulated with software in a manner similar to other computer storage devices. In 1985 a subsidiary of Blue Cross-Blue Shield in Maryland announced the use of a laser optical card that could hold up to 800 pages of personal medical information and could be carried in wallets or pocketbooks by members of their plan. The cards were designed to facilitate patients' hospital admissions and to provide information to patients' physicians about prior clinical care received, whether in the hospital, the emergency room, or the physician's office. The portable card reader-writer unit was connected to the bus of an IBM personal computer [111].

Vallbona [173] used a laser optical card capable of storing 1.76 megabytes of digitized data, which was equivalent to about 700 pages of text. This Health Passport collected and made available for retrieval, the identification data, medical problems, medications, laboratory and x-ray results, and medical history items of each card-carrying patient. Vallbona reported that patients did indeed carry their cards with them when they visited the clinic, and that the optical card reader-writer functioned without problems. Since information once written onto the card could not be removed, the card was a good mechanism for recording historical information, such as a patient's medical history.

Historically, telecommunications go back to 1844, when near-instantaneous communication across long distances began in the United States with the inauguration of public telegraph services between Washington and Baltimore. In 1876 Bell patented the telephone for the electronic transmission of voice [53]. Telemedicine, in the general meaning of the word, began with the use of telephone lines to transmit voice.

Telemedicine was defined by Grigsby [64] as the use of communications technology to provide health care services for persons who are at a distance from the health care provider. Merrell [123] defined telemedicine as the use of transmitted text, images, voice, and other signals to permit consultation, and education in medicine over a distance. Houtchens et al. [84] also defined telemedicine as medicine at a distance, and described its role in influencing the development of standards and protocols for the transfer of patients' records that contained images. They outlined the requirements for image size, storage, transmission, resolution, and viewing, as well as requirements for linking images to textual or coded data.

Field [53] defined telemedicine as the use of electronic information and communications technologies to provide and support health care when distance separates the participants. Field differentiated between the site that organized and provided the telemedicine services (the central or consulting site) and the site at which the patient being served was located (the remote, satellite, or distant site). The earliest description of a tele-radiology system in the United States was reported in 1950 [53].

A frequently cited early telemedicine system linked a nurse practitioner located at the Logan Airport with physicians at the Massachusetts General Hospital in Boston, using a two-way, audio/video, slow-scan microwave system to transmit x-ray images [129]. Moore [128] described the Cambridge Telemedicine Project, which employed audio-visual links to support consultations from physicians at Cambridge Hospital to nurse practitioners at three satellite neighborhood health clinics.

Dunn [46] described an evaluation of the efficacy of four, two-way telemedicine systems – black and white television, color television, hand-free telephone, and regular telephone – in a community health center caring for more than 1,000 patients. The investigators concluded that in their study the ordinary telephone was just as effective as the other forms of communication tested.

Bennett [11] and Fasano [48] defined telehealth as the use of technology to support long-distance clinical health care and distinguished this from telemedicine, which from their perspective gave a more narrow definition to the delivery of patient care through telecommunications. Field [53] suggested that telehealth, when used as electronic house calls, had the potential to serve patients without the inconvenience or discomfort of office visits, and that such telehealth might help some patients avoid hospitalization, or help some hospitalized patients be discharged sooner than would otherwise have been advisable.

Bennett [11] also published a telehealth handbook that described the functional and technical requirements for telehealth systems, and that provided a list of systems developed in the 1970s. Bennett pointed out that properly functioning telehealth systems can benefit patients by bringing to them the expert care of physicians who are located remotely.

With the advent of the Internet and the World Wide Web, telemedicine permitted health care providers to have access to patients' medical records no matter where the patients were seen. In addition, this technology can enable clinicians to have online access to medical knowledge and bibliographic databases, and to provide follow-up advice to patients in their homes. In the 1990s telemedicine via the Internet was used for the transmission of digitized radiology and pathology images, and for dermatological consultation.

Vaughan [176] described a client-server telemedicine system developed at the Medical College of Ohio. It used a private communications network centered in Toledo, and connected to the Medical College by a high bandwidth transmission line. The Toledo network center was connected to each rural and urban client site by leased telephone lines. Multiple servers within the medical departments of the Medical College transmitted encrypted telemedicine consultations to the client sites, and provided these sites with access to the Internet and to the World Wide Web.

Electronic mail was reported by Worth [192] as an effective and low-cost way of providing telemedicine reports for laboratory test results, for responding to patients' simple questions, for cancelling appointments, and for routine patient care communications.

In the 2000s, wireless, hand-held, mobile smart phones became available. The Apple iPhone was introduced in 2007, and electronic tablets, such as Apple's iPad soon followed. These devices began to function as mobile terminals that permitted caregivers to enter and retrieve a patient's data anywhere within range of their medical facility.

Also in the 2000s, Verizon and other information technology vendors announced cloud server storage using Web-based technology that could communicate relatively secure, protected patient data between collaborating health care providers. An increasingly common and efficient use of telemedicine was for mobile, health monitoring in the homes of patients with chronic diseases, such as diabetes, advanced heart disease, and renal disease. Such monitoring could be supported by personal portable patients' records [64].

In 2003, PubMed for Handhelds (PubMedHh) was released by the National Library of Medicine to provide MEDLINE access at the point of patient care by means of smartphones, wireless tablet devices, netbooks, and portable laptops (NLM Programs and Services 2012). In 2010 physicians and nurses in hospitals were using hand-held smart phones and iPads to download patients' electronic records, and to retrieve and enter clinical data [124, 134].

In the 2010s, commercial vendors of electronic health care systems, with the financial stimulus of the federal government, produced a diffusion of their system installations in the United States, with an associated rapid growth of mobile health care. Halvorson [71] and Fasano [48] referred to the Veterans Administration and Kaiser Permanente as excellent examples of places where telehealth was used effectively in the direct support of patient care.

5.7 Summary and Commentary

Lindberg [99] outlined the degrees of difficulty in the development of medical innovations: the easiest is the automation of a simple function, such as providing a patient's billing for services; more difficult is the automation of a more complex function, such as collecting and storing a patient's medical history; more difficult still is the complex process of constructing a medical database; and the most difficult is developing the highly complex, medical information and database management system for a hospital. This highest degree of difficulty is in keeping with Starr's [158] apt ranking of the hospital as the most complex organizational structure created by man.

There were relatively few office information systems in the United States in the 1960s. Those that were operational were mostly in ambulatory clinics that shared time on mainframe computers with affiliated hospitals. In the 1970s, some stand-alone OISs in larger groups began to function on minicomputers. With the advent of low-cost microcomputers in the 1980s, OISs began to diffuse rapidly throughout the United States. By the end of the 1980s, about 80 % of physicians had some type of computer in their offices, primarily for administrative and business functions. Although OISs were simpler than hospital information systems, computer-based patient records and other OIS clinical applications were still infrequently used, even at the end of the 1980s. When they admitted a patient to the hospital, few physicians could transfer data from their OIS to the information system of the hospital.

The review of 17 OISs in the mid-1970s by Henley's group Henley and Wiederhold [81] demonstrated that each had developed its own distinct design, hardware, software, and applications; for the most part, lack of standardization made the interchange of data difficult or impossible. Although government support had contributed to most of these pilot OISs, government neither coordinated, nor exercised leadership in their development – an example of a national "bottom-up" approach to a basic medical technology.

On the other hand, COSTAR, the Duke TMR, and the Regenstrief system were three outstanding, comprehensive, and successful OISs in the 1970s and 1980s. Each satisfied most of the basic requirements for a successful information system. Throughout the two decades, each was led by one competent and committed physician (Barnett, Stead, and McDonald, respectively), who were supported by a team with a high level of medical and computing expertise. The teams were capable of exploiting the currently available hardware and of developing their own software for a medical database management system together with a computer-based patient record and many of the required medical applications.

COSTAR, TMR, and the Regenstrief system were developed in an academic environment with a supportive organization, a cooperative group of health professional users, and a sizable outpatient population with which to test the prototype. Each program found adequate and continued funding over the 1970s and 1980s from multiple sources – the developers' own institutions, the federal government, and private industry. Although all used some paper input and output documents, each developed what Stead called a "chartless" record, meaning that the primary, continuously updated patient record was stored in the computer. COSTAR was almost entirely focused on OIS applications, whereas the Regenstrief and Duke systems had linkages to large affiliated hospitals.

For OIS applications, the few evaluations published were insufficient to be convincing as to their benefits. That few physicians used computer-based patient records in their offices provides evidence that physicians did not consider computer-based records to be more efficient for their office practice than their paper-based records. It was expected that, in the 1990s, requirements for electronic claims reporting would produce major changes in OIS requirements. It was also expected that the increasing prevalence of OISs would lead to increased monitoring of the quality of patient care in office practice.

In 2009 the U.S. Congress passed the American Recovery and Reinvestment Act that directed about $150 billion in new funds to the healthcare industry, including $19.2 billion for health information technology. The Federal government announced it would subsidize qualifying institutions and their physicians who purchased electronic health record systems that met Federal certification requirements that demonstrated their compliance with the Federal definition of "Meaningful Use" between 2011 and 2015.

References

1. Arellano MG, Simborg DW. A probabilistic approach to the patient identification problem. Proc SCAMC. 1981;852–6.
2. Ausman RK. Automated storage and retrieval of patient data. Am J Surg. 1967;114:159–66.
3. Barnett GO. The application of computer-based medical record systems in ambulatory practice. In: Orthner HF, Blum BI, editors. Implementing health care information systems. New York: Springer-Verlag; 1989. p. 85–99.
4. Barnett GO. Computer-stored ambulatory record (COSTAR). US Department of Health, Education, and Welfare, Public Health Service, Health Resources Administration, Washington, DC: National Center for Health Services Research; 1976.
5. Barnett GO, Souder D, Beaman P, Hupp J. MUMPS: an evolutionary commentary. Comput Biomed Res. 1981;14:112–8.
6. Barnett GO. The modular hospital information system. In: Stacy RW, Waxman BD, editors. Computers in biomedical research. New York: Academic Press; 1974. p. 243–5.
7. Barnett GO, Greenes RA, Grossman JH. Computer processing of medical text information. Methods Inf Med. 1969;8:177–82.
8. Barnett GO, Justice NS, Somand, et al. COSTAR: a computer-based medical information system for ambulatory care. Proc SCAMC. 1978;486–7.
9. Barnett GO, Justice NS, Somand ME, et al. COSTAR:a computer-based medical information system for ambulatory care. Proc IEEE. 1979;67:1226–37.
10. Barnett GO, Zielstorff RD, Piggins J, McLatchey J, Morgan MM, Barrett SM, et al. COSTAR: a comprehensive medical information system for ambulatory care. Proc SCAMC. 1982;8–18.
11. Bennett AM. Telehealth handbook. A guide to telecommunications technology for Rural Health Care. DHEW Pub No (PHS). 1978;79–3210.
12. Blois MS. Information and medicine: The nature of medical descriptions. Berkeley: University of California Press; 1984.
13. Bloom SM, White RJ, Beckley RF, Slack WV. Converse: a means to write, edit, administer, and summarize computer-based dialogue. Comput Biomed Res. 1978;11:167–75.
14. Blum BI. A history of computers. In: Blum B, editor. Clinical information systems. New York: Springer; 1986. p. 1–32.
15. Blum BI, Lenhard RE. An oncology clinical information system. Computer. 1979;12:42–50.
16. Blum RL. Automating the study of clinical hypotheses on a time-oriented data base: the RX project. Proc MEDINFO. 1979;456–60.
17. Bolt, Beranek, Newman. The CAPO project: phase 1 evaluation of an automated medical history in office practice. Boston: BB 1972.
18. Bouchard RE, Tufo HM, Van Buren H, Eddy WM, Twitchell JC, Bedard L. The patient and his problem-oriented record. Applying the problem-oriented system. New York: Medcom Press; 1973. p. 42–6.
19. Bowie J, Kerlin BD. A multi-clinic implementation of COSTAR V. Proc MEDINFO. 1980;862–6.
20. Braunstein M. The computer in a family practice centre: a "public" utility for patient care, teaching, and research. Proc Int Symp IRIA. 1976;761–8.
21. Braunstein ML, Schuman SH, Curry HB. An on-line clinical information system in family practice. J Fam Pract. 1977;5:617–25.
22. Brodman K, van Woerkom AJ, Erdmann AJ, Goldstein LS. Interpretation of symptoms with a data-processing machine. AMA Arch Int Med. 1959;103:776–82.
23. Brodman K, Erdmann AJ, Lorge I, Wolff HG, Broadbent TH. The Cornell medical index-health questionnaire as a diagnostic instrument. JAMA. 1951;145:152–7.
24. Brodman K, Erdmann AJ, Lorge I, Wolff HG, Broadbent TH. The Cornell medical index: an adjunct to medical interview. JAMA. 1949;140:530–4.

25. Brunjes S. An anamnestic matrix toward a medical language. Comput Biomed Res. 1971;4:571–84.
26. Buchan RRC. Low cost comprehensive microcomputer-based medical history database acquisition. Proc SCAMC. 1980;2:786–93.
27. Budd M, Bleich H, Sherman H, Reiffen B. Survey of automated medical history acquisition and administering devices. Part I, questionnaires, Project report ACP-4 (Ambulatory care project). Lexington: Lincoln Laboratory, MIT; 1969.
28. Capozzoli E. An automated approach to medical record tracking. Top Health Rec Manage. 1981;2:27.
29. Carlstedt B, Jeris DW, Kramer W, Griefenhage R, McDonald CJ. A computer-based pharmacy system for ambulatory patient care. Indiana Pharm. 1977;58:92–8.
30. Castleman PA, Bertoni P, Whitehead SF. An ambulatory care center support system. In: van Egmond J, de Vries Robbes PF, Levy AH, editors. Information systems in patient care. Amsterdam: North Holland; 1976. p. 45–56.
31. Chen TT, Williams BT, Levy AH. Graphically enhanced medical information system network. In: Hinman EJ, editor. Advanced Medical Systems: the 3rd century. Miami: Symposia Specialists; 1977. p. 135–44.
32. Coleman JR, Lowry CE. A computerized MIS to support the administration of quality patient care in HMOs organized as IPAs. J Med Syst. 1983;7:273–84.
33. Collen M. A guide matrix for technological system evaluation. J Med Syst. 1978;2:249–54.
34. Collen M. Hospital computer systems: reasons for failures and factors making for success. In: Public Health in Europe 1. Copenhagen: World Health Organization; 1972. p 91–7.
35. Collen MF. A history of medical informatics in the United States, 1950 to 1990. Indianapolis: American Medical Informatics Association; 1995.
36. Collen MF. Computers in preventive health services research. 7th IBM Medical Symp. 1965;331–44.
37. Collen MF. Patient data acquisition. Med Instrum. 1977;12:222–5.
38. Collen MF. Automated multiphasic screening and occupational data. Arch Environ Health. 1967;15:280–4.
39. Collen MF. Periodic health examinations using an automated multitest laboratory. JAMA. 1966;195:830–3.
40. Collen MF, Linden C. Screening in a group practice prepaid medical care plan as applied to periodic health examinations. J Chronic Dis. 1955;2:400–8.
41. Collen MF, Cutler JL, Siegelaub AB, Cella RL. Reliability of a self-administered medical questionnaire. Arch Intern Med. 1969;123:664–81.
42. Collen MF, Rubin L, Neyman J, Dantzig GB, Baer RM, Siegelaub AB. Automated multiphasic screening and diagnosis. Am J Publ Health Nations Health. 1964;54:741–50.
43. Conrath DW, Bloor WG, Dunn EV, Tranquada B. A clinical evaluation of four alternative telemedicine systems. Behav Sci. 1977;22:12–21.
44. Cordle F. The automation of clinical records: an overview with special emphasis on the automation of office records in the primary medical care setting. Med Care. 1972;10:470–80.
45. Cross HD. The problem-oriented system in private practice in a small town. In: Hurst JW, Walker HK, editors. The problem-oriented system. New York: MEDCOM Learning Systems; 1972. p. 143–72.
46. Dunn EV, Conrath DW, Bloor WG, Tranquado B. An evaluation of four telemedicine systems for primary care. Health Serv Res. 1997;19–29.
47. Evans LA, Vallbona C, Speck CD. An ambulatory care system for a network of community health centers. Proc MEDINFO. 1980;871–5.
48. Fasano P. Telehealth for one-stop care. In: Fasano P, editor. Transforming health care: the financial impact of technology, electronic tools, and data mining. Hoboken: Wiley; 2013. p. 87–103.
49. Feinstein AR. Quality of data in the medical record. Comput Biomed Res. 1970;3:426–35.
50. Felts WR. Choosing office practice systems for billing, accounting, and medical record functions. MD Comput. 1984;1:10–7.

51. Felts WR, Kirby Jr WH. Overview: need and demand. Proc SCAMC. 1979;709–15.
52. Fiddleman RH. Proliferation of COSTAR: a status report. Proc SCAMC. 1982;175–8.
53. Field MJ. Telemedicine: a guide to assessing telecommunications for health care. Washington, DC: National Academies Press; 1996.
54. Friedman C. A broad-coverage natural language processing system. Proc AMIA. 2000;270–4.
55. Friedman GD, Ury HK, Klatsky AL, Siegelaub AB. A psychological questionnaire predictive of myocardial infarction: results from the Kaiser-Permanente epidemiologic study of myocardial infarction. Psychosom Med. 1974;36:327–43.
56. Friedman RB, Huhta J, Cheung S. An automated verbal medical history system. Arch Intern Med. 1978;138:1359–61.
57. Friedman RB, McDonald CJ. A buyer's guide to microcomputers for the home of office. Medcomp.1983;1:60–71.
58. Fries JF. Alternatives in medical record formats. Med Care. 1974;12:871–81.
59. Fries JF. Time-oriented patient records and a computer databank. JAMA. 1972;222:1536–42.
60. Gabrieli ER. Planning a health information system. Symposium on use of computers in clinical medicine. Buffalo: State University of New York, Buffalo; 1968.
61. Giebink GA, Hurst LL. Computer projects in health care. Ann Arbor: Health Administration Press; 1975.
62. Goldstein SS. Assisted recording of the medical history (ARM): a method of recording the medical history during the interview. Comput Biol Med. 1974;4:215–22.
63. Greenes RA, Pappalardo AN, Marble CW, Barnett GO. Design and implementation of a clinical data management system. Comput Biomed Res. 1969;2:469–85.
64. Grigsby J. Current status of domestic telemedicine. J Med Syst. 1995;19:19–27.
65. Grossman JH, Barnet GO, McGuire MT, Swedlow DB. Evaluation of computer-acquired patient histories. JAMA. 1971;215:1286–91.
66. Grossman JH, Barnett GO, Koepsell TD, Nesson HR, Dorsey JL, Phillips RR. An automated medical record system. JAMA. 1973;224:1616–21.
67. Haas RE, Fleishl G. Medical time sharing on a small business computer. Proc San Diego Biomed Symp. 1972;11:359–62.
68. Haessler HA. The interactive, self-administered medical history: automated multiphasic health testing. Eng Found Res Conf. 1970;276–86.
69. Haessler HA, Holland T, Elshtain EL. Evolution of an automated database history. Arch Intern Med. 1974;134:586–91.
70. Hall WD. Introduction of the problem-oriented record into an outpatient subspecialty clinic. In: Hurst JW, Walker HK, editors. The problem-oriented system. New York: MEDCOM Learning Systems; 1972. p. 131–6.
71. Halvorson G, Goldsbrough P, Kennedy S, Close K, Becker D. The digital dimension of healthcare. Report of the digital innovation in healthcare working group 2012. Imperial College, London: Global Health Policy Summit; 2012.
72. Hammond W, Stead W, Straube M, Kelly M, Winfree R. An interface between a hospital information system and a computerized medical record. Proc SCAMC. 1980;3:1537–40.
73. Hammond WE, Stead WW, Snow JL, et al. Clinical applications of a minicomputer information support system. In: Proceedings 27th ACEMB; 1974. p 73.
74. Hammond WE, Snow JL, Dorsey FC. A primary care medical record system. Proc 27TH ACEMB. 1974;326.
75. Hammond WE, Stead WW, Straube MJ, Jelovsek FR. Functional characteristics of a computerized medical record. Methods Inf Med. 1980;19:157–62.
76. Hammond WE, Stead WW, Feagin SJ, Brantley BA, Straube MJ. Data base management system for ambulatory care. Proc SCAMC. 1977;173–87.
77. Hammond WE, Stead WW, Straube MJ. Adapting to the day to day growth of TMR. Proc SCAMC. 1983: 101–5.

78. Hammond WE, Brantley BA, Feagin SJ, Lloyd SC, Stead WW, Walter EL. GEMISCH: a minicomputer information support system. Proc IEEE. 1973;61:1575–83.
79. Haug PJ, Warner HR, Clayton PD, Schmidt CD, Pearl JE, Farney RJ. A computer-directed patient history: functional overview and initial experience. Proc MEDINFO. 1986;2:849–52.
80. Henke J, Whiting-O'Keefe Q, Whiting A, Schaffner R, Schnake R, Goldstein R, et al. STOR: from pilot project to medical center implementation. Proc SCAMC. 1988: 733–7.
81. Henley RR, Wiederhold G. An analysis of automated ambulatory medical record systems. San Francisco: University of California; 1975.
82. Hershberg PI, Englebardt C, Harrison R, Rockart JF, McGandy RB. The medical history question as a health screening test: an assessment of validity. Arch Intern Med. 1971;127:266–72.
83. Hinman EJ. The patient-carried personal health record. In: Hinman EJ, editor. Advanced medical systems: the 3rd century. Miami: Symposia Specialists; 1977. p. 55–62.
84. Houtchens BA, Allen A, Clemmer TP, Lindberg DA, Pedersen S. Telemedicine protocols and standards: development and implementation. J Med Syst. 1995;19:93–119.
85. Jelovsek FR, Deason BP, Richard H. Impact of an information system on patients and personnel in the medical office. Proc SCAMC. 1982:85–8.
86. Jelovsek FR, Hammond WE, Stead WW, Deason BP, Straube MA. Computer based reports for ambulatory care administrative management. Proc AMIA. 1982;10–3
87. Jessiman AG, Erat K. Automated appointment system to facilitate medical-care management. Med Care. 1970;8:234–46.
88. Johns CJ, Blum B, Simborg D. The minirecord approach to continuity of care for large populations of ambulatory patients. Proceedings of the 3rd Illinois conference on medical information systems; 1976. p. 121–32.
89. Johns CJ, Simborg DW, Blum BI, Starfield BH. A minirecord: an aid to continuity of care. Johns Hopkins Med J. 1977;140:277–84.
90. Juergens JL, Kiely JM. Physician entry of cardiac physical findings into a computer-based medical record. Mayo Clinic Proc. 1969;44:361–6.
91. Kanner IF. Use of computers in an outpatient clinic. In: Rose J, Mitchell J, editors. Advances in medical computing. New York: Churchill Livingstone; 1975. p. 143–7.
92. Kanner IF. Programmed medical history-taking with or without computer. JAMA. 1969;207:317–21.
93. Kerlin BD. Dissemination of COSTAR. J Med Syst. 1986;10:265–9.
94. Kiely JM, Juergens JL, Hisey BL, Williams PE. A computer-based medical record: entry of data from the history and physical examination by the physician. JAMA. 1968;205:571–6.
95. Knight BP, O'Malley MS, Fletcher SW. Physician acceptance of a computerized health maintenance prompting program. Am J Prev Med. 1987;3:19–24.
96. Kuhn IM, Wiederhold G, Rodnick JE, Ransey-Klee D, Benett S, Beck DD. Automated ambulatory record systems in the US. NTIS Publication (1982, August); 1982. p. 178–89.
97. Lindberg D. The computer and medical care. Springfield: CC Thomas; 1968.
98. Lindberg D. Collection, evaluation, and transmission of hospital laboratory data. Methods Inf Med. 1967;6:97–107.
99. Lindberg DAB. The development and diffusion of a medical technology: medical information systems. In: Medical technology and the health care system: a study of the diffusion of equipment-embodied technology. Washington, DC: National Academy of Sciences; 1979. p. 201–39.
100. Lloyd SC, Hammond WE. The physician computer interface. DECUS Proc. 1972; 18:355–9.
101. Lloyd SC, Brantley BA, Hammond WE, Stead WW, Thompson Jr H,K. A generalized medical information system (GEMISCH) for practicing physicians. Proc ACM. 1971;684–92.
102. Long JM. On providing an automated health record for individuals. Proc MEDINFO. 1986;805–9.

103. Luciani F. Do you need an appointment? Using a computerized system to match patient needs with provider resources. In: Eimeren W, Englebrecht R, Flagle C, editors. 3rd Int Con on system science in health care. New York: Springer; 1984. p. 1338–41.

104. Lunde AS. The birth number concept and record linkage. Am J Public Health. 1975;65:1165–9.

105. Martin MJ, Mayne JG, Taylor WF, Swenson MN. A health questionnaire based on paper-and-pencil medium individualized and produced by computer: II. Testing and evaluation. JAMA. 1969;208:2064–8.

106. Mayne JG, Weksel W. Use of automation in collecting medical history data: a feasibility study. Proc in 20th Annual Conf on Engineering in Med and Biol. 1967;17: 1.

107. Mayne JG, Weksel W, Sholtz PN. Toward automating the medical history. Mayo Clin Proc. 1968;43:1.

108. Mayne JG, Martin MJ, Taylor WF, O'Brien PC, Fleming PJ. A health questionnaire based on paper-and-pencil medium, individualized and produced by computer. III. Usefulness and acceptability to physicians. Ann Intern Med. 1972;76:923–30.

109. Mayne JG, Martin MJ, Morrow GW, Turner RM, Hisey BL. A health questionnaire based on paper-and-pencil medium individualized and produced by computer: I. Technique. JAMA. 1969;208:2060–3.

110. McColligan E, Blum B, Brunn C. An automated care medical record system for ambulatory care. In: Kaplan B, Jelovsek FR, eds. Proc SCM/SAMS Joint Conf on Ambulatory Med. 1981;72–6.

111. McDonald CJ. Medical records on a credit card. MD Comput. 1986;3:8–9.

112. McDonald C, Wiederhold G, Simborg DW. A discussion of the draft proposal for data exchange standards for clinical laboratory results. Proc IEEE. 1984;406–13.

113. McDonald C, Blevins L, Glazener T, Haas J, Lemmon L, Meeks-Johnson J. Data base management, feedback control, and the Regenstrief medical record. J Med Syst. 1983;7:111–25.

114. McDonald CJ, Tierney WM. Computer-stored medical records: their future role in medical practice. JAMA. 1988;259:3433–40.

115. McDonald CJ, Murray R, Jeris D, Bhargava B, Seeger J, Blevins L. A computer-based record and clinical monitoring system for ambulatory care. Am J Public Health. 1977;67:240–5.

116. McDonald CJ, Siu LH, Smith DM, et al. Reminders to physicians from an introspective computer medical record. Ann Intern Med. 1984;100:130–8.

117. McDonald CJ. The medical gopher – a computer-based physician workstation. Proc SCAMC. 1988;5:34–47.

118. McDonald CJ, Wilson G, Blevins L, Seeger J, Chamness D, Smith D, et al. The Regenstrief medical record system. Proc SCAMC. 1977;168–9.

119. McDonald CJ, Overhage JM, Tierney WM, Dexter PR, Martin DK, Suico JG, et al. The Regenstrief medical record system: a quarter century experience. Int J Med Inf. 1999;54:225–53.

120. McLean ER, Foote SV, Wagner G. The collection and processing of medical history data. Methods Inf Med. 1975;14:150–63.

121. McLean ER. Automated medical history systems. J Clin Comput. 1977;7:59–74.

122. McLean, Rockart J, Hershberg P. The Lahey clinic automated medical history system. AIS working paper No. 72–17. Los Angeles: University of California; 1972. pp 1–42.

123. Merrell RC. Telemedicine in the 90's: beyond the future. J Med Syst. 1995;19:15–8.

124. Mies G. Best cell phones by carriers. PC World. 2010;28:38–40.

125. Miller OW, Adams GE, Simmons EM. The automated physician's assistant. Proc San Diego Biomed Symp. 1972;11:47–55.

126. Mishelevich DJ, Kesinger G, Jasper M. Medical record control and the computer. In: Topics in health record management. Computers and the Medical Record Department. Germantown: Aspen Systems Corp; 1981. p. 47–55.

127. Moore FJ. Mechanizing a large registers of first order patient data. Methods Inf Med. 1965;4:1–10.
128. Moore GT, Willemain TR, Bonanno R, Clark WD, Martin AR, Mogielnicki RP. Comparison of television and telephone for remote medical consultation. N Engl J Med. 1975;292:729–32.
129. Murphy RLH, Fitzpatrick TB, Haynes HA, Bird KT, Sheridan TB. Accuracy of dermatologic diagnosis by television. Arch Dermatol. 1972;105:833–5.
130. Nelson EC, Bise B, Gagne R, Ohler J, Kirk J, Sarro J, et al. A computerized medical information network for small practices. Proc SCAMC. 1980;2:861–6.
131. O'Desky R, Petroski SP, Ball M. Computerized physician's office practice. Health Care Comput Commun. 1985;2:25. 8,45.
132. Polacsek RA. The fourth annual medical software buyer's guide. MD Comput. 1987;4:23–136.
133. Pryor DB, Stead WW, Hammond WE, Califf RM, Rosati RA. Features of TMR for a successful clinical and research database. Proc SCAMC. 1982;79–84.
134. Puskin DS, Sanders JH. Telemedicine infrastructure development. J Med Syst. 1995;19:125–9.
135. Roach J, Lee S, Wilcke J, Ehrich M. An expert system for information on pharmacology and drug interactions. Comput Biol Med. 1985;15:11–23.
136. Rockart JF, Herschberg PI, Harrison R, Stangle BE. A method of scheduling patients in a multi-specialist medical group practice using a statistically-based symptom scoring technique. Cambridge, MA: Alfred Sloan School of Management, MIT; 1972. p. 1–25. Working Paper 1972.
137. Rockhart JF, McLean EF, Hershberg PI, Harrison R. Some experience with an automated medical history questionnaire. In: Proceedings 10th IBM medical symposium. Yorktown Heights: IBM;1971. pp 125–43.
138. Rockart JF, McLean ER, Hershberg PI, Bell GO. An automated medical history system: experience of the Lahey Clinic Foundation with computer-processed medical histories. Arch Intern Med. 1973;132:348–58.
139. Schenthal JE. Clinical concepts in the application of large scale electronic data processing. Proceedings of the 2nd IBM Medical Symposium. Endicott, NY: IBM. 1960;391–9.
140. Schenthal JE, Sweeney JW, Nettleton W. Clinical application of electronic data processing apparatus. II. New methodology in clinical record storage. JAMA. 1961;178:267–70.
141. Schenthal JE, Sweeney JW, Nettleton WJ, Yoder RD. Clinical application of electronic data processing apparatus. III. System for processing of medical records. JAMA. 1963; 186:101–5.
142. Schulman J, Wood C. Flow sheets for charts of ambulatory patients. JAMA. 1971;217:933–7.
143. Schwichtenberg AH. The development and use of medial machine record cards in the astronaut selection program. Proceedings 1st IBM medical symposium. Endicott, IBM; 1959. pp 185–216.
144. Schwichtenberg AH, Flickinger DD, Lovelace I, Randolph W. Development and use of medical machine record cards in astronaut selection. US Armed Forces Med J. 1959;10:1324–51.
145. Shapiro AR. Exploratory analysis of the medical record. Inf Health Soc Care. 1983;8:163–71.
146. Slack WV. Medical interviewing by computer. South Med Bull. 1969;57:39–44.
147. Slack WV. A history of computerized medical interviews. MD Comput. 1984;1:52–9.
148. Slack W, Porter D, Witschi J, Sullivan M, Buxbaum R, Stare FJ. Dietary interviewing by computer: an experimental approach to counseling. J Am Diet Assoc. 1976;69:514–7.
149. Slack WV, Van Cura L. Computer-based patient interviewing. 1. Postgrad Med. 1968;43:68–74.
150. Slack WV, Van Cura LJ. Computer-based patient interviewing. Postgrad Med. 1968;43:115–120.

151. Slack WV, Hicks GP, Reed CE, Van Cura LJ. A computer-based medical-history system. N Engl J Med. 1966;274:194–8.
152. Slack WV. Patient counseling by computer. Proc SCAMC. 1978;222–6.
153. Slack WV, Slack CW. Patient-computer dialogue. N Engl J Med. 1972;286:1304–9.
154. Slack WV, Van Cura LJ. Patient reaction to computer-based patient interviewing. Comput Biomed Res. 1986;1:527–31.
155. Slack WV, Peckham BM, Van Cura LJ, Carr WF. A computer-based physical examination system. JAMA. 1967;200:224–8.
156. Smith RE. You know my name, look up the number. Datamation. 1985;31:108–14.
157. Stacy RW, Waxman BD. Computers in biomedical research. New York: Academic; 1974.
158. Starr P. The social transformation of American medicine. New York: Basic Books; 1982.
159. Stead WW, Hammond WE. Computer-based medical records: the centerpiece of TMR. MD Comput. 1988;5:48–62.
160. Stead WW, Heyman A, Thompson HK, Hammond WE. Computer-assisted interview of patients with functional headache. Arch Intern Med. 1972;129:950.
161. Stewart SP, Arellano MB, Simborg DW. Optimal patient identification system. J Am Med Rec Assoc. 1984;55:23–7.
162. Stoneburner LL. Survey of computer systems for the physician's office: current systems. Proc MEDINFO. 1983;164–9.
163. Strong RM. Survey of automated medical history acquisition and administering devices. Part 2. Administering devices, Project Report ACP-5. Lexington: Lincoln Lab, MIT; 1969. p. 1–75.
164. Strong R. The QUARK: concept and demonstration. Lexington: Lincoln Lab, MIT; 1970.
165. Swedlow DB, Barnett G, Grossman JH, Souder DE. A simple programming system (driver) for the creation and execution of an automated medical history. Comput Biomed Res. 1972;5:90–8.
166. Templeton J, Bernes M, Ostrowski M. The financial impact of using TMR in a private group practice. Proc SCAMC. 1982;95–7.
167. Thompson HK. Acquisition and reporting of medical history data. In: Proceedings 10th IBM med symposium. Yorktown Heights: IBM; 1971. pp 117–24.
168. Thompson HK, et al. Medical history and physical examination. In: Haga E, editor. Computer techniques in biomedicine and medicine. Philadelphia: Auerbach Publishers; 1973. p. 209–25.
169. Tufo HM, Eddy WM, Van Buren H, et al. In: Walker H, editor. Applying the problem-oriented system. New York: Medcom Press; 1973. p. 19–28.
170. Tufo HM, Bouchard RE, Rubin AS, Twitchell JC, VanBuren HC, Weed LB, et al. Problem-oriented approach to practice. I. Economic impact. JAMA. 1977;238:414–7.
171. Vallbona C. Computerized information systems for ambulatory care. Proc MEDINFO. 1980;852–6.
172. Vallbona C, Spencer WA. Texas Institute for research and rehabilitation hospital computer system (Houston). In: Collen MF, editor. Hospital computer systems. New York: Wiley; 1974. p. 662–700.
173. Vallbona C, Brohn J, Albin J. Pilot test and preliminary evaluation of an optical card medical record system. Proc MEDINFO. 1989;809–12.
174. Vallbona C, Schade CP, Moffet CL, Speck CD, Osher WJ, Tristan MP. Computer support of medical decisions in ambulatory care. Methods Inf Med. 1975;14:55–62.
175. Van Brunt E, Collen MF, Davis LS, Besag E, Singer SJ. A pilot data system for a medical center. Proc IEEE. 1969;57:1934–40.
176. Vaughan BJ, Torok KE, Kelly LM, Ewing DJ, Andrews LT. A client/server approach to telemedicine. Proc SCAMC. 1994;776–80.
177. Wakefield JS, Yarnall SR. The history database: computer-processed and other medical questionnaires. Seattle: Medical Computer Services Association; 1975.

178. Walter EL, Hammond WE. An information retrieval language: P ISAR. In: Proceedings 27th ACEMB; 1974. p 81.
179. Walters RF. File structures for database management systems. MD Comput. 1987;5:30–41.
180. Warner HR. A computer-based patient monitoring. In: Stacy RW, Waxman B, editors. Computers in biomedical research. New York: Academic; 1972.
181. Waxman BD, Yamamoto WS, Rockoff ML. Recent trends in health care technology. In: Stacy RW, Waxman BD, editors. Computers in biomedical research, vol 4. New York: Academic Press; 1974. pp 1–13.
182. Weed LL. Problem-oriented medical records. In: Driggs MF, editor. Problem-directed and medical information systems. New York: Intercontinental Medical Book Corp; 1973. p. 15–38.
183. Weed LL. Medical records, medical education, and patient care: the problem-oriented record as a basic tool. Cleveland: Press of Case Western Reserve University; 1971.
184. Weed LL. Medical records, medical education, and patient care. Chicago: Year Book Pub; 1969.
185. Weed LL. Special article: medical records that guide and teach. N Engl J Med. 1968;278:593–600.
186. Whiting-O'Keefe QE, Simborg DW, Epstein WV. A controlled experiment to evaluate the use of a time-oriented summary medical record. Med Care. 1980;18:842–52.
187. Whiting O'Keef QU, Simborg DW, Warger A, et al. Summary Time Oriented Record (STor): a node in a local area network. Proc SCAMC. 1983;322–5.
188. Wiederhold G. Summary of the findings of the visiting study team on automated medical record systems for ambulatory care: visit to Duke University Medical Center. CDD-5, HRA Contract, June 29, 1975.
189. Wiederhold G, Fries JF, Weyl S. Structural organization of clinical data bases. Proc AFIPS Conf. 1975;479–85.
190. Williams BT. Computer aids to clinical decisions. Boca Raton: CRC Press; 1982.
191. Williams BT, Foote CF, Galassic C, Schaeffer RC. Augmented physician interactive medical record. Proc MEDINFO. 1989;779–83.
192. Worth ER, Patrick TB, Klimczak JC, Reid JC. Cost-effective clinical uses of wide-area networks: electronic mail as telemedicine. Proc SCAMC. 1995;814–18
193. Yarnall SR, Samuelson P, Wakefield JS. Clinical evaluation of an automated screening history. Northwest Med. 1972;71:186–91.
194. Yoder RD, Swearingen DR, Schenthal JE, Sweeney JW, Nettleton W. An automated clinical information system. Methods Inf Med. 1964;3:45–50.
195. Yoder RD, Dreyfus RH, Saltzberg B. Identification codes for medical records. Health Serv Res. 1966;1:53.

Chapter 6
The Early History of Hospital Information Systems for Inpatient Care in the United States

Morris F. Collen and Randolph A. Miller

Abstract In the 1960s, large hospital systems began to acquire mainframe computers, primarily for business and administrative functions. In the 1970s, lower-cost, minicomputers enabled placement of smaller, special purpose clinical application systems in various hospital departments. Early time-sharing applications used display terminals located at nursing stations. In the 1960s and 1970s, a small number of pioneering institutions, many of them academic teaching hospitals with federal funding, developed their own hospital information systems (HISs). Vendors then acquired and marketed some of the successful academic prototypes. In the 1980s, widespread availability of local area networks fostered development of large HISs with advanced database management capabilities, generally using a mix of large mini- and microcomputers linked to large numbers of clinical workstations and bedside terminals. When federal funding for HIS development diminished in the mid-1990s, academic centers decreased, and commercial vendors increased their system development efforts. Interoperability became a main design requirement for HISs and for electronic patient record (EPR) systems. Beyond 2010, open system architectures and interconnection standards hold promise for full interchange of information between multi-vendor HISs and EPR systems and their related subsystems.

Keywords Hospital information systems • Electronic patient records • Academic and vendor systems • Clinical applications • Evolution of clinical information systems

Author Collen was deceased at the time of publication. R.A. Miller edited the original work of Dr. Collen.

M.F. Collen (deceased)

R.A. Miller, M.D. (✉)
Department of Biomedical Informatics, School of Medicine, Vanderbilt University Medical Center, Nashville, TN, USA
e-mail: randolph.a.miller@vanderbilt.edu

© Springer-Verlag London 2015
M.F. Collen, M.J. Ball (eds.), *The History of Medical Informatics in the United States*, Health Informatics, DOI 10.1007/978-1-4471-6732-7_6

In his Pulitzer Prize winning book, *The Social Transformation of American Medicine*, Paul Starr commented extensively on the extraordinary complexity of health care, and was widely credited with ranking the hospital as the most complex organizational structure created by man [146]. Hospital Information Systems (HIS) function to collect, store, process, retrieve, and convey relevant administrative and clinical information to support healthcare professionals engaged in inpatient care [38, 39]. The primary users of a HIS comprise the physicians, nurses, unit staff, pharmacists, administrators, and technologists in the hospital. Each HIS integrates an (often unique) array of computer hardware, software, protocols, standards, and communications equipment. By linking HISs with associated medical offices and ambulatory outpatient information systems (OISs), developers can create comprehensive medical information systems (MIS).

This chapter focuses on the early history of HIS development in the United States. It includes examples of major HISs that underwent initial development between 1959 and 1980. Other chapters of this book cover HIS subcomponent systems in greater depth – for example, laboratory, pharmacy, and imaging systems. This chapter consequently omits description of HIS subsystems, except where relevant to the overall history of HIS. A discussion of the evolution of admission-discharge-transfer systems appears below as an example of the cross-pollination of ideas among early developers of HISs.

6.1 Overview of Early HIS Development

In the 1950s, users of large mainframe computers began to explore the applicability of time-sharing computers to information processing in hospitals. In the early 1960s, Baruch [24] at Bolt, Beranek, and Newman observed that the digital computer could already support many hospital functions. Roach [124] at the Systems Development Corporation (SDC) described the system components necessary for implementing an HIS.

In the 1960s, only the largest hospitals could afford the enormous capital expenditures associated with acquisition of large mainframe computers. As pioneering hospitals developed their own in-house HISs, they connected the central mainframe computer to key sites throughout the institution using a number of terminals in a simple star network. Most early HIS implementations followed a modular implementation approach of the sort advocated by Barnett [20]. The hospitals typically developed or acquired one HIS module at a time. The various modules and departmental subsystems (laboratory, radiology, and pharmacy) required often difficult and complex linkages (typically, one-of-a-kind, pre-Health Level 7). When connected to an affiliated outpatient information system, the HIS could function as part of an evolving total medical information system (MIS). In the mid-1960s, Flagle [55] at the Johns Hopkins University cited the paucity of literature on medical and hospital data processing, stating that the subject remained a fertile area for empirical development.

In 1962, the American Hospital Association surveyed more than 7,000 registered hospitals regarding their usage of computer data processing applications. They found that only 7 % of hospitals used data processing equipment. Fewer than 1 % of smaller hospitals (<100 beds) used computer data processing, and 33 % of larger hospitals (at least 500 beds) used it. Among hospitals with electronic data processing capabilities, 63 % used it for payroll, 53 % for inventory control, and 44 % for patient billing. Only 28 % of such hospitals used data processing for patients' medical records; and 14 % used it for medical research [61].

During the 1960s and 1970s, most American HISs focused on automation of hospital administrative services. Ball [6] categorized the earliest (1960s) operational HISs as the First Generation Level-1 HIS. These encompassed a basic set of inpatient-oriented computer applications, including: an ADT (admission-discharge-transfer) application with bed status and census reporting; an order/requisition entry, communication, and charge collection application; and an inquiry application for today's charges for demand bill purposes. Ball characterized changes in the 1970s as Second Generation Level-1 systems, with enhancements that included: computer-assigned patient identification; nursing order-set entry, nursing notes and care plans, medication schedules and medication monitoring; laboratory-specimen collection lists and labels; order entry and results reporting; scheduling for patients, radiology procedures, and the operating room; medical records indexing, abstracts, and chart locations; diet-list preparation; utilization review; and doctors' registries. An advanced Level-1 HIS provided control functions to monitor routine procedures and activities, such as inventories of supplies.

Ball [4, 11] noted that some HIS vendors planned their basic HIS designs around activities that occur at the nursing station. Those activities focused directly on patient care and were therefore the most important. Nurses constituted the largest group of health care professionals in any hospital; they accessed the HIS more often than any other category of health care professional. Nursing functions were always central to the care of hospital patients, and nurses' services to patients directly complemented those of physicians. Nursing information systems (NISs) were defined by Saba and McCormick [129] as computer systems to collect, store, retrieve, display, and communicate timely information needed to administer nursing services and resources; to manage patient information for the delivery of nursing care; and to link nursing practice, research, and education. Nursing systems have become integral components of HIS since the 1980s.

Summerfield and Empey [153] at Systems Development Corporation in Santa Monica, California, reported a survey of computer-based information systems in medicine, and listed 73 ongoing projects attempting to develop components of, or full-scale HISs. In a historical review, Jacobs [73] noted that commercial vendors first began in the mid-1960s to realize the significant potential of the hospital data processing market. In 1966 Honeywell announced the availability of a business and financial package, acquired from Blue Cross of Minnesota, for a shared hospital data processing center. The next year, IBM followed with the Shared Hospital Accounting System (SHAS). Lockheed and National Data Communications, Inc. (then known as REACH, Inc.) began the development of HISs to be offered to hospitals on a turnkey basis. In the late 1960s MEDELCO, Inc. brought a simplified HIS to the market and met with immediate success.

In 1968 the National Center for Health Services Research and Development (NCHSR&D) conducted and published a survey of 1,200 hospitals regarding their information systems. About one-half of all hospitals with more than 200 beds used computers for some business functions. Of these facilities, only about 15 % had operational medical or medical research computing applications [70].

Another NCHSR&D report published in 1969 noted although that a total, complete operational HIS did not yet exist, there were some working HIS subsystems, listed as follow [115]: (1) Data Automation Research and Experimentation by Lake at Memorial Hospital of Long Beach, California; (2) Demonstration of a Hospital Data Management System by Spencer at the Texas Institute for Rehabilitation and Research, Houston, Texas; (3) Hospital Computer Project by Barnett at the Massachusetts General Hospital, Boston, Massachusetts; (4) Demonstration of a Shared HIS by Huff at the Sisters of the Third Order of St. Francis, Peoria, Illinois; (5) Computer Technics in Patient Care by Clark at the University of Tennessee School of Medicine, Memphis, Tennessee; (6) Computer Facilitation of Psychiatric In-Patient Care by Gluek at the Institute of Living, Hartford, Connecticut; (7) Psychiatric Data Automation by Graetz at the Camarillo State Hospital, Camarillo, California; and (8) the Pilot AHIS at the Veterans Administration Hospital in Washington, DC. This report stated that for the research and development of HISs, the Department of Health, Education, and Welfare had obligated and committed funds totaling about $10 millions for ten projects. The report identified four government-funded HIS projects that had major relevance to medical records: (1) Experimental Medical Records Systems by Ausman at Roswell Park Memorial Institute, Buffalo, New York; (2) Demonstration of the Integration of Active Medical Records by Robinson at Bowman-Gray School of Medicine, Winston-Salem, North Carolina; (3) Automation of a Problem Oriented Medical Record by Weed at Cleveland Metropolitan General Hospital, Cleveland, Ohio; and (4) A System for Computer Processing of Medical Records by Schenthal at Tulane University, New Orleans, Louisiana.

After reviewing the history of the diffusion of HISs to the early 1970s, Jacobs et al. [74] concluded that there had been a rapid growth in the number of hospitals with on-site computers, especially in the larger, general, not-for-profit, non-governmental hospitals. In a smaller survey (with approximately 100 U.S. hospitals responding), 75 % of hospitals indicated they used at least some computer applications for administrative functions; and about one-third reported clinical laboratory and/or other patient care applications [143]. Ball and Jacobs [6] reported that Level-1 HISs, which provided primarily administrative, business, and communication applications, had begun to be accepted in the second half of the 1960s. A 1974 survey showed that the majority of hospitals still subscribed to out-of-hospital, shared computing services. However, the percentage of short-stay general hospitals with in-hospital computers had increased from 30 % for small hospitals to 75 % for hospitals with 500 or more beds. Other surveys found that 80 % of U.S. hospitals in 1975, and 90 % in 1976 used some sort of data processing for business applications [1]. In the mid-1970s, the availability of lower-cost minicomputers enabled placement of small, special-purpose computers in various hospital departments, all linked to one or more large mainframe computers. Ball [7] considered this distributed approach a major change in the implementation of HISs, in that the use of minicomputers in specific areas such as laboratory and pharmacy was not new, but what was new was expanding the concept into a network of inter-related, modular, functional subsystems.

In the 1970s, as HISs included more computer applications and clinical subsystems, the HIS data management and communications software became more complex. This required more computer core memory and increased ancillary storage. Edwards [48] and associates published guidelines for shared computer services. They cited the advantages to hospitals of their reduced outlay of capital funds, elimination of duplicated facilities, extended scope and improved quality of available services, better containment of operating costs, and improved ability to conduct research and long-range planning. Nevertheless, they also noted that the main disadvantage to a hospital of a shared-service program for its HIS was some loss of administrative control over its services. As de la Chapelle [43] observed that in an environment with as many varied computer applications as those of the hospital, the central processor soon became large, expensive, and less flexible. In addition, as applications were added to the central processor, the impact of a system failure on the operation of the hospital became increasingly severe. Disaster prevention through access to a local or remote duplicate system became generally less possible. As a result, with the availability of lower-cost minicomputers in the late 1960s, many hospital departmental applications used minicomputers to carry out most of the required data processing independently from a central mainframe computer. In the larger hospitals, by using an expanded star communications network, the patient data for the medical record that originated from different minicomputers were usually stored in a central processor.

Beginning in the late 1970s, hospitals began to station computer terminals at or near patients' bedsides. This enabled concurrent display of the patient's record at multiple terminals [119]. The first bedside terminals were "dumb" extensions of the mainframe host computer. Hospital personnel used the display terminals for data selection from displayed menus of information. This allowed them to enter data (via keyboards) directly into the computer, at the time of caring for the patient. The printouts from the computer terminal might then include the patient's vital signs, nursing observations, administered medications, and a variety of useful reports. In the 1980s intelligent, quasi-autonomous microcomputer-based terminals appeared. Those terminals ran internal programs that facilitated entry, analysis, and display of patient data. The data were transferred into the patient's mainframe-based (or minicomputer-based) electronic patient record (EPR). Clinicians could access patients' computer-based records directly at the point of care. This, for example, improved the documentation, quality, and efficiency of nursing care [150].

In the 1980s, local area networks (LANs) permitted their hospital-based users with many inexpensive microcomputers to integrate their various individual databases into large, shared databases; or to develop efficient database management systems. Multiple computers in affiliated hospitals began to use communication networks to link their hospital databases. Lund and associates [99] at the Henry Ford Hospital in Detroit, Michigan, reported the installation of a broadband, cable-television LAN that connected a variety of computers located in seven buildings; the system was capable of transmitting digital computer data, as well as analog video information. By 1987 almost all hospitals with more than 100 beds had a HIS financial system, and 44 % had a nursing station, order entry system [150]. More advanced HISs linked clinical data to the financial database, and permitted the association of quality assurance measures with cost data, in order to provide guidelines for more cost effective procedures [172]. About 20 % of U.S. hospitals had computer links between their HISs and affiliated physicians' offices. Some had workstation terminals that enabled data to be exchanged, copied, and modified; and some permitted direct access to laboratory and radiology reports from an outpatient information system [116]. Such linkage required additional security procedures to protect patient confidentiality and to prevent unauthorized access to patient data. Linkage of a HIS to staff physicians' offices was encouraged because it facilitated transfer of the results of diagnostic tests to the physicians who ordered them [105].

While in the 1980s Leonard and associates [85] at the University of Missouri-Columbia had published a catalog describing 112 commercially available components that could be used in the design of HISs, by the end of that decade, not a single vendor had designed and developed a comprehensive HIS that could provide all the necessary clinical and administrative subsystems. Accordingly, a main design requirement in the 1990s for HISs, and in the 2000s for an EHR, was the capability of interfacing and integrating multiple vendor components interoperably.

Those HIS requirements mandated creation of common data coding and transmission standards. Data sharing requirements expanded to include linkages to affiliated hospitals for transfer of patient care data, and linkages to outside factual databases (for example, for information on medications, poisons and toxic substances), and to online medical literature databases such as the NLM's MEDLINE.

The hardware required for HISs began with large mainframe computers in the 1950s and 1960s, then was replaced or added to by minicomputers in the 1970s, and replaced or added to by microcomputers in the 1980s and beyond. Typical HIS software evolved from using punch card inputs for data processing in the 1950s, to providing administrative information systems in the 1960s, to decision support systems in the 1970s, to networked database management systems in the 1980s, to Internet-based systems in the 1990s, and to Web-based, cloud-based systems in the 2000s.

The advent of innovations in specialized technology for medical subsystems required the appropriate enhancement of HISs. In the 1980s, the increasing costs of medical care resulted in national legislative changes that altered the organizational and operational structure of hospitals and brought about the merger of some hospitals, which in 1990s required their HISs to install Internet-based communications networks, and to develop interoperability of their database management systems.

6.2 External Forces Influencing HIS Development

Ball [9] described the basic business applications for a HIS as including: patient admission, discharge, and transfer; bed control and inpatient census; billing, accounts receivable, accounts payable, and general ledger; purchasing; payroll and personnel; inventory control; budgeting; and planning. Ball also included as basic administrative patient care functions the nursing services, dietary services, the medical records department; and patients' procedures scheduling. Hospitals used HIS administrative data for financial analyses, resource utilization, and productivity analyses; they used patient care data for administrative planning and forecasting [36]. The HIS data supported studies of inpatients' length of stay for utilization review and quality assurance monitoring for adverse medical events or inappropriate procedures. An Informatics Technology (IT) Officer is often responsible for administrating the information processing requirements for a large HIS.

In 1983, Medicare, which accounted for about 40 % of total hospital revenues, began a phased transition in its methods of payments. In contrast to the usual method of reimbursing hospitals on the basis of their costs for individual services and procedures, the financing of hospital care began a significant transformation when the U.S. Congress enacted the Medicare Prospective Payment System (PPS). In order to then process Medicare payments, every HIS had to accommodate to new accounting requirements based on 470 diagnosis related groups (DRGs) that were derived from 23 major organ-system groupings of similar International Classification of Diseases (ICD) codes. In contrast to prior methods of reimbursement of hospitals on the basis of the costs for individual services and procedures, with the advent of the PPS and DRGs, hospitals were faced with the need for tightening fiscal operations, and for maintaining better information concerning their case mix and use of resources. This required more sophisticated information systems capable of providing such information for each department, service, and nursing unit in the hospital; and the development of effective cost-containment measures [52, 125, 163]. Within 1 year of the enactment of the PPS/DRG regulations, about one-half of all U.S. hospitals were operating under these new regulations. The Medicare PPS served as an impetus for developing new databases that could be used as administrative planning tools for controlling both production costs and quantities of services provided. Because the medical record became the main source for generating the hospital bills, medical records were being linked to financial data [46]. These regulations affected a large state like California, for example, where the California Medical Review, Inc., was organized in 1984 to perform peer review of Medicare medical services in the state. A system was developed that converted 800,000 existing case records, and processed and stored on disk one-million new cases per year for medical review and statistical analyses. Hospital personnel completed work sheets for data entry that included patients' demographic and clinical information, coded clinical decisions on the need for admission, and the patient's condition on discharge. The coded information on the work sheets was entered using microcomputer workstations and stored on diskettes that were sent to the central office. In addition to permitting review of individual cases, the large databases allowed analyses of physicians' practice patterns and trends of patient care [128]. Ertel [50] wrote of some adverse consequences to a hospital's financial status caused by inaccurate reporting of clinical data by DRGs, since inappropriate DRG assignments could produce under- or over-payments to hospitals; and he listed some specific functions that automated systems could do to improve the accuracy of reported data. McPhillips [111], the director of the Bureau of Data Management and Strategy of the Health Care Financing Administration (HCFA) that administrated the Medicare and Medicaid programs, estimated that in 1986 HCFA would spend $112 billion, at the rate of $12.8 million per hour. The Medicare Statistical System (MSS) of HCFA established a database that contained a Master Enrollment Record for each person enrolled in Medicare; a Provider of Service Record for information on every hospital (about 6,700) and other institution that provided services to Medicare patients; a Utilization Record of services billed for Medicare patients by hospitals and physicians; and a Provider Cost Report Record for cost data for the hospital services provided. In addition, a Utilization and Special Program contained procedure-specific data for samples of Medicare patients and of their hospital and physician providers.

Following the changes in 1983 for payments to hospitals by diagnostic related groups (DRGs), in 1984 Congress also began a series of actions that changed physicians' payment by Medicare's Supplementary Medical Insurance Program [84]. For payments to physicians for their services provided to Medicare patients in hospitals, Congress had initially adopted a system of payment based on the customary, reasonable, and prevailing charges. Nevertheless, in 1984, Congress limited the amount that physicians could charge Medicare patients; and in 1988 it established a relative-value fee scale, based on resource costs for providing services, taking into account the medical specialty, regional location, and the severity of disease factors [126]. By the end of the 1980s, HCFA and other insurers were considering incentives to health care providers for submitting their claims for payments electronically, using magnetic tape, diskettes, or computer-to-computer input to speed up claims processing, and to give the insurers a database for better assessment of future claims. Some large hospitals with advanced HISs, such as Boston's Beth Israel Hospital, had already developed automated patient record summaries and claims processing as a spinoff to online patient care transactions [130]. By the 1990s the hospital information processing became so complex and challenging that some large hospitals appointed a chief information officer (CIO) to administer their HIS services.

In the 2000s and 2010s HCFA and the Centers for Medicare and Medicaid Services (CMS) distributed large sums of money to eligible HISs to support the diffusion of electronic health record (EHR) systems. Web-based data-exchange permitted, in the 2010s, for a great federal financial stimulus to support the diffusion of enhanced electronic health record (EHR) systems that greatly increased HIS requirements.

6.3 Examples of Early HIS Development, 1959–1980

6.3.1 Texas Institute for Rehabilitation and Research (TIRR)

In the mid-1950s, Spencer and Vallbona reported use of a digital computer for research purposes [142, 144, 145]. In 1959, Spencer and Vallbona at the Texas Institute for Rehabilitation and Research (TIRR) began development of an HIS for TIRR, a private, non-profit, 81-bed, special-purpose hospital in the Texas Medical Center in Houston. Their extended-stay hospital delivered comprehensive rehabilitation services to patients having a wide variety of physical disabilities. At TIRR, the patient care plans were relatively stable over long periods of time, in contrast to shorter-stay hospitals where care activities change rapidly. The patient care planning functions in TIRR, however, were appropriate to both long- and short-stay institutions. Vallbona and Spencer [158] reported that the major objectives of the TIRR system were to: expedite the flow of information between the physician and the patient and between the physician and the rehabilitation team; enhance efficient hospital management; provide data for the study of cost of rehabilitation; improve the outcome of disability; and facilitate utilization of clinical data for research. The 1959 TIRR HIS included several clinical support subsystems: nurses' notes, clinical laboratory reports, and physiological test data. At the end of each shift and at the end of the day, keypunch clerks transformed manually recorded nurses' notes into batch-processed, computer-generated reports. Similarly, clinical staff initially manually recorded on specially designed forms the clinical laboratory reports and physiological test data. Clerks then coded and keypunched the data in the forms, and processed the results on a batch basis with unit-record equipment.

In the 1960s, the TIRR began to extend its HIS with additional patient care functions [156, 157, 159–162]. In 1961, the acquisition by TIRR of International Business Machines (IBM) computers models 1401 and of 1620 with magnetic-tape storage allowed for enhanced data processing, storage, and data retrieval capabilities. In 1964, TIRR installed an IBM 1050 typewriter and card-reader terminal on one hospital ward to allow nursing personnel to enter data in response to queries using prepunched cards. Initially, this terminal was connected by a telephone line to a remote, paper-tape punch machine located at Baylor medical school, where data were batch processed on an IBM 1410 computer [28]. In 1965 the problem of errors in data entry by punched paper tape and cards required TIRR to switch to on-line computing with an IBM 1410 computer. A clerk entered data via the remote typewriter terminal located at TIRR.

With the establishment of a conversational mode between the terminal and the computer, error detection and correction by staff personnel became feasible. Magnetic tapes and random-access disk drives stored the data. Online recording of vital signs, obtained by physiological monitors, was effectively carried out using this system [158]. In 1967, acquisition of an IBM 360/50 computer enhanced the system. The new implementation used Baylor University software and CRT display and typewriter terminals located in the Institute, connected by telephone lines to the

IBM 360/50. After a larger core memory storage unit was installed in 1968, decision support became available for laboratory procedures involving pulmonary function tests and blood gas analysis; the mainframe improvements enhanced data
retrieval and analysis [158]. Physicians began to enter orders into the HIS, using
IBM 2260 cathode ray tube (CRT) display terminals located in various clinical
departments [25].

In 1969, a patient-scheduling system became operational. It used eight IBM CRT
visual display terminals connected to the Baylor IBM/360 computer. It scheduled
an average of 30 patients (54 % of the hospital's inpatients) for physiotherapy and
occupational therapy daily; and generated updated reports for each patient [63]. In
1970, TIRR initiated its pharmacy information system. In 1971, a new Four-Phase
Systems minicomputer supported the new clinical laboratory system. The evolving
TIRR Information System (TIRRIS) now provided administrative functions that
included patient identification and registration; admissions and discharge; billing,
accounting, and payroll; and a medical records statistical and reporting system. At
that time, clinical support units included the clinical laboratory; a program that performed calculations on raw data derived during pulmonary-function evaluation testing from spirometers and other equipment used in the cardiopulmonary laboratory;
arterial blood-gas analysis; occupational-therapy and physical-therapy patient status reports; and, vocational services reports [158].

By the 1970s, the TIRRIS database contained approximately 48,000 records,
averaging 167 characters in length. This database was maintained as a partially
inverted file, and involved approximately 4,000 transactions per week [158]. The
functioning electronic patient record included such data as: patient descriptors and
demographic data; medical problems represented by a description of the pathology,
the functional impairments and any associated complications; detailed care plans
that facilitated the coordination of ordered care events; results of all laboratory and
functional capacity tests; details of types and quantities of various forms of therapy;
and the abstracted summary report prepared from the complete hospitalization record
following the patients' discharge. Frequently required patient information was available to the care staff as computer-printed documents. These comprised parts of the
regular paper-based patient record. While there was no single integrated computer
file which contained all of a patient's information, programs could readily extract and
combine data from individual reports with other information as needed [158].

Despite the limitations of its early display terminals, TIRR was able to develop
relatively sophisticated computer-assisted patient care planning functionality. That
subsystem provided a care plan listing the major goals that the medical staff intended
to achieve for the patient; and the corresponding care plans and activities specified
to achieve these goals. The activity lists appeared in chronological order for a 24-h
period, and indicated which department was responsible for the performance of
each task. When the patient arrived at the nursing station, the basic plan of care was
already there. Valbonna (1974) reported that this automated process reduced by as
many as 3 days the time lag between the admission of a patient and the start of the
care plan. During a patient's stay, the basic plan was updated with orders written by
the physician, the nurse, and the therapists to fit the patient's specific needs and the

doctor's particular mode of practice. Other clinical departments added their activities to the patient's plan list, which became an event schedule in addition to being a care plan. The reports and CRT displays generated from the care plans and schedules were used daily by all professionals involved in patient care, including the nurses, aides, orderlies, ward clerks, clinic personnel, social workers, laboratory technicians, vocational counselors, social service counselors, x-ray technicians, dietician, transportation personnel and therapists.

The TIRR IS was one of the earliest HISs developed in the United States. Beginning with batched, punched-card processing of patient data in 1959, TIRR initiated online interactive computer processing in 1967 and had a fairly comprehensive HIS operating by the early 1970s. The system continued to operate thereafter and was exported to other sites. Versions of the system were installed at Baylor College of Medicine by Baylor's Institute of Computer Science (where it was called *BIAS*), to support research departments and a cervical cancer registry, and at the University of Missouri-Columbia, where it was called GISMO for General Information System, Missouri [3].

6.3.2 *Fairfax Hospital in Falls Church, Virginia*

In 1961, the Fairfax Hospital in Falls Church, Virginia, began to use unit-record, punch-card tabulating equipment for business and administrative functions. In January 1962, the Fairfax Hospital began to time-share a single computer with the Alexandria Hospital; and employed a unified staff for both data processing operations and systems development [44].

6.3.3 *Children's Hospital in Akron, Ohio*

In 1962, Children's Hospital in Akron, Ohio installed an IBM 1401 computer for scheduling nursing personnel and for processing doctors' orders. After physicians wrote orders for patients, clerks keypunched the orders for data processing. The keypunched information included patient identification and admission data, as well as orders for medications, laboratory tests, x-ray examinations, and diets. The resulting data underwent statistical analysis [49]. In 1964, the hospital discontinued using punched cards, and installed at every nursing station an electric typewriter. The latter served as both an output printer and a data entry unit. Using a matrix of 120 buttons, all data were numerically coded, including the patients' identification numbers, orders for medications, laboratory tests, x-ray studies, diets, and other procedures. Data entry clerks turned a scroll on the data-entry unit to show the type of entry to be made. The first two columns of buttons indicated the type of order; the next three columns of buttons served to enter the patient's number; the next four columns designated the order number; the remaining three columns of buttons were used to enter modifiers, such as the type of order and frequency. The printer then provided the printouts for use as requisitions, which were also used as laboratory report slips to be filed in the patients' charts. All data were stored on a random-access device. Schedules for surgery and personnel, as well as for administrative and business reports, were provided by the system [34].

6.3.4   LDS Hospital in Salt Lake City, Utah

In the early 1960s, Warner and associates at the University of Utah affiliated LDS Hospital (formerly known as the Latter Day Saints Hospital) in Salt Lake City began to use a Control Data Corporation (CDC) 3300 computer to support clinical applications. They used Tektronix 601 terminals capable of displaying 400 characters in a 25-column by 16-row pattern, or graphical data with a capability of 512 horizontal and 512 vertical dots. Each terminal had a decimal keyboard, and two 12-bit, octal thumbwheel switches for coding information into the computer [164]. In the 1970s they developed one of the most effective hospital information systems of the early HIS era. Their Health Evaluation through Logical Processing (HELP) System at the LDS Hospital had terminals located at its nursing units. Those allowed the nurses to select new orders from displayed menus, to review previous orders, and to examine reported results. In the early 1970s, they created MEDLAB to market the clinical laboratory system they had developed that was directly interfaced to automated laboratory equipment. Special coding systems were devised to enter data from radiology. In 1971, use of the Systematized Nomenclature of Pathology (SNOP) coding system enabled entry of diagnoses via a video terminal [60]. In 1975, the LDS subsystems included the clinical laboratory, multiphasic testing for patients admitted to the LDS Hospital, and computerized electrocardiogram analysis [80]. By 1978, the LDS hospital information system had outgrown its centralized computer system. During the 1980s, the LDS HELP system formed the center of a series of networked minicomputers interfaced to the existing central computer. A central database stored data imported from all hospital sources. From the central store, data were transmitted data to-and-from microcomputers located in each of the intensive care units [59]. By the 1980s, items stored in the integrated patient record database included reports from the clinical laboratory, from pathology biopsies, radiology, electrocardiography, multiphasic testing, and pharmacy [122]. In the 1990s, the HELP system expanded to provide comprehensive clinical support services in nine affiliated Intermountain Health Care Hospitals in Utah [58].

6.3.5   University of Missouri in Columbia, Missouri

The University of Missouri medical center had 441 hospital beds and admitted 60,000 patients in 1964. In 1963, Lindberg [93] and associates at the University of Missouri in Columbia installed an IBM 1410 computer. While their overall objective was to support the practice and teaching of medicine, the initial project was development of one of the first systems that reported all clinical laboratory results through the computer [93]. Keypunch operators entered laboratory data on approximately 500,000 tests per year into the computer. Additionally, the computer processed patient information including the tumor registry, hospital discharge diagnoses, and data on operations and related surgical pathology findings. The system grew to support the hospital's admission, discharge, and patient census programs; patient billing and accounting; nightly nursing report sheets; the dietary department inventory; periodic hospital statistics; and, personnel records.

In 1965, the University of Missouri replaced the laboratory punched card system with IBM 1092/1093 matrix-keyboard terminals. A limits program categorized results entered into the computer as reasonable, abnormal, or as unreasonable. The system recognized patterns of laboratory test results and correlated the patterns with other findings recorded in the patient's record. It could thus advise physicians about potential patient care actions to consider. Lindberg [96], using the Standard Nomenclature of Diseases and Operations (SNDO), between 1955 and 1965 coded patients' discharge diagnoses and surgical operative procedures and stored these on magnetic tape. The system also accumulated SNDO coded diagnoses for all autopsy and surgical pathology specimens, and coded interpretations for each radiology and electrocardiogram tests. Computer-based records for 1,200 active patient cases with thyroid disease included all laboratory test results, the patient's history and physical examination, progress notes, prescribed therapies, and evaluations of the effects of therapy [91, 92]. The system also processed patient' data from pulmonary function tests, adjusted the results for age and body stature, and provided a differential diagnosis of possible diseases. By 1968, Lindberg had added an information system for the department of surgery to provide patient identification, admission, and discharge functions; listing of all surgical complications while in the hospital; operating room procedure entries made by the surgeon, anesthesiologist, and circulation nurse; laboratory, surgical-pathology, and autopsy reports; a daily operating room log; and individual patient summary reports [88].

Lindberg's system also supported 34 research projects and was used in the teaching of medical students [95]. They used the Standard Nomenclature of Diseases and Operations (SNDO) for the coding of patients' discharge diagnoses and surgical operative procedures [96], and stored these on magnetic tape for all patients admitted to the hospital (1955–1965). Other categories of patient data in the system included a patient master reference file with identification data stored on a random-access disk file. All SNDO-coded diagnoses for autopsy and surgical-pathology specimens, and all coded radiology and electrocardiogram interpretations, were stored on magnetic tape in fixed-field format. Computer routines were available for recovery of all categories of data stored. All were aimed at medical student and physician inquiries [95]. To query the system, the user keypunched a control card with the code number of each diagnosis about which the user was inquiring. The computer system read the punched cards and searched the magnetic tape records containing all patients' diagnoses. When a record with the specified diagnosis code was found, the system identified the unit numbers of the patients associated with the diagnosis, and assigned a 'flag' in the random access working storage corresponding with each patient who had the diagnosis [33]. Lindberg [89] used this approach to combine multiple diagnoses to flag unique diagnoses. He also used laboratory test patterns to aid clinicians in the recognition of a possible abnormal or premorbid state. For example, Lindberg [92] studied the patterns found in almost 6,000 electrolyte determinations for serum sodium, potassium, chlorides, and carbonate; and was able to not only identify important combinations of abnormal test values, but also to recognize new patterns; and to predict the state of kidney function.

Lindberg [89] also developed his CONSIDER program, which used the American Medical Association (AMA) publication, *Current Medical Terminology*, to provide the signs, symptoms, and findings for common diagnoses. If the user submitted a set of signs and symptoms, the computer would then list the diseases the physician should consider. With Kingsland, Lindberg initiated a fact bank of biomedical information for use by practicing physicians, and also by scholars and students, that contained information from diverse origins such as text-books, monographs, and articles. In 1969 Lindberg operated for the Missouri Regional Medical program a computer dedicated to electrocardiogram interpretation by using the 12-lead scalar system developed by Caceres within the United States Public Health Service (USPHS) Systems Development Laboratory. The electrocardiograms were transmitted over dial-up telephone lines to the computer center; and automated interpretations were returned to teletype printers in the hospital or in doctor's offices. Lindberg also provided computer services to the Missouri State Division of Health for all births, deaths, divorces, and hospital diagnosis records for the state of Missouri; and provided periodic analysis to the Missouri Crippled Children's Service for diagnoses, therapy, costs, and patients' statistics. By 1969 they had collected 12 years of coded hospital discharge, autopsy, and surgical diagnoses. They also used a differential diagnosis x-ray program developed by Lodwick for the x-ray interpretation of bone tumors, coin lesions in chest films, and suspected gastric cancer [94]. Lindberg [98] also reported using cathode ray tube (CRT) display terminals for taking automated patient histories.

Lindberg [90] introduced the addition of a seventh-place check digit to each patient's unique six-digit identification. The computer calculated the check digit from the sum of the preceding six digits using the modulo-11 arithmetic. The check digit helped to detect and prevent transmission of incorrect patient identification numbers due to transcription errors by enabling the computer system to only accept patient information with valid check digits.

In the 1970s, teams from 45 medical institutions in the United States and abroad visited and inspected Lindberg's system. Lindberg et al. distributed many copies of their system and its design documents [87]. In 1984, Lindberg left the University of Missouri – Columbia to become the Director of the U.S. National Library of Medicine (NLM), where he became an international leader in medical informatics. Medical informatics at the University of Missouri-Columbia continued under the direction of J. Mitchell.

6.3.6   National Institutes of Health (NIH), Bethesda, Maryland

In 1963, the National Institutes of Health (NIH) initiated a central computing facility to provide direct data processing support to its various Institutes and laboratories. By 1964, this central facility contained two Honeywell series-800 computers [77]. In 1965, the NIH established its Division of Computer Research and Technology (DCRT), with Pratt as its director for intramural project development. In 1966, DCRT began to provide computer services with an IBM 360/40 machine; and then rapidly expanded to four IBM 360/370 computers that were linked to a large number of peripherally located computers in NIH clinics and laboratories [120].

6.3.7   El Camino Hospital in Mountain View, California

In 1964, the Information Systems Division of the Lockheed Missiles and Space Company in Sunnyvale, California, began to apply their aerospace expertise to develop a Lockheed hospital information system. In 1969, the Lockheed management decided to carry out the development of its information system in the El Camino Hospital in Mountain View, California, a 464 bed, general community hospital with a medical staff of 340 physicians without interns or resident physicians [56, 57]. In 1971, Lockheed sold its system to the Technicon Corporation, which had come to dominate automation in the clinical laboratory. The company's new owner, Whitehead, saw an opportunity to extend automation from the clinical laboratory into the entire hospital and develop the Technicon Medical Information System. In March 1971, El Camino Hospital signed a contract for the installation of the Technicon HIS. The hospital information system operated with an IBM 370/155 time-shared computer located in Technicon's Mountain View offices [132]. In December 1971, the first step in installing the computer-based HIS brought the Admissions Office at the El Camino Hospital online. Nine months later, the entire hospital, with few exceptions, converted to using the system [165]. By early 1973, the hospital had installed terminals throughout, and had abandoned most traditional paperwork. Significant medical staff concerns developed. One third of the medical staff initially expressed dissatisfaction [32]. Most of the medical staff concerns focused on deficiencies in the initial system, and anticipated problems with altering the traditional practice modes of fee-for-service physicians. Nevertheless, the nursing staff comprised the majority of the professional use of the system, and three-fourths of hospital nurses reported favorably regarding the Technicon HIS. The nurses specifically noted that they liked using the light-pen selectors on the display terminals.

Considerable effort to refine the system's basic operating features during 1975 and 1976 resulted in greater user acceptance [32]. System improvements included better clinical support services and subsystems, improved laboratory test scheduling, and the ability to order medications from the pharmacy. In 1977, a total of 60 display terminals, each consisting of a television screen with a light-pen data selector, a keyboard, and a printer were located throughout the El Camino Hospital; with two terminals installed at most nursing stations. The terminal's display screen presented lists of items, for example, a list of orders for laboratory tests. The user selected a specific displayed item by pointing the light-pen at the desired word (or phrase), and pressing a switch on the barrel of the pen. The Technicon HIS was one of the first systems designed to allow the physicians to enter orders and review the results [30].

Using the light-pen, a physician could select a specific patient, and then enter a full set of medical orders for laboratory work, medications, x-rays, and other procedures. The computer then stored the orders and sent appropriate laboratory requisitions, pharmacy labels, x-ray requisitions, and requests for other procedures to the appropriate hospital departments. Some departments provided standard "routine" sets of orders, such as for patients admitted for coronary artery disease. In addition, physicians could generate personal order sets for particular conditions and write the complete order with a single light-pen selection [60]. By 1977, 75 % of all orders were entered into the computer by the physicians. Physicians, nurses, and other hospital personnel used the light-pen technique extensively, and employed the keyboard only occasionally [72, 165]. Computer-produced printouts included medication-due time lists, laboratory specimen-pickup time lists, cumulative test-result summaries, radiology reports, and hospital discharge summaries [23]. Physicians, on retrieving a patient's data from the display terminals, also received clinical reminders and alerts. In 1978, El Camino developed a computer-based library that contained information on diagnoses, recommended treatments, laboratory interpretation aids for test results, and indications for ordering diagnostic tests for certain diseases. Laboratory test results and radiology interpretations were available at the terminals as soon as someone entered them into the system. A daily cumulative laboratory summary report showed the last 7 days of each patient's tests results [140].

At El Camino, paper-based medical charts existed to encompass all handwritten and dictated documents. Physicians primarily used the Technicon system as an order entry and results reporting system. Upon a patient's discharge, the system printed a complete listing of all tests and procedures results, including any graphic charts, at the medical records department, to be filed in the patients' paper charts.

El Camino Hospital physicians also developed a Medical Information Library for the Technicon system designed to provide physicians with a comprehensive and current collection of clinical diagnostic and therapeutic information. Physicians could access this information from any display terminal in the hospital. In 1978, this library contained information on effective antibiotics for specific organisms; antipsychotic agents; and recommended treatments; laboratory interpretation aids for test results, for diagnosis, and for drug levels. For example, the library could provide a hyperlipemia workup with recommended tests and their interpretation; a thyroid-radioisotope ordering aid; indications for ordering tests and therapy for patients with pulmonary disease; and, an index to surgery articles with the capability of printing out any indexed article [140].

The pharmacy received all drug orders as they were entered into the system, and printed dispensing labels including known drug allergies. The system also provided daily patient drug profiles of all medications being taken by each patient. Dietary orders entered by physicians and nurses printed out in the dietician's office prior to each meal. The system supported all nursing functions, including nursing care plans, charting, scheduling, and supply ordering.

Technicon developed an online database management system called MATRIX, which allowed hospitals to modify their clinical applications to meet their own needs locally [140]. About 30 % of patient discharge summaries were generated from a sequence of displays, without requiring any dictation [165]. The patient's file was removed from computer disk storage 2 days after the patient's discharge from the hospital; and the file was then transferred to magnetic tape.

The Technicon MIS was installed also at the Ralph E. Davies Medical Center in San Francisco in 1972; it operated via the Technicon regional time-sharing computer center. In 1973, the first in-hospital Technicon computer installation occurred at the Nebraska Methodist Hospital in Omaha. From Technicon's second regional center in Fairfield, New Jersey, Technicon next installed a system at St. Barnabas Hospital in Livingston, New Jersey, and at the Maine Medical Center in Portland. In 1975, Technicon installed its system at the Clinical Center of the NIH, initially operated from a time-shared computer at the Technicon Fairfield Center, but transferred later to the NIH computer facility in Bethesda, Maryland [71]. The El Camino Hospital continued through the 1980s to operate with a time-shared computer.

In 1980, Revlon, Inc. acquired the Technicon Data Systems Corporation. It was repurchased in 1986 by a new company, called TDS Healthcare Systems Corporation, headed by Whitehead, the son of the founder of the Technicon Corporation. In 1987, it announced its enhanced TDS 4000 system [35]. By 1986 the Technicon MIS had been installed in about 40 hospitals [30]. By the end of the 1980s, there were 85 TDS system installations across the United States, Canada, and the United Kingdom. These installations included major teaching institutions such as New York University, Temple University, Medical College of Virginia, University of Illinois, Loyola, University of Chicago, Baylor University, and the University of California at Irvine [71].

The Lockheed HIS, initiated in 1966, became the Technicon MIS in 1971 and the TDS in 1986. It was probably the best commercially developed HIS in the United States throughout the 1970s and 1980s. It had some deficiencies, such as a discontinuous patient record that did not integrate patient data collected over multiple admissions, and it did not support clinicians' office automation. By the end of the 1980s, enhancements added to the TDS 4000 system partially corrected these deficiencies. The modifications expanded the computerized patient record and provided linkages of the hospital system to attending physicians' offices.

6.3.8 Henry Ford Hospital in Detroit, Michigan

In 1965 Stobie [151] at Henry Ford Hospital in Detroit, Michigan, reported beginning the implementation of an HIS with files for some medical applications in addition to administrative and business functions.

6.3.9 Memorial Sloan-Kettering Cancer Center, New York, New York

Financial management systems are essential for every HIS administration. Zucker [174] at Memorial Sloan-Kettering Cancer Center reported that their HIS began operation in 1964 with an administrative management system that included a patient admission and discharge application, accounts receivable, patient invoices, financial reports, payroll, and personnel files.

6.3.10 Massachusetts General Hospital in Boston, Massachusetts

In 1966, Barnett and associates at the Laboratory of Computer Science (LCS) initiated a pilot project in the Massachusetts General Hospital (MGH) for a computer-based, clinical laboratory reporting system. The LCS was a unit of the Department of Medicine of the MGH and the Harvard Medical School. Barnett [15, 16] reported that the MGH system enabled entering and printing of any selected groupings of laboratory test results. Weekly summaries appeared in a format designed by the users that displayed tests in associated groups, such as by serum electrolytes or by hematology.

In 1967, Barnett also developed a medications ordering system at the MGH. Every hour on each MGH patient care unit, the computer generated a list of medications to be administered at that hour. By 1974, the system encompassed clinical laboratory and medication order functions, and modules for hematology, pathology, x-ray scheduling, x-ray film folder inventory control, and x-ray reporting. These modules were all written in the MUMPS language (MGH Utility Multi-Programming System), an operating system developed at MGH [17, 22, 65]. The modules were implemented on several different vendors' computer systems, but were functionally identical. Barnett's MGH system soon expanded into nine patient care areas covering about 300 beds, and three laboratories in the hospital. It used more than 100 standard model Teletype terminals. Computer programs were interactive, whereby the computer asked a question and the user entered a response.

Barnett recognized that the order entry systems generally available at that time allowed the physicians to write their orders and notes in the routine fashion, and then use clerical personnel to enter the information into the computer system. He felt that the inherent weakness in this strategy was that the computer interaction was then not with the physician who was generating the order, but with a clerical staff member who had no decision making power [19]. The Teletype terminals could support interactive order entry by any healthcare worker. Nevertheless, Barnett [15, 19] was reluctant to use clerical personnel to enter physician's orders. He believed that physicians should enter orders so as to not eliminate the system's clinical decision support capabilities. Physicians were most qualified to benefit from feedback from a system that checked their orders for completeness, accuracy, and acceptability of an order. An online, interactive system could check an order against the data in the computer record for drug-drug interactions, for drug-laboratory test value interactions, or known allergic reactions to drugs. If this information was not given back immediately to the physician at the time of the creation of the order, Barnett felt that it was less useful. He believed that if there was a significant time delay between the writing of the order and its entry into the computer system, the responsible physician might have left the care unit and any needed clarification of the order would then be more difficult and time-consuming to obtain.

In 1971, the Massachusetts General Hospital initiated a nurse-practitioner project to allow nurses access to computer-stored medical records. Using a video terminal with a light-pen data selector, after entering the patient's identification number, a nurse could retrieve and review current medication orders, recent progress notes, and laboratory test results. Nursing progress notes were entered by selecting appropriate data items from a series of displayed frames. A Teletype printer could print out a data flow sheet for that office visit. The project used the computer and software of Barnett's Laboratory of Computer Science at MGH [60]. In 1971 Barnett also initiated the Computer-Stored Ambulatory Record (COSTAR) system for the Harvard Community Health Plan (HCHP) in Boston. Health professionals in their offices manually completed paper-based structured encounter forms at the time of each patient visit. Printed templates were used for the first visit, and then computer-generated forms for subsequent visits. On these forms, the physicians recorded diagnoses, orders for tests, and treatments. Clerks, using remote terminals connected by telephone lines to the computer located at the Laboratory of Computer Science, entered completed forms that had been collected in the medical record room. After the entry of new data into the patient's record, the system generated a an updated status report summarizing the patient's current information, including current medications and latest laboratory test results. Barnett [14] wrote that in its design and implementation, a central objective of COSTAR was to provide information-processing support for communication of laboratory, x-ray, and electrocardiogram reports. COSTAR operated under the MUMPS language. By the late 1970s, COSTAR had gone through four revisions in its system design at the HCHP [18]. By the end of the 1980s, the COSTAR system was widely disseminated in the United States, being used in more than 120 sites [13].

6.3.11   Roswell Park Memorial Institute in Buffalo, New York

Ausman and associates [2] at Roswell Park Memorial Institute in Buffalo, New York, reported in 1966 a prototype HIS operating in one 42-bed nursing station that provided care to patients with malignant diseases. They collected all data for the patient's history and nurses' and physicians' notes on punched cards or by transcription to punched paper tape for entry into the computer.

6.3.12   Monmouth Medical Center Hospital in Long Branch, New Jersey

In 1966, the Monmouth Medical Center Hospital in Long Branch, New Jersey installed a system with an IBM 360/30 computer and using similar matrix-button input terminals. These input terminals, along with keyboard typewriters, were located in 14 nursing stations, admitting office, business office, pharmacy, laboratory, x-ray, dietary, central supply, and operating-room supervisor's office [113].

6.3.13   University of Vermont Medical Center in Burlington, Vermont

In 1967, Weed and associates began to develop their Problem-Oriented Medical Information System (PROMIS) at the 450-bed University of Vermont Medical Center, Burlington. In 1971, the PROMIS system was installed in a 20-bed obstetrics-gynecology ward at the University Hospital, with linkages to radiology, clinical laboratory, pharmacy, and to the doctors' lounge for entering of surgeons' notes. This hospital ward averaged from 75 to 80 inpatient admissions per month. After 1 year of operation, Weed [167] concluded that PROMIS provided the guidance of the logical power of the computer to the structured selection of medical-content displays in the context of the problem-oriented record. As a result of the implementation of PROMIS in the obstetrics-gynecology ward, a major reorganization of nursing duties transpired; with a reduction in the number of nurse aides and some addition to the nursing staff, the nurse took on a different role and became responsible for accurate patient record keeping. The PROMIS project was primarily financed by a grant from the National Center for Health Services Research (NCHSR) of the U.S. Department of Health, Education, and Welfare [118], with additional resources provided by the Robert Wood Johnson Foundation and the University of Vermont College of Medicine.

By 1975, Weed's PROMIS system used two Control Data Corporation (CDC) 1700 series computers with CDC's operating system, and used 14 Digiscribe touch-sensitive video terminals. Five terminals were located in the obstetrics-gynecology ward, one in surgery, one in the conference room for demonstration purposes and system development, one in the pharmacy, and one in the x-ray department [51]. The terminals could display 1,000 characters of information in 20 lines of 50 characters each, and had 20 touch-sensitive fields. The user selected an item by touching the screen at the position of that choice. The user could enter textual data by typing on the keyboard attached to the terminal. Weed's basic approach to using PROMIS was through a collection of computer-based clinical displays called "frames", which helped to guide and teach the health professionals who interacted with the system as they entered the patient's data. Physicians' entries were stored in the patient's record. The system branched to various decision points where the physician could elect courses of action selected from the stored frames, or selected other appropriate action [121].

Weed [168] described the prototype system after it had been in operation for almost 4 years in the gynecology ward, and for 6 months on a general medical ward. The system at that time supported 30 touch-sensitive display terminals connected to a single minicomputer. Each user had a distinct password, which allowed access to data in accordance with the user's classification. After health care professionals selected a patient from a ward census, they chose one of four actions: (1) the DataBase, (2) Problem Formulation, (3) Initial Plans, or (4) Progress Notes to add to or retrieve specific parts of the patient's record. A nurse usually entered into the database the patient's chief complaint, the patient's profile, general appearance, and vital signs. The patient could enter a self-administered inventory-by-systems history, which included a series of up to 275 questions. After completion of the first DataBase phase, clinicians entered physical examination findings using up to 1,410 branching displays. Next, the physician formulated the patient's problems by making a series of selections from displays that contained frames and tables. Excluding the initial DataBase section, every entry into a patient's computer-based record was associated with a particular patient problem. An Initial Plan was entered for each problem, followed by intermittent Progress Notes. The system contained problem-specific information for more than 700 disease entities. The above four sections comprised the basic electronic record for each patient. No written records were maintained in parallel [168].

By 1979, PROMIS used a network of minicomputers [131] and contained more than 45,000 frames and tables that structured the decisions and actions of health care providers [52]. By the early 1980s, Weed et al. had a well-developed software system for generating and displaying frames. Application programming was done entirely by the PROMIS staff. Programmers used a special-purpose language, called PROMIS Programming Language (PPL). The PPL supported functions specific to PROMIS, such as interacting with touch-screen terminals [51].

On a single ward at the University of Vermont Hospital where PROMIS had been implemented from 1971 to 1975, a vote took place on the gynecology service. All of the nurses and a majority of the house officers, who were the primary users of the system, voted to keep it. However, attending physicians voted eight to six to discontinue its use [118]. In a 1979 evaluation of PROMIS, supported by the NCHSR, a study compared two similar wards at the Vermont Medical Center Hospital. One ward used PROMIS. The control ward used a manual, paper-based, problem-oriented medical record. Compared to the manual system, PROMIS provided slightly better documentation. No significant differences occurred in the mean cost of provided patient services or in the time physicians spent using the two record systems. The study noted that the PROMIS developers believed that effective and committed leadership was an essential need for PROMIS to succeed [152]. Subsequent evaluations of PROMIS showed that nurses accepted PROMIS more readily than did doctors. The physicians felt coerced rather than attracted to using the system. They believed they were expected to adapt to the system rather than the converse [54]. A similar sentiment was that PROMIS users perceived that they were working for the system rather than vice versa [30]. In 1981, when Weed's grants expired, a group of PROMIS developers formed PROMIS Information Systems, and continued the system's development activities in South Burlington, Vermont. Its marketing unit, PROMIS Health Care Systems, established its headquarters in 1984 in Concord, California [114]. In the mid-1980s Weed began to develop a series of commercially available computer programs that he called "problem-knowledge couplers" to apply his methods in the care of specific medical problems [169].

Although PROMIS, as a system, failed to gain general acceptance, Weed's influence on HISs and the conceptual organization of the patient record was substantial. The PROMIS system was one of the first to use in-hospital network linkages, and pioneered use of touch screen technology long before commercial touchscreens were generally available. Weed [166] had defined methods for recording data in a problem-oriented medical record (POMR). He continually emphasized that the whole thrust of PROMIS was to first create the structures and the four phases of medical action. From that basis, one could then determine what basic data was needed to make first approximations, calculate probabilities as experience accumulated, modify the approximations, and slowly create a better plan. Blum [30] lauded PROMIS as a complete and well-organized medical record system with a sophisticated user interface; but observed that no major hospital was using PROMIS for the main reason that PROMIS users perceived that the system was too controlling.

6.3.14 New York-Downstate Medical Center in Brooklyn, New York

In 1968, Siegel [133], at the New York-Downstate Medical Center described a hospital information system (HIS) that used an IBM 1440-1410 computer complex connected to 40 remote typewriter-terminal printers. They entered data using punched cards, paper tape, and IBM 1092 matrix-overlay keyboards; and they used magnetic tape and disk for data storage. Terminals were placed in the specialty clinics, as well as in the clinical laboratories, radiology, pharmacy, and central stores. Their initial hospital applications included patient admission-discharge-bed assignment, outpatient appointment scheduling, accounting and administrative functions, and developing an electronic medical records system.

6.3.15 University of California Hospitals in Los Angeles, California

In 1968, Lamson and associates at the University of California Hospitals in Los Angeles acquired their first computer and built a clinical laboratory and surgical pathology reporting system [82]. Their initial information system was gradually expanded, and by 1975 it provided summary reports that included data received from a large number of clinical laboratory computers, computers and from the coronary care unit, a pulmonary-function computer, and an anesthesia-monitoring computer. The system also included a tumor registry [81]. In 1969, the nine Los Angeles County hospitals initiated a centralized information system. Beginning with an IBM 360/40 computer connected by telephone cable to remote display terminals and printers, located initially in the admitting offices and pharmacies, centralized patient records were established. Pilot testing was conducted at that time by nurses for the order entry of medications, diets, and laboratory tests [127]. Lamson [83] noted that a HIS with a full financial management system changed the accounting department from a basic bookkeeping operation to a data-gathering and report-analyzing unit. The *financial management system* facilitated detailed cost accounting. It set charges for and tracked each item and service used by a patient, and could bill the patient on either a fee-for-service basis or a third-party payer reimbursement basis.

6.3.16 University of Southern California School of Medicine in Los Angeles, California

In 1969, Jelliffe and associates [75] at the University of Southern California School of Medicine initiated at the Los Angeles County General Hospital a series of programs for clinical pharmacology to analyze dosage requirements for a variety of medications, antibiotics, and inhalational anesthetics. In 1972, programs were added to analyze data from their cardiac catheterization laboratory, from echocardiograms, and from the pulmonary-function laboratory.

6.3.17 Beth Israel Hospital in Boston, Massachusetts

In 1969, the Beth Israel Hospital in Boston began an ambulatory patient care project, funded by grants from the U.S. Department of Health, Education, and Welfare. Slack and associates [135, 137, 138] described the project's objectives as to develop computer-supported, problem-oriented protocols to help non-physician practitioners to provide care for patients who had common medical problems, such as headaches, low back pain, upper-respiratory infections, and lower-urinary-tract infections. The computer-supported system was discontinued after a few years because it was more expensive than was a manual, paper-based flowchart system [60].

In 1976, Bleich, Slack, and associates at Beth Israel Hospital initiated a new hospital information system. In 1982, they expanded the HIS into the Brigham and Women's Hospital. By 1984, the HIS ran on a network of Data General Eclipse minicomputers that supported 300 video display terminals located throughout the hospital. The system permitted users to retrieve data from the clinical laboratories, to look up reports from the departments of radiology and pathology, look up prescriptions filled in the outpatient pharmacy, and to request delivery of patients' records. In 1983, a survey of 545 physicians, medical students, and nurses reported that they used the computer terminals most of the time to look up laboratory test results; and 83 % of users said that the terminals enabled them to work faster [26]. In the 1990s, their HIS provided results from all laboratories and clinical departments [134]. In 1994, Brigham and Women's Hospital joined with Massachusetts General Hospital to form Partner's Health Care System that included 10 hospitals and more than 250 practice sites [154].

6.3.18   Johns Hopkins Hospital in Baltimore, Maryland

In 1970, the Johns Hopkins Hospital (JHH) initiated a prototype HIS to process physicians' written orders, produce work lists for ward nurses, and generate daily computer-printed, patient drug profiles for the patients' records. In 1975, a "Minirecord" (minimal essential record) system was also initiated for an outpatient information system (OIS) in the JHH Medical Clinics. The latter used encounter forms with an area for recording medications and procedures. Forms were filled out at each patient visit [101]. Work also began on a prototype Oncology Clinical Information System (OCIS) for their cancer patients. The OCIS contained patient care data for both hospital and clinic services, and also captured clinical laboratory test results and pharmacy data [29, 31, 76].

In 1976, the JHH implemented a radiology reporting system using a terminal that permitted the radiologist to select phrases with which to compose descriptions and interpretations for their x-ray reports. Its output was a computer-printed report that became available as soon as the radiologist completed his report [170]. By 1978, a clinical laboratory information system was also operational, which supported the internal working processes for the laboratory, and also produced the patient's cumulative laboratory report [76]. During the 1980s, a network gradually evolved in the JHH information system. By 1986, the JHH system included IBM 3081 and 3083 computers that also supported an inpatient pharmacy system with a unit dose distribution system. The radiology system and clinical laboratory system ran on three PDP 11/70 computers [155].

6.3.19   Shands Hospital in Gainesville, Florida

In 1972, Grams and associates at the University of Florida in Gainesville and the 500-bed Shands Hospital, with its outpatient clinic and emergency room, began to formulate a computer-based laboratory information system that provided some clinical decision support capabilities. Initially the system did not have any reporting capabilities. The test results were manually recorded on a cumulative report form. In 1975, a single computer began to service their subsystems for hospital admissions functions, the clinical laboratory, anatomic pathology, microscopy, and blood banking. In 1977, they installed a network to integrate their laboratory functions, hospital admissions service, and nursing stations. They used one computer for the nursing and admissions functions, and linked it to a second computer in the laboratory.

6.3.20   Regenstrief Institute for Health Care and the Indiana University School of Medicine in Indianapolis, Indiana

In 1973, McDonald and associates at the Regenstrief Institute for Health Care and the Indiana University School of Medicine developed the Regenstrief Medical Record (RMR) system for the care of ambulatory patients. It was initially installed in the diabetes clinic of Wishard Memorial Hospital in Indianapolis. By 1977, the general medicine clinics, the renal clinic, and two community-based clinics located three miles from the central computer site had been added. The system supported electronic medical records for 19,000 ambulatory patients who had 40,000 office visits per year [109]. The RMR system was intended to complement, rather than to replace, the paper-based patient record. For each patient served, RMR contained a core medical record, which included patient data such as treatment records; and reports from laboratory tests, x-ray studies, and electrocardiograms. By 1982, RMR's medical database contained 60,000 patients' records, of variable length, with the data coded or stored as free-text narrative reports.

The RMR system used a PDP11/45 computer, which ran under the RSTS/E operating system. The computer programs were initially written in BASIC-PLUS. The system provided time-sharing services 24 h per day, 7 days per week. The RMR database contained the medical record file and RMR's associated language, CARE. Patients' records within the medical record file contained patient data that was most often stored in a coded (structured) format, although some free-text entry occurred. Patients records were of fixed-field and fixed-format; that is, within a given file, all records had the same length. Correspondingly, data fields appeared in the same location in every patient's record [103]. A set of utility programs supported storing, editing, sorting, and reporting data, as well as aggregate batch-processing and administrative analyses. Database files existed for the clinical laboratory subsystem, the pharmacy subsystem, the patient registry file, patient appointments, the physician registry, and physicians' schedules. A metathesaurus provided a dictionary of terms. It defined the kinds of data that could be stored in the medical record files.

The RMR system initially focused on supporting physicians' decision making in the office. It presented clinical information in compact reports, and reminded physicians about clinical conditions requiring corrective action. For each patient, the RMR produced three reports that constituted a core medical record, and/or provided protocol-based feedback "reminders" or "alerts" to the physician about important clinical conditions [107]. Physician-authored protocols controlled generation of these computer reminders and alerts. Each protocol defined the clinical condition (trigger), and the content of the corresponding reminder that would result when triggered [104].

McDonald et al. [109] reported that the RMR system used paper-based reports, rather than visual displays as its primary mechanism for transmitting information to the physician, as this mode of data transfer was preferred since it was inexpensive, portable, easier to browse, and paper reports could be annotated by pencil. In addition to printing paper encounter forms to be used for the next patient visit, the RMR system provided cumulative summary reports of the information stored in the computer-based patient record [109]. With the time-oriented view of the patient's data, the physician could readily find and compare the most recent data to prior data, such as for repeated laboratory tests. An asterisk appeared beside each abnormal value for emphasis.

For most patients, an electronic paper-chart abstract formed the initial body of the computer-based record. In the RMR system, clinical laboratory information was acquired directly from the laboratory computer system. The pharmacy prescription information was captured from both the hospital and outpatient pharmacy systems. For each patient's return visit a patient summary report was generated which included historical and treatment information; and reports from laboratories, radiology, electrocardiography, and nuclear medicine in a modified flow sheet format. At each subsequent encounter visit, additional data were added to the record electronically. A two-part patient encounter form was generated for each patient's return visit. The physician could readily identify the returning patient, note the active problems from the last visit, and see the active treatment profile. The physician recorded numeric clinical data, such as weight and blood pressure, for later optical machine reading into the computer. The problem list was updated by drawing a line through problems that had been resolved and by writing in new problems that had arisen. Progress notes were entered in the space beside the problem list; and a space was also provided for writing orders for tests and for return appointments. Essential information from hospital stays, such as diagnoses, was transferred from hospital case abstract tapes. A space was provided on the form for writing orders for tests. Within the space for orders, the computer suggested certain tests that might be needed. The patient's current prescriptions were listed at the bottom of the encounter form in a medication profile. The physician refilled (by writing "R") or discontinued (by writing "D/C") after each drug, and wrote new prescriptions underneath this prescription list. The patients took a carbon copy of this section of the encounter form to the pharmacy as their prescription. Thus the encounter form performed many recording and retrieving tasks for the physician. Data recorded by physicians on the encounter forms were entered into the computer by clerks.

The patient summary report was the second report generated for each patient's return visit. This report included laboratory data, historical information, treatment, radiology, EKG, nuclear medicine, and other data in a modified flow sheet format [107]. It also listed the patient's clinic, hospital, and emergency room visits and the results of x-ray and laboratory tests, with test results presented in reverse chronological order. With this time-oriented view of the data, the physician could quickly find the most recent data (for example, blood pressure or blood glucose) and compare them to the previous levels. The objective of the patient's summary report was to facilitate data retrieval and to perform some data-organization tasks for the physician.

The patient's surveillance report was the third report generated for each patient's return visit. This report represented the most sophisticated processing of data in the OIS, and assisted the physician in clinical decision making. McDonald et al. [109] developed a computer program called CARE, which permitted non-programmers to perform complex queries of the medical records. It could also provide health care practitioners with aspects of clinical decision support for the diagnosis or treatment of a patient, as well as some quality assurance metrics regarding care delivery. The patient's surveillance report contained statements that served as clinical reminders to physicians regarding diagnostic studies or treatments. These statements were programmed by physicians in terms of, "IF-THEN-ELSE statements" called "protocols" that were written in the CARE language [109]. In 1 year, the CARE program generated more than 70,000 reminders for 30,000 patient visits [108].

In the early 1980s, the RMR system contained medical records for more than 60,000 patients, with data regarding inpatient, outpatient, and emergency room care [104]. The shared clinical laboratory and pharmacy systems used a microcomputer-based workstation to display forms on "windows." The user could enter data using a mouse to select data from menus such as problem lists [106]. McDonald applied the term gopher work to the functions of recording, retrieving, organizing, and reviewing data. In the 1980s, the RMR system was operational in the general medical clinic and in the diabetes clinic, and included a hospital and a pharmacy module.

In the early 1980s, the RMR system shared a DEC VAX 11/780 computer between the clinical laboratory and pharmacy systems, and used a microcomputer-based workstation to display forms, in which the user could enter data using a mouse to select data from menus [108]. By the mid-1980s, any patient seen by the General Medicine Service in the emergency room, in the outpatient clinics, or in the hospital wards had been registered with the Regenstrief computer-based medical record system. After a patient was registered, the computer record included most of the patient's diagnostic studies, treatments, hospital discharge and clinic visit diagnoses, problems lists, imaging studies, EKGs, and laboratory and medication data that were entered automatically from computerized laboratory and pharmacy systems [102]. In 1988, the RMR system was also linked to the laboratory, radiology, and pharmacy within the local Veterans and University hospitals [106]. By the end of the 1990s the RMR system served a large network of hospitals and clinics [110]. It had become a leading HIS and OIS model in the United States.

Two RMR modules, the database management system and the pharmacy system, could be purchased from the Digital Equipment Corporation [79]. The Digital Equipment Corporation planned to market the Regenstrief Data Base System [103].

6.3.21 Duke University Medical Center in Durham, North Carolina

In 1976, Hammond and Stead at Duke University Medical Center began to develop The Medical Record (TMR). The Duke University hospital used an IBM computer with display terminals located in the hospital nursing stations for obstetrics patients. When a pregnant woman entered the hospital, the hospital system sent a message to the TMR system, and the patient's prenatal record was transferred into the hospital's computer-stored record [66]. The initial Duke HIS transmitted the outpatient prenatal records to the inpatient obstetrics department when a woman in labor was admitted [68].

In 1983, TMR was installed in the Kenneth Norris Cancer Research Hospital that had a 60-bed inpatient service and an outpatient clinic. To satisfy the requirements for this hospital information system, TMR was modified to conform with this hospital's admission and discharge functions, billing and claims processing, and 24-h-a-day patient encounters [148, 149]. In 1984, the Duke HIS serviced 52 nursing stations with an aggregate of 1,008 beds. It was linked to 18 clinical service departments and 64 specimen laboratories [149]. Microcomputers were used as departmental workstations linked to the central computer. By 1985, the Duke TMR system had increased in size to require a local area network (LAN); and it was also linked to its clinical laboratory system by an Ethernet connection so that the laboratory could query a patient's record directly on the main TMR system through the network [67, 147].

The TMR system became a prototype for IBM's Patient Care System (PCS) for obstetrics patients. In 1976, a prototype of IBM's Patient Care System (PCS) began to be implemented as a joint project with Stead and Hammond's group in Durham. The Duke HIS ran on an IBM 3033 computer with IBM's IMS database management system and its CICS terminal handler. It used IBM 3278 visual displays with light-pen selectors, and terminals were available at each nursing station and in each service department. It stored all clinical information in its database and was interfaced with Duke's outpatient information system using Duke's The Medical Record (TMR). In 1987, the Duke HIS central computer was upgraded to an IBM 3090-200 that serviced 550 display terminals. It used an application generator program called the Application Development System (ADS), which was also marketed by IBM. IBM's PCS was also developed to run under ADS [78].

6.3.22   Commercial (Vendor) Hospital Information Systems

At the end of the 1970s, Maturi and DuBois [100] conducted a survey for the National Center for Health Services Research (NCHSR) of the state of commercially available, hospital department-specific information systems, including their relationship to hospital-wide communication systems. The department-specific applications that they reviewed were medical record room functions (tracking charts, coding diseases, and similar record librarian activities), laboratory, radiology, and pharmacy systems. The survey did not include computer-based patient records or general clinical applications. They reported that the department-specific systems were usually acquired by the hospital before a hospital-wide communication system was in place. However, many department-specific systems soon became part of a network as industry provided expanded interfacing capabilities. This trend which encouraged development of distributed systems involving department-specific and hospital-wide systems.

Young and associates [173] at the University of Southern California also conducted a survey of minicomputer-based HISs in medium-sized hospitals (those with 100–300 beds). They identified 75 different applications that were grouped into five levels in steps of complexity comprising a modular implementation of a HIS. All hospitals had step-1 applications which included billing and accounting, payroll, and inpatient census), and step-2 applications that included admission-discharge-transfer, patient-record data collection, patient identification-number assignment, general ledger interface, and credit and collections. Only about one-half of the hospitals had step-3 applications that used online data entry terminals for order-entry, message communication, patient's identification number retrieval, discharge abstract preparation, and various inventory applications. Less than one-fourth had step-4 applications, which included patient identification-number assignment, discharge analysis and reports, clinical laboratory worksheets and schedules, budget preparation and expense reports, and labor time collection. Few hospitals in this survey had step-5 applications with two-way data transmission and clinical functions which included test results reporting, medical chart reports, personnel history, and utilization review. They concluded that, as of that date, the smaller HISs based on minicomputers fell short of the more sophisticated HISs in larger hospitals with mainframe computers. The larger systems provided a greater variety of patient care and clinical applications.

In the early 1970s, Ball authored a series of reviews of the status of the vendor systems that attempted to provide comprehensive HIS services. Brief descriptions of those vendors follow. Biomedical Computer Services focused on the medical record and used a variety of computers linked to touch-screen terminals. The Control

Data Corporation (CDC) MEDICOM system used CDC computers connected to CDC touch-screen terminals. Medelco's Total HIS (T.H.I.S.) used prepunched cards for each order, service, or product available in the hospital; these were read into a hard-wired, preprogrammed machine. The McDonnell-Douglas Automation Company (MCAUTO) offered the HIS acquired in 1970 from the Sisters of the Third Order of St. Francis (briefly mentioned above). The Medical Information Technology, Inc (MEDITECH) was initiated in the late 1960s by MUMPS co-developer Neil Pappalardo; it initially used DEC or Data General minicomputers with display terminals and MEDITECH's own software for a relatively comprehensive integrated HIS. The National Data Communications Real-Time Electronic Access Communications for Hospitals (REACH) System used Honeywell and other computers; they were connected to Raytheon CRT display terminals with 20 selector push buttons (located along the left side of the display) for the entry of orders and routine tasks and a keyboard for entering textual data. The Searle Medidata System had touch terminals that used sets of overlays (for example, one for laboratory, another for pharmacy, and so on), each of which presented 320 order choices, in addition to display terminals and keyboards; Searle offered this system for only a few years, when it was taken over by Mediquip, a subsidiary of Quanta System Corporation. The Spectra Medical Systems offering used a Data General Nova minicomputer connected to color display terminals with a keyboard and light-pen selector for data entry. It was designed to be used by physicians [5, 7–9].

In 1976, a Spectra 2000 system for 800 beds was installed at Rush-Presbyterian-St. Lukes Medical Center in Chicago. It was replaced by a Spectra 3000 system in 1980, linked to minicomputers. It used visual display terminals with light-pens for users to select items from displayed, predefined data sets. Physicians entered their orders directly, and a nursing module was well accepted [123].

IBM's PCS/ADS (originally developed at Duke; see above) included development tools enabling install sites to make modifications after the delivered applications had been installed. It thus served as an application-enabling system for large mainframe HISs. In 1987, IBM announced PCS/ADS as a licensed product for ADS-based application development [69]. In parallel with the development of the Duke HIS, IBM also began in 1976 to install its PCS using an IBM 370 computer at Parkland Memorial Hospital in Dallas, Texas, where it was called the Parkland Online Information System (POIS) and was under the direction of Mishelevich and associates. By 1978 a relatively comprehensive HIS was operational, with terminals at all 40 nursing stations [112].

Barker [12] observed that in the 1970s about 90 % of all hospital charges were paid by third parties; therefore it was important that the business applications of the HIS not only reported revenues produced by each cost center for each type of procedure, but also generated statistical reports that analyzed units of service. Through the 1980s, IBM continued to provide most of the mainframe-based HISs in the United States. In the 1980s, the infusion of minicomputers and microcomputer-based clinical workstations resulted in the application of a variety of specialized local area networks (LANs) to support distributed data processing systems connecting different vendor's computers.

As increasing competition resulted from the new hardware and software that evolved in the late 1970s and 1980s, vendor-provided HISs underwent constant changes. Correspondingly, the dramatis personae of HIS vendors evolved and diversified.

6.4 Evolution of ADT Systems: Concept Sharing During HIS Development

Many fields of scientific inquiry and engineering begin with isolated pioneers working "in the wilderness" before next-generation concepts evolve through sharing of ideas. The foregoing history of the early HISs exemplifies this pattern. The cross-institutional history of ADT design and evolution follows below as an example of how shared ideas across institutions accelerated progress after the early days of the isolated pioneers.

6.4.1 Overview of ADT System Functions

Admission, discharge, and transfer (ADT) functions are used when a patient enters a hospital. The hospital admitting department has usually received from the referring physician a tentative diagnosis and a request for admission to an appropriate nursing unit, such as to medicine, surgery, obstetrics, pediatrics, or other specialty units. The ADT functions, and billing and accounting, were among the earliest HIS applications. ADT functions included patient identification, preparation of identification wristbands, and bed management capabilities that supported admission to a nursing unit. As in any MIS, the entry of a patient to the HIS required a set of identification data that included the patient's name, gender, birthdate, and the assignment of a unique medical record number that served as the basic linkage for all the computer-processed patient data, so that data generated by every service received by the patient during the hospital stay could be linked and stored in the patient's computer-based record. After the admitting office had notified the appropriate nursing unit of the admission of the patient, the ADT system (or the nursing unit in some cases) assigned the patient to a suitable room and bed. The ADT system maintained a record of bed assignments, of any transfers of patients to other beds, and of patients' discharges from the hospital. ADT had to notify all relevant hospital departments of any changes in bed assignments, since laboratory personnel, for example, had to be kept informed where to find patients in order to collect blood specimens and where to send test results. The ADT system maintained a registry of all hospital patients and prepared a variety of patient census and management reports, including periodic listings of admissions and discharges, and listings of patients by nursing units. ADT bed control and census reports monitored the number of patients in the hospital, their clinical service, their nursing unit with patient's bed locations, and their attending physicians. Patients were often transferred to different nursing units, such as when a medical patient required an operation and became a surgical patient. Housekeeping services were notified when a bed was vacated to prepare the bed for the next patient.

6.4.2   History of Early ADT System Development

The earliest admission, discharge, and transfer (ADT) systems in the 1950s used paper forms and punch cards to enter data. In the early 1960s, some hospitals used keyboards with rows of push-button precoded keys to enter data into their computers, including the patient admission data, as was reported at Children's Hospital in Akron, Ohio [45]. With the advent of visual display terminals in the 1960s, data were entered by keyboard and were displayed for verification and retrieval. On April 1, 1966, Boston's Children's Hospital claimed to have the first ADT system with display terminals in the United States [42, 139]. In the fall of 1966, Massachusetts General Hospital (MGH) initiated its own ADT system [64]. Both of these systems were similar in that they used visual display terminals with keyboards for data entry and teletypewriters for printers in the admitting office, which communicated to 16 terminals at the nursing stations in the Children's Hospital, and to nine terminals in the nursing units in the MGH. In both hospitals, ADT had links to the clinical laboratory for communication of admitting laboratory test orders and for collection of test samples; and both provided similar comprehensive ADT functions with associated reports.

Elsewhere, Dunn [47] at the Henry Ford Hospital, reported beginning to use a computer as a communication system for ADT functions to relieve the large backlog of patients waiting for admission to the hospital. Wood [171] at the Massachusetts Eye and Ear Infirmary in Boston, reported a computer-based ADT system programmed to schedule patient admissions 2 months in advance of elective surgery procedures. A physician's request for admission of a patient resulted in the completion of a preadmission form with the names of the physician and the patient, the patient's diagnosis and anticipated surgical procedure, the time needed for the procedure and the anesthesia requirements, and the anticipated length of the patient's stay in the hospital. These data were punched into cards and entered into the computer. Using statistical data accumulated at the hospital from past years, the computer estimated: (1) the number of beds to be available on any given day; and (2) a projection of the total number of beds to be available on a given day 2 months in the future. The discharge functions of the HIS ADT program were activated when a nursing unit notified the ADT system that the physician had entered the order for a patient's discharge from the hospital. This affected the ADT bed control and census data, and initiated requests for any other discharge instructions for the patient, such as medications to take home or follow-up ambulatory visits and procedures. Discharge instructions for a patient's home care were taken over generally by the

HIS nursing department as these became increasingly more sophisticated in the 1970s and 1980s.

For example, by 1987 the Johns Hopkins Hospital patients at their discharge received computer-printed Discharge Instructions for Health Management from a prestructured format, completed by a nurse using displayed menus for data entry, and custom-tailored to each patient [117].

6.5 HIS Functional Requirements and Technical Designs

As noted above, specialized domains of scientific inquiry and engineering begin with isolated pioneers working "in the wilderness." For such early systems, the general rule was "if you've seen one, you've seen one" – that is, commonalities in design and generally accepted requirements can only occur after many disparate approaches exist. Only later do next-generation concepts evolve. The development of shared functional requirements and technical designs for HISs followed upon the development of early HISs described in preceding Sect. 6.3.

Technical experts must specify functional requirements for each HIS installation, describing how to harness various technologies available to accomplish what designers and users expect the HIS to do. Through the decades, the functional requirements for HISs have changed less than have their technical specifications. From the 1950s to the present time, the individual expectations of healthcare professionals for HISs have not evolved substantially regarding inpatient care. Nevertheless, technology innovations in each decade modified the potential capabilities, and enhanced the desired functionality of a HIS. In parallel, the somewhat different expectations of hospital administrators have also not changed much over time.

The HIS functional requirements developed for the care of hospital inpatients are generally more complex than those developed for an outpatient system (Chap. 5), even though their basic functional requirements are somewhat similar. Before a HIS can be implemented, the future users of the HIS must first develop the detailed specifications regarding what they wanted the HIS to do – that is, to fully define its functionality. These HIS functional requirements needed to describe all the specific applications and tasks that the HIS was to perform for each hospital component, for each department, service, and procedure; as examples, for admitting a patient, ordering and giving a medication, or requesting and reporting a clinical laboratory test at a nursing station. Flagle [55] proposed that the general functional requirements for a HIS needed to satisfy specific work levels of a hospital on each of its clinical services, from the intensive care unit (ICU) to the convalescent care services, based on assessments of workloads and associated information requirements. The HIS needed to: (1) provide information to support hospital decision processes; (2) satisfy needs for completeness as to all required information elements; (3) maintain timeliness such that orders would be made in time to permit appropriate responses; (4) maintain accuracy and reliability of data so that information would be transmitted without error; (5) encourage economy of cost and avoidance of repetitive handling of data elements; and (6) permit manipulation of data, and its retrieval in a useful format.

Barnett [15] described the functions of an HIS from the viewpoint of its various users. To the physician, a HIS should provide accurate and legible communication of reports; reliable scheduling of procedures; and timely, precise implementation of activities ordered for patients' care. To the nurse, a HIS should lighten the load of communications, and of preparing requisitions, and of transcribing and charting patients' information. To the administrator, a HIS should help to use resources more effectively, help to gather the data necessary for appropriate decisions, and to ensure that the information necessary for the patient billing process was readily available and accurate. To the medical research investigator, a HIS should offer the potential of a database of patient care activities that was not only accurate, but was also organized so data could be retrieved and analyzed easily. Barnett [21] further grouped the functional components of HISs into four generic forms: (1) the transactional system that is primarily concerned with financial management; (2) the ancillary support systems aimed at improving the information-related activities of individual administrative subsystems including patient identification, business and financial, inventory management, admission, discharge, and transfer (ADT), and bed census; patient and staff scheduling; dietary services; utilization review, and quality assurance; patient record systems; clinical specialty subsystems; outpatient clinics; nursing services; clinical support systems; service units such as the clinical laboratory, pharmacy, (3) the communications system that focuses on transmitting data among various personnel in different clinical support units of the hospital; and (4) the overall system that integrates information from all shared databases related to patient care.

Blois [27] defined the functions of a HIS as including: (1) data processing involving a single hospital or medical function related to the management of a given patient; (2) data communication from one location to another for patient care; and (3) studies involving compilations of data for research purposes. Spencer [141] described information processing in a general hospital as comprising the admission process, the evaluation of the patient status, the need for identification of various diagnostic and therapeutic problems, the ordering of patient care events, the coordination of those events by the physician and other professionals, and the periodic evaluation of changes in the patient's status. Finally, there was the need for discharge care planning, outcome evaluation, and patient disposition. Surveillance of how the care system was performing for quality assurance was based on information on patients' needs and outcomes. Lincoln [86] described the general activities of the various departments of a hospital as functioning both as individuals and as part of a team focused on the care of each patient. Services by these departments were provided by care units, such as the nursing stations and emergency rooms; the demand for these services was generated primarily by physicians concerned with the patients' problems. The informational tools of a hospital were its medical records which stored data on the procedures provided to patients.

As the general goal for a HIS, Collen [37–41] advocated that HISs use computers and communications equipment to collect, store, process, retrieve, and communicate patient care and administrative information for all activities and functions within the hospital, its outpatient medical offices, its clinical support services (laboratories, radiology, pharmacy, and others), and to communicate to and from any of its affiliated medical facilities. Such an integrated information system should have the abilities for communicating and integrating all patient data during the patient's lifetime of health care, and should provide appropriate clinical and administrative decision support. More specifically, the HIS functional requirements included the ability to: (1) Establish files and communicate information for identification and scheduling of patients and personnel; establish a database for business and administrative functions; and provide administrative decision support. (2) Provide an integrated computer-based patient record that had a high utility for the individual patient and for all involved health care professionals. (3) Facilitate entry of all orders for patient care, and display all results from ordered tests and procedures. Support nursing functions, and monitor the prescribing and administering of prescribed medications. Communicate patient data to-and-from all health care professionals, to-and-from the patient's computer-based medical record, and to-and-from all clinical support services (such as the laboratory and radiology). (4) Establish a database that can support clinical, epidemiological, and health services research; and satisfy legal requirements for patient data confidentiality and security. (5) Provide to health care professionals appropriate clinical decision support, including reminders and warning alerts of potential adverse events; and support utilization-review and quality-assurance procedures. (6) Have the capacity for an increasing number of patients and personnel, and for progressive expansion of the health care system's components. (7) Support continuing education of staff and patients; and provide linkage to outside bibliographic databases such as the NLM's MEDLINE. (8) Assure system reliability for 24-h a day, 7 days a week, year-round.

Lindberg [89] described HIS technical requirements, specifications, and system designs as needing to fully meet the administrative and clinical requirements of HIS users. He advised that if an HIS was well-designed to function in its medical requirements, it would by default supply much of the information required for hospital management. However, the reverse was not true, since a system designed to do administrative and business functions could rarely be converted into doing anything clinically meaningful. The hardware and software specifications for a comprehensive HIS always included a patient-record database, a variety of linked databases with specialized data sets, and a database management system.

The database management system was designed to support hospital administrative-level functions and departmental service functions, as well as to satisfy the clinical requirements of all health professionals (doctors, nurses, technicians). A management system configuration needed to be designed to operate all applications and subsystem modules so as to create and maintain functionally separate subsystem databases for managerial, clinical, operational, and investigational activities (for example, for utilization review and quality assurance, for operational clinical subspecialties and disease registries, and for research and ad hoc investigational studies); and to integrate all the data generated for each patient into a patients' medical records database and provide computer-based patients' records with format and content that satisfied the health care professionals in the hospital. The patient record database needed to be large enough to store all data entered for every patient during their stay in the hospital, including all essential medical data from prior hospitalizations. Basic was the need to integrate all HIS data and to make relevant active data available at the user interface to avoid the need for repetitious re-entry of the same data. The computer system analysts who were designing the HIS with a computer-based patient record had to satisfy the clinician's requirements for an integrated display or printout of any part or all of the data in a patient's record. Thus, the engineer had to design one computer-stored database to contain all of the patient's data; or provide an integrating database-management system that would bring together all the patient's data that had been originally collected and stored in multiple, subsystems, distributed databases; and present to the clinician what appeared to be an integrated patient record. The user would not need to know how this task was performed by the system, as long as the patient's medical record data that was displayed or printed did indeed present all the relevant data in an integrated and usable format.

Data quality control procedures need to be instituted for every HIS – with data error-checking techniques, and validity limits for physiological and test procedure measurements. A HIS needed to be designed so that computer-based patient data would comply with legal regulations for patient data confidentiality and security at least equal to those applied to paper-based patient records in the traditional hospital record room. Since many patient care functions in a hospital needed an online communications system with essentially 100 % reliability, the HIS needed to have: an uninterruptible electric power supply, an appropriate mix of backup equipment for replacement of failed components, and backup procedures to permit an acceptable, even if degraded, mode of operation until the full normal operating system was restored. With the advent of low cost minicomputers, maintaining duplicate computers for essential functions became a common backup mode. A backup system capable of the prompt reconstruction of a patient record by the linkage to, and the integration of information from distributed databases to always be able to provide an integrated electronic patient record from distributed databases, was an important requirement.

The detailed functional and technical requirements for a HIS were given to systems analysts and engineers, who then developed a set of detailed computer and communications technical specifications and a system design [62]. These were followed with plans for a HIS that hopefully would satisfy the users' specified needs. The HIS was then built either in-house or purchased from a vendor, and installed and operated in accordance with its functional and technical specifications. Human factors studies have demonstrated that meeting technical requirements is a necessary but not a sufficient condition to guarantee successful HIS installation.

6.6 Summary and Commentary

Lindberg [97] described the degrees of difficulty in the development of medical innovations in terms of the degrees of their complexity: (1) The easiest was the automation of a simple function such as providing a patient's billing for services. (2)

More difficult was the automation of a more complex function such as collecting and storing a patient's medical history. (3) Very difficult was constructing a complex function such as a medical database. (4) The most difficult was developing the highly complex medical information and database management system for a hospital.

The daunting complexity of a large hospital and the enormous number of functional and technical requirements for a comprehensive HIS were clearly evidenced by the relative lack of major achievements in the development of HISs during the early decades of medical informatics in the United States. Although successful subsystems were implemented for hospital administrative and business functions, as well as for some clinical departmental subsystems (such as nursing, clinical laboratory, and pharmacy), patient care clinical subsystems and the integrated computer-based patient record were still only incomplete prototypes that satisfied few physicians.

In the 1960s users of large mainframe, time-sharing computers began to provide services for some applications of information processing in hospitals, almost exclusively for hospital business and administrative functions. In the 1970s lower-cost minicomputers introduced the capabilities of locating smaller, special purpose computers in various hospital departments; they supported some clinical applications using display terminals located at nursing stations. In the 1980s, LANs permitted users of multiple, inexpensive microcomputers to interface with various individual local databases. Computers in affiliated hospitals began to use communication networks to link their information systems. By the end of the 1980s, large HISs with more advanced database management systems generally used a mix of large mini- and microcomputers linked by LANs, and some supported large numbers of clinical workstations and bedside terminals.

The major developmental work on early clinical applications of electronic patient record (EPR) systems and HISs were carried out primarily in academic centers, as described above. The successful academic prototypes were then acquired by vendors and marketed. As was the case for most medical technology in the United States, innovation followed funding. When federal funding decreased following the 1970s and 1980s, EPR and HIS development in academic centers decreased, and commercial EPR and HIS system development increased.

With the evolution of automated generation of summaries of electronic patient records and of electronic claims reporting as an automatic byproduct of EPR systems, patient care transactions, and data from a patient's different records of services received from a variety of separate healthcare providers would need to be linked by a common patient identification (ID) number. In the past, each health care provider assigned to each patient a different ID number. It would be ideal to give every person a unique health record ID number for nationwide use, and that would not be the same as the Social Security number. If pragmatists and economists were to prevail in using the Social Security number for health records, it would be unlikely that an electronic patient identification (EPI) system would then be able to fully protect the privacy and confidentiality of its patients' medical information.

Nursing information systems generally became the most widely used HIS modules, even as they evolved through the decades from punched-card data processing of medication orders to bedside computer terminals, with expert systems for guiding nursing diagnoses and patient care management. In contrast to physicians, most nurses readily accepted HIS and EPR systems.

Because HIS and EPR systems comprise complex aggregates of many continually changing clinical subsystems, it seems unlikely that any single vendor in the coming decades would develop a comprehensive EPR system that would satisfy the needs of every user and department. Hopefully in the 2010s the emerging open-systems architecture and the evolving interconnection standards for multivendor hardware and software will permit full flow and interchange of information between all multi-vendor EPR systems and subsystems and computer-based patients' records.

The evaluations of EPR systems were never fully satisfying, since data were always collected in a changing system within a changing environment; and controlled comparisons were not feasible because researchers could not find two hospitals that were the same in patients or providers or services. The installation of an EPR system meant the operation of a hybrid system during the transition; the initial period of operation meant using relatively untrained personnel. After an EPR system reached steady-state operation, the long-term benefits expected included access at all times to patient data by multiple users, improved retrievability and legibility of data, faster transmission of orders and results, decreased hospital information-handling costs, and better clinical decision support that would hopefully improve the quality of patient care. Few of these benefits were achieved in the 2000s. More frequently, the negative effects of EPR systems were documented as physicians found the methods of data entry to computers to be unfamiliar, burdensome, and more time-consuming than using pen and paper.

Installation of integrated, comprehensive, HIS and EPR systems in medical centers has become an achievable objective. Even in successful installations, the costs are not merely technical. The substantial impact of system installation, of end-user training, of workflow redesigns, and of system utilization and maintenance on end users, compounded by the requirement of keeping up with two rapidly evolving technologies – computer systems and clinical practice – takes a far larger toll than the simple costs of hardware and software acquisition.

References

1. Abdelhak M. Hospital information systems applications and potential: a literature review. In: Topics in health record management: hospital information systems. Germantown: Aspen Systems; 1982:3(1). p. 8–18.
2. Ausman RK, Baer GD, McGuire MR, Marks RA, Ewart R, Carey J, et al. Clinical data management. Ann N Y Acad Sci. 1966;128:1100–7.
3. Baker RL. An adaptable interactive system for medical and research data management. Methods Inf Med. 1974;13:209.
4. Ball MJ. An overview of total medical information systems. Methods Inf Med. 1971;10:73–82.
5. Ball MJ. EDP terminals: speed, legibility, control. Mod Hosp. 1971;117:119–22.

6. Ball MJ, Jacobs SE. Information systems: the status of level 1. Hospitals. 1980;54:179–86.
7. Ball MJ, Hammon GL. Overview of computer applications in a variety of health care areas. CRC Crit Rev Bioeng. 1975;2:183.
8. Ball MJ, Jacobs SE, Colavecchio FR, Potters JR. HIS: a status report. Hosp JAHA. 1972;46:48–52.
9. Ball MJ. Fifteen hospital information systems available. In: Ball MJ, editor. How to select a computerized hospital information system. New York: S Karger; 1973. p. 10–27.
10. Ball MJ, Jacobs SE. Hospital information systems as we enter the decade of the 80's. Proc SCAMC. 1980;1:646–50.
11. Ball MJ, Hannah KJ, Browne JD. Using computers in nursing. Reston: Reston Pub. Co; 1984.
12. Barker WD. Management reports can help control costs. Hospitals. 1977;51:165–70.
13. Barnett GO. The application of computer-based medical record systems in ambulatory practice. In: Orthner HF, Blum BI, editors. Implementing health care information systems. New York: Springer; 1989. p. 85–99.
14. Barnett GO. Computer-stored ambulatory record (COSTAR). US Department of Health, Education, and Welfare, Public Health Service, Health Resources Administration, National Center for Health Services Research; 1976.
15. Barnett GO. Computers in patient care. N Engl J Med. 1968;279:1321–7.
16. Barnett GO, Castleman PA. A time-sharing computer system for patient-care activities. Comput Biomed Res. 1967;1:41–51.
17. Barnett GO, Souder D, Beaman P, Hupp J. MUMPS: an evolutionary commentary. Comput Biomed Res. 1981;14:112–8.
18. Barnett GO, Justice NS, Somand ME, Adams JB, Waxman BD, Beaman PD, et al. COSTAR: a computer-based medical information system for ambulatory care. Proc IEEE. 1979;67:1226–37.
19. Barnett GO. The modular hospital information system. In: Stacy RW, Waxman BD, editors. Computers in biomedical research, vol. IV. New York: Academic; 1974. p. 243–85.
20. Barnett GO. Massachusetts General Hospital computer system. In: Collen MF, editor. Hospital computer systems. New York: Wiley; 1974. p. 517–45.
21. Barnett GO, Zielstorff RD. Data systems can enhance or hinder medical, nursing activities. Hospitals. 1977;51:157–61.
22. Barnett GO, Greenes RA, Grossman JH. Computer processing of medical text information. Methods Inf Med. 1969;8:177–82.
23. Barrett JP, Hersch PL, Caswell RJ. Evaluation of the impact of the implementation of the Technicon Medical Information System at El Camino Hospital, Part II: Economic Trend Analysis. Columbus: Battelle Columbus Labs; 1979. NCHSR&D, NTIS No. PB 300 869.
24. Baruch JJ. Hospital research and administration with a digital computer. Circ Res. 1962;11:629–36.
25. Beggs S, Vallbona C, Spencer WA, Jacobs FM, Baker RL. Evaluation of a system for on-line computer scheduling of patient care activities. Comput Biomed Res. 1971;4:634–54.
26. Bleich HL, Beckley RF, Horowitz GL, Jackson JD, Moody ES, Franklin C, et al. Clinical computing in a teaching hospital. N Engl J Med. 1985;312:756–64.
27. Blois MS, Henley RR. Strategies in the planning of hospital information systems. Journee D'Informatique Medicale. 1971;11:89–98.
28. Blose WF, Vallbona C, Spencer WA. System for processing clinical research data. System design. Proc 6th IBM Symp. 1964.
29. Blum BI, Lenhard RE J, McColligan EE. An integrated data model for patient care. IEEE Trans Biomed Eng. 1985;32:277–88.
30. Blum B. Ambulatory care systems. In: Blum BI, editor. Clinical information systems. New York: Springer; 1986. p. 253–93.
31. Blum BI. Design of an oncology clinical information system. Proc Annu Conf ACM. 1977:101–7.
32. Buchanan NS. Evolution of a hospital information system. Proc SCAMC. 1980;1:34–6.

33. Buck CR J, Reese GR, Lindberg DA. A general technique for computer processing of coded patient diagnoses. Mo Med. 1966;63:276. 9 passim.
34. Campbell CM. Information system for a short-term hospital. Hosp JAHA. 1964;38:71–80.
35. Childs BW. TDS is changing to meet the challenges of the future. Healthc Comput Commun. 1987;4:12–3.
36. Clark WE, Clark VA, Souder JJ. Data for planning from health information system sources. Inquiry. 1968;5:5–16.
37. Collen M. General requirements. In: Collen M, editor. Hospital computer systems. New York: Wiley; 1974a. p. 3–23.
38. Collen MF. HIS concepts, goals and objectives. In: Towards new hospital information systems. Amsterdam: North Holland; 1988. p. 3–9.
39. Collen MF. General requirements for clinical departmental systems. Proc MEDINFO. 1983;736–9.
40. Collen MF. The functions of a HIS: an overview. Proc MEDINFO. 1983;61–4.
41. Collen MF. General requirements of a medical information system (MIS). Comput Biomed Res. 1970;3:393–406.
42. Cronkhite LW. Patient location control as a first step toward a total information system. Hospitals. 1967;41:107–12.
43. de la Chapelle, Ball MJ, Wright DJ. Networked minicomputers for hospital information management. Med Instrum. 1974;8:281–4.
44. de la Chapelle NF. Automatic data processing in hospitals: one system serves two hospitals. Hospitals. 1964;38:77–80.
45. DeMarco P. Automating nursing's paper work. Am J Nursing 1965;65:74–7.
46. Dobson A. The medicare prospective payment system: intent and future directions. Proc SCAMC. 1984:497–501.
47. Dunn RG. Scheduling elective admissions. Health Serv Res. 1967;2:181.
48. Edwards SA. Guidelines for health services research & development: shared services. NCHSR&D DHEW Pub. No. (HSM) 72-3023. 1972.
49. Emmel GR, Greenhalgh RC. Hospital information system study (part I), Proc 4th IBM Med Symp. Endicott: IBM; 1962. p. 443–58.
50. Ertel PY. Accuracy in the reporting of clinical data: proper roles for the physician and the computer. Proc SCAMC. 1984:484–6.
51. Esterhay R, Foy JL, Lewis TL. Hospital information systems: approaches to screen definition: comparative anatomy of the PROMIS, NIH and Duke systems. Proc SCAMC. 1982:903–11.
52. Estherhay RJ, Walton PL. Clinical research and PROMIS. Proc SCAMC. 1979:241–54.
53. Felts WR. Classification standards for billing databases and health-care reimbursement. MD Comput. 1987;5:20. 6, 53.
54. Fischer PJ, Stratmann WC, Lundegaarde HP, Steele DJ. User reaction to PROMIS: issues related to acceptability of medical innovations. Proc SCAMC. 1980;1722–30.
55. Flagle CD. On the requirements for information systems in hospitals. Proc Conf on ADP in Hospitals. Elsinore: 1966.
56. Gall J. Computerized hospital information system cost-effectiveness: a case study. In: van Egmond J, de Vries Robbe PF, Levy AH, editors. Information systems for patient care. Amsterdam: North Holland; 1976. p. 281–93.
57. Gall J. Cost-benefit analysis: total hospital informatics. In: Koza RC, editor. Health information systems evaluation. Boulder: Colorado Associated University Press; 1974. p. 299–327.
58. Gardner RM, Pryor TA, Warner HR. The HELP hospital information system: update 1998. Int J Med Inform. 1999;54:169–82.
59. Gardner RM, West BJ, Pryor TA. Distributed data base and network for ICU monitoring. IEEE Computers in Cardiology, Salt Lake City: 1984. 305–7.
60. Giebink GA, Hurst LL. Computer projects in health care. Ann Arbor: Health Administration Press; 1975.

61. Giesler RH. How many hospitals use automatic data processing equipment. Hospitals. 1964;38:49.
62. Goldman J, Leonard MS. A strategy for the design of automated information systems. Proc MEDINFO. 1983:744–7.
63. Gotcher SB, Carrick J, Vallbona C, Spencer WA, Carter RE, Cornell S. Daily treatment planning with an on-line shared computer system. Methods Inf Med. 1969;8:200.
64. Grossman JH, Thoren B. Census operation: technical memorandum. Boston: Laboratory of Computer Science, Massachusetts General Hospital; 1966.
65. Grossman JH, Barnett GO, Koepsell TD, Nesson HR, Dorsey JL, Phillips RR. An automated medical record system. JAMA. 1973;224:1616–21.
66. Hammond WE, Stead WW, Straube MJ et al. An interface between a hospital information system and a computerized medical record. Proc SCAMC. 1980:1537–40.
67. Hammond WE, Stead WW, Straube MJ. Planned networking for medical information systems. Proc SCAMC. 1985:727–31.
68. Hammond WE, Stead WW, Straube MJ. Adapting to the day to day growth of TMR. Proc SCAMC. 1983:101–5.
69. Helppie R. Superior insight. Comput Healthc. 1987;20:53–65.
70. Herner & Co. The use of computers in hospitals: Report III-Survey analysis; Report IV-Descriptions of computer applications. Bethesda: National Center for Health Services Research; 1968.
71. Hodge MH. History of the TDS medical information system. In: Blum BI, Duncan KA, editors. A history of medical informatics. New York: Addison-Wesley; 1990. p. 328–44.
72. Hodge MH. Medical information systems: a resource for hospitals. Germantown: Aspen Publishers; 1977.
73. Jacobs SE. Hospital-wide computer systems: the market and the vendors. MUG Q. 1983;12:1–12.
74. Jacobs SE, Reeves PN, Hammon GL. A historical review of hospital surveys on computerization. In: Ball MJ, editor. How to select a computerized hospital information system. New York: S. Karger; 1973. p. 62–70.
75. Jelliffe RW, Schumitzky A, Rodman J, Crone J. A package of time-shared computer programs for patient care. Proc SCAMC. 1977:154–61.
76. Johns RJ, Blum BI. The use of clinical information systems to control cost as well as to improve care. Trans Am Clin Climatol Assoc. 1979;90:140–51.
77. Juenemann HJ. The design of a data processing center for biological data. Ann N Y Acad Sci. 1964;115:547–52.
78. Kirby JD, Pickett MP, Boyarsky MW, Stead WW. Distributed processing with a mainframe-based hospital information system: a generalized solution. Proc SCAMC. 1987:764–70.
79. Kuhn IM, Wiederhold G, Rodnick JE, Ransey-Klee D, Benett S, Beck DD. Automated ambulatory record systems in the US. NTIS Publication; 1982:178–89.
80. Kuperman GJ, Gardner RM, Pryor TA. The pharmacy application of the HELP system. In: HELP: a dynamic hospital information system. New York: Springer; 1991. p. 168–72.
81. Lamson BG. Mini-computers and large central processors from a medical record management point of view. Int Symp Med Inf Syst. 1975:58–65.
82. Lamson BG, Russell WS, Fullmore J, Nix WE. The first decade of effort: progress toward a hospital information system at the UCLA Hospital, Los Angeles, California. Methods Inf Med. 1970;9:73–80.
83. Lamson BG. Present possibilities for realizing HIS. Comput Prog Biomed. 1976;5:215.
84. Lee PR, Ginsburg PB. Building a consensus for physician payment reform in Medicare. The Physician Payment Review Commission. West J Med. 1988;149:352–8. 1026440.
85. Leonard MS, Ashton WB, Blackwell PW. Automated Hospital Information System (AHIS) component catalog. Columbia: Health Services Research Center, Health Care Technology Center, University of Missouri-Columbia; 1980.
86. Lincoln TL. Hospital information systems: what lies behind friendliness and flexibility? Inform Health Soc Care. 1984;9:255–63.

87. Lindberg D. The growth of medical information systems in the United States. Lexington: Lexington Books; 1979.
88. Lindberg D. CONSIDER: a computer program for medical instruction. N Y State J Med. 1969;69:54.
89. Lindberg D. The computer and medical care. Springfield: CC Thomas; 1968.
90. Lindberg D. Collection, evaluation, and transmission of hospital laboratory data. Methods Inf Med. 1964a;6:97–107.
91. Lindberg D. Operation of a hospital computer system. J Am Vet Med Assoc. 1965;147:1541–4.
92. Lindberg D. Electronic retrieval of clinical data. J Med Educ. 1965;40:753–9.
93. Lindberg D. A computer in medicine. Mo Med. 1964b;61:282–4.
94. Lindberg D, Schroeder JJ, Rowland RR. Experience with a computer laboratory system. In: Benson ES, Strandjord PE, editors. Multiple laboratory screening. New York: Academic; 1969. p. 2245–55.
95. Lindberg D, Vanpeenen HJ, Couch RD. Patterns in clinical chemistry. Low serum sodium and chloride in hospitalized patients. Am J Clin Pathol. 1965;44:315–21.
96. Lindberg D, Reese GR, Buck C. Computer generated hospital diagnosis file. Mo Med. 1964;61:581–2. passim.
97. Lindberg DAB. The development and diffusion of a medical technology: medical information systems. In: Medical technology and the health care system: a study of the diffusion of equipment-embodied technology. Washington, DC: National Academy of Science; 1979. p. 201–39.
98. Lindberg DAB. A statewide medical information system. Comput Biomed Res. 1970;3:453–63.
99. Lund SR, Ackerman LV, Martin JB, Somand ME. Distributed processing with a local area network. Proc AAMSI. 1984:52–6.
100. Maturi VF, DuBois RM. Recent trends in computerized medical information systems for hospital departments. Proc SCAMC. 1980;3:1541–9.
101. McColligan E, Blum B, Brunn C. An automated care medical record system for ambulatory care. Proc SCM/SAMS Jt Conf Ambul Med. 1981:72–6.
102. McDonald CJ. The medical gopher: a microcomputer based physician work station. Proc SCAMC. 1984:453–9.
103. McDonald C, Blevins L, Glazener T, Haas J, Lemmon L, Meeks-Johnson J. Data base management, feedback control, and the Regenstrief medical record. J Med Syst. 1983;7:111–25.
104. McDonald CJ. Standards for the transmission of diagnostic results from laboratory computers to office practice computers: an initiative. Proc SCAMC. 1983:123–4.
105. McDonald CJ, Tierney WM. Computer-stored medical records: their future role in medical practice. JAMA. 1988;259:3433–40.
106. McDonald CJ, Blevins L, Tierney WM, Martin DK. The Regenstrief medical records. MD Comput. 1987;5:34–47.
107. McDonald CJ, Murray R, Jeris D, Bhargava B, Seeger J, Blevins L. A computer-based record and clinical monitoring system for ambulatory care. Am J Public Health. 1977b;67:240–5.
108. McDonald CJ, Hui SL, Smith DM, Tierney WM, Cohen SJ, Weinberger M, et al. Reminders to physicians from an introspective computer medical record: a two-year randomized trial. Ann Intern Med. 1984;100:130–8.
109. McDonald CJ, Wilson G, Blevins L, Seeger J, Chamness D, Smith D, et al. The Regenstrief medical record system. Proc SCAMC. 1977a:168–9.
110. McDonald CJ, Overhage JM, Tierney WM, Dexter PR, Martin DK, Suico JG, et al. The Regenstrief medical record system: a quarter century experience. Int J Med Inform. 1999;54:225–53.
111. McPhillips R. Keynote address: the health care delivery system. Comput Nurs. 1987;5:89–93.

112. Mishelevich DJ, Hudson BG, Van Slyke D, Mize EI, Robinson AL, Brieden HC, et al. The POIS (Parkland on-line information system) implementation of the IBM health care support/patient care system. Proc SCAMC. 1980;1:19–33.
113. Monmouth. Monmouth medical shapes a total system. Systems. 1966;12–48.
114. Myers E. Shot in the arm. Datamation. 1985;31:75–83.
115. NCHSR&D. Summary Report on Hospital Information Systems. Springfield: National Center for Health Services Research and Development. NTIS PB 189 174. 1969.
116. Newald J. Hospitals look to computerization of physician office linkage. Hospitals. 1987;61:92–4.
117. Nichols KJ, Ardolino M, Kahane SN, Richmond D. The Johns Hopkins Hospital discharge instructions application. Proc SCAMC. 1987:401–3.
118. OTA. Office of Technology Assessment. Policy implications of medical information systems. 1977:58–63.
119. Pesce J. Bedside terminals: MedTake. MD Comput. 1988;5:16–21.
120. Pratt AW. Progress towards a medical information system for the research environment. In: Fuchs G, Wagner G, editors. Deutsche Gesellschaft Medizinische Dokumentation und Statistik. New York: Schattauer; 1972. p. 319–36.
121. PROMIS Laboratory. Representation of medical knowledge and PROMIS. Proc SCAMC. 1978:368–75.
122. Pryor TA, Gardner RM, Clayton PD, Warner HR. The HELP system. J Med Syst. 1983;7:87–102.
123. Reynolds RE, Heller EE. An academic medical center experience with a computerized hospital information system: the first four years. Proc SCAMC. 1980;1:13–6.
124. Roach CJ. Patient data processing – the key to hospital automation. Am J Med Electron. 1962;1:51.
125. Rogerson CL. Towards a case-mix information system for the emergency department. Proc SCAMC. 1984;514–7.
126. Rosko MD. DRGs and severity of illness measures: an analysis of patient classification systems. J Med Syst. 1988;12:257–74.
127. Runck HM. Computer planning for hospitals-large-scale education and involvement of employees. Comput Autom. 1969;18:33.
128. Rusnak JE. The CMRI PRO medicare review information system. Proc MEDINFO. 1986:448–50.
129. Saba VK, McCormick KA. Essentials of computers for nurses. Philadelphia: Lippincott; 1986.
130. Safran C, Porter D, Lightfoot J, Rury CD, Underhill LH, Bleich HL, et al. ClinQuery: a system for online searching of data in a teaching hospital. Ann Intern Med. 1989;111:751–6.
131. Schultz JR, Davis L. The technology of PROMIS. Proc IEEE. 1979;67:1237–44.
132. Shieman BM. Medical information system, El Camino Hospital. IMS Ind Med Surg. 1971;40:25–6.
133. Siegel SJ. Developing an information system for a hospital. Public Health Rep. 1968;83:359–62.
134. Slack WV, Bleich HL. The CCC system in two teaching hospitals: a progress report. Int J Med Inform. 1999;54:183–96.
135. Slack WV, Van Cura LJ. Computer-based patient interviewing. Postgrad Med. 1968;43:115–20. concl.
136. Slack WV, Van Cura L. Computer-based patient interviewing. Postgrad Med. 1968;43:68–74.
137. Slack WV, Hicks GP, Reed CE, Van Cura LJ. A computer-based medical-history system. N Engl J Med. 1966;274:194–8.
138. Slack WV. Patient counseling by computer. Proc SCAMC. 1972:222–6.
139. Smith JW. A hospital adverse drug reaction reporting program. Hospitals. 1966;40:90.
140. Sneider RM. Using a medical information system to improve the quality of patient care. Proc SCAMC. 1978:594–7.

141. Spencer WA, Baker RL. Accomplishing the transition to computers in medicine. In: Flagle CD, editor. Advanced medical systems: issues and challenges. New York: Stratton Intercontinental Medical Book Corp; 1975. p. 37–63.
142. Spencer WA, Vallbona C. Digitation of clinical and research data in serial evaluation of disease processes. IRE Trans Med Electron. 1960;ME-7:296–308.
143. Spencer WA. An opinion survey of computer applications in 149 hospitals in the USA, Europe and Japan. Inform Health Soc Care. 1976;1:215–34.
144. Spencer WA, Vallbona C. Application of computers in clinical practice. JAMA. 1965;191:917–21.
145. Spencer WA, Baker RL, Moffet CL. Hospital computer systems: a review of usage and future requirements after a decade of overpromise and underachievement. Adv Biomed Eng. 1972;2:61–138.
146. Starr P. The social transformation of American medicine. New York: Basic Books; 1982.
147. Stead WW, Hammond WE. Computer-based medical records: the centerpiece of TMR. MD Comput. 1988;5:48–62.
148. Stead WW, Hammond WE. Functions required to allow TMR to support the information requirements of a hospital. Proc SCAMC. 1983:106–9.
149. Stead WW, Hammond WE, Winfree RG. Beyond a basic HIS: work stations for department management. Proc SCAMC. 1984:197–9.
150. Stefanchik MF. Point-of-care information systems: improving patient care. Comput Healthc. 1987;4:7–8.
151. Stobie G. Medical data processing in a large hospital environment. Proc 7th IBM Med Symp. 1965:365–70.
152. Stratmann WC. A demonstration of PROMIS: the problem oriented medical information system at the Medical Center Hospital of Vermont, NCHSR Research Summary Series. Hyattsville: National Center for Health Services Research; 1979. DHEW Publication No (PHS) 79-3247.
153. Summerfield AB, Empey S. Computer-based information systems for medicine: a survey and brief discussion of current projects. Santa Monica: System Development Corporation; 1965.
154. Teich JM, Glaser JP, Beckley RF, Aranow M, Bates DW, Kuperman GJ, et al. The Brigham integrated computing system (BICS): advanced clinical systems in an academic hospital environment. Int J Med Inform. 1999;54:197–208.
155. Tolchin SG, Barta W. Local network and distributed processing issues in the Johns Hopkins Hospital. J Med Syst. 1986;10:339–53.
156. Vallbona C. Ten years of computers in medicine: a retrospective view. Proc 9th IBM Med Symp. 1968:189–94.
157. Vallbona C. Processing medical information at the bedside. Proc 4th IBM Med Symp. 1962:405.
158. Vallbona C, Spencer WA. Texas Institute for Research and Rehabilitation Hospital computer system (Houston). In: Collen MF, editor. Hospital computer systems. New York: Wiley; 1974. p. 662–700.
159. Vallbona C, Spencer WA, Moffet CL. The patient care centered information system of the Texas Institute for Rehabilitation and Research. Proc Int Conf Health Technol Syst. ORSA. 1973:232–60.
160. Vallbona C, Blose WF, Spencer WA. Systems for processing clinical research data. Part 1. Experience and problems. Proc 6th IMB Symp. 1964:437–48.
161. Vallbona C. Preparing medical record data for computer processing. Hospitals. 1967;41:113.
162. Vallbona C. Application of computers for hospital usage. J Chronic Dis. 1966;19:461–72.
163. Vladeck BC. Medicare hospital payment by diagnosis-related groups. Ann Intern Med. 1984;100:576–91.
164. Warner HR. A computer-based patient monitoring. In: Stacy RW, Waxman B, editors. Computers in biomedical research. New York: Academic; 1972.
165. Watson RJ. A large-scale professionally oriented medical information system – five years later. J Med Syst. 1977;1:3–21.

166. Weed LL. PROMIS Laboratory. Representation of medical knowledge and PROMIS. In: Blum BI, editor. Information systems for patient care. New York: Springer; 1984. p. 83–108.
167. Weed LL. Problem-oriented medical records. In: Driggs MF, editor. Problem directed and medical information systems. New York: Intercontinental Medical Book Corp; 1973. p. 15–38.
168. Weed LL. PROMIS Laboratory. Automation of the problem-oriented medical record. DHEW, Health Resources Administration, National Center for Health Services Research. 1977.
169. Weed LL, Hertzberg RY. The use and construction of problem-knowledge couplers, the knowledge coupler editor, knowledge networks, and the problem-oriented medical record for the microcomputer. Proc SCAMC. 1983;831–6.
170. Wheeler PS, Simborg DW, Gitlin JN. The Johns Hopkins radiology reporting system. Radiology. 1976;119:315–9.
171. Wood CT, Lamontagne A. Computer assists advanced bed booking. Hospitals. 1969;43:67–9.
172. Yeh S, Lincoln T. From micro to mainframe. Am J Perinatol. 1985;2:158–60.
173. Young EM, Brian EW, Hardy DR, Kaplan A, Childerston JK. Evaluation of automated hospital data management systems (AHDMS). Proc SCAMC. 1980;1:651–7.
174. Zucker LW. An integrated information system for hospital financial operations. Hospitals. 1965;39:55–8.

Chapter 7
Nursing Informatics: Past, Present, and Future

Morris F. Collen and Patricia Hinton Walker

Abstract Early hospital information systems (HISs) placed computers at nursing stations, and the passage of Medicare in 1965 set reimbursement rules that required documentation, first met by nurses using precoded cards and forms. In the 1970s, interactive terminals with visual displays became available; in the 1980s, microcomputers custom-tailored for nursing functions began to be installed at the patient's bedside. Handheld portable devices began to appear for use at the point of care, and hospitals began to use bar codes for identification purposes. Nurses became increasingly involved in specifying information requirements for nursing services. In the 1980s, nursing information systems (NISs) were probably the most widely used HIS subsystem. They were used for bed assignment and control, nurse staffing recommendations based on patient classification systems, quality assurance programs, nursing care planning, and decision support. The 1980s also saw advances toward implementation of the Nursing Minimum Data Set and development of nursing education programs. In the 1990s, the American Nurses Association published documents defining the scope and standards of nursing informatics practice, and the American Nurses Credentialing Center had established a certification in nursing informatics as a practice specialty. In the 2000s, an international nursing terminology summit brought nurses and standards experts together to integrate nursing concepts and map nursing

---

The views expressed are those of the author Walker and do not reflect official policy or position of the USUHS, the Department of Defense, or the United State Federal Government.

Author was deceased at the time of publication.

M.F. Collen (deceased)

P.H. Walker (✉)
Strategic Initiatives and Graduate School of Nursing,
Uniformed Services University of the Health Sciences, Bethesda, MD, USA
e-mail: phintonwalker@comcast.net

© Springer-Verlag London 2015   385
M.F. Collen, M.J. Ball (eds.), *The History of Medical Informatics*
in the United States, Health Informatics, DOI 10.1007/978-1-4471-6732-7_7

interface terminologies to SNOMED-CT, ultimately creating what in 2007 became an international reference terminology standard. The 2000s also saw the establishment of the Alliance of Nursing Informatics (ANI) and TIGER (Technology Informatics Guiding Education Reform); both continue to be active today.

Keywords Nursing informatics • Nursing information systems • Nursing terminology • Nursing minimum data set • Professional certification • Nursing practice • Professional associations • Direct patient care • Nursing management

Technological advances in society and in the delivery of health care, governmental policy implementation and funding, private investment/funding, and subsequent accreditation requirements in practice and education settings set the stage for many of the documented advances in nursing informatics. Other drivers of nursing informatics include changing health needs of populations such as an increasing elderly population with more chronic diseases; renewed emphasis on the individual's responsibility for health maintenance and self care; the need for improved efficiency, patient safety and evidence-based care; and requirements for economic data related to nurses, still the largest health profession impacting health, wellness and wellbeing.

This chapter highlights these drivers and the expanding roles for nurses as administrators, educators, scientists, and leaders in industry and government. In these roles and in all their varied roles in practice settings, including those of advanced practice nurses and nurse researchers, they represent the voice of their profession – in hospital-based acute care, ambulatory care, home health, schools, the workplace, community centers, home health, public health, and nursing homes. Finally this chapter explores the emerging and future impact of new technologies on patients and families, such as provider-driven dashboards populated with data from electronic health records, personal health records, and mobile health devices. Their impact, combined with society's changing health and medical care needs, gives rise to changing requirements and roles for nurses in relation to nursing informatics.

Despite the fact that nurses in different roles have been involved in modern informatics for over 25 years with some of the first contributions recorded in the 1970s, the term "nursing informatics" was not seen in the literature until 1984 [34]. A major reason was that nursing informatics was included in the broader, overarching term "medical informatics," a term used since the mid-1970s, referring to information technologies that concern patient care and medical decision making [84]. According to Saba and McCormick [66], nursing, medical, dental informatics overlap in several important areas including, but not limited to, information retrieval, patient care, decision support, human-to-computer interactions, information systems, computer security, and computerized patient records. Recently, the term "health care informatics" emerged to describe the "integration of health sciences, computer science, information and cognitive science to assist in the management of health care information" [66].

7.1 Nursing Informatics: A Historical Overview

In any historical discussion of informatics, it must also be acknowledged that major elements of nursing informatics are a significant part of nursing's roots going back to Florence Nightingale, the first nursing informatician [34]. Considered the founding mother of modern nursing and a very early patient safety advocate, Nightingale pushed for hospital reform with statistical analysis by collecting, tabulating, interpreting and graphically displaying data to improve patient care during the Crimean War [55]. According to Ozbolt and Saba [57], 137 years before the Institute of Medicine reported that medical errors were killing up to 98,000 in American hospitals, "Nightingale called for standardized clinical records that could be analyzed to assess and improve care processes and patient outcomes." Foster and Conrick [28] agree that "Florence Nightingale began gathering the first minimum health data over a century ago." Yet over 100 years would pass before Harriet Werley became the first designated nurse researcher at Walter Reed Army Research Institute. In the late 1950s, she was one of a few people who consulted with IBM regarding possible uses of computers in health care; these experiences led her to recognize the need for what would be known as the minimum set of standardized nursing data to be collected on every patient [82]. This resulted in a committee being appointed by the American Nurses Association (ANA) focused on nurses' use of information for communication and decision making [1]. Going forward, modern nursing informatics continued to build on this seminal work. The advances recorded in the 1970s in subsequent decades expanded the influence and contributions to health care, patient safety, and care across the continuum to persons, families, and communities [37].

7.1.1 The 1960s

Computer terminals located at the nursing stations were critical to the nurses' acceptance of a hospital information system (HIS). In the early 1960s, Spencer and Vallbona [73] at the Texas Institute for Rehabilitation and Research (TIRR) used specially designed source documents for recording at the patient's bedside the nursing notes and the patient's vital signs. The data were then keypunched and read into the computer, following which progress notes were printed, and vital signs were plotted for filing in the patient's paper-based chart [68]. At the University of Missouri-Columbia Hospital, IBM 1092 terminals with multiple function buttons and plastic overlay mats to define different data sets were placed at nursing stations [44]. At the Children's Hospital in Akron, Ohio, DeMarco [19] reported the installation of an IBM 1710 system with data entry terminals with keyboards consisting of rows of push buttons that served as code keys for order entry, admissions, dietary services, and census reports. This system completely replaced the Kardex file system in which orders had been manually written. To enter an order for penicillin, for example, the nurse started at the left side of the keyboard, entered the type of order (its function code) in the first two rows, the patient's code number in the next three columns, the order number (of the medication and its strength) in the next four columns, how frequently the order should be carried out in the next two rows, and the type of order (modifier) in the last row on the right. Instantly, the order was decoded and printed back on the output printer. However, push-button, key-coded type terminals were soon found to be too slow and inflexible.

The United States Congress amended the Social Security Act to include Medicare and Medicaid in 1965. This federal law now required nurses to document care and be provided to Health and Human Services in order for the hospital to qualify for reimbursement. Addressing this requirement in 1965, nurses at San Jose Hospital recorded their observations on a checklist form that could be read by a mark-sense reader that produced punched cards. The cards were then processed through an IBM 1441 computer, which created the records necessary to print out the nurses' notes. Forms were developed for medical, surgical, pediatric, and maternity nursing units [56]. In 1966 the Institute of Living in Hartford, Connecticut, reported that its nurses checked off statements on a machine-readable form that described their patient's status. The completed forms were picked up daily and read into a computer. The computer, in turn, printed out a checklist that incorporated the additional written observations, and thus created a narrative statement [63]. The precoded cards and forms were too inflexible, however, and were replaced by interactive terminals in the 1970s when nursing information systems began to include visual display terminals at the nursing stations. These interactive terminals permitted the selection of data from menu listings. Some terminals had light-pen or touch-sensitive data selectors; all had keyboards for entry of other non-displayed, pre-formatted data [8]. It was the hope that one of the main benefits of interactive display terminals would be that it would encourage physicians to enter their orders directly, without any nurse or clerk intermediaries, to eliminate transcription errors and to provide online clinical decision support to physicians. However, nurses accepted these display terminals more than did physicians.

Stimulated by the advances in technology, the need for data/information input and the growing need to utilize the data for research and decision-making, a national working conference was held in 1969 to "develop a 'minimum basic set' of data elements to be collected from all hospital records at the point of patient discharge from hospitals" [35]. At the same time, advances in computer design made it feasible to manage data using computers. Thus the problem was the need to identify available and reliable data elements that would be consistent across multiple users and settings.

7.1.2   The 1970s

In 1974, a Uniform Hospital Discharge Data Set (UHDDS) was adopted by Health and Human Services; however, the items focused on medical diagnosis and treatments. Nurses provided much of the clinical care 24-7, yet there was no nursing clinical data in the dataset. In 1977, this prompted nurses to build on Werley's earlier work (REF) and to move forward with the development of the Nursing Minimum Data Set (NDMS). This work was not completed until the mid-late 1980s.

During this important decade, according to Ozbolt and Saba [57], the "first reports of computer applications in nursing began to appear in the scholarly literature." Zielstorff was hired into the Laboratory of Computer Science at Massachusetts General Hospital (MGH), where she contributed a nursing perspective to funded grants. In 1971 Massachusetts General initiated a nurse-practitioner project designed to allow nurses access to computer-stored medical records. Using a video terminal with a light-pen data selector, after entering the patient's identification number, a nurse could retrieve and review current medication orders, recent progress notes and laboratory test results. Nursing progress notes were entered by selecting appropriate data items from a series of displayed frames. A teletype printer could print out a data flow sheet for that office visit. The project was based on Barnett's pioneering work in his laboratory at MGH [29]. Later in the 1970s, Zielstorff edited the first monthly column on computer applications in nursing in the *Journal of Nursing Administration* and subsequently complied/edited one of the first textbooks, *Computers in Nursing* [85].

Ball [5] also wrote that some vendors of hospital information systems (HIS) planned their basic philosophy in HIS design on the concept that activity at the nursing station is the activity most directed to patient care and therefore the most important. Ball and associates [6] further wrote that nurses constituted the largest group of health care professionals in any hospital and accessed the HIS more often than any other category of health care professional. Nursing functions were always central to the care of hospital patients, and nurses' services to patients directly complemented those of physicians. Two early developments reflected this reality. At the El Camino Hospital in Mountain View, California, nurses assisted in the development of an integrated system for nursing care planning, documentation, and feedback working with Technicon Medical Information Systems [17]. At the Clinical Center of the National Institutes of Health, McCormick and Romano were among nurses focused on interdisciplinary efforts to include documentation of nursing data when implementing Technicon there [57].

Federal funding from a predecessor of the Agency for Research and Quality, the National Center for Health Services Research (NCHSR) helped support the development of HIS that included nursing care planning. In addition, computer vendors contributed substantially to the development of information systems (NISs). Saba and McCormick [66] defined NISs as computer systems to collect, store, retrieve, display, and communicate timely information needed to administer nursing services and resources; to manage patient information for the delivery of nursing care; and to link nursing practice, research, and education.

The technical design of a NIS was generally similar to that for any clinical department. The NIS had to be able to support all nursing functions, to have computer terminals acceptable to nurses, to be integrated into the overall HIS, and to provide data security and integrity [87]. However, the detailed functional requirements of a NIS were sufficiently different that nurses had to actively participate in determining the NIS requirements [22].

Special considerations were needed for database and knowledge-based requirements to satisfy nursing diagnoses, interventions, and evaluations [58]. Furthermore, specifying the information system requirements for the nursing services was critical for the overall HIS. Ball [4] advised that a nursing information expert, a crucial role in nursing, must take a leading role on the selection team in search of an effective computer-based HIS. As the importance of nursing services to direct patient care became increasingly recognized, larger HISs worked closely with nurses to design and develop specialized NISs. Saba [68] wrote that the functions of a hospital NIS were to classify patients for nurse staffing, to schedule nurses, manage nursing personnel, and administer quality assurance programs. Ball [3] and Hannah wrote that the broad goal of a NIS was to free nurses to assume the responsibility for systematic planning of nursing care for patients and their families, for continual review and examination of nursing practice for quality assurance, for applying basic research to innovative solutions to patient care problems, and for devising creative new models for the delivery of nursing care.

Beyond the focus on NISs for hospitalized patients, in the 1970s another source of federal support was the Division of Nursing within Health and Human Services which funded nursing research as well as education. Beginning in 1975, a series of grants to the Visiting Nurse Association of Omaha, Nebraska resulted in the development of the Omaha system by Simmons, Martin and colleagues (Martin and Simmons). Consistent with the need for federal reporting related to Medicare and Medicaid, the initial purpose of this system was to use computer-based data in record systems to meet reporting requirements and to improve the quality of care.

In 1973, Gebbie and Lavin organized the first conference focused on standardizing nursing diagnosis. Subsequently, a professional association was developed, known as the North American Nursing Diagnosis Association. Chaired by Gordon, this group developed standardized nursing terminology and further refined the criteria and taxonomy that were presented as an organizing framework for nursing diagnoses in 1982 [54].

7.1.3   The 1980s

In the 1980s, significant progress was made in nursing informatics not only in technology that directly impacted practice, in education, research and advances in nursing professions and interdisciplinary associations, in education and research. During this important decade, significant attempts continued to be advanced to capture nursing's unique contributions to patient care and ability to track those contributions to outcomes. Also, continued significant attempts to standardize nursing language and data elements and legitimate nursing informatics as a specialty in the profession of nursing.

With the advent of the personal computer in 1980, vendors also began to develop specialized, microcomputer-based video display terminals with simplified keyboards custom-tailored for nursing functions to be used at the patient's bedside. These bedside terminals were connected to nursing-station units that were linked by LANs into the HIS [61]. This allowed nurses to record directly into the computer, at the time of caring for the patient, the patient's vital signs, the nursing observations, and the medications given. Printouts from the terminal located at the bedside included graphs of the vital signs and a variety of useful reports.

The 1981 Fifth Annual Symposium on Computer Applications in Medical Care (SCAMC) held what was its first full session on nursing applications of computers, organized by Virginia Saba [70]. McNeely [50] emphasized the importance of nurse participation in the planning of the NIS for the Clinical Center of the National Institutes of Health (NIH). Zielstorff [86] reviewed the status of Nursing Information Systems (NIS) administrative applications in hospitals. Charters described the use of microcomputers to automate 80 % of nursing service paperwork [15].

At a conference held in 1981 at the Clinical Center of the National Institutes of Health and attended by more than 700 nurses, it was agreed that nurse administrators needed to have a voice in purchasing and implementing decisions, authority for controlling nursing database development, a stake in the development of content and standards of nursing documentation, and an agreed-upon taxonomy for the nursing process, including nursing diagnoses [83].

In 1984 a distributed system of microcomputers was installed at the LDS Hospital in Salt Lake City, with four display terminals and one printer at each 48-bed nursing division; and a group of 30 display terminals were connected to each microcomputer. Patient data were entered and reviewed at each local terminal, and eventually were transferred from the microcomputer into the central Tandem computer. Through menu selection from the displays, nurses had access to order-entry and review, results review, and discharge and transfer functions. The system generated nursing care plans and performed some charting functions [41]. The system automatically measured patient acuity or degree of dependency based on nursing time spent with each patient, in accordance with preassigned time factors as the nurse entered aspects of patient care during a work shift [42]. Nurses wanted to capture source data as close to the patient's bedside as feasible; so with the advent of lower-cost minicomputers connected to smart terminals, these terminals were placed at the patient's bedside. In 1984 LDS Hospital placed such terminals at the bedsides in their ICU [14]; by 1987 the hospital had 400 such terminals in their general nursing divisions. They performed a study that compared on-line nurse charting on one nursing unit where nurses used terminals located at the bedside with charting by nurses using similar terminals located at the nursing station. The researchers evaluated nurses' satisfaction, amount of use of each terminal, and the number of items being double charted (written down and then entered later). The results were so favorable that by the end of the 1980s the LDS hospital was installing bedside terminals throughout all nursing units [40].

By the mid-1980s portable handheld terminals appeared that permitted the nurse to enter patient data at the point of care. The ability of nurses to access the patient's computer-based record directly at the point of care was expected to improve the quality and documentation of nurses' bedside care and to save nursing time [75]. The patient's vital signs and the medications given were entered directly into the patient's computer-based record, eliminating the paper charting process and allowing nurses more time for other nursing functions. At the end of the 1980s a medical information bus was developed, that was a standardized connection, so any vendor's bedside technology could take data from the bedside terminals and integrate the data into the HIS database. This bus was a standardized connection, so any vendor's bedside technology could communicate with the HIS database [21].

Hospitals began to use bar codes to identify patients, using bar-coded wristbands, bar-coded medical records, blood-bank samples, laboratory samples, and x-ray folders. For clinical applications that allowed the use of bar-code labels, using a wand bar-code reader connected to, or communicating by radio to, a computer was a much faster method for nurses than was typing to enter the data contained on the label, and it was more accurate [30]. In 1986 M. Monahan and associates at the University of Hospitals of Cleveland, Ohio, reported the use of handheld terminals that, after manual entry of the patient's identification, used barcode readers to scan and enter automatically nurse identification and relevant patient conditions from a listing of 61 possible nursing diagnoses. After all patient and nursing data were entered into the terminal for the day, the data were transmitted to the hospital computer via any telephone, since a modem was located in the back of the terminal. Advantages of the technology included its affordability and a data entry procedure that was reported to be easily learned by 1100 nurses on 33 inpatient units for its rapid data entry [52]. However, because there was not a two-way link to the hospital computer, patient identification numbers could not be verified to determine whether they were correct. This deficiency was corrected when the vendors (1) provided portable handheld terminals with barcode readers that communicated with a base unit via radio frequency and (2) set up communications between the base units and nursing-station terminals linked to the HIS over existing telephone lines [36]. In 1988 Childs [16] described how a nurse, with a handheld terminal containing a barcode reader, read the patient's identification number from the code stripes on the patient's wristband before giving a medication to verify that the patient was due at that time for that specific medication. When the computer identified matching bar codes, it authorized giving the medication and recorded the date and time. By the end of the 1980s, bedside systems were available from a variety of vendors, so a hospital could select a system with bedside terminals connected to the main HIS, bedside terminals connected to the nursing station in the HIS, or portable point-of-care terminals interfaced by radio frequency to the nursing system of the HIS.

Nursing services have their own administrative and managerial responsibilities, in addition to direct patient care functions [69]. Nursing management functions include: staffing and scheduling the nursing staff, maintaining personnel records, administering quality-assurance programs, managing resources used, and preparing nursing-service budgets. Traditionally, nurse staffing had been based primarily on the ratio of hospital patients to nursing personnel. A group at Johns Hopkins Hospital reported studies that indicated that functional activity planning and budgeting for nursing services improved these activities [72]. In the 1980s NISs began to provide nurse staffing recommendations based on some classification system of patients' status. Nurses assessed their patient's acuity level and entered the appropriate data by selecting descriptors from a displayed list (or menu); patients were then categorized as to the probable hours of nursing care they would require, and then staffing requirements for the nursing shift were recommended [66, 68]. Also in the 1980s reports appeared that described automated nurse-scheduling and nurse-staffing systems using personal computers. At the Milwaukee County Medical Complex, Flanders [27] reported that an IBM personal computer (PC) had been operational for 20 months preparing schedules for 1500 nurses, generating 4–6-week schedules for several classifications of nursing staff. The developmental and operational costs of the system were favorable due to the system being microcomputer-based and totally under the nursing department's control. Kogut [45] at the Montefiore Medical Center in the Bronx, New York, reported the installation in 1983 of a patient acuity and nurse-staffing system for 28 nursing units using a personal computer with a series of displayed menus for item selection.

Saba [71] reported that, as a result of the Joint Commission on Accreditation on Hospitals (JCAH) recommendation that nurse staffing should be based on patient cuity/classification systems instead of the traditional nurse-to-patient ratios, such systems became the major method to administrate nursing services in hospitals in the 1980s. Saba [68] described four patient classification systems then being used for nurse staffing:

• The San Joaquin System, which used nine indicators of patient care requirements
• The Medicus Patient Classification Module of Nursing Productivity and Quality of Patient Care System (NPAQ), which used 36 indicators of patient care
• The Grace Reynolds Applications and Study of PETO (GRASP), which used time requirements for 60 nursing activities
• The Halloran and Kiley Nurse Management System based on nursing diagnoses.

Nursing Information Systems (NISs) also had a role in bed assignment and control. Nurses regularly confirmed bed census with the admitting service; assigned beds on request of the admitting service; notified housekeeping when a bed needed to be prepared; notified dietary service on bed changes and dietary requirements; and notified the business office when a patient was discharged, so that a bill could be prepared. NISs were also used to administer the quality assurance programs of nursing services on patient care, and to monitor adherence to predefined quality assurance standards [68].

According to Saba [68], the steps of the nursing process in direct patient care could be classified as collecting data, diagnosing, setting objectives (with priorities and target dates for achievement), choosing and implementing interventions, and evaluating the effectiveness of care. The patient care nursing functions that required the entry, retrieval, and communication of data in the nursing system of a HIS included: physicians' orders, patient status reports, medication administration, nursing diagnoses, and patient care plans [77]. The Nursing Information System (NIS) database containing the data documenting what nurses did in their practice, included patient interventions in response to medical orders; and relatively independent nursing interventions based on nursing diagnoses relating to patient needs, which encompassed air, circulation, food and fluid, elimination, sleep and rest, comfort and pain, hygiene and skin, and others [62].

As had users of other NIS systems, nurses recognized the importance of developing their own standard sets of data for nursing practice. By the mid-1980s, Gordon [31], at the Boston College of Nursing in Chestnut Hill, Massachusetts, had proposed a standard nursing data set that included 17 data items. Werley [81], Lang, and associates at the University of Wisconsin-Milwaukee School of Nursing tested a standard nursing minimum data set of 16 data items. These data sets included: items representing patient demographic variables (age, gender, ethnicity, marital status, next of kin, and residence); provider variables (facility providing care, primary nurse identification, admission and discharge dates, disposition, anticipated source of payment); and care provision variables (functional health status, nursing diagnoses, projected and actual outcomes, nursing treatment orders, medical diagnoses, medical treatment orders, diagnostic and surgical procedures). This data set was to be applied to nursing practice in at least five settings including hospitals, ambulatory care, home care, community, and long-term care. Assisted by funding from the Hospital Corporation of America (arranged by Simpson) and sponsored by IBM (contacted by Werley based on early consulting relationships) and the University of Wisconsin – Milwaukee School of Nursing, the Nursing Minimum Data Set became a reality in 1985–1986.

Ball and Hannah [6] described two general approaches to the automated recording of nurses' notes on their observations of patients. The first method employed the development of a group of frequently used descriptive terms, and the earliest nursing systems used machine-readable forms from which the nurse selected the appropriate statements that applied best to the patient. The marked forms were batch processed, and the data were read into the computer. Later, display terminals connected to the computer permitted online processing of nurses' notes with a computer-based library of frequently used phrases arranged in subject categories. For example, if the nurse chose the phrase, patient's sleeping habits, a displayed menu of standard descriptions appeared, additional comments were allowed; and when completed the nursing station printer immediately printed a complete narrative that could then be attached to the patient's paper chart.

The second method used a branching questionnaire for data entry. The computer terminal displaced an initial list of subjects from which the nurse would select the one most appropriate for the patient. For example, if describing skin conditions, the nurse then would be led through a series of questions, such as skin intact, yes, no? If answered yes, then other questions followed until completion of the desired observation. The computer then processed the information and provided a narrative printout for the patient's chart.

Nurses needed to enter data describing the patient's status as to mental acuity, physical abilities, vital signs, fluid balance, and other data. They also entered terms representing nursing diagnoses, which classified the patients' problems that nurses were licensed to treat. Like medical diagnoses, nursing diagnoses were based on patients' signs and symptoms. The North American Nursing Diagnosis Association (NANDA) [54] developed a classification for nursing diagnoses using a four-character code modeled after the International Classification of Diseases (ICD); examples at that date were: Y.20.3 for diarrhea, Y.25.1 for hyperthermia, and Y.50.4 for impaired physical mobility [26]. Following the establishment of their patients' diagnoses, nurses prepared nursing care plans for each patient; then carried out these plans, and documented all results as a part of the traditional nurses charting activities. Computer-based patient care management plans were built into some of the earliest HISs, such as those used at TIRR. In the late 1960s, the TIRR information system prepared treatment plans and generated department lists of tasks to be carried out by the nursing units [76].

Saba [68, 71] described two types of nursing care planning systems that were available in the second half of the 1980s:

- Traditional systems focused on medical diagnoses or diseases; these consisted of elements that addressed signs and symptoms, and contained protocols that reflected the medical orders for nursing care for each diagnosis.
- New nursing care planning systems that focused on nursing diagnoses; these set forth the nursing process that consisted of assessing and diagnosing the nursing problems for care of the patient and then planning, intervening, and evaluating the outcome of care.

Although Ozbolt and Saba [57] found agreement on how to operationalize nursing data elements consistently across systems, other systems were developed in addition to NANDA. One of these was the Omaha System, which provided a practical approach to recording nursing diagnosis, interventions and outcomes. Another was the Home Health Care Classification System developed by Saba and research colleagues at Georgetown University in the late 1980s, which classified home health Medicare patients as a method to predict resource requirements and measure outcomes [67]. Later known as the Clinical Care Classification (CCC), Saba's system was expanded from home health and ambulatory care settings into other settings and was accepted by the Department of Health and Human Services as the first national nursing terminology that allowed nurses, allied health professionals, and researchers to determine care needs (resources), workload (productivity), and outcomes (quality).

Crosley [18], at Long Island Jewish-Hillside Medical Center in New Jersey, and Light [47], at Crouse-Irving Memorial Hospital associated with Syracuse University, reported on the use of IBM's computer-based nursing care plan developed as a separate application module in its HIS, developed earlier at Duke University and announced at IBM in early 1978. This nursing system displayed a set of screens labeled as nursing diagnostic category, signs and symptoms, related factors, patient outcomes, nursing orders, and evaluation. Selections were made from items listed in the series of displays by use of a light pen selector, supplemented by keyboard data entry when needed. The computer printed out a copy of the aggregated data that had been entered, and this printout constituted the patient's care plan and was placed in the patient's paper chart [18]. Jenkins [38], at the University of Tennessee in Knoxville, described the McDonnell Douglas Patient Care System, which permitted nurses to develop care plans with four elements: the problem description; the etiologies; the goals of treatment; and the interventions. If the system did not include desired information, nurses could modify the plan using a free-form comment function. Saba [68] reported that HISs in which the nursing subsystem was primarily used for nursing care planning included Shared Medical Systems, Ulticare, the LDS Hospital's HELP System, and the NIH's Technicon System.

After physicians began to develop expert systems to aid them in their clinical decisions for patients' medical problems, some nurses began to develop nursing expert systems to provide decision support in care plans for patients' nursing problems. Such nursing expert systems usually required using a computer terminal that permitted the user to ask the system specific questions about the patient's problems, and to receive relevant information. As in any expert system, such responses required a knowledge base of information obtained from the literature or from experts in the field and a mechanism for applying the expert knowledge to the specific questions asked about the patient's problem. A common technique was for the computer to ask the nurse a series of questions about the patient. With the information thus obtained about the patient and using the knowledge base, the program suggested diagnoses and alternative managements [46].

By the early 1980s, some NISs were available that provided a baseline assessment guide using information that included the patient's perceptions of: chief complaint, health history, medications, neurological status, mobility, activities of daily living, sleep/rest, comfort/pain, nutrition, psycho-social status, respiratory, circulatory, elimination-bowel and urinary, reproductive, and integumentary items [2]. After guiding the nurse through the collection of these data, the system suggested diagnoses to consider. Once a diagnosis was established, the nurse developed a care plan selected from a list of suggested alternative actions. Lombard [49] at Crouse-Irving Hospital in Syracuse, New York, described their nursing system, which had patient care plans developed by a consensus of nursing experts for such common diagnoses as anxiety, pain, decreased mobility, dependency, disorientation, impaired self concept, impaired skin integrity, impaired transport, respiratory impairment, and others.

The Creighton Online Multiple Modular Expert System (COMMES) was developed by Evans [23] at Creighton University as an educational tool for different health professionals; but the system found its best application as a consultant clinical nursing expert system. Using Creighton's time-sharing computer, a nurse could request a protocol for the care of a specific condition (such as emphysema) and then use the protocol consultant of COMMES to tailor a set of recommendations into an actual care plan for the specific patient. By guiding the nurse through the patient's signs and symptoms, the system's nursing diagnosis consultant would aid in arriving at a diagnosis and possible etiologies [24]. In addition, the system could provide a general nursing plan by medical diagnosis or by a diagnosis related group (DRG). Ryan [64, 65] described COMMES as an expert system that involved the structure of the domain of nursing, with a semantic network based on the conceptual relationships of more than 20,000 terms; having the ability to search heuristically based on if, then rules that explored their relationships. Bloom [10] reported a prototype system for COMMES that used an IBM PC computer. Evans [25] reported that care plans devised by nurses using COMMES were thorough and appropriate. Ozbolt and associates [59] at the University of Michigan also reported developing a prototype expert system for nursing practice. To derive nursing diagnoses from client data, they designed algorithms that consisted of "if, then" decision rules. The decision rules were based upon knowledge derived from the clinical literature, as for example, about normal and abnormal patterns of elimination and self care when applied to bowel elimination problems.

In 1985 a survey of 28 hospital information system vendors found that approximately 86 % of the vendors offered a product to support nursing activities; 88 % of the products supplied featured needs of the nursing manager; 83 % provided a patient classification system; and 25 % provided support for quality assurance activities [60]. A survey conducted in 1988 found 16 vendors who offered a nursing information system (NIS) that supported nurse functions in general medical and surgical units; nurse charting was provided by ten vendors; intake/output calculations and tracking vital signs by nine vendors; results reporting, nurse care planning and graphic charting by seven; interfacing to the HIS and other departmental systems by six; and nurse assessment, medication administration, admission-discharge-transfer, order entry functions, and standard shift reporting by five vendors [20]. Nurses generally accepted HISs better than did physicians. A survey of registered nurses at the 1150-bed Methodist Hospital of Indiana that had used the Technicon MIS for 5 years found that 86 % of the nurses agreed they liked working with the HIS [12]. In the 1980s NISs were probably the most widely used HIS subsystem in the United States.

During the late 1980s, McCloskey, Bulecheck, and colleagues from the University of Iowa began development of what would become known as the NIC, or Nursing Intervention Classification [13]. The first identified comprehensive classification of treatments that both nurses and physicians perform, the NIC was developed with research funding from the National Institute for Nursing Research (NINR) and includes physiological and psychosocial aspects of illness treatment, prevention, and health promotion.

With advances in technology and increased activity in the development of nursing classification systems to standardize nursing data, the American Nurses Association formed a Council in 1984 and adopted a resolution identifying the need for nurses to use information systems for the purposes of collecting and utilizing data in practice, education administration and research, with the specific recommendation that the Nursing Minimum Data Set be tested and implemented [51]. Additionally, the National League for Nursing created a Computers in Nursing forum in 1985 to influence the development of educational materials and advance educational nursing informatics related programming. In 1988, the first graduate education program in nursing was opened at the University of Maryland, led by Gassert and Mills under the leadership of Heller, the school's dean. Subsequently, nurse leaders introduced informatics courses were introduced elsewhere: Ronald, at the State University of Buffalo; Saba, Georgetown University; and Skiba, at Boston College [57].

During the 1980s, definitions of nursing informatics began to clarify the role of nurses with regard to computer technology. Ball and Hannah [35] modified an early definition of medical informatics to acknowledge that all health care professionals are part of medical informatics. Graves and Corcoran [32] defined nursing informatics as a scientific discipline bringing together nursing science, information science, and computer science. Subsequently, in late 1980s the ANA Council of Computer Applications in Nursing expanded previous definitions by incorporating the role of the informatics nurse specialist into Graves and Corcoran's definition [32].

7.1.4   The 1990s

Advances in technology such as the introduction of the internet, the emergence of Web-based applications, and the availability of smaller, lighter computers including personal data assistants (PDAs) shifted the emphasis of nursing informatics beyond hospital walls. According to Staggers and Thompson [74], conceptually-oriented definitions of nursing informatics gained acceptance and began to replace earlier technology-focused definitions. Nurses in informatics roles gained prominence, and in 1994 the ANA published the first versions of the Scope of Nursing Informatics Practice and the Standards of Informatics Practice. By 1995 a certification in nursing informatics as a practice specialty was established by the American Nurses Credentialing Center (ANCC).

During this time, the growing interest in nursing language, data, and standardization led nursing leadership to change the name of the ANA Data-base Steering Committee to the Committee on Nursing Practice Information Infrastructure. Although there was a drive towards a Unified Language System, several nursing languages continued to grow, including Saba's Clinical Care Classification, the Omaha language which was adopted by some home care and community health nursing agencies across the nation, and Grobe's Nursing Interventions Lexicon and Taxonomy, published in 1990. During this time, a pilot project in a Rochester Community Nursing Center SBHC (school-based health clinic) where care was provided by Advance Practice Nurses collected data using the Omaha System, ICD-9, and Current Procedural Terminology (CPT codes) "to determine if whether a nursing taxonomy is more sensitive in predicting number, type and costs of health care encounters for population-based care of adolescents in SBHCs" [80]. Additionally, the Nursing Outcomes Classification (NOC) joined the NANDA and NIC classification to complete a varied set of clinical nursing languages [80]. The number of languages, the lack of consensus, combined with varied licensing fees so complicated choices that many health care organizations chose vendor-provided non-standard terms for nursing's contribution to care, thus hampering the ability to collect data across systems to measure quality or conduct research.

Community Nursing Centers (CNCs), which were an important approach to providing community-based, nurse-managed care in the 1990s, also had informatics challenges specific to nursing documentation without a unified nursing language system. Centers affiliated with the University of Rochester and the University of Wisconsin were challenged by the need to collect, track, and analyze clinical data. In the NLN published book *Nursing Centers: the Time Is Now* [53], Lundeen and Walker, directors at the two centers, discussed challenges specific to clinical data collection and management for research, health professions education (faculty practice), and health policy purposes. Both leaders identified the need for relational databases for CNC management, staffing, tracking costs and quality of care. Walker and Walker [78] clarified the need for "information engineering" to address six critical success factors for CNCs: "1. Development of diverse revenue streams; 2. Cost control; 3. Providing and documenting quality services (care); 4. Client and faculty practitioner satisfaction; 5. Development of practice-based research; and 6. Integration of the CNC into the educational activities of the School of Nursing."

In 1990, the American Medical Informatics Association (AMIA) was founded through a merger of three existing informatics associations, one of which was the Symposium on Computer Applications in Medical Care (SCAMC). Since nurses had been involved, a Nursing Informatics Working Group (NI-WG) was formed with Ozbolt as the first chair. Nurses subsequently assumed interdisciplinary leadership roles in AMIA and have continued to current times. The College of American Pathologists worked to integrate nursing concepts into the Systematic Nomenclature of Medicine (SNOMED). Also in 1999, Ozbolt brought together nurse informaticians, experts on terminology, members from the federal government and vendor community, and representatives of professional organizations to attempt to interface languages with semantic interoperability. Although imperfect, the Unified Medical Language System (UMLS) and SNOMED – CT did incorporate nursing concepts. To date, this remains a challenge for progress in nursing informatics.

Nursing informatics was also gaining acceptance and growing influence with educators and nurse researchers. The University of Utah, University of Colorado, Duke University, and other schools also established graduate programs, and the University of Maryland awarded the first PhD in Nursing Informatics to Staggers. In 1997 at the University of Colorado, Walker, the new dean Walker named Skiba the first Associate Dean for Informatics and Academic Innovations to help develop a new curriculum focused on theory-guided, evidence-based practice with a increased focus on informatics.

Also, with the significant advances in technology identified earlier in the 1990s, Patricia Brennan initiated a new focus on the health benefits that new technologies could provide to consumers and the need for increased computer-based education and support to patients and caregivers in their homes. This emphasis on consumer engagement in care in the turn of the century continues to gain momentum with federal policy initiatives, technological advances, and increasing digital-oriented populations of all ages.

7.2   The New Millennium: 2000–2014

In 2000, leading developers of nursing terminologies from the U.S., Europe, Latin America, Australia and Asia gathered at a Nursing Terminology Summit conference to try to resolve issues related to nursing terminology with the International Standards Organizations Technical Committee (ISO-TC). Subsequently, the ISO work combined with the work of the Nursing Terminology Summit resulted in integration of nursing concepts and nursing interface terminologies mapped to concepts in SNOMED-CT, ultimately in 2007 becoming SNOMED, an international reference terminology standard.

The need for informatics advancement became an imperative when two reports from the Institute of Medicine related to patient safety were published. *To Err is Human* (1999) and *Crossing the Quality Chasm* (2001) created a mandate for improving the quality of care. In 2004, President Bush called for every American to have an electronic health record by 2014 and established the office of the National Coordinator of Health Information Technology. These actions stimulated the need for adopting standards for interoperability of health information transactions across settings. This policy decision resulted in the formation of the Health information Technology Standards Panel (HITSP) in partnership with the American National Standards Institute (ANSI). The other organization created from this federal policy decision was a private, not-for-profit Certification Commission for Healthcare Information Technology (CCHIT) to review and ensure hardware and software products meet adopted standards. The first nursing language adopted was Saba's Clinical Care Classification System, and nurses have been well-represented on HITSP, CCHIT and involved in other standards setting organizations including SNOMED, Health Level 7 (HL7) and Logical Object Names, Identifiers and Codes (LOINC). After serving in leadership roles in SNOMED and HL7, Warren became the first nurse appointed to the National Committee on Vital and Health Statistics.

Other nurses continue to make contributions related to consumer-driven health care. Continuing her work done in the 1990s on consumer-driven health care, Brennan became the national director of a multi-site research program funded by the Robert Wood Johnson Foundation to develop innovative approaches to personal health records and tools for health management [11]. At the University of Maryland, Nahm and colleagues are conducting research related to the use of personal and family health records to assist family caregivers to manage care of older adults [43].

In 2004, with the leadership of Delaney from AMIA board and Sensmeier at Health Information Management and Systems Society (HIMSS), 18 national and regional nursing informatics groups established the Alliance of Nursing Informatics (ANI), with the AMIA and HIMSS boards of directors agreeing to provide ongoing support, coordination and leadership [33].

In 2004, after President George Bush created the Office of the National Coordinator (ONC), several nurses attending the first HIT summit convened by Brailer, then National Coordinator for Health IT. Since there were no nurses included at the table nor were nurses even mentioned, a group of leaders met and resolved to strengthen the voice of the nursing profession at this important time in history [78]. In 2005, the group held a strategy session to plan for an invitational summit that would bring nurses together from academia, government, and industry in what became the TIGER Initiative, an acronym for Technology Informatics Guiding Education Reform. In 2006, over 100 nurses representing all walks of the profession (not just nursing informatics specialists) met at the Uniformed Services University of the Health Sciences. Together they articulated a vision that would interweave nursing informatics technologies into nursing practice and education. In what they designated as Phase I of TIGER, they identified seven pillars:

- Management and Leadership
- Education
- Communication and Collaboration
- Informatics Design
- Information Technology
- Policy
- Culture

To gain top level support for nursing informatics, the TIGER leadership scheduled the summit to coincide with the annual fall meeting of the American Association of Colleges of Nursing (AACN) and invited deans from schools of nursing to a reception and "gallery walk" that exhibited a number of emerging technologies.

During Phase II, initiated 6 months after the summit, TIGER reorganized its action plan into nine key areas and formed nine collaboratives. Volunteers in each group reviewed the literature, developed strategies/recommendations for implementation and integration of nursing informatics across all groups within the profession. With grassroots involvement of more than 1500 nurses, the nine collaboratives generated reports in their areas of focus:

- Standards and Interoperability
- Health Policy
- Informatics Competencies
- Education and Faculty Development
- Staff Development
- Leadership Development
- Usability and Clinical Application Design,
- Consumer Empowerment and Personal Health Record
- Virtual Learning Environment.

TIGER Phase III involved dissemination through numerous webinars across professional organizations, universities, clinical settings, and presentations at national and international meetings. Progress made through the TIGER initiative formed the core of the fourth edition of *Nursing Informatics: Where Technology and Caring Meet*, as reflected in the new subtitle that took the place of *Where Caring and Technology Meet* used in previous editions [7].

In 2011, TIGER became the TIGER Initiative Foundation connected to the Health Information Management and Systems Society (HIMSS). The TIGER Board of Directors and it director, Schlak, continued to advance competencies through continued dissemination and outreach to nursing specialty and interprofessional groups. The Virtual Learning Environment was launched and a TIGER Newsletter kept nurses active in the initiative informed. In 2014, TIGER became part of the HIMSS organization and continues to offer grass roots nurses and individuals from other disciplines advancement in informatics and opportunities for participation.

During the period of 2005 and 2014, two federal policy initiates have had and will continue to have significant influence on informatics. The American Recovery and Reinvestment Act (ARRA) signed by President Obama in 2009 authorized the Centers for Medicare and Medicaid Services (CMS) to provide incentive payments to eligible professionals and hospitals who adopt, implement, upgrade or demonstrate "meaningful use" of certified electronic health records. ARRA funding continued the race begun by President George Bush for every American to have an electronic health record by 2014 with evolving technologies and interoperability creating both challenges and opportunities for nursing and interprofessional informaticists. The Patient Protection and Affordable Care Act (PPACA), commonly called the Affordable Care Act (ACA), was signed into law by President Barack Obama in 2010 and represents significant change impacting health systems and consumers. This act has increased the focus on reducing hospitalization by improving outcomes of care. Also, with growing knowledge and access to health related information and a shift to emphasis on healthy lifestyles and self management of chronic illnesses/conditions, nursing informatics has the potential to rapidly moving to the forefront in coordination and management of individuals, families and communities through care coordination and coaching using both system and person/family generated data and dashboards [39].

According to Klasnja and Pratt [44], mobile phones are increasingly valuable tools for improving health and managing chronic conditions. With the capability to self monitor healthy behaviors (exercise, food intake) and key measures (glucose, blood pressure), consumers can become actively engaged in improving their own health. Combined with coaching, these mobile platforms combined can help individuals make positive changes in their behaviors [44].

Health coaching enabled by mobile health applications allow coaches to communicate with patients/persons real-time allowing tracking of health and wellness measures such as nutrition, diet, exercise and mood integrated with traditional medical data. Also, mobile health applications enable patients with chronic diseases to focus on more precise, personalized self-management resulting in improved quality of life and fewer hospital visits. Coaching presumes a collaborative paradigm (asking patients what changes they are willing to make) rather than a directive paradigm (telling patients what to do). Nurse informaticists and nurses with an understanding of the use of data and information along with coaching skills can assist persons, caregivers and families in choosing healthy lifestyles, managing chronic conditions and transitioning from health care settings to home with the increased availability and use of personal health records and mobile devices [9].

Future advances in genomics and genetics combined with increasing access by patients/persons and families to the knowledge realtime will increasingly challenge providers and the health care systems and empower patients with just-in-time access to information and decision-support tools for address preferences and personalized care.

References

1. ANA (American Nurses' Association). Committee on research and studies: ANA blueprint for research in nursing. Am J Nurs. 1962;62(8):69–71.
2. Aveni S. Nursing and computer technology – information overload or structured information? Comput Hosp. 1982;3:26.
3. Ball M. Integrating information systems in health care. In: Bakker AR, et al., editors. Towards new hospital information systems. Amsterdam: IOS Press; 1988. p. 39–44.
4. Ball M, Hannah KJ. Hospital information systems: the nursing role in selection and implementation. In: Hannah KJ, Guillemin E, Conklin D, editors. Nursing uses of computer and information and information science. Amsterdam: Elsevier Science; 1985. p. 121–6.
5. Ball MJ. An overview of total medical information systems. Methods Inf Med. 1971;10(2):73–82.
6. Ball MJ, Hannah KJ, Browne JD. Using computers in nursing. Reston: Reston Publishing; 1984.
7. Ball MJ, Douglas JV, Hinton WP. Nursing informatics: where technology and caring meet. 4th ed. London: Springer; 2011
8. Barnett GO, Zielstorff RD. Data systems can enhance or hinder medical, nursing activities. Hospitals. 1977;51:157–61.
9. Bennett HD, Coleman EA, Parry C, Bodenheimer T, Chen EH. Health coaching for patients with chronic illness. Fam Pract Manag. 2010;17:24–9.
10. Bloom KC, Leitner JE, Solano JL. Development of an expert system prototype to generate nursing care plans based on nursing diagnoses. Comput Nurs. 1986;5:140–5.
11. Brennan PF. Health informatics and community health: support for patients as collaborators in care. Methods Inf Med. 1999;38:274–8.
12. Brown A. A computer generated aid for scheduling operating rooms. Proc AAMSI Congress. 1984;259–99.
13. Bulechek GM, Butcher HK, Dochterman JMM, Wagner C. Nursing Interventions Classification (NIC). Amsterdam: Elsevier Health Sciences; 2013.
14. Chapman R, Ranzenberger J, Killpack AK, Pryor TA. Computerized charting at the bedside: promoting the nursing process. Proc SCAMC. 1984;8:700–2.
15. Charters K. Computers as management tools: acceptance by nursing personnel. Proc SCAMC. 1981;725–7.
16. Childs BW. Bedside terminals – status and the future. Healthc Comput Commun. 1988;5:12–4.
17. Cook M, McDowell W. Changing to an automated information system. Am J Nurs. 1975;75:46–51.
18. Crosley JM. Computerized nursing care planning utilizing nursing diagnosis. Proc SCAMC. 1984;642–5.
19. DeMarco JP. Automating nursing's paper work. AJN: Am J Nurs. 1965;65:74–7.
20. Drazen EL. Bedside computer systems overview. In: Abrami PF, Johnson JE, editors. Bringing computers to the hospital. New York: Springer Publishing; 1990. p. 1–15.
21. ECRI (Emergency Care Research Institute). Clinical information systems improve with new standard. Health Technol Trends. 1989;1:3–6.
22. Edmunds L. Computers for inpatient nursing care. What can be accomplished? Comput Nurs. 1984;2:102.

23. Evans S. Nursing applications of an expert system. Proc MEDINFO. 1983;182–5.
24. Evans S. A computer-based nursing diagnosis consultant. Proc SCAMC. 1984;658–61.
25. Evans S. A clinical tool for nursing. Comput Healthc. 1988;9:41–4. 2.
26. Fitzpatrick JJ, Kerr ME, Saba VK, Hoskins LM, Hurley ME, Mills WC, et al. Nursing diagnosis: translating nursing diagnosis into ICD code. Am J Nurs. 1989;89(4):493–5.
27. Flanders J, Lutgen T. The development of a microcomputer-based nurse management system. Proc SCAMC. 1984;618–21.
28. Foster C, Conrick M. Nursing informatics: an international overview for nursing in a technological era. In: Grobe SJ, editor. Nursing informatics: combining clinical practice guidelines and patient preferences. Amsterdam: Elsevier Science and Technology; 1994. p. 150.
29. Giebink GA, Hurst LL. Computer projects in health care. Ann Arbor: Health Administration Press; 1975.
30. Glazener TT, McDonald CJ. Putting doctors behind bars. MD Comput. 1986;3:29–33.
31. Gordon M. Practice-based data set for a nursing information system. J Med Syst. 1985;9:43–55.
32. Graves JR, Corcoran S. The study of nursing informatics. Image J Nurs Sch. 1989;21:227–31.
33. Greenwood K. The alliance for nursing informatics: a history. Comput Inform Nurs. 2010;28:124–6.
34. Guenther JT. Mapping the literature of nursing informatics. J Med Libr Assoc. 2006;94:E92–8.
35. Hannah KJ, Ball MJ, Edwards MJA. Introduction to nursing informatics. New York: Springer; 1994. p. 61.
36. Hughes S. Bedside terminals: cliniCom. MD Comput. 1988;5:22.
37. Institute of Medicine. To err is human: building a safer health system. Washington, DC: National Academy Press; 2000.
38. Jenkins C. Automation improves nursing productivity. Comput Healthc. 1988;9:40–1.
39. Jimison H, Pavel M, Larimer N, Mullen P. A general architecture for computer based health coaching. Proceedings of the international conference on technology and aging, Toronto; 2007.
40. Johnson D. Decisions and dilemmas in the development of a nursing information system. Comput Nurs. 1986;5:94–8.
41. Johnson D, Ranzenberger J, Pryor TA. Nursing applications of the HELP system. Proc SCAMC. 1984;703–8.
42. Killpack AK, Budd MC, Chapman RH, Ranzenberger J, Johnson DS, Pryor TA. Automating patient acuity in critical care units from nursing documentation. Proc SCAMC. 1984;709–11.
43. Kim KS, Nahm ES. Benefits of and barriers to the use of personal health records (PHR) for health management among adults. Online J Nurs Inform (ONJI). 2012;16(3). http://onji.org/issues/?p=1995
44. Klasnja P, Pratt W. Healthcare in the pocket: mapping the space of mobile-phone health interventions. J Biomed Inform. 2012;45:184–98.
45. Kogut GG, Hazen EB, Heffner RE. Automating a patient acuity system: application development on a personal computer. Proc SCAMC. 1984;629–31.
46. Laborde JM. Expert systems for nursing? Comput Nurs. 1983;2:130–5.
47. Light NL. Developing a hospital system nursing data base: a pragmatic approach. Proceedings of the 2nd national conference computer technology and nursing; 1984. p. 7–12.
48. Lindberg D. Electronic retrieval of clinical data. J Med Educ. 1965;40:753–9.
49. Lombard N, Light N. On-line nursing care plans by nursing diagnosis. Comput Healthc. 1983;4(11):22–3.
50. McNeely LD. Concerns for nursing administration: planning for implementation of the NIH clinical center medical information system. Proc SCAMC. 1981;713–6.
51. Milholland KD. The role of the professional association in policy development related to information standards. In: Mills ME, Romano CA, Heller BR, editors. Information management in nursing and health care. Springhouse: Springhouse Corp; 1996. p. 272–9.

52. Monahan ML, Kiley M, Patterson C. Bar code technology: its use within a nursing information system. Proc MEDINFO. 1986;26–30.
53. Murphy B. Nursing centers: the time is now. Washington, DC: National League for Nursing; 1995.
54. NANDA. Defining the knowledge of nursing. Available at http://www.nanda.org/nanda-international-history-1973-9.html. Accessed August 9, 2015.
55. Nightingale F. Notes on hospitals. London: Longman; 1863.
56. Olsson DE. Automating nurses' notes: first step in a computerized record system. Hospitals. 1967;41:64.
57. Ozbolt JG, Saba VK. A brief history of nursing informatics in the United States of America. Nurs Outlook. 2008;56:199–205.e2.
58. Ozbolt JG. Designing information systems for nursing practice: data base and knowledge base requirements of different organizational technologies. Comput Methods Programs Biomed. 1986;22:61–5.
59. Ozbolt JG, Samuel Schultz I, Swain MAP, Abraham IL, Farchaus-Stein K. Developing an expert system for nursing practice. Proc SCAMC. 1984;654.
60. Partin MH, Monahan ML. Computer-based information systems models. J Med Syst. 1985;9:5–18.
61. Pesce J. Bedside terminals: medTake. MD Comput. 1988;5:16.
62. Romano CA. Computer technology and nursing: 1st national conference. 1983;26–33.
63. Rosenberg M, Carriker D. Automating nurses' notes. AJN: Am J Nurs. 1966;66:1021–3.
64. Ryan SA. An expert system for nursing practice. Clinical decision support. J Med Syst. 1985;9:29–41.
65. Ryan SA. An expert system for nursing practice. Clinical decision support. Comput Nurs. 1985;3:77–84.
66. Saba VK, McCormick KA. Essentials of computers for nurses. Philadelphia: Lippincott; 1986.
67. Saba VK, O'Hare PA, Zuckerman AE, Boondas J, Levine E, Oatway DM. A nursing intervention taxonomy for home health care. Nurs Health Care. 1991;12:296–9.
68. Saba VK. Nursing information systems. In: Saba VK, Rieder KA, Pocklington DB, editors. Nursing and computers, an anthology. New York: Springer; 1989. p. 3–12.
69. Saba VK. Computer applications in nursing. Proc SCAMC. 1983;467–8.
70. Saba VK. Introduction. Proc SCAMC. 1982;515.
71. Saba VK. Nursing diagnosis in computerized patient classification systems. In: Carroll-Johnson RM, editor. Classification in nursing diagnoses. New York: Lippincott; 1989. p. 84–8.
72. Simborg DW. Rational staffing of hospital nursing services by functional activity budgeting. Public Health Rep. 1976;91:118.
73. Spencer WA, Vallbona C. A preliminary report on the use of electronic data processing technics in the description and evaluation of disability. Arch Phys Med Rehabil. 1962;43:22–35.
74. Staggers N, Thompson CB. The evolution of definitions for nursing informatics: a critical analysis and revised definition. JAMIA. 2002;9:255–61.
75. Stefanchik MF. Point-of-care information systems: improving patient care. Comput Healthc. 1987;8:7–8.
76. Vallbona C. The influence of computer technology in nursing care. Proc AMIA 1982;140–4.
77. Van Brunt E, Collen M. Hospital computer systems. In: Collen MF, editor. Hospital computer systems. New York: Wiley; 1974. p. 114–47.
78. Walker PH. The TIGER initiative: a call to accept and pass the baton. Nursing. 2010;28:352.
79. Walker PH, Walker J. Community nursing center informatics for business, practice, research and education. In: Murphy B, editor. Nursing centers: the time is now. Washington, DC: National League for Nursing; 1995.
80. Walker PH, Baker JJ, Chiverton P. Costs of interdisciplinary practice in a school-based health center. Outcomes Manag Nurs Pract. 1998;2:37–44.
81. Werley HH, Devine EC, Westlake SK, Manternach CA. Testing and refinement of the nursing minimum data set. Proc MEDINFO. 1986;816–7.

82. Werley HH, Lang NM. Preface. In: Werley HH, Lang NM, editors. Identification of the nursing minimum data set. New York: Springer. pp xix–xxii.
83. Wiener F, Weil MH, Carlson RW. Computer systems for facilitating management of the critically ill. Comput Biol Med. 1982;12:1–15.
84. Young KM. Informatics for healthcare professionals. Philadelphia: FA Davis; 2000.
85. Zielstorff RD. Computers in nursing. Germantown: Aspen Publishers; 1980.
86. Zielstorff RD. Computers in nursing administration. Proc SCAMC. 1981:717–20.
87. Zielstorff RD, McHugh ML, Clinton J. Computer design criteria for systems that support the nursing process. Kansas City: American Nurses' Association; 1988.

Chapter 8
Specialized High-Intensity Clinical Settings: A Brief Review

Morris F. Collen and Marion J. Ball

Abstract In the early 1960s, some medical centers began to develop intensive care unit (ICU) information systems to monitor critically ill patients. These used a combination of devices to obtain measurements and derive variables. One generated a severity index to guide treatment and compute the probability of survival; another saved data to use in analysis and educational simulations. Studies of the clinical effectiveness of such systems were mixed, despite findings that variations in hospital death rates were associated with variations in care processes. While few hospitals had emergency department (ED) subsystems installed by the end of the 1980s, some participated in community emergency medical systems that routed patients to hospitals for treatment. Despite progress in intervening years, recent studies find that both settings face continued challenges. The data-intensive ICU faces interoperability issues arising from incompatible piece of monitoring equipment. For the ED, exchange of patient information from other settings remains difficult and evidence as to the impact of health information technology remains limited.

Keywords Intensive care unit information systems • Emergency department information systems • Specialized information systems • Interoperability • Clinical effectiveness • Medical devices • Community emergency medical systems

Two hospital settings have an undeniable hold on the mass media and the public imagination: the intensive care unit (ICU) and the emergency department (ED). Both of these specialized high-intensity environments rely on health information technology (IT) and an array of health informatics applications to treat patients who are severely ill or injured and potentially at risk of death. Beyond those commonalities, there are significant differences. The ICU treats critically ill patients transferred in from other care settings; the ED admits patients from the community to treat

---

Author was deceased at the time of publication.

M.F. Collen (deceased)

M.J. Ball, Ed.D. (✉)
IBM Research, Baltimore, MD, USA

Johns Hopkins University, Baltimore, MD, USA
e-mail: marionball@us.ibm.com

© Springer-Verlag London 2015
M.F. Collen, M.J. Ball (eds.), *The History of Medical Informatics in the United States*, Health Informatics, DOI 10.1007/978-1-4471-6732-7_8

problems ranging from minor (but urgent) to life-threatening. Intensely patient-focused, the ICU care team uses multiple technology-based medical devices to monitor and treat the patient; length of stay is measured in days. The ED communicates with multiple entities – from emergency medical technicians, police officers, and insurance company representatives, to parents, spouses, and children – to treat patients who walk in or are brought by ambulance; length of stay in the ED is measured in hours.

This chapter opens by reviewing key decades in the development of systems for the ICU and ED. It concludes by offering insights from two recent assessments of the status of information technology in each setting, highlighting the challenges that health IT adoption must overcome in order to improve care.

8.1 Key Decades in the Development of Specialized Systems

8.1.1 Intensive Care Unit Information Systems

Patients in shock, such as from serious trauma or from an acute myocardial infarction, usually are admitted to a specialized ICU where they are attached to appropriate life-support and monitoring systems. Intensive care unit is a term applied to coronary care units, shock units, postoperative recovery rooms, and similar highly specialized facilities for the care of critically ill patients; and ICUs were designed for adults, children, and newborns. The primary function of the computer in the ICU is to collect the data from the physiological monitoring instruments, integrate all the patient data collected from all sources into a computer-stored patient database, interface the local ICU database with the MIS computer-stored patient record, furnish alarms for abnormal measurements, and aid in the selection of treatments for the ICU patient.

In the early 1960s some medical centers in the United States began to report the development of ICU information systems. In 1962 at the Texas Institute for Research and Rehabilitation (TIRR), the ICU system recorded the chemical composition of gases (oxygen, carbon dioxide, and nitrogen) in inspired and expired air; lung-function monitors (pneumogram for pulmonary ventilation, pneumotachogram for respiratory rate, and spirogram for respiratory volume); cardiovascular monitors (electrocardiogram, phonocardiogram, cardio-tachometer, and vectorcardiogram); and neuromuscular phenomena (electromyogram and nerve impulses) [14, 39]. TIRR developed a bedside computer terminal system for monitoring the physiologic variables in postoperative patients. In 1962 they reported beginning the development of an automated monitoring system for the acquisition of temperature, blood pressure, pulse (heart) rate, and respiratory rate. In 1965 their bedside monitor collected data from sensors that continued to measure the four vital signs described and that provided graphic plots of these variables, along with displays of the patient's electrocardiogram and an impedance pneumogram of pulmonary ventilation [41]. In 1966, with an analog-to-digital computer interfaced to an IBM 1410 computer, they recorded analog signals on analog tape and then entered the digitized data into punched cards. They developed computer programs for the automatic computation of results, and the computer printout of reports. They also developed an online computer program to calculate the fluid and electrolyte needs of critically ill patients [42]. In the second half of the 1960s, their monitoring system was an integral part of their TIRR HIS.

In 1965 Weil and associates at the University of Southern California began to use in the Los Angeles County General Hospital's critical care ward, an IBM 1710 computer equipped with an analog-to-digital converter to concurrently monitor multiple signals collected from critically ill patients in circulatory shock. They used a combination of devices to obtain 11 primary measurements and 25 derived variables. On request, or at desired intervals, the system automatically reported heart and respiratory rates, arterial and venous pressures, cardiac output, peripheral vascular resistance, mean circulation time, central blood volume, total work of the heart and stroke work, and urine output. In addition to these online measurements, when blood was sampled, the plasma volume, red-cell mass, blood pH value, and oxygen and carbon dioxide pressures were determined off-line. Data were manually entered for the patient's age, height, and weight, as were nurses' notes for fluid intake and medications received. Summary reports were generated on request, as well as routinely at the end of each 8-h shift and every 24 h. Reports were printed automatically by typewriter, and also were transmitted by closed-circuit television for display at the patient's bedside. Trends of selected parameters were graphed by an online plotter. The data were also punched into cards, which were used for investigational purposes [37, 46].

In 1967 they transferred their unit to the Hollywood Presbyterian Hospital which had a six-bed coronary care unit, a nine-bed ICU, and a shock ward [47]. They upgraded their ICU system with a Xerox Data Systems Sigma 5 computer with an analog-to-digital converter connected to the various monitoring instruments, and used five visual display terminals with keyboards and a line printer. A larger television display in the ICU permitted users to read current significant information from any location within the room. They developed a statistical program that derived a severity index of the patient's status to guide treatment, as well as a predictive formula for the probability of survival; and the index and the probability of survival were computed online. By 1978 they had advanced their data management system so that at the core of the system was the computer-based patient record that contained all of the data generated during the entire stay in the ICU. Laboratory tests, x-ray reports, and progress notes in free text were all entered; so the complete record of each patient was available for online retrieval. By the early 1980s they had one of the most advanced ICU systems for the time, with improved electronic preprocessing to increase the efficiency and speed of data acquisition, signal analysis, and online computer accessibility to patient records [49]. Weil and Rackow advised that a pressing problem was the rapid increase in the numbers and complexities of procedures that were performed in ICUs, and with a high cost. By the late 1960s computer-based pulmonary function tests were also being performed routinely in the ICUs of the LDS Hospital in Salt Lake City [9] and at the Los Angeles County

General Hospital. In 1966 Lewis and associates at Northwestern University Medical School reported the use of an IBM 1710 computer to collect and integrate the data that they had been collecting from their postoperative recovery-room patients. They obtained respiratory, circulatory, and blood-sample measurements separately from a variety of physiological monitoring devices. They collected the analog data on magnetic tape and transmitted the data via telephone lines to an analog-to-digital converter that digitized the data and entered them into the computer memory. The test results were printed out and also were punched into cards for later studies.

In 1970 the group began to use a DEC PDP-12 computer with an analog-to-digital converter, disk storage, and bedside television display terminals; they wrote all their systems and applications programs in PDP-12 assembler language. They monitored four patients continuously. In addition to the task of monitoring all the physiological instrumentation, they now received an updated report of the patient's status every 30 s, with a display of the current value for all patient data collected. On request, the computer furnished a graphic display of past monitoring data. If desired, it also would type out a copy of the graphic output [8, 24] and Lewis reported that their ICU system functioned around the clock, day in and day out.

In 1967 an ICU monitoring system became operational at the LDS Hospital. It was developed in the cardiac catheterization laboratory by Warner and associates at the University of Utah, Department of Biophysics. After heart surgery, the patient was transferred to the ICU; and when the nurse pressed the appropriate button on the remote console, the computer sampled the next 64 heart beats of the patient and determined the mean value of each of the variables calculated from the central aortic pulse pressure. The nurse could review the course of the patient over any desired period of time. Any data that differed significantly from the patient's baseline values were saved in the patient's computer record, and a warning red light was turned on. The data could also be reviewed by a plot on the oscilloscope presented as a series of bar graphs representing the averages of any desired number of measurements for each variable. At the end of each 8-h shift, a summary report was printed for each patient, which showed the values of each variable, and the comments entered by the nurses. When a patient was discharged from the ICU, the data were copied from computer disk to magnetic tape and were saved for subsequent analysis [44–45].

Warner also used his system as a teaching and testing program for ICU nurses. The program simulated the rhythm disturbances that patients with an acute episode of heart disease might develop during their stay in the ICU; and it displayed an electrocardiogram in the same way the nurses saw it in the ICU [45]. In 1973 A.D. Little, under a contract from the NCHSR&D, reviewed the LDS ICU unit used as the recovery room for thoracic surgery patients; where patients were monitored by what was now called the MEDLAB ICU system, which collected physiological parameters on a fixed schedule from 2- to 15-min intervals. Two computer terminals in the ICU unit were used to enter and retrieve data on its ten patients, whose ICU records were kept partially on paper and partially in the computer. Nurses used the monitoring system to obtain blood pressures and heart rates; and followed cardiac output values on the monitor to alert the physician if the values indicated something was wrong.

In 1973 the estimated cost for patient monitoring using this system was $75 per patient day (excluding the cost of computer technicians) [26]. By 1974 in the LDS Hospital they were monitoring a thoracic surgery operating suite, a ten-bed thoracic surgery unit, a four-bed coronary care unit, a six-bed general surgery unit, and a three-bed pulmonary ICU [10]. In 1980 the LDS ICU system consisted of a group of four Tandem computers in their computer center linked to minicomputers located within the ICU [5]. In 1982 they had increased to six Tandem computers and six minicomputers in the ICU, serving 67 ICU beds [12]. In each patient's room, they placed a computer terminal with adequate memory to store several pages of the patient's data to gain the added benefits of providing nurses with bedside terminals. Since they had found that clinical laboratory test findings made up almost one-half of the data reviewed by physicians at the ICU patient's bedside, they expected the installation of bedside terminals would improve the data acquisition and charting process, and would result in saving nurses' time. However, contrary to their expectations, a study that used work sampling to measure the time spent by nurses in all activities related to patient care before and after the implementation of computer-based charting did show a 12 % decrease in time the nurses spent in direct patient care, but a 33 % increase in charting after the computerization [4].

In 1967 Osborn and associates at the Pacific Medical Center in San Francisco initiated an ICU system using an IBM 1800 computer. They monitored two patients simultaneously for their heart rates with the electrocardiogram, and for the arterial pressure and pulse rate. With their first prototype they found the problem of false alarms disturbing [31]. In 1969 they reported that they had enlarged the size of their ICU, and added more equipment to provide full online monitoring capabilities for circulatory, respiratory, blood, and gas measurements, with oscilloscope and television displays and a variety of printouts. They solved the problem of excessive false alarms by requiring the coincidence of exceeding alarm-limit settings in both ECG and vascular channels, which effectively reduced false alarms from 330 to 8 in a similar period of study [29]. As a test in 1973, using a remote terminal attached by phone line they began to monitor a patient in the post-operative cardiac surgical unit at the Mt. Sinai Hospital in New York City. In 1973 they moved into a new hospital where their system served five beds in the cardiopulmonary ICU. However, they did not yet have a full database management system with a computer-based patient record integrated with the remainder of the hospital database. They evaluated the effectiveness of their ICU system as to death rates, length of stay in the unit, days on the respirator, days with an arterial line, number of arterial blood gases; and nurse-to-patient ratio per-day. The results showed essentially no difference between the monitored and control groups; however, the nurses and the doctors felt that the system was useful in patient care, and they felt more secure with the more comprehensive, timely data obtained from the system [22].

In 1967 Sheppard [35, 36] and associates at the University of Alabama in Birmingham initiated an ICU system for two beds in their cardiac surgery postoperative care unit, where they employed an IBM 1800 computer to monitor their patients and to implement rules and logic for the treatment of the patients. The computer was programmed to acquire automatically, at 5-min intervals, a variety of signals and to digitize and display the measurements at the patient's bedside. A metering pump measured the medications that were administered intravenously and the amount of blood infused. They developed rules for the infusion of blood in patients after open-heart surgery, and blood was infused by the system automatically using these rules. Approximately 1,800 patients were treated with the automated system between July 1967 and April 1972 [34]. Sheppard was the first to do what was called closed-loop control and showed a significant effect on the time to normalize patient's fluid balance when the infusion of blood was automatically controlled by the computer system in a closed loop feedback mode based on left atrial pressure which is related to stroke volume and cardiac output. In 7 years the automated care system was used in the postoperative observation and treatment of 4,624 patients [2]. By 1979, 14 cardiac surgical beds in their ICU were instrumented for measurement and monitoring; ten beds were connected to a Hewlett-Packard 2112 computer, and four beds were connected to a DEC PDP 11/20 computer [35]. A similar computer-controlled, automatic closed-loop, blood replacement system was used for the postoperative care of patients who had undergone coronary-artery bypass surgery at Heineman Medical Research Center in Charlotte, North Carolina [28]. Westenskow [48], who used a closed-loop control system for anesthesia at the University of Utah, found that only eight universities in the United States had published reports of applications that used closed-loop systems for control of fluid replacement (blood or intravenous medications), blood pressure, or anesthesia delivery.

In the 1970s some use of minicomputers was reported for ICU systems, such as the LINC-8 computer at the Medical College of Wisconsin [1] and the DEC PDP-11 computer at the Naval Regional Medical Center in Portsmouth, Virginia [6]. A good review of the status of computer monitoring in patient care in the early 1970s was written by Glaeser and Thomas [16]. In 1976 A.D. Little evaluated ICUs by comparing units with-and-without computer-based monitoring. They reported there was no definitive, quantitative evidence to indicate that computer-based patient monitoring systems changed overall patient mortality or morbidity; however, the report concluded that automated computer systems could save significant staff time amounting to one nurse-per-shift in an 8–12 bed unit. Furthermore, when the computer performed calculations for the staff, these calculations could save considerable physician time, and promote accurate measurement and better understanding of the patient's status [25]. It soon became apparent that in an ICU system a data management system was essential to integrate all the local data collected and processed in the ICU, and to interface with the MIS to use any patient data collected in other MIS subsystems. Although the ICU information subsystem was basically similar to any other clinical specialty information subsystem, the database management program was more difficult to develop than was the physiologic monitoring component. In 1974 the coronary care unit at the University of Chicago established a computer-based patient record based on the data-collection techniques developed by Slack (see Sect. 5.4). Patient data were recorded on a multipage form, which a clerk used to enter the data into a minicomputer by answering the questions displayed on the screen. The system was cumbersome and soon was revised to be compatible with other clinical subsystems in the HIS and clinics [50].

Kezdi and associates at the Cox Heart Institute initiated a cardiac ICU monitoring system for a six-bed coronary care unit at the affiliated Kettering Memorial Hospital. They used an IBM 1800 computer to help with the enormous volume of measurements coming from all of their monitor equipment. Analog preprocessors conditioned the signals before the data were transmitted to the digital computer; and this processing greatly reduced the number of computations performed by the computer. In addition to the usual variables monitored in an ICU, their computer also provided trend analyses, and allowed a prediction of future trends. They also used LINC and PDP-8 computers for the development and testing of their programs [40].

In the 1980s more ICU systems began to use microcomputers. The Methodist Hospital in Houston, Texas, with 12 ICU beds, implemented a Mennen Medical Bedside Monitoring System that used microprocessor interfaces linked by a local network to a central minicomputer [30]. The National Institutes of Health (NIH) Clinical Center ICU had four computer systems operating: one for patient monitoring and the others for software development, research, and instrumentation. In 1980 they reported installing Hewlett-Packard minicomputers for their ICU overall data management [27]. Microcomputers in the ICU were reported at the Johns Hopkins Hospital using a Radio Shack Color Computer [15]; at the University of Missouri Health Sciences Center in Columbia using an IBM PC/XT [17]; and also at the Cleveland Clinic using an IBM PC/XT [38].

In 1980 Greenburg [18] reviewed the status of computers in ICUs, and wrote that then current research focused on the design of effective man-machine systems with particular emphasis on data acquisition, the database, and adjuncts for medical decision making. ICU terminals with improved graphical reports and video images provided combined digital, pictorial, bivariate, and bar displays of complex hemodynamic data [33]. Siegel and Coleman and associates at the University of Maryland Institute for Emergency Medical Services Systems developed a method of displaying the large volume of data so that the rapidly changing status of patients in the ICU could be monitored more readily. The computer output of data from a portion of their cardiovascular program was arranged in a circle rather than in the usual tabular or linear, graphic formats. The various test measurements were all normalized by comparison to normal persons' values, so that all normal values would arrange themselves around a zero-value circle. Any variations from normal would then project above or below the zero circle; thus patterns for different abnormal states could be easily recognized.

In 1986 Gardner at the University of Utah School of Medicine wrote a comprehensive review of ICU systems. He described their role in monitoring and providing alarms for important physiologic variables in critically ill patients. He emphasized the need for a total integrated data management system to provide adequate alerts and suggestions for treatment based on the total clinical database. He reported that all of the estimated 75,000 adult, pediatric, and neonatal *intensive care beds* operating in the United States were equipped with some type of physiological monitor [11]. Few institutions, however, used microcomputer-based monitoring systems to provide alarms, arrhythmia monitors, and digital data processing. Although Gardner found 11 manufacturers in the United States that sold ICU bedside monitors, the number of commercial computer-based ICU patient data-management systems in routine use in 1986 was only 14–20 manufactured by Hewlett-Packard and 15 made by Mennen Medical; with each system for 16 beds costing about $100,000. He cited only nine institutions in the United States that used such ICU computer-based data-management systems.

Knaus reported that by 1988, there were 6,556 ICUs in the United States with a total of 86,543 beds. Intensive care accounted for approximately 7 % of all hospital beds, 15–20 % of hospital expenses, and approximately 1 % of the gross national product. To evaluate the effectiveness of ICUs, Knaus developed a prognostic scoring system for critically ill patients, which he called the Acute Physiology and Chronic Health Evaluation (APACHE). Using APACHE, he found substantial variations in hospital death rates which appeared to be associated with distinct variations in the process of care.

By the end of the 1980s, the technology for ICU systems had evolved to only partially satisfy its two major functional requirements: (1) the need for physiologic monitoring devices that would also automatically administer medications and blood, using closed-loop feedback algorithms; and (2) the need to be integrated into an HIS subsystem with a comprehensive patient computer-based record. There was still a need to learn how to better aid the extremely complex clinical decision processes involved in the minute-to-minute care of the critically ill patient.

8.1.2 Emergency Department Information Systems

Just as in the surgery suite, the emergency department (ED) and the intensive care unit (ICU) in a hospital have a common need to provide urgent care for critically ill patients. These departments use computer technology both for their monitoring instrumentation and for data processing. When a patient was admitted to the emergency department of a hospital, clinical decisions often had to be made without adequate information about the past history of the patient. An MIS had the advantage of being able to immediately provide to the emergency room staff any relevant past information as to prior hospital or outpatient care received at that medical center. To achieve the desired 24-h availability of patients' records, Ayers and associates [3] at Georgetown University School of Medicine adapted their pediatric department's computer-based patient record for use as an emergency room record. Using their experience with self-administered patient histories, Greist and associates [19] at the University of Wisconsin placed a computer interviewing terminal in the emergency room. They reported that about 85 % of the patients entering their emergency room were not urgently ill and could use the terminal for self-administered histories as they had in their office practice.

Although it was evident that the emergency room could benefit from an MIS subsystem, even by the end of the 1980s few hospitals had installed an information system for their emergency room. Some hospital emergency departments participated in community emergency medical systems that directed ambulances to transport emergency patients to the nearest available hospital emergency room. In the 1970s some cities (for example, Philadelphia with 37 emergency rooms scattered throughout the city) used a computer model to assist in the planning of their emergency care system. The model considered the severity rating of the emergency, the time of day, the known patient load and past experience for each emergency room, and the estimated transit time [20]. In 1976 with the increasing use of emergency rooms by patients who did not need immediate care, the De Paul Hospital in Norfolk, Virginia, placed at the entrance to their emergency room a nurse who performed a triage assessment of each patient. Those patients who were not acutely ill were interviewed by a clerk who used a display terminal to enter the patient data for storage on magnetic tape. The data were later batch processed into their MIS mainframe computer and were used to establish a medical record such as for an office patient. The more acute and critically ill patients were admitted and treated immediately, and their medical records were completed later [23]. In 1977 Tri-City Hospital in Oceanside, California, used a portable computer to create and store a patient record on floppy disks for each emergency-room patient. Their database was linked to clinical support knowledge bases for differential diagnosis, poisoning problems, and others [13].

8.2 Current Status and Challenges

8.2.1 Intensive Care Information Systems

In 2015 De Georgia [7] and colleagues at University Hospitals Case Medical Center in Cleveland, Ohio, reviewed the status of information technology in the ICU and identified the areas that remain challenging. Their review of efforts to introduce computers into the ICU focused on work beginning in the mid 1960s [37]. Advances followed in the 1970s and 1980s, with significant improvements in the 1990s as clinical functionality increased and access to the Internet became available. By 2015, several vendors marketed clinical information systems that offered "end-to-end platforms for the ICU," yet serious limitations remained, including "incompatibilities among monitoring equipment, proprietary limitations from industry, and the absence of standard data formatting." They conclude that the integration of large amounts of data, both numeric and waveforms, will require the development of a critical care informatics architecture [7] in order to realize the full benefits that health information technology offers.

8.2.2 Emergency Department Information Systems

In 2011 Handel [21] and associates reviewed the findings of a 2002 consensus conferenc on the use of information technology to improve the quality and safety of emergency room care and presented a research agenda. In 2015 Selck and Decker reported on the adoption of health information technology in hospital emergency departments and its impact, citing findings from the 2007–2010 National Hospital Ambulatory Medical Care Survey conducted by the Centers for Disease Control and Prevention's National Center for Health Statistics [32]. Their analysis showed that the percent of visits seen in an ED with "at least a basic health IT system more than doubled from 25 % in 2007 to 69 % in 2010, and the percent of visits seen in an ED with an advanced system increased tenfold from 3 to 31 %." EDs in urban areas, with high visit volumes, and in teaching hospitals were more likely to have advanced systems. They found that waiting times decreased in EDs with advanced systems, while the number of tests ordered increased, and concluded that advanced health IT systems in the ED may improve efficiency, but were unable to determine whether such systems reduced costs or improved patient outcomes.

8.2.3 Concluding Comments

While the ICU has experienced a proliferation of technological devices in the ICU, the ED is a relatively late adopter of specialized information systems. Each setting faces challenges posted by the need for interoperability among multiple devices within the ICU and across myriad health and community systems for the ED, and integration with their patients' electronic health records.

References

1. Ackmann JJ. A computer system for neurosurgical patient monitoring. Comput Programs Biomed. 1979;10:81–8.
2. Acton JC, Sheppard LC, Kouchoukos NT, Kirklin JW. Automated care systems for critically ill patients following cardiac surgery. In: Kemper K, editor. Computers in cardiology. Long Beach: IEEE Computer Society; 1974. p. 111–5.
3. Ayers WR, Murray DB, Aller JC, Montgomery EE. Mobilizing the emergency room record: a case study in the capture of technology developed elsewhere for use in health care delivery. Comput Biol Med. 1973;3:153–63.
4. Bradshaw KE, Sittig DF, Gardner RM, Pryor TA, Budd M. Computer-based data entry for nurses in the ICU. MD Comput. 1988;6:274–80.
5. Clemmer TP, Gardner RM, Orme Jr J. Computer support in critical care medicine. Proc SCAMC. 1980;3:1557–61.
6. Comerchero H, Thomas G, Shapira G, Greatbatch M, Hoyt JW. A micro-computer based system for the management of the critically ill. Proc SCAMC 1978;634–44.
7. DeGeorgia MA, Kaffashi F, Jacono FJ, Loparo KA. Information technology in critical care: review of monitoring and data acquisition systems for patient care and research. Sci World J. 2015; Article ID 727694. http://dx.doi.org/10.1155/2015/727694.
8. Deller SE, Lewis FJ, Quinn ML. Utilization of a small computer for reat-time continuous patient monitoring. Proc 1971 ACM Annual Conf. 1971;622–39.
9. Dickman ML, Schmidt CD, Gardner RM, Marshall HW, Day WC, Warner HR. On-line computerized spirometry in 738 normal adults. Am Rev Respir Dis. 1969;100:780.
10. Gardner RM. Computerized intensive care monitoring at LDS hospital: progress and development. In: Kemper K, editor. Computers in cardiology. Long Beach: IEEE Computer Society; 1974. p. 97–105.
11. Gardner RM. Computerized management of intensive care patients. MD Comput. 1986;3:36–51.
12. Gardner RM, West BJ, Pryor TA, Larsen KG, Warner HR, Clemmer TP, et al. Computer-based ICU data acquisition as an aid to clinical decision-making. Crit Care Med. 1982;10:823–30.

13. Garrick RM. What's a computer doing in the ER? Am Med News. 1978;21(suppl 9).
14. Geddes LA, Hoff HS, Spencer WA, Vallbona C. Acquisition of physiologic data at the bedside. A progress report. Am J Med Electron. 1961;1:62–9.
15. Gladen HE. ICU Microcomputing on a shoestring: decisions when resources are limited. Proc SCAMC. 1984;238–41.
16. Glaeser DH, Thomas LJ. Computer monitoring in patient care. Annu Rev Biophys Bioeng. 1975;4:449–76.
17. Goldman D, Rodey G. Microcomputer monitor in the neurosurgery ICU. Proc MEDINFO. 1986;459–61.
18. Greenburg AG. Computers in emergency systems, surgery, and intensive care units: an overview. Proc MEDINFO. 1980;26:1184–9.
19. Greist JH, Van Cura LJ, Kneppreth NP. A computer interview for emergency room patients. Comput Biomed Res. 1973;6:257–65.
20. Hamilton WF. Systems analysis in emergency care planning. Med Care. 1974;12:152–62.
21. Handel DA, Wears RL, Nathanson LA, Pines JM. Using information technology to improve the quality and safety of emergency care. Acad Emerg Med. 2011;18:e45–51.
22. Hilberman M, Kamm B, Tarter M, Osborn JJ. An evaluation of computer-based patient monitoring at Pacific Medical Center. Comput Biomed Res. 1975;8:447–60.
23. Hilton DH. Intelligent terminal expedites emergency room patient care. Comput Med. 1976;5:1–2.
24. Lewis FJ, Deller S, Quinn M, Lee B, Will R, Raines J. Continuous patient monitoring with a small digital computer. Comput Biomed Res. 1972;5:411–28.
25. Little AD. Computer-based patient monitoring systems. Washington, DC: National Center for Health Services Research; 1976.
26. Little AD. Evaluation of computer-based patient monitoring systems: final report. Appendix D. A review of the MEDLAB system in the thoracic surgery intensive care unit at the Latter Day Saints hospital. Washington, DC: National Center for Health Services Research; 1973.
27. Martino RL, Kempner KM, McClellan JR, McLees BD. Automation of a medical intensive care environment with a flexible configuration of computer systems. Proc SCAMC. 1980;3:1562–8.
28. Masters TN. Beneficial aspects of computer-controlled blood replacement in cardiac surgical patients. Coll Works Cardiopulm Dis. 1982;23:23.
29. Osborn JJ, Beumont JO, Raison JCA, Abbott RP. Computation for quantitative on-line measurements in an intensive care ward. In: Stacy RW, Waxman BD, editors. Computers in biomedical research. New York: Academic; 1969. p. 207–37.
30. Pollizzi III JA, Stega M, Comerchero H, Milholland AV, Fox F. A structured network for the clinical management of the critically ill. Proc SCAMC. 1980;3:1611–7.
31. Raison JCA, Beaumont JO, Russell JAG, Osborn JJ, Gerbode F. Alarms in an intensive care unit: an interim compromise. Comput Biomed Res. 1968;1:556–64.
32. Selck FW, Decker SL. Health information technology adoption in the emergency department. Health Serv Res. 2015. doi:10.1111/1475-6773.12307 [Epub ahead of print].
33. Shabot MM, Carlton PD, Sadoff S, Nolan-Avila L. Graphical reports and displays for complex ICU data: a new, flexible and configurable method. Comput Methods Programs Biomed. 1986;22:111–6.
34. Sheppard LC, Kirklin JW, Kouchoukos NT. Computer-controlled interventions for the acutely ill patient. In: Stacy RW, Waxman B, editors. Computers in biomedical research. New York: Academic; 1974. p. 135–48.
35. Sheppard LC. The computer in the care of critically ill patients. Proc IEEE. 1979;67:1300–6.
36. Sheppard LC, Kouchoukos NT, Kurtts MA, Kirklin JW. Automated treatment of critically ill patients following operation. Ann Surg. 1968;168:596.
37. Shubin H, Weil MH. Efficient monitoring with a digital computer of cardiovascular function in seriously ill patients. Ann Intern Med. 1966;65:453–60.
38. Sivak ED, Gochberg JS, Fronek R, Scott D. Lessons to be learned from the design, development, and implementation of a computerized patient care management system for the intensive care unit. Proc SCAMC. 1987;614–9.

39. Spencer WA, Vallbona C. A preliminary report on the use of electronic data processing technics in the description and evaluation of disability. Arch Phys Med Rehabil. 1962;43:22–35.
40. Stacy RW. Comprehensive patient monitoring at Cox Heart Institute. Proc San Diego Biomed Symp 1980;48–52.
41. Vallbona C, Geddes LA, Harrison GM, Hoff HE, Spencer WA. Physiological monitor: experience, clinical value and problems. Proceedings of the national telemetering conference, Instrument Society of America; 1965. p. 126–9.
42. Vallbona C. Application of computers for hospital usage. J Chronic Dis. 1966;19:461–72.
43. Warner HR. Computer-based patient monitoring. In: Stacy RW, Waxman BD, editors. Computers in biomedical research. New York: Academic; 1969. p. 239–51.
44. Warner HR, Morgan JD. High-density medical data management by computer. Comput Biomed Res. 1970;3:464–76.
45. Warner HR, Budkin A. A "link trainer" for the coronary care unit. Comput Biomed Res. 1968;2:135–44.
46. Weil MH. Experience with the use of a digital computer for the study and improved management of the critically ill, and especially patients with circulatory shock. Proc on automated data processing in hospitals. Elsinore, Denmark. 1966. p. 276–87.
47. Weil MH, Shubin H, Cady LD. Use of automated techniques in the management of the critically ill. In: Bekey GA, Schwartz MD, editors. Hospital information systems. New York: Marcel Dekker; 1972. p. 333–81.
48. Westenskow DR. Automating patient care with closed-loop control. MD Comput. 1986;3:14–20.
49. Wiener F, Weil MH, Carlson RW. Computer systems for facilitating management of the critically ill. Comput Biol Med. 1982;12:1–15.
50. Yanowitz F, Fozzard HA. A medical information system for the coronary care unit. Arch Intern Med. 1974;134:93–100.

Chapter 9
Information Systems for Clinical Subspecialties

Morris F. Collen and Nancy M. Lorenzi

Abstract Some of the earliest applications of computers in clinical medicine were in the clinical subspecialties, including cardiology, pulmonary, nephrology, gastroenterology, pediatrics, and the surgical sciences. But health professionals found these prototypes difficult to use; data entry devices were awkward and inefficient, and order entry functions were often not integrated. Each information system for a clinical subspecialty (ISCS) evolved differently, with its own specialized functional and technical requirements. In the 1960s mainframe computers were limited in their ability to meet all the processing requirements of all the ICSCs in a large hospital. By the 1970s each ISCS could have its own minicomputer-based system linked directly to the central mainframe. Health care professionals used terminals connected to the central computer to enter orders and to receive test results; the central computer transferred the orders to the appropriate ISCS subsystems and integrated the data coming back from the ISCSs into the patients' records stored in the mainframe computer. In the 1980s local area networks linked multiple lower-cost minicomputers; with distributed minicomputers and interactive visual display terminals, clinicians could begin to benefit from the ISCSs in direct patient care and each ISCS could develop its own system to meet its own requirements. In the 1990s distributed information systems allowed physicians to enter orders and retrieve test results using clinical workstations connected to client-server minicomputers in the local area network that linked the entire hospital, and patient data from all of the distributed ISCS databases were integrated in a computer-based patient record.

Keywords Clinical subspecialties • Direct patient care • Medical subspecialties • Surgical subspecialties • Computer-based patient record • Distributed information systems • Clinical information subsystems

Author was deceased at the time of publication.

M.F. Collen (deceased)

N.M. Lorenzi, Ph.D., M.A., M.S. (✉)
School of Medicine, Department of Biomedical Informatics, School of Nursing,
Vanderbilt University, Medical Center, Nashville, TN, USA
e-mail: nancy.lorenzi@vanderbilt.edu

© Springer-Verlag London 2015   419
M.F. Collen, M.J. Ball (eds.), *The History of Medical Informatics*
in the United States, Health Informatics, DOI 10.1007/978-1-4471-6732-7_9

Lindberg [111] described the evolution of the various information systems for clinical subspecialties (ISCSs) as the response to the need to keep in contact with the evergrowing mass of new medical knowledge. The rapid development of so many medical subspecialties strongly suggested that the growth of significant medical knowledge outpaced the ability of most individuals to master it. Although some of the earliest applications of computers to clinical medicine were in the clinical subspecialties, health professionals found these prototypes difficult to use since their data entry devices were awkward and inefficient, their order entry functions were not integrated, and their computer-based patient records lacked adequate standardization, so their information system did not fulfill the functional and technical requirements.

In 1968 a survey conducted for the National Center for Health Services Research and Development reported that in the United States about half of the 1,200 hospitals with more than 200 beds used computers for some business functions; but only about 15 % of these had some operational clinical subsystem or medical research computing applications [78]. Until the mid-1970s. the majority of hospitals subscribed to out-of-hospital shared computing services. In the mid-1970s, lower-cost, smaller, special-purpose minicomputers were introduced with the capabilities of being located in different clinical departments, all linked to one or more central, large mainframe computers [6]. In the mid-1970s a survey of computer applications in approximately 100 hospitals in the United States reported that only about one-third had clinical laboratory or other patient care applications [172]. In the 1980s the advent of local area networks that linked multiple lower-cost minicomputers permitted distributed information systems to be implemented in hospitals. Although information systems for clinical subspecialties (ISCSs) were some of the earliest and most advanced computer-based information systems in medicine, it was not until the advent of distributed minicomputers equipped with interactive visual-display terminals, that clinicians began to benefit from the ISCSs in direct patient care. Minicomputers allowed each ISCS to develop its own internal information system that best satisfied its own functional requirements.

9.1   Functional and Technical Requirements

Information systems for clinical subspecialties need to satisfy the many similar functional and technical requirements for all clinical information systems, including patient identification, registration and scheduling; and administrative and business functions. However, their clinical applications comprised a more limited domain of medical knowledge and clinical practice that varied with the clinical subspecialty and its specialized diagnostic and treatment procedures. The ISCS's primary objective is to provide the computer processing of information in support of the direct care of patients in that subspecialty. As for any module in a system, the users of an ISCS needed to first define exactly what they wanted the ISCS to do. Since an ISCS usually operated as a referral service within a clinical department located within a larger medical information system (MIS), the functional requirements of the ISCS had to be compatible with those of the MIS and of the clinical department of which it was a part. Thus an ISCS usually has the general functional requirements to: (1) Identify and register the patient, identify the reason for the visit and for any specialized procedure requested. (2) Record the date and time, and the location of every patient care transaction. (3) Collect and store all data collected from the patient and from all procedures performed. (4) Fulfill billing and accounting procedures for all services provided to each patient. (5) Provide capabilities for data linkages to other medical sites for the transfer of patient data [37, 38, 102].

In the 1980s the advent of local area networks that linked multiple lower-cost minicomputers permitted distributed information systems to be implemented in hospitals. Although information systems for clinical subspecialties were some of the earliest and most advanced computer-based information systems in medicine, it was not until the advent of distributed minicomputers equipped with interactive visual display terminals, that clinicians began to benefit from ISCSs in direct patient care. Minicomputers allowed each ISCS to develop its own internal information system that best satisfied its own functional requirements. When lower-cost, smaller, special-purpose minicomputers that could be located in different departments and linked to large mainframe computers were introduced, separate information subsystems were developed for different clinical subspecialties within a hospital that needed to have compatible information systems technology, even though the functional requirements and the information domain were specific for the particular subspecialty, and interoperability of data was essential. Jenkin [92] pointed out that the clinical subspecialty systems, as functional parts of a MIS, do not represent separate information systems as much as they are separate knowledge bases; and the same technical information system can often function in different clinical subspecialties, even though the clinical data collected, the diagnoses made, and the treatments provided could vary.

When linked to, or functioning within a MIS, an ISCS needed to: (1) interface to an order entry (OE) module that communicated all requisitions for procedures that the patient was to receive, provided any special instructions to the patient and to relevant personnel that included the time the procedure was to be done, and noted any restrictions as to the patient's physical activity and food intake prior to the procedure; (2) interface to a results reporting (RR) module and be able to communicate to one or more desired locations the time of completing the procedure, and the results of the procedure including any interpretive comments; (3) be able to transmit the data into a computer-based patient record; (4) support the decision-making processes involved in the patient care; (5) provide reliable and rapid turn-around services for urgent and emergency medical conditions; (6) include specific functional and technical requirements to support any unique procedures that the subsystem provides; (7) and provide the flexibility needed to meet future service requirements, adapt to changes in medical technology and knowledge, and accommodate an increasing volume and variety of procedures.

In the early 1990s distributed information systems allowed physicians to enter orders and retrieve test results using clinical workstations connected to client-server minicomputers in the local area network that linked the entire hospital. Patient data from distributed ISCS databases were integrated in a computer-based patient record. The advent of clinical workstations linked by local area networks to the clinical support services made a computer provider order entry (CPOE) program more acceptable for clinicians to use. Each ISCS had its own specialized functional and technical requirements; each evolved differently.

Requirements for the various clinical subspecialties have some important differences in their functional requirements due to differences in the clinical information processed and the different technical procedures provided to patients. In contrast to the surgery subspecialties, the internal medicine subspecialties perform primarily noninvasive procedures. The medical subspecialties include cardiology, pulmonology, endocrinology, nephrology, neurology, gastroenterology, oncology, rheumatology, physiatry and rehabilitative services, and others. The surgery specialties include head and neck surgery; eye, ear, nose, and throat (EENT) surgery; cardiothoracic surgery; abdominal surgery; orthopedics; proctology; urology; gynecology and obstetrics; and others. Pediatrics provides care to children. General medicine and family practice have the broadest domain of information, whereas urology and EENT have the most limited. Yet all clinical subspecialty systems require a uniform method for patient identification, a common data dictionary, and a communications network to enter patient data from their subspecialty or departmental databases into the central computer-based patient record. All specialty subsystems require the same degree of system reliability as that of the overall MIS; the acute and intensive care services have the highest rate of data processing and transfer, and cannot tolerate any system downtime. All clinical subsystems require the same level of security and confidentiality, except that psychology/psychiatry subsystems require even more severe requirements for security and data confidentiality protection, with the capability to lock out all other health professionals so that access to psychiatric data is permissible only to eligible psychiatrists and psychologists.

From the functional requirements developed for an information system for a clinical subspecialty, the technical design specifications had to be prepared by the system developer or by the vendor. The ISCS had to be designed to: (1) have acceptable computer terminals for entering patient and procedure data, and for reporting the results of the completed procedures; (2) provide appropriate interfaces between specialized instruments, data-acquisition equipment, and the ISCS computer; (3) include computer programs for processing order entry requisitions for services, for providing quality control measures, and for processing and reporting procedure or test results; (4) provide for a ISCS computer database adequate in capacity to store all of the patients' data, and the information associated with and resulting from all procedures; (5) have a computer-stored data dictionary that described all tests and procedures performed, with any special instructions for conducting the procedures, and the normal and alert boundary limits for each procedure; (6) provide communication links to the information systems in affiliated medical offices and hospitals from which the patient came, and also provide links to any needed external databases; (7) provide a reliable computer system with an uninterruptible power supply; (8) have a flexible information system design that could meet changing and expanding requirements for technical and medical innovations; and (9) employ a vocabulary of standard terms to facilitate exchange of information with other information systems.

Since the exchange of clinical data between different databases required the use of standard terms, in 1983 standards for the transmission of clinical data between computers began to be developed [124]. The proposed standards addressed what items of information should be included in defining an observation, what data structure should be employed to record an observation, how individual items should be encoded and formatted, and what transmission media should be supported. Formal attempts to improve the standardization of medical information were carried out by collaborating committees, including the subcommittees on Computerized Systems of the American Standards for Testing Materials (ASTM) that is the oldest of the nonprofit standard setting societies and a standards-producing member of the American National Standards Institute (ANSI) [153].

The ASTM technical subcommittee E31.12 on Medical Informatics considered nomenclatures and medical records [61]. In 1988 ASTM's subcommittee E31.11 on Data Exchange Standards for Clinical Laboratory Results published its specifications E1238 for clinical data interchange, and set standards for the two-way digital transmission of clinical data between different computers for laboratory, office, and hospital systems; so that, as a simple example, all dates would be recorded as an eight-character-string, YYYYMMDD. Thus the date January 12, 1988 would always be transmitted as 19880112.

Health Level Seven (HL7), an organization made up of vendors, hospitals, and consultants was formed in 1987 to develop interface standards for transmitting data between applications that used different computers within hospital information systems [165]. The message content of HL7 was to conform to the International Standards Organization (ISO) standards for the applications level 7 of the Open Systems Interconnection (OSI) model. The HL7 standard used the same message syntax, the same data types, and some of the same segment definitions as ASTM 1238 [123]. The Medical Data Interchange (MEDIX) P1157 committee of the Institute of Electrical and Electronics Engineers (IEEE), formed at the Symposium on Computer Applications in Medical Care (SCAMC) in 1987, was also developing a set of standards, based on the ISO application-level standards, for the transferring of clinical data over large networks from mixed sources, such as from a clinical laboratory and a pharmacy, for both intra- and inter-hospital communications [154]. Every ISCS had to accurately identify each patient; and link or integrate all patient data and reports that were collected on that patient. ISCSs located within a hospital or its associated clinics usually used the same patient identification (ID) number that had been assigned to the patient on the first outpatient visit or admission to the hospital; and that same patient's ID number was recorded for each and all subsequent services received by that patient.

9.2   Internal Medicine

In 1959 the evolution of ISCSs began when Schenthal [158, 159] and Sweeney at Tulane Medical School, used an IBM 650 computer equipped with magnetic tape storage to process medical record data for their internal medicine office patients. They used a mark-sense card reader that sensed marks made with high-carbon content pencils on special formatted cards. The marks were converted into punched holes in standard punch cards. They read these punched cards into the computer, which then processed and stored the data for the clinic's physicians. Internal medicine requires a relatively broad domain of medical knowledge, so internists often limited their practices to the internal medicine subspecialties of cardiology, rheumatology, endocrinology and metabolism, diabetes, pulmonology, nephrology, oncology, geriatrics, and others.

9.2.1   Cardiology

Cardiology information subsystems were developed to support the care of patients with heart disease; provide computer-based patient records; collect data from computer-supported cardiac catheterization procedures; generate diagnostic cardiac stress-test reports; and furnish computer interpretations of electrocardiograms. Starting in the mid-1960s, Warner and associates at the LDS Hospital in Salt Lake City applied their cardiovascular research computer to provide a cardiology information system for patient care. By the mid-1970s their data input programs used for cardiology patients included admission data, a self-administered history, clinical laboratory test-results, blood gas laboratory data, spirometry and pulmonary function data, electrocardiographic data, pharmacy records, and catheterization laboratory data [34]. Their cardiology system functioned as an integral component of their cardiac catheterization unit and of their intensive care unit (ICU), and integrated its patient data into the LDS HIS.

In the late 1960s, Crouse and associates at Stanford University reported the use of their Advanced Computer for Medical Research (ACME) by their Division of Cardiology to analyze online cardiac catheterization data for diagnostic purposes. By 1974 this cardiac catheterization system was reported to have a simplified user interface, flexible data-sampling sequence, immediate display of results of computer analysis for physician review, and hard-copy output of computer measurements [1]. In 1969 the Division of Cardiology at Duke University Medical Center in Durham, North Carolina, began to collect data on patients hospitalized with coronary artery disease. The information collected included each patient's history, physical examination data, and the results of laboratory and diagnostic tests and of cardiac catheterization. Users entered data from cardiac catheterization by using a coding algorithm that displayed a series of questions, and the user entered the responses. A total of ten keystrokes was used to describe the coronary artery anatomy of a patient. The database was used in their clinical practice to provide automated reports of the testing procedures and results, and to provide diagnostic and prognostic profiles of new patients based on their previous experience [145]. These data on cardiac catheterization results and patients' outcomes were aggregated into the Duke Databank for Cardiovascular Disease and used to support clinical research in this field [146].

In 1970 the Cardiovascular Clinic in Oklahoma City initiated an office information system (OIS) for six physicians providing care for about 14,000 cardiology patients. This system included medical records, patient scheduling, and business office functions. On entering the clinic, the patient completed an automated, interactive, branching, self-administered medical history. The physician then completed an encounter form containing physical examination findings, patient's symptoms, medical problems, and diagnoses all focused on the cardiovascular system. Using a video display terminal with keyboard entry, clerks entered the data from the encounter forms into the computer. For follow-up clinic visits, appropriate information was added using additional encounter forms. This OIS was entirely funded by the clinic; the PDP-15 computer and its software were acquired from Meditech [64, 204].

For the care of ambulatory hypertension patients, a Data General Nova computer, with CRT terminals for data input and retrieval, was programmed to provide algorithms to support a non-physician practitioner's clinic at the Naval Regional Medical Center in Oakland, California. It was used to maintain a computer-based patient record for more than 2,000 office patients with hypertension. Patients completed a self-administered questionnaire form at the initial visit. Nurse practitioners and hospital corpsmen completed a physical examination, and recorded the patient's blood pressure and other findings. All the data were entered into the computer, which provided printout reports. Using computer-directed therapy algorithms, the paramedical staff maintained a large hypertensive population with a satisfactory degree of blood pressure control in the majority of patients [80]. Whenever abnormalities were evaluated by the nurse practitioners to be significant, a physician would be called in to see the patient. An evaluation of the first year's experience showed that the operational costs of the computer-supported clinic were 13 % less than those for their general internal medicine clinic, primarily due to a 25 % savings in physicians' time.

Similarly, in the hypertension clinic at the Wayne State University Medical School in Detroit, a nurse practitioner provided full services to patients being treated for hypertension. The nurse used forms to record data for entry by key punch to a time-sharing computer. For follow-up visits, using a CRT display terminal, the nurse could access the computer-stored patient record to enter new data, to retrieve prior data, to query the clinical laboratory file for test results, and to generate flow sheets of blood pressure and clinical laboratory data. In their first 30 months of operation the clinic processed almost 8,000 office visits [104].

9.2.2 Pulmonology

Pulmonary diseases require special pulmonary function studies that are greatly facilitated by computer analysis in a special pulmonary function laboratory that can provide a variety of procedures to quantify patients' breathing deficiencies. In 1964 a group of investigators led by Caceres at the Heart Disease Control Program at the Department of Health, Education, and Welfare developed a method for computer analysis of pulmonary function curves. Using an analog-to-digital converter, they digitized the vital-capacity curves obtained from a spirometer to provide values for 1-, 2-, and 3-s measures of volume and expiratory air-flow rates; and the capacity of the lungs to diffuse oxygen from the pulmonary alveoli into the blood capillaries, and to diffuse carbon dioxide from the blood back into the lungs. Patients with severe pulmonary insufficiency could accumulate an excess of carbon dioxide in their blood, which disturbed their blood acid-base balance and produced respiratory acidosis [164].

In the late 1960s, Osborn's group at the Pacific Medical Center in San Francisco began to develop their pulmonary function monitoring system. In 1974 they reported the use of the data obtained from the pulmonary function tests and the cardiac catheterization procedure done on patients before and after surgery, along with chest x-ray reports and clinical laboratory tests. This helped to determine when patients on automated ventilation following cardiac surgery could be weaned from the respirator and returned to spontaneous breathing [79]. By the mid-1970s Caceres' laboratory was providing a service to other providers. Providers would submit the required data and in return would receive patient's vital capacity and ventilation measurements, plus gas analysis and arterial blood data, before and after exercise. The computer generated a printout that showed the patient's values for ventilation, diffusion and gas exchange, and blood gas measurements; the printout also compared the patient's values to age- and gender-specific normal ranges [152].

Spencer and Vallbona at the Texas Institute for Research and Rehabilitation (TIRR) in Houston provided arterial blood-gas analysis in their respiratory center for patients with respiratory insufficiency. They developed a computer program that assisted the technician in the automatic calculation of blood pH, blood gases, and acid-base balance; and provided the physician with an automatic interpretation of the results as well as with recommendations on the treatment to correct acidosis if present [200]. Menn et al. [128] described the clinical subsystem for the respiratory care unit at the Massachusetts General Hospital (MGH), where the data on the patient's medical status were entered into the computer in a conversational interactive mode. The clinician entered the patient's data by replying to a series of questions with "Y" (yes) or "N" (no), or the numerical value. Additional data were entered concerning arterial blood gases, the patient's state of consciousness, and certain laboratory test values. The computer then printed out a summary of the patient's respiratory data in a tabular form, with an interpretation of the information.

In the 1970s more advanced techniques were available to provide pulmonary function tests, such as were instituted in 1976 at the University of Nebraska Medical Center. That computer-based system, written in FORTRAN and using a PDP 11/03 computer, processed patient data to provide lung volumes, breathing mechanics, diffusing capacity, arterial blood gases, and capillary blood volume [65]. Similarly at the Veterans Administration (VA) Medical Center in Washington, DC, a pulmonary function test was written in the MGH Utility Multi-Programming System (MUMPS) language, and used a PDP 11/34 computer to process pulmonary function and arterial blood-gas data. A printed report with test results and an interpretation of the test data was produced in letter form for transmission to the physician [95]. By the late 1980s spirometry test modules for office information systems (OISs) were available to permit physicians in their offices to conduct pulmonary function tests, to store the data in the patient's OIS record, and to complete the test reports while the patient was still in the office for the immediate consideration of diagnosis and treatment [135].

9.2.3 *Nephrology*

Kidney diseases in patients often require long-term care ending with renal dialysis. Pryor et al. [147] employed the HELP system at the LDS Hospital in Salt Lake City, and reported that its nephrology information system assisted in planning the management of patients with end-stage renal disease. The program gave advice as to the best mode of dialysis (either hemodialysis or peritoneal dialysis), best location (home dialysis versus hospital dialysis), and best treatment (dialysis or kidney transplant).

In 1977 Stead and Hammond [179] began to use an OIS when treating patients with kidney diseases in the nephrology service at the VA Medical Center in Durham. Developed at the Duke renal outpatient clinic in 1977, the system was written in the GEMISCH language and operated on a DEC PDP-11 minicomputer with a display terminal and printer available in the clinic area for interactive data entry and printouts. The system stored in its computer-based records the patient's demographic data, a medical problem list, and a time-oriented summary of subjective and physical data, laboratory and therapeutic data. Data was collected from the physician, nurse, or technician using either computer-generated paper encounter forms, or interacting with a video terminal where the data could be displayed graphically [182]. By 1980 the Stead-Hammond nephrology service was responsible for over 300 active patients. About one-third of these patients required renal dialysis therapy. The initial transfer of legacy medical data from the old paper-based charts to the computer-based records involved the extraction by the physicians of selected information for up to two prior years of care, and averaged 1.5 h per record for about 200 patients. The clinical acceptability of the computerized records was judged to be 93.2 % [62]. In 1981 the computer record was the only record used for a patient's encounter with the nephrology service. The physician could supplement the record with textual notes, either handwritten or entered as text into the computer record. The intensity of data collection on the nephrology service was indicated by the facts that these patients were seen as often as three times a week. The patients had an average of 11 medical problems, at least 18 laboratory tests were performed every 1–4 weeks, and each patient took an average of nine different medicines [180, 183]. It was from Stead's and Hammond's experiences with this subsystem that they went on to develop their TMR system.

Pollak and associates [142] at the University of Cincinnati Medical Center reported a nephrology system for inpatients with acute and chronic renal diseases; their patient care included renal transplants, renal dialysis, and outpatient follow-up. They developed a time-oriented record similar to that used by Fries for his rheumatology clinic. They used a program written in BASIC+, for a PDP 11/70 computer. Visual display terminals were located in the clinic for ambulatory patients and in the hospital for the care of renal patients admitted for kidney transplants or other reasons. Data were entered using the display terminal keyboard. Visual display terminals permitted access to the system over telephone lines protected with password security. Data were entered in a conversational mode, and the computer prompted the user for items to be entered. Each data item was coded in their data dictionary. A single patient's daily, time-oriented, data could be entered in 2–4 min, depending on the number of items; up to 11 different visits, usually the most recent, could be displayed simultaneously. Computer printouts supplemented the paper-based patient record. The first page of their computer-based record system contained a problem list that displayed a continuous summary of major clinical events and problems. Flow sheets displayed time-oriented data, and the progress notes recorded the serial interpretations of the data.

In 1983 Levy and Say [109] at the Henry Ford Hospital in Detroit, described their large nephrology information system for five clinics that provided 10,200 patient visits per year. These clinics used a central IBM time-sharing computer system with telecommunications that supported, in the clinics, light-pen visual display terminals and printers for data entry and information retrieval. Although this was primarily a batch-processing operation, online data entry and retrieval of reports were obtainable. A single patient's daily, time-oriented data could be entered in 2–4 min, depending on the number of items; up to 11 different visits, usually the most recent, could be displayed simultaneously. Levy and Say chronicled their 8-year experience and described the many lessons learned in implementing their vendor-provided system. The first vendor went bankrupt after completing only 30 % of the system; and the authors concluded from their experience that implementing a nephrology dialysis subsystem could be almost as difficult as installing a medical information system.

9.2.4 Metabolic

Metabolic disorders occur in patients with a variety of diseases; they appear as disorders of body fluids electrolytes and acid-base balance, and as abnormalities of nutrition. The assessment of metabolic disorders required a complicated set of calculations. In 1968 Vallbona et al. [199] at TIRR first reported using their computer to support calculations of doses of medications, and of fluid and electrolyte requirements of such patients. The tabular printout of the fluid-balance report provided calculations of water, glucose, sodium, and potassium requirements; and recommended parenteral fluid therapy for a 24-h period to meet the calculated requirements. The computer process took into account the data obtained on the patient including specific gravity, blood urea nitrogen, and an estimate of the patient's dehydration by the physician.

Bleich [16] at the Beth Israel Hospital in Boston wrote a program in the MUMPS language that asked the physician to enter the values obtained for the patient of the serum electrolytes, carbon-dioxide tension, and hydrogen-ion activity. The computer then evaluated the patient's acid-base balance, recommended appropriate therapy, and cited relevant references. Bleich [17] soon reported that the program had been used about 1,500 times. With the later implementation of the Beth Israel hospital information system (HIS), the electrolyte and acid-base program automatically obtained clinical laboratory data from the HIS; it then directed a dialogue in which the physician supplied clinical information; upon completion of the interchange, the program produced an evaluation note that resembled a consultant's discussion of the problem [156]. Kassirer and associates [97] at Tufts University School of Medicine in Boston described an integrated information system that was programmed for reading and punching into cards the data from an automated chemical analyzer and from other laboratory equipment; using these data supplemented by the patient's weight and urine volumes, the program completed the required calculations and printed out the final and full fluid balance study. Thompson [192] wrote a program in the BASIC language using a Radio Shack TRS handheld, pocket computer designed for nurses to monitor total parenteral nutrition. A series of displays directed the nurse to enter the quantities of urine output, and of the fluids and nutrients that the patient had received during the 24-h period. The program then calculated the patient's fluid balance, caloric intake, percentage of calories provided by each energy source, nitrogen balance, calorie ratio, and catabolic index.

9.2.5 Endocrine

Endocrine disorders are common and include diabetes mellitus, obesity, and thyroid disorders. In 1964 a diabetes clinic was developed at the University Hospitals of Cleveland, Ohio, by Levy and associates. They used encounter forms for recording patients' data. The data were then keypunched into cards, which periodically were read into the computer and stored on magnetic tape. Printed reports of the patient records were available prior to a follow-up visit. In 1964, 209 patients had their records in the system. In 1973 McDonald's Regenstrief Medical Record (RMR) system initiated its diabetes clinic, which evolved to provide a comprehensive ambulatory care system that served as one of the model office information systems (OISs) in the United States [125]. In the mid-1970s, an OIS for patients with diabetes mellitus became operational and was reported by Thomas and Moore [191] in the diabetes clinic at the University of Texas Medical School in Houston. Using paper encounter forms and keypunched cards for data entry, they provided services to 500 patients who received continuing care that resulted in voluminous medical records. After 4 years of experience with 6,000 patient visits, the contents of the records had evolved to entering only the significant data necessary for each physician to make medical decisions in this clinic; and they had developed algorithms that selected, for their routine office practice, about 20 % of the data specific to diabetes and its complications.

By the early 1980s, OISs in diabetes clinics were using display terminals with keyboard entry of data to microcomputers [63, 195]. Lomatch and associates [112] at the University of Michigan, used a relational database system to collect information on 1,200 patients with diabetes to monitor their care and to support clinical research in diabetes. By the end of the 1980s a fully interactive diabetes management system on a personal computer was reported by Zviran and Blow [212] at the Naval Postgraduate School in Monterey, California. It provided a computer-based patient record, a log display of trends of the patient's blood glucose levels, decision support reminders as to diet and exercise, and instructions with a dictionary of common terms for patient education.

9.2.6 Rheumatology

Rheumatology and immunology services were initiated in the late 1960s by Fries at Stanford University Medical Center using their Time Oriented Database (TOD) System to collect data over long-time periods on their patients who had chronic arthritis. The objectives of their OIS were to support both patient care and clinical research and to provide a research database. In the 1970s the Stanford group joined with other rheumatology centers in the United States and Canada to form the American Rheumatism Association Medical Information System (ARAMIS), which became a model for national chronic disease research databases [59, 60]. By 1974 this clinic served 900 patients with 4,000 visits per year; most of the patient data were stored in the immunology and rheumatology OIS [77]. At this time in its development, computer time-sharing services were obtained from the Stanford University Center for Information Processing, which maintained the software for TOD, which was also used by other Stanford medical services. Patient data were collected by physicians, clerks, and technicians on formatted pages and on flow sheets with tabulated data. Then the data were entered into the computer by using modems and telephone lines. The paper-based patient record remained the primary medical record; the computer-based patient record provided backup and was also the research database. The medical record contained patient identification, medical history, a problem list, treatments specific to rheumatology and immunology, and selected follow-up data. The system permitted retrieval of the complete computer-stored patient record, or an abstract of the last visit. Statistical analysis of the data with scatter plots and bar graphs were available. Computer-generated prognostic summaries of patients' records could be obtained that selected a population comparable to the patient, and displayed the group experience as to morbidity and mortality. A password system controlled user access to the system. Administrative and business functions for the clinic were provided by other Stanford systems. According to [77], the development of this OIS involved about eight person-years of effort at an estimated cost of $100,000. Fries' system was so successful that it became the basis for *ARAMIS*, a national database for rheumatoid diseases.

9.2.7 Neuromuscular

Neuromuscular and locomotor disabilities in patients were often treated in specialized rehabilitation services. Spencer and Vallbona [171, 173] at the Texas Institute for Research and Rehabilitation developed a HIS for a specialized hospital that provided rehabilitation services. As early as 1960, they reported the use of electronic data processing techniques in the description and evaluation of disabilities in their patients. They placed data pertaining to the patient's physical activities and functional limitations on a punch card. Records of treatments and exercises, and other routine HIS data, were also added. By 1969 they had computer programs that could suggest plans of care and specific treatments for disabled patients, and a computer model for the prediction of recovery of muscle strength in patients with paralytic disease [196]. By the early 1970s, they used a set of programs in which therapists evaluated and graded 94 muscle groups of the patient. A computer algorithm then computed the total score for different body parts as well as for the whole patient. The system generated a report that represented the patient's ability to perform the basic tasks related to normal living. It also provided a profile of the disability for each patient that described the primary pathology with its related impairments and complications, and any operative procedures performed [198].

In the early 1980s, bioengineers began to interface microprocessors with electro-mechanical devices to aid severely physically handicapped people. Sanders and associates [157] at the Georgia Institute of Technology devised a system using a personal computer (PC) interfaced with a robot arm. Commands could be entered by (1) touch selection with a finger, or with an instrument held in the mouth, from a display of numbers; or (2) words spoken to a speech-recognition unit with a 200-word vocabulary. The robot arm could turn pages, pick up a cup, dispense medications, operate an electric bed, and turn on a radio or television. By the end of the 1980s computers were providing increasing independence to physically handicapped persons. Quadriplegics could operate wheelchairs controlled by microprocessors. The hearing impaired could use a computer-based, electromechanically powered, aluminum hand that could engage in sign language and finger spelling, and provide their interpretations [66].

9.2.8 Oncology

Oncology information systems for patients with cancer required a wide variety of hospital medical, surgical, chemotherapy, and radiation services. One of the earliest, large, oncology information systems was developed at Johns Hopkins Hospital (JHH) that provided comprehensive care to adult cancer patients in a 56-bed oncology center that also served 500 outpatients per week [20]. In 1970 at the Johns Hopkins Hospital (JHH), a prototype information system was initiated to process physicians' written orders, produce work lists for ward nurses, and generate daily computer-printed, patient drug profiles for the patients' records. In 1975 a Minirecord (minimal essential record) system was initiated in the JHH Medical Clinic that used encounter forms that were filled out at each patient visit; and they contained an area for medications and procedures [119]. Work also was begun on a prototype Clinical Oncology Information System (OCIS). The OCIS contained patient care data for both hospital and clinic services, and also captured clinical laboratory test results and pharmacy data [19, 20, 22].

In 1976 a radiology reporting system was implemented at JHH using a terminal that permitted the radiologist to select phrases with which to compose descriptions and interpretations of x-ray studies. Its output was a computer-printed report which became available as soon as the radiologist completed his interpretation [202]. In 1978 a clinical laboratory information system was operational; it provided the internal working documents for the laboratories, and produced the patient's cumulative laboratory report [94]. During the early 1980s, a network gradually evolved in the JHH information system. By 1986 the JHH system included IBM 3081 and 3083 computers that supported an inpatient pharmacy system with a unit dose medication distribution system, a clinical laboratory system which ran on three PDP 11/70 computers, and a radiology system [194]. At any one time, 2,000 patients were being treated with one or more of several hundred established treatment plans called oncology protocols. Their prototype Oncology Clinical Information System (OCIS) used a remote computer located at the Johns Hopkins Applied Physics Laboratory. It also operated a tumor registry that ran in batch mode and was used for searches, tumor reports, abstract preparation, and quality assurance.

In 1976 JHH purchased a PDP-11 computer with a MUMPS operating system [20] to support the development of a larger system for their Oncology Center. By 1979 their enhanced OCIS organized the clinical data to produce plots and tabulations that assisted in decision making. Since they often collected as many as 100 different clinical and laboratory values for a single patient each day, it was useful for the data to be organized in the form of plots and flow sheets (time-sequenced tabulation of data) to assist physicians in handling large amounts of data [25]. In addition daily care plans were implemented, with protocols (treatment sequences) processed by their OCIS that provided printed plans for ordering tests and procedures, with warnings and reminders of potential adverse clinical events.

Because of the complexity of the treatment plans for many cancer patients, much of the therapy followed predefined protocols that often involved the use of antitumor drugs in multi-drug combinations and administered using complex time-sequenced relationships; and therapy that could extend for months or years [24]. A daily care plan generally contained patient status data, summary of therapy protocols, treatment sequence-generated comments, tumor measurements, clinical findings, chemotherapy orders, history of chemotherapy administered, and tests and procedures [121]. In 1979 JHH acquired a second computer and a new programming tool, TEDIUM, was used to provide database management system functions, and the old MUMPS-based system was retired in 1982 [108]. The two computers were linked with distributed database software, and a direct link was made to the computer system in the department of laboratory medicine so that all test results were transferred automatically to the OCIS.

The computer also supported an oncology center pharmacy with a common database. Blum [23] reported on the data model, which described their database at that time, as containing patient identification data, patient clinical data, patient protocol assignments, patient standing orders, patient recommended orders, treatment sequence, clinical actions (such as tests and procedures), and protocol-descriptive text and flowchart schema that defined the protocols. Since the system now managed a large and comprehensive database, they implemented an enhanced system that provided the tools to manipulate the database for retrospective analysis. Online access was provided to the data required by the health care team by means of a summary abstract that contained identification and administrative data; and for each primary tumor site, the diagnosis, a summary of treatment, and a summary of the pathology report. Clinical data were displayed as a chronological tabulation for a specifically defined time period.

These flow sheets presented the desired data in columnar format, according to the date the data were collected. In addition, graphic plots were provided when a display was desired of changes in data through time. Daily care plans were designed to assist the physician who treated many patients over long periods of time using complex treatment modalities in both an inpatient and an ambulatory setting. Patients treated for their cancer, as well as for other disease or therapy related medical complications, often followed one or more predefined protocols that detailed treatment sequences. A daily care plan provided printouts for each patient every day, with changes resulting from the entry of new orders [23]. The cumulative OCIS database permitted increasingly useful analyses to aid physicians in making clinical decisions and to evaluate the clinical management of cancer patients [106, 107]. In 1986 they reported the active use of 125 formal cancer therapy protocols [22]. Blum [21] published a historical review of the development of the OCIS at Hopkins; and Enterline and associates [52] reviewed its clinical applications. McColligan [118] reported that the Hopkins OCIS had also been implemented in 1989 at Ohio State University's Cancer Hospital. Friedman [58] and Horwitz [83] and associates at the Boston University Medical Center described Cancer Data Management System (CDMS), which operated on a PDP-11 computer with a MUMPS operating system. Their CDMS provided the functions generally necessary for the care of cancer patients, including computer-generated medical records, and supported their oncology research. Serber and associates [162] at the Memorial Sloan-Kettering Cancer

Center, New York, also implemented an information system for clinical oncology using a Data General Eclipse C330 computer and MUMPS programming, designed largely to support research. Marciniak and associates [116] at the National Cancer Institute in Bethesda and the VA Medical Center in Washington, DC, reported on the activities of VA hospitals tumor registry using their HIS; they cited the use of the VA File Manager program by the MD Anderson Hospital in Houston for their protocol data management system. In the mid-1980s, the National Cancer Institute made Physician Data Query (PDQ) available, a cancer information database of active oncology protocols, accessible to hospital cancer units through the NLM's MEDLINE [84].

9.2.9   Gastroenterology

Gastroenterology patients were treated by Kahane and associates [96] at JHH who employed a clinical workstation that permitted them to use a variety of data input methods, including voice-recognition technology, to record observations made of the inner surface of the gastrointestinal tract during endoscopy.

9.2.10   Geriatrics

Elderly patients received care in an ambulatory clinic with an OIS specially designed in 1988 for their care in the VA Medical Center in Tacoma, Washington, and appropriately called GRAMPS (Geriatric Record and Multidisciplinary Planning System). This interactive MUMPS-based application operated off of the VA's File Manager-based record system. It allowed physicians to document patient care in a problem-oriented format with structured narrative and free text, eliminating handwritten input [73]. Sets of data were developed for 38 geriatric syndromes that could be displayed as menus for data selection to facilitate data entry.

9.3   Surgery, Obstetrics, and Gynecology

Surgery specialties have administrative and business requirements for their patients similar to those for the medical specialties. However, the clinical data collected by neurosurgeons, head and neck surgeons, chest surgeons, abdominal surgeons, obstetricians, gynecologists, and urologists are more limited to office surgery procedures and to pre- and postoperative follow-up care of patients whose surgical procedures had been performed in the hospital or specialty surgery clinics. Surgery specialties in a hospital are characterized by their application of invasive procedures, which usually require specialized technology. In addition to the general information processing requirements similar to those for any HIS department, surgery services require records of anesthetics given and detailed reports that document the operative procedures. The operating room is the basic workshop for the surgeon, and each surgery specialty requires some equipment in the operating room tailored to its needs.

9.3.1   Operating Rooms and Surgicenters

The operating room is an expensive resource in the hospital [13], so the operating room supervisor is continually challenged to improve its efficiency. Most operating rooms are busiest in the morning; some rooms are often idle in the afternoon, so optimal scheduling of operating room staff can significantly affect hospital costs. As early as 1968, Barnoon and Wolfe [10] developed a computer simulation model to test the effectiveness of various configurations of schedules by analyzing the use of its facilities and manpower. Ausman and associates at Roswell Park Memorial Institute began to use precoded operative record and report forms on which the surgeons noted the appropriate information after completing an operation [3, 4]. Clerks transferred the codes to punch cards; these were read into an IBM 1401 computer that stored the data on magnetic tape that generated printouts for insertion in the patients' charts. Michas and associates [130] at the University of California in Davis reported that their surgery services were using a special form to record patient's diagnoses, operative procedures, and other relevant data, which were then typed onto magnetic cards using the IBM Magnetic Card/Selectric Typewriter (MC/ST). The data on the cards were then transmitted to a time-sharing mainframe computer that stored the data, and provided printout reports for the patients' charts. Brown [27], at the University of Michigan in Ann Arbor, wrote that since 1976, for each patient undergoing a surgical operation, clinical data had been collected, punched into cards, and computer processed. Yearly data were abstracted from the surgery database, analyzed, and compared to the prior year's data to improve operating room scheduling and utilization.

In the 1970s the appearance of free standing surgical centers for ambulatory patients generated a need for their information systems to provide hospital-type patients' records, including any laboratory, x-ray, and pathology data as well as to maintain extensive records of the surgeons, of the anesthesiologists, and of the insurance carriers. As an example, the Salt Lake Surgical Center reported providing services to 500 patients per month using four operating rooms; and maintained a computer-based patient record on a Texas Instruments minicomputer that was accessed by eight visual display terminals. Their computing applications included interactive preoperative scheduling of surgical procedures, and storing the scheduled procedure codes. Also included were patients' preoperative diagnoses, identification of the surgeons and referring physicians, and the type of anesthesia to be given. Data stored on postoperative patients included the code number of the actual procedure performed, length of time of the procedure, the anesthesia given, and any postoperative complications. Pre- and postoperative instructions for each patient were personalized and were printed out by the computer [99].

Computerized Operating Room Management System (CORMIS) was developed by Nault and associates [137] to assist surgery personnel in scheduling and staffing, as well as in using operating room facilities. Data were collected on forms and key-punched into cards for time in and out, by procedure, for surgeons, anesthetists, and surgical nurses. Any causes for delay also were noted. A time-sharing computer service then prepared summary reports for scheduling and staffing requirements. Schmidt and associates [160] at the University of Michigan Hospitals in Ann Arbor described a computer model for predicting a surgeon's operating room time for a specific scheduled procedure based on 5 years of experiential data stored in their hospital's mainframe computer database. Other investigators developed computer programs for operating room scheduling. Hancock and associates [74] at the University of Michigan divided their experiential database into many subsets to improve the reliability of predicting the operating room time to be scheduled for a specific surgeon for a specific procedure.

By the early 1980s many hospitals had operating room management information systems. Some of these used minicomputers, such as at Johns Hopkins Hospital [120, 122]; but most used microcomputers, as reported by the University of California in San Diego [86] and the Thomas Jefferson University Hospital [209]. By the end of the 1980s, microcomputer-based surgical suite management systems were available that provided case scheduling, the surgeons' preference lists of instrument and supply needs with automatic inventory control, and a posting and log program to monitor surgeon and staff activities and performance [5]. More advanced minicomputer-based operating room information systems were beginning to offer real time clinical patient record data acquisition and retrieval from terminals located in each operating room, in addition to anesthesia and recovery room infor-mation, infection control, and incident reporting [105]. Building on the industrial experience with computer-aided systems design, software was being developed that would assemble two-dimensional x-ray scans into three-dimensional x-ray images for computer-aided surgery performed in complex orthopedic and neurosurgical procedures [155]. The monitoring of patients who were critically ill was usually done in an intensive care unit.

9.3.2 Anesthesiology

Anesthesiology became a prime target for patient safety concerns by the second half of the 1980s. The Joint Commission for Associated Hospital Organizations (JCAHO) chose anesthesiology as one of the first areas in which to incorporate outcome indicators into its hospital accreditation standards. Some states began to require that, when general anesthesia was used, there must be continuous monitor-ing of the patient's blood oxygen content and of changes in exhaled carbon dioxide [49]. Monitoring anesthesia administration to surgical patients required as great a variety of technology as any other medical specialty. It had many of the same requirements as monitoring patients in intensive care units (ICUs). A surgery anesthesia monitoring system developed by Michenfelder and associates [131] at the Mayo Clinic with IBM monitored and stored the vital physiological variables for an anesthetized patient. These data included measurements of arterial and venous blood pressures, heart rate and electrocardiogram, respiratory rate, airway pressure, and body temperature. The digitized data were stored on magnetic tape; displays of the data appeared on television-type monitors.

Through the years the anesthetist became somewhat comparable to the airplane pilot in the cockpit surrounded by myriad instrument and computer displays. The surgery and the anesthetic affected many organ systems, so the anesthetist had to continually monitor the anesthetic and oxygen-gas intake and their blood concentrations, the depth of anesthesia and the brain function, the cardiac and pulmonary functions, intravenous fluid intake, body temperature, and degree of muscle relaxation. The anesthetist usually determined a patient's blood-gas levels during surgery by periodically testing blood samples for dissolved oxygen, carbon dioxide, and pH value. In 1968 Warner [201] and associates at the LDS Hospital inserted into the patient, prior to surgery, a central aortic-pressure catheter that was connected to a pressure transducer. The anesthetist obtained measurements of arterial pressure, stroke volume, heart rate, and cardiac output by pressing buttons on the console; and the results were displayed on the oscilloscope of the console. Other pertinent data, such as drugs administered and comments about the status of the patient, were entered in the computer-based record and printed out at the end of the operation in the form of an integrated anesthesiology record.

Crouse and Wiederhold [44] reported the use of their ACME system for monitoring patients under anesthesia by recording measured concentrations of carbon dioxide during respiration, and continuously analyzing data obtained from their electrocardiogram and carotid pulse monitors. Chodoff and Gianaris [32] at Johns Hopkins University School of Medicine and Gianaris at Northwestern University Medical Center reported using a preoperative anesthesia *management system* in which a nurse anesthetist interviewed the patient scheduled for surgery, and recorded on mark-sense forms the patient's history and physical examination findings. The data were then read into the computer and were subjected to a clinical decision support system (CDSS) developed by IBM, which suggested significant anesthetical abnormalities and their possible causes, orders for further study, and anesthesia recommendations. However, when the researchers compared data from the system to data recorded from the physicians, they found little agreement between the computer and the physicians.

Shaffer and associates [163] at the George Washington University Medical Center used handwritten forms to record the anesthesiologist's preoperative summary of the patient's condition and of the postoperative course; the nurse's notes on the operative course; and the recovery-room course. From these forms, data items were coded and keypunched into cards for batch processing by an IBM 370 computer. Monthly statistics were provided of operating room utilization. By the end of the 1970s, system developers began to use microcomputers for surgery information systems. Cozen [43] at the California Hospital Medical Center in Los Angeles, used a microcomputer connected to a monitor to measure and display the patient's blood pressure and pulse rate; the data were then transmitted to a minicomputer database.

At the University of California in San Francisco, Young [209] used a DEC minicomputer-controlled mass spectrometer to analyze samples of both inspired gases and expired air, and thus eliminated the need for drawing blood samples. Similarly, Harbort and associates [75] at Emory University used a Hewlett Packard minicomputer for the management and display of data from a Perkin-Elmer microcomputer-controlled mass spectrometer used to monitor and plot, every 5 min, the flow of anesthetic gases administered and the levels of oxygen, carbon dioxide, nitrogen, and argon in the patient's respired air.

At Yale University School of Medicine, Miller [132] developed a program called ATTENDING that received a list of the patient's problems, a planned surgical procedure, and a proposed anesthetic plan. The system critiqued this plan from the standpoint of the patient's underlying problems and their inherent risks, suggested alternative approaches, and discussed the risks and benefits of different approaches for the patient's problems.

In the 1980s integrated technologies began to be developed for noninvasive monitoring of both the gas anesthetics and a patient's physiologic measurements. Lewis and associates [110] at the Eastern Virginia Medical School reported the use of a desktop-sized Hewlett Packard microcomputer to store the data entered by clerks in a coded format from the operative records of patients who had undergone vascular surgery. As the preoperative evaluation of a patient is an important procedure, Keating and associates [98] at Jefferson Medical College developed a Computer-Assisted Preoperative Evaluation (CAPE) system to help identify risks associated with the patient's diagnosis and with the planned surgical procedure. The system also provided estimates of mortality, and specific recommendations for decreasing risks for the patient. In the 1980s operating room information systems were reported by Ball et al. [7] to be available in 18 software packages, each of which provided some of the 21 important functions, including operating room scheduling, anesthesia and surgery logs, equipment control, medical records, staff records, inventory control, resource use, infection control, and patient care plans. Of the 18 vendors, only two software packages offered all 21 of these functions. Berg [13] estimated that only 10 % of U.S. hospitals used some type of computer support in their operating rooms.

9.3.3 Oral Surgery and Dentistry

Oral surgeons and dentists began to explore the use of computers in their offices in the late 1960s. According to Tira et al. [193], in the 1970s an increasing number of journal articles began to appear describing computer applications in clinical dentistry, and dentists began to employ computer batch-processing using time-sharing service bureaus for office administrative and business applications. Diehl [47, 48], at the Naval Dental Research Institute in Great Lakes, Illinois, noted that in the 1970s microcomputers and floppy discs brought computer capabilities to dentist's office staff. Some computer-based simulation models were developed to assist dentists in planning and operating their offices by studying their practice mix for tooth fillings, crowns, extractions, and other procedures; by evaluating the effects of adding auxiliary personnel or altering office configuration [100]; and by planning a new dental practice [148]. In the 1980s there were available several hundred dental office software packages, many had been custom written by dentists. By the end of the 1980s, computer-assisted imaging systems were available to make dental prostheses such as crowns; so rather than making a physical model or a die of the tooth to be replaced, an electro-optical scanning method obtained the necessary three-dimensional information, which was digitized by camera and entered into the computer [14].

In the second half of the 1980s, Zimmerman [211] at the University of Maryland at Baltimore that a survey of 628 dentists showed about one-fourth had some type of computer system in their offices. Two-thirds of these were microcomputers or minicomputer inhouse systems used mostly for billing and accounting applications; only about one-third had some patient record-keeping applications. In 1986 Southard and Rails at the Naval Dental Research Institute in Great Lakes, Illinois, described a computer-based dental record system that collected, stored, and displayed in a standard clinical format, the information generated during a comprehensive general dental examination. They used a microcomputer with a keyboard, visual display, and a dot matrix printer with high-resolution graphics capabilities for printing symbols, markings, and text, to print a copy of the computer-stored examination record in the same textual and graphic format as standard, manually recorded dental charts [170]. Using preprinted examination charts showing all 32 teeth, their computer program overprinted on each of the teeth appropriate marks and symbols for missing teeth, existing restorations, root-canal treatments, partial dentures, and caries; it also gave recommendations for extracting any teeth. In 1986 Rails and associates also developed a computer-assisted dental diagnosis program to operate on a microcomputer; it was written in the BASIC language. After taking a dental history and completing an examination of the teeth, the user would answer a series of computer-displayed questions. Using algorithms and rules such as, if this … then do this …, if the answers representing the dental findings fit a diagnostic pattern, the computer classified the patient's dental abnormality and recommended treatment if requested [170].

In the 1970s some computer-based simulation models were developed to assist dentists in planning and operating their offices by studying their practice mix for tooth fillings, crowns, extractions, and other procedures; by evaluating the effects of adding auxiliary personnel or altering office configuration [100]; and by planning a new dental practice [148]. By the end of the 1980s, computer-assisted imaging systems were available to make dental prostheses such as crowns; rather than making a physical model or a die of the tooth to be replaced, an electro-optical scanning method obtained the necessary three-dimensional information, which was digitized by camera and entered into the computer [14]. Simulated surgery on three-dimensional models became available in the 1980s when interactive computer graphics introduced the capabilities of preoperative planning for difficult operations. Using x-ray scans that focused on the abnormality, the surgeon could simulate operating on an abnormality, and refine and repeat the process until the appropriate surgery was planned properly [45].

9.3.4   Obstetrics and Gynecology

Obstetricians use the general surgery suite for surgical procedures such as Cesarean sections; otherwise, obstetrical deliveries were completed in separate delivery rooms to minimize the risk of contamination. Since most pregnancies resulted in the collection of similar patient data for around 9 months, in the 1970s the American College of Obstetricians and Gynecologists (ACOG) and the American Academy of Pediatrics (AAP) developed standard data collection obstetrics data forms for the prenatal visits, for the delivery and hospital course of the infant, and for the first post-partum visit of the mother [88].

Obstetricians have the special requirement of maintaining a continuing record of the prenatal care of a pregnant woman, and having this record available at the time of delivery. In 1971 Jelovsek and associates [91] at the Duke University Medical Center initiated an OIS with a computer-based patient record using the Duke GEMISCH database management system, the precursor to Duke's TMR system. Stead et al. [178] reported that the patient's record for an entire pregnancy was gathered on 50 pages of check sheets, resulting in a printout that averaged 10 pages. A set of paper forms was used to collect a self-administered patient history, a physician's physical examination, and clinical laboratory test results. These forms were then entered into the database using an optical scanner and an interactive video display. A complete printout of this data was then placed on the patient's paper chart within 48–72 h [26]. An updated printout was always available from a Teletype printer located in the delivery suite. After several revisions of the data collection forms and printout reports, in 1974 the computer-based obstetrics record was implemented using a separate PDP 11/40 computer and two visual display terminals, and programmed as an application of the GEMISCH system. The records of approximately 10,000 pregnant women had been processed by the system by the end of 1975 [178].

In 1980 their Women's Clinic began to use the Duke TMR system. Physicians still recorded patient data and orders on encounter forms that were given to a clerk to enter into the computer using visual display terminals with keyboards while the patient was still present. The computer printed out laboratory requisitions and billings that were then given to the patient. They concluded that their information system in which data transactions were captured in realtime in the presence of the patient, had a significant effect on office personnel and patient flow. Jelovsek [91] reported its advantages included improved data quality, control, and timely availability; its disadvantages included increased hardware requirements, major retraining of personnel, and more rigid adherence to organizational policy.

In the late 1970s, Wirtschafter and associates [205] in Birmingham, Alabama, initiated the development of a computer-based medical record system serving the obstetrics services of two hospitals and several clinics located in the county. In 1982 they provided care to more than 4,000 pregnant women per year, and generated more than 40,000 encounter forms. In 1977 they acquired an IBM 370/158 computer and used the Time Oriented Database (TOD) system, developed at Stanford University; the system was operational in all clinics by the end of 1979. Data input paper forms from the various prenatal clinics were transmitted to their computer center where a prenatal summary report was generated and made available online at the two hospitals for the patient's delivery. Labor and delivery data were handled similarly from physicians' recorded data on forms, and a perinatal discharge summary was prepared at the time of the patient's discharge.

In 1986 Gonzalez and Fox [67] at the Columbia University College of Physicians and Surgeons implemented a complete computer-based obstetrics record. All patient encounters were recorded directly into the system by the health care providers; all of the information was stored in the computer and was available in real time. Personal computers acting as terminals were placed in all examination rooms, consultation rooms, physicians' offices, and in the labor and delivery rooms; and all were connected to a central microcomputer. Even into the late 1980s, most obstetricians still used paper forms to record their patient data, which clerks then entered into the computer-stored medical record. Since the time of delivery was usually unpredictable and often occurred at night when there was not easy access to paper-based records, the main advantage of a computer-based obstetric record was that of assured availability of prenatal patient data at the time of delivery, night or day.

Listening to the fetal heart during a delivery by placing a stethoscope on the mother's abdomen is a routine procedure for obstetricians to monitor the fetal heart rate for evidence of fetal distress. Electronic fetal monitoring by recording the fetal electrocardiogram was introduced in the 1960s [103] for the purpose of detecting fetal distress. Hon [81] at the Loma Linda School of Medicine in Los Angeles, used electrodes placed in the mother's vagina to pick up the fetal signals and to record them on magnetic tape. These analog signals were then digitized and analyzed by an IBM 7094 computer, which permitted monitoring of the fetal electrocardiogram and the fetal heart rate. In the 1970s continuous electronic monitoring of the fetal heart rate became increasingly common in the United States; and computers began to be used to apply techniques developed for automated monitoring of the electrocardiogram in ICUs, with alarms that sounded when preset normal values were exceeded [151]. However, an evaluation by Banta and associates [8, 9] at the National Center for Health Services Research reported that monitoring of the fetal electrocardiogram was no better than auscultation by the stethoscope; this report somewhat dampened for a time the diffusion of electronic fetal monitoring in the United States.

9.4 Pediatrics

Pediatricians provide care to children from birth through teenage years. The data processing requirements vary considerably for newborns, preschool and school-aged children. Important medical procedures include immunizations and body measurements for identifying growth and developmental problems. In contrast to the data collection process in adult patients, pediatricians in most cases acquire the medical histories from parents. The hospital information system functional requirements for children in the hospital pediatric services are generally similar to those for adults in the medical and surgical services. However, newborns require very different specialized care. The first data relevant to a pediatric patient are those recorded for the yet unborn baby in the mother's obstetrics prenatal record. At birth, the newborn is transferred to the nursery service and assigned an identification code; and the baby's pediatric record is initiated. Monitoring the growth and development of infants and children is important since these variables were closely related to children's health; and these data required comparisons to standard charts.

In 1969 a pediatric information system was initiated by Lyman and Tick for the pediatrics department of Bellevue Hospital in New York Medical Center that supported 30,000 patients with 70,000 clinic visits per year. Since the traditional paper-based record had been available for only 20–30 % of visits, a major objective of the outpatient information system (OIS) was to provide realtime access to the patients' records. In 1975 the clinic was staffed by eight to ten physicians; and a relatively comprehensive computer-stored patient record was maintained for the patients' initial and follow-up visits. Data collection mostly used free-text encounter forms for data organized by categories. All data were entered via Teletype terminals connected by telephone lines to a large mainframe, time-sharing UNIVAC computer at New York University. In 1975, 35,000 children were registered, receiving about 75,000 encounters a year. The central Univac computer provided both online and batch processing services via telephone lines to terminals located in the hospital and clinics [64]. Retrieval of patient records could be initiated within a few seconds; but printing the reports in the 1970s on teletypewriters could take several minutes depending on the length of the record. Patients were seen with a traditional paper-based record, supplemented by attached computer printouts of abstracts of the computer-stored record of recent data, such as diagnoses and medical problems, laboratory test results, and hospitalization discharge summaries. The system was also used by Tick and associates for research in the computer processing of natural language free text [77].

In 1976 the obstetrics medical record implemented by Jelovsek [89] at Duke University Medical Center in 1971 was modified to collect newborns' data from the nursery. A data sheet for each infant was entered into the computer and combined with the maternal information to generate automatically an infant discharge summary). A computer-based perinatal data system was developed at the St. Josephs Hospital in Phoenix, Arizona, that served as the basis for the statewide Arizona Perinatal Program [93]. Wasserman and Stinson [202] at the University of California

San Francisco and Stinson at the University of Rochester Medical School developed detailed specifications for their perinatal records, that included information collected from the mother and fetus during pregnancy and delivery, and for the first 28 days postpartum or until the baby left the hospital. Pediatricians at the Medical University of South Carolina developed a computer-based system that provided information on the growth of infants and children, and compared the height and weight of the patient with those of a child of the same age, race, and sex in a standard population. In addition visual warnings were included on a computer terminal screen of any possibility that measurement errors had occurred or that the patient was experiencing abnormal growth [149].

Newborns with a low birth weight (2,500 g or less) or with a very low birth weight (1,500 g or less) were mostly premature infants and were usually placed in incubators in a neonatal intensive care unit (NICU) for their first week or two of life. With the advent of neonatal specialists in the 1970s, a NICU was established in many pediatric hospital services [29]. Initially the Primary Children's Hospital in Salt Lake City used the computer at the LDS Hospital, with which it was affiliated [33]. However, it soon employed a dedicated PDP-8 computer to process all the patient data generated in the NICU and used the LDS time-sharing computer for compiling and printing reports [54]. Maurer and associates [117] at Washington University in St. Louis developed a data management system for neonatology which they defined as the hospital-based subspecialty of pediatrics devoted to the care of sick infants from birth to generally 1–2 months of age, but in cases involving hospitalization might extend to 8–9 months. Cox and associates [42] at Washington University proposed the design for a formal model of a database system for neonatology based on Maurer's database. Neonatal information systems often shared the HIS central computer, as did the one at the Loma Linda University Medical Center in California [87].

In the 1970s and 1980s, many pediatric services installed information subsystems. With increasing use of the newer technology, Ertel and associates [53] at the Children's Hospital in Columbus, Ohio, initiated an outpatient information system for their pediatric clinics, which at that time provided more than 100,000 outpatient visits per year. Initially, their primary objectives were to support administrative functions and to automatically generate the detailed external reports that were required. They developed encounter forms for data input for family and child demographics, and for the basic clinical data summarizing each patient's visit as to diagnosis and treatment. Copies of these paper forms were transmitted to a central computer, which entered and batch processed the data; and periodically generated individual patient reports and tabulations of data for frequency of diagnoses, clinic visits, of immunizations given, and other statistical analyses. After nearly 2 years of full operation and the processing of more than 187,000 documents, they concluded that their data system met all major design specifications; and the effect on service operations included a significant increase in efficiency at administrative, clerical, and clinical levels.

In 1970 Haessler and associates at Searle Medidata in Lexington, Massachusetts, extended their automated self-administered history taker to provide a pediatric database history. Their branching history questions included the child's current symptoms and diagnosed illnesses as well as perinatal, developmental, family, social, and school history data. After a period of testing the system, they added more questions covering the first 2 years of life, provided the option of abbreviated histories for children with a single problem, and added encounter forms for return visits. With these modifications, they reported that their new Pediatric Database Questionnaire was acceptable to both physicians and patient responders [50].

The pediatricians at Duke University Medical Center also developed a specialized, online, computer-based, self-administered, tree-structured questionnaire for use in their well baby clinic, which provided services to children up to 27 months of age. This was an application of their Generalized Medical Information System for Community Health (GEMISCH) program. Their questionnaire was administered on a visual display terminal to the mothers. Computer printouts provided to the clinic pediatricians contained alerts to certain identified problems, such as problems with feeding the baby. They concluded that the computer could take much of the patient history for the physician, could make "suggestions" depending on the data acquired, and allowed the physician more time to attend to the patients more pressing problems [139].

In 1976 a group of pediatricians in the Boston City Hospital and its seven affiliated Neighborhood Health Centers implemented a computer-based Medical Record Communications (MARCO) system for the care of 30,000 pediatric patients. This system operated on a DEC PDP 11/45 computer using a MUMPS/11 based operating system, which supported seven terminals. During a patient's visit, the physician recorded the patient's data on a structured paper encounter form, from which a clerk entered the data into the computer using the computer terminal. The computer then generated a report for the physician, and printed a copy as part of the chart for the patient's next visit. By 1978, 55,000 encounters had been processed by the system [134].

Newborn screening information systems were established to track babies from their first screening test through their last follow-up test [46]. In 1980 the University of New Mexico Hospital employed two DEC PDP-11 computers to provide an information system for its newborn ICU. Codes were used to enter data in response to sets of menus shown on display screens asking for specific information. Daily updated summaries of patients' information and discharge summaries were provided by display or by printouts to be filed in the patients' charts [169]. In 1980 the First National Conference on Perinatal Data Systems was held in Milwaukee [76]. In the 1980s large perinatal databases, such as the University of Illinois Regional Perinatal Network Database, were used to support decision making by clinicians, administrators, and research epidemiologists [70]. Systems such as the Maryland Perinatal Database used a series of forms for recording and entering data to provide a comprehensive repository of the clinically significant information during the perinatal period; the data were retrievable for both patient care and research purposes [136]. In the early 1980s some states began to mandate newborn screening tests for certain metabolic disorders, such as phenylketonuria and hypothyroidism. The proceedings of a conference on computer-based newborn screening programs were reported in the April 1988 issue of the *Journal of Medical Systems*. In the early 1980s, perinatal and neonatal computer-based systems were becoming common, often using minicomputers: Chicago Lying-in Hospital installed a DEC PDP-10 computer l [113]; the Medical University of South Carolina used a Prime 550 computer [133]; and the Los Angeles County Hospital used a PDP-11/40 computer [208]. Soon microcomputers became more widely used to acquire data from monitoring equipment, and to process and display of patient data in graphic and textual formats [82]. A microcomputer-based perinatal and neonatal information system using a Radio Shack TRS computer for interactive processing of patient data was used at the East Carolina University School of Medicine [51].

In 1983 narrative discharge summaries of some pediatric patients in the New York University Medical Center were being analyzed by a computer system for the processing of natural language records [114]. Due to the large population served, the Los Angeles County Hospital modified its perinatal system by using an Apple II Plus computer for data entry; when the data file was completed, it was transmitted using a telephone line to an IBM 370/168 mainframe computer [207]. The University of Minnesota used a microcomputer for its neonatal system and linked it to the clinical laboratory system for other patient data [41]. Budd and associates [28] at the University of Minnesota Medical School described a medical information relational database system (MIRDS) for their division of pediatric pulmonology; the system accessed their clinical database by using microcomputers. By the late 1980s, large, multiuser pediatric office information systems were available that provided patient management with specialized sets of display screens for programs requiring clinical calculations, for administrative and business functions, word processing for report writing, and electronic mail [144]. In the 1990s, some placed an interactive terminal in the patient's home, with access to a pediatric mobile database in their system, which was programmed to provide advice to a patient's family in response to queries when a child had certain common symptoms [206].

9.5 Mental and Behavioral Health

Not all hospitals will admit patients with mental disorders since these patients require special facilities for their care and security. Patients who require long-term psychiatric care usually are in psychiatric hospitals. When hospitals with a computer-based patient record system have psychiatrists and psychologists on their staff, all data processed for psychiatric patients require extraordinary protection for the security, privacy and confidentiality of the patients' data; only the patient's personal psychiatrists and psychologists are legally permitted access to that patient's records. Otherwise, the information processing requirements for a psychiatric service are similar to those for a general medical service. Interviewing and history taking constitute a prominent part of a psychiatric patient's medical record, and are generally similar for hospital and for office patients.

Beckett [11] noted that psychiatrists collected a vast amount of clinical information in lengthy interviews with patients, and proposed that this information could be reliably recorded in a form suitable for high-speed data processing. Since most data in the practice of psychiatry and psychology were collected by interviews with patients, a great amount of effort was directed to the development of computer-based questionnaires and programs for interpreting their results.

In 1971 Slack developed and used a computer-based psychiatry history system based on an automated history taker [168]. However, processing of data from patients with mental disorders required not only a specialized data dictionary for terms used in psychology and psychiatry, but also extraordinary measures for the security and protection of the confidentiality of the patients' data.

Rome [150] at the Mayo Clinic in Rochester, Minnesota, reported the initiation in 1961 of a joint project with IBM to test an automated version of the then widely used paper-and-pencil-based Minnesota Multiphasic Personality Inventory (MMPI). This test, was developed to help distinguish between functional and organic disease, consisted of 550 statements to which the patient responded by checking each statement as "true" or "false". The responses were then scored to generate 14 scales that predicted personality patterns, such as hypochondriasis, hysteria, depression, paranoia, schizophrenia, and others, in addition to "normal". The test was modified for computer processing so that the 550 statements were printed on 23 standard-sized punch cards. The patient used a special electrographic pencil to fill in the space at the left of the statement if "true", or to the right of the statement if "false". The patient's identifying data were keypunched into a header card, which was then processed with the test cards by a mark-sensing machine that read the marks and punched them into cards readable by the computer. The patient's responses were automatically scored and scaled into personality patterns by the computer program, and a printed report of descriptive diagnostic statements was provided to the patient's psychiatrist or psychologist [188]. By 1964 the Mayo group reported the evaluation of the automated MMPI for the testing of 50,000 patients; they concluded that the automated MMPI was well tolerated by patients and provided meaningful information to psychologists to motivate its continued use [140].

The data derived from this large group of patients permitted them to refine the personality patterns, and the automated MMPI began to be used by others [39, 187, 189]. Finney [55] at the University of Kentucky Medical Center in Lexington advanced this work by combining the automated MMPI with another test, the California Psychological Inventory. Finney's program counted patient's responses and converted them into scores; the scores were combined into indices for which designated statements were put into proper order and into paragraphs. Rather than providing a series of statements, this program generated a report that read as if it had been spontaneously composed by a professional looking at the results of testing. The report described the various processes going on in a person and how they are related to each other. As a variance to using patients' responses to predict psychiatric diagnoses, Overall [138] at the University of Texas Medical Branch in Galveston used the responses of psychiatric patients with known diagnoses who were receiving multiple medications to develop a program that advised which particular drug would be best suited for a given patient.

Starkweather [177] at the University of California in San Francisco addressed the more difficult problem of developing automated text processing from the psychiatric interview, and concluded that analyzing *psychotherapeutic interviews* introduced the problem of processing immense amounts of verbal and textual material. Starkweather first developed a listing of all words used by patients in their recorded interviews, and wrote a program to build a vocabulary and an organized summary of the patient's usage of words. He studied ways of grouping words, and counting word frequency of use as related to categories of meaning and psychologic diagnoses, and developed a program he called COMPUTEST, which simulated a psychiatric interview. The program had questions that were typically used by a psychologist interviewer; the questions and answers were transcribed on an electric typewriter and entered into the computer. The computer program recognized individual words and groups of words, and varied subsequent questions in accordance with the occurrence of "right" or "wrong" answers, and whether the word "yes" was found in the answer. The program could simulate and take the part of either the interviewer or the patient [176]. Starkweather applied factor analysis to the rate of occurrence of words in patients' responses, and applied labels, such as "denial" or "self- aggression" to factors produced from such analysis [175]. As an example, the occurrence of the word "discouraged" in a response was one of a group of words found to suggest a depression of mood [174]. Starkweather's group went on to develop a computer-based medical record system for the Langley Porter Neuropsychiatric Institute, with a System for Efficient Automated Retrieval and Checking of Hypothesis (SEARCH) program to retrieve text on the basis of criteria that included psychiatric terms [186]. The system was first developed to include the psychiatry department's outpatients; later it also included their inpatients [115].

In the 1960s studies were also reported of computer interpretations of unstructured tests, such as the Rorschach, Figure Drawing, and Thematic Apperception tests, which depended on the clinical experience and judgment of the interpreter rather than on statistical scores and rules of interpretation [56]. A relatively advanced program was developed by Piotrowski [141] for interpreting the Rorschach inkblot test by using the detailed scores derived from experts experienced with the test to develop several hundred decision rules to print out a series of interpretive statements based on configurations of scores. In addition to developing methods for computer-assisted assessment of patients with mental disorders, computer-aided psychology therapy was evaluated for conditions that could be helped through behavior modification by processes similar to computer-assisted education [185]. In the early 1970s, a survey of 243 responding psychologists showed that two-thirds were using minicomputers, and one-third used remote-terminal systems attached to a central processing unit. Of those using minicomputers, 57 % wrote their own computer programs mostly using the FORTRAN language, and mainly for clinical and research purposes. Primary applications of users of central processing computers were for statistics and large-scale data reduction [190].

Computer-aided counseling was employed for psychological problems [165] for patients with dietary problems; and a program offered education and altered dietary behavior for overweight patients [143]. Stillman and associates [184] at Stanford University Medical Center developed a Computer Assisted Special Enquirer (CASE) to elicit and record mental status, psychometric, and personal history information directly from patients without the aid of an interviewer. They found that even severely disturbed patients could answer computer-presented questions without assistance. Slack and Slack [167] also evaluated the computer as an interviewer for patients with emotional problems; suggested that the computer-based interview, a "psychology soliloquy", encouraged the patient talking to one-self; and hoped that it would be therapeutic to proceed with questions to encourage relevant soliloquy.

Angle and Ellinwood [2] at Duke University Medical Center reported that their computer interview system routinely gathered extensive patient pretreatment or baseline problem data in a number of psychology treatment programs, and also patient progress information and outcome results. In the 1970s reports of activity in developing computer-based information systems for hospital psychiatry patients were published by professionals at the University of California in San Francisco [115], Forest Hospital in Des Plaines, Illinois [127], Duke University Medical Center [2], West Virginia University Medical Center [161], and the University of Michigan [101]. Black and Saveanu [15] published a comprehensive analysis for the entire decade of the 1970s of the admissions into the Ohio State Mental Health hospitals, using his group's computer-based patient data systems. He identified high-risk groups of patients and emphasized the need to integrate community and hospital data for more accurate evaluations.

In the 1980s microcomputer programs were developed for interactive display and data processing of the mental status examination, the past history, treatment plans, progress notes, real time psychological testing, biofeedback training, and accounting and billing. Because of their low cost, these instruments could be useful in the psychiatrist's office practice [126]. The MMPI was reported to be administered on the TRS-80 computer [31]. A portable microcomputer was used to administer tests, store responses, and view results for psychiatry patients at several locations in Dallas, Texas [30]. The Computer-Stored Ambulatory Record (COSTAR) system was modified to meet the needs of clinicians and administrators in the Outpatient Navy Mental Health Clinics [40]. Greist and associates [69] at the University of Wisconsin developed a computer-based Lithium Library, which in 1983 contained 9,000 citations, and provided online access by free-text entry for information requests by clinicians or investigators on diagnosis, pretreatment work-up, and possible complications of lithium treatment. In the 1980s many information systems for psychiatry departments were reported, using minicomputers, including the University of Pittsburgh School of Medicine [35, 129] and the VA Hospital in Loma Linda, California [72]; and using microcomputers at Northwestern University Medical School [71].

9.6   Other Clinical Specialties

9.6.1   Ophthalmology

Ophthalmologists began to exploit the capabilities of the computer in their office practice in the 1980s, primarily through advances in bioengineering and instrumentation. Jacobs [85] reviewed the then-current applications of computers in ophthalmology and described computer-controlled perimeter devices that detected the absence of vision in automated testing devices of visual fields, with the test results stored in microcomputers. Jacobs also reported a microprocessor-controlled, automated refractometer that measured infrared light reflected back from the retina of the eye, converted the signals to a digital format, and measured the refractive power of the eye. Similarly, automated keratometers with photosensors detected infrared light reflected from the cornea, and measured the curvature of the cornea. Jacobs also described automated lens analyzers that measured deviations of light beams through the lens of the eye.

9.6.2   Physical Medicine and Rehabilitation

Physiatrists and physiotherapists in rehabilitation centers, such as Spencer and Vallbona at the Texas Institute for Rehabilitation and Research (TIRR) developed a fairly comprehensive medical information system (MIS) with several clinical subspecialty systems for patients' rehabilitation. TIRR was a private, non-profit, special-purpose hospital in the Texas Medical Center at Houston that delivered comprehensive rehabilitation services to patients having a wide variety of physical disabilities. In February 1959 physiological test data were manually recorded on specially designed source documents. The data were then coded, keypunched, and processed on a batch basis with unit-record equipment. The software consisted of diagrams of complex patch boards. In 1961 the acquisition of IBM 1401 and 1620 computers with magnetic tape storage provided for data processing, storage, and data retrieval capabilities [18]. In 1965 the problem of errors in data entry associated with the use of punched paper tape and cards required TIRR to advance to online computing with an IBM 1410 computer. Data entries were made by a clerk at TIRR via a remote typewriter terminal. With the establishment of a conversational mode between the terminal and the computer, error detection and correction by staff personnel became feasible.

In 1967 the system was enhanced by the acquisition of an IBM 360/50 computer [197]. In 1968 physicians' orders began to be entered into their medical information system; and appropriate displays were accessed on IBM 2260 cathode-ray-tube terminals located in various clinical departments [12]. In 1969 using these display terminals connected to the Baylor University IBM/360 computer, updated reports were batch-processed daily for each patient [68]. By the mid-1970s, TIRR had an information system with several operational modules, including the provision of results of all patients' laboratory and functional capacity tests [197].

9.7 Summary and Commentary

Although some of the earliest applications of computers in clinical medicine were in the clinical subspecialties, health professionals found these prototypes difficult to use since their data entry devices were awkward and inefficient, and their order entry functions were often not integrated. Each information system for a clinical subspecialty had its own specialized functional and technical requirements; each evolved differently. In the 1960s hospitals information systems with ISCSs used large mainframe computers that served all computer applications within the hospital. It was soon found that although a single mainframe computer could readily integrate patient data into a single patient record database, it could not adequately support the information processing requirements of all of the multiple departmental and clinical support systems within a large hospital.

In the 1970s, the advent of minicomputers permitted each ISCS to have its own computer-based information system; and the computers in the various departmental information systems were directly linked to the central mainframe computer. Healthcare professionals used terminals connected to the central computer to enter orders and to receive test results. Directly linked to the departmental minicomputers, the central computer transferred the orders to the appropriate ISCS subsystems and integrated the data coming back from the ISCSs into the patients' records stored in the mainframe computer. In the 1980s the advent of local area networks that linked multiple lower-cost minicomputers permitted distributed information systems to be implemented in hospitals. Although ISCSs were some of the earliest and most advanced computer-based information systems in medicine, it was not until the advent of distributed minicomputers equipped with interactive visual-display terminals, that clinicians began to benefit from the ISCSs in direct patient care. Minicomputers allowed each ISCS to develop its own internal information system that best satisfied its own functional requirements.

In the 1990s, distributed information systems allowed physicians to enter orders and retrieve test results using clinical workstations connected to client-server minicomputers in the local area network that linked the entire hospital. Patient data from all of the distributed ISCS databases were integrated in a computer-based patient record. The advent of clinical workstations linked by local area networks to the ISCSs made the clinical subsystems, and applications such as a computer provider order entry (CPOE) program more acceptable for clinicians to use [36, 57].

These achievements, and more since, stand on the "shoulders of giants" who had the foresight and innovation to move forward in a new way of supporting clinical care through the use of digital information within computer systems. Today the technology has evolved to allow the goals of early ISCS creators to be easily implemented. As the technology has become more sophisticated, the computer based programs have grown richer and richer.

References

1. Alderman EI, Spitz AL, Sanders WJ, Harrison DC. A cardiologist's evaluation of a computer cardiac catheterization system. In: Cox J, editor. Computers in cardiology. Long Beach: IEEE Computer Society; 1974. p. 81–3.
2. Angle HV, Ellinwood EH. A psychiatric assessment-treatment-outcome information system: evaluation with computer simulation. Proc SCAMC. 1978;149–59.
3. Ausman RK, Baer GD. Machine processing of the operative record. Proc 6th IBM Med Symp. 1964;553–8.
4. Ausman RK, Moore GE, Grace JT. An automated operative record system. Ann Surg. 1965;162:402.
5. Austin H, Laufman H, Zelner L. Strategic automation for surgery. Comput Healthc. 1987;8:44–9.
6. Ball MJ. Computers-prescription for hospital ills. Datamation. 1975;21:50–1.
7. Ball MJ, Douglas JV, Warnock-Matheron A, Hannah KJ. The case for using computers in the operating room. West J Med. 1986;145:843.
8. Banta HD, Thacker SB. Costs and benefits of electronic fetal monitoring: a review of the literature. Hyattsville: National Center for Health Services Research; 1979a.
9. Banta HD, Thacker SB. Policies toward medical technology: the case of electronic fetal monitoring. AJPH. 1979;69:931–5.
10. Barnoon S, Wolfe H. Scheduling a multiple operating room system: a simulation approach. Health Serv Res. 1968;3:272–85.
11. Beckett PGS. Computers and clinical psychiatry. Med Electron IRE Trans. 1960;ME-7:248–50.
12. Beggs S, Vallbona C, Spencer WA, Jacobs FM, Baker RL. Evaluation of a system for on-line computer scheduling of patient care activities. Comput Biomed Res. 1971;4:634–54.
13. Berg CM, Larson D. Operating room systems software. In: Ball MJ, Hannah KJ, Gerdin Jelger U, Peterson H, editors. Nursing informatics: where caring and technology meet. New York: Springer-Verlag; 1988. p. 146–59.
14. Biesada AM. Tooth Tech. The new dentistry. High Technol Bus. 1989(April);28–31.
15. Black GC, Saveanu TI. A search for mental health output measures. Proc SCAMC. 1980b;3:1859–71.
16. Bleich H. Computer evaluation of acid-based disorders. J Clin Invest. 1969;48:1689–96.
17. Bleich HL. The computer as a consultant. N Engl J Med. 1971;284:141–7.
18. Blose WF, Vallbona C, Spencer WA. System for processing clinical research data. II. System design. Proc 6th IBM symposium. Poughkeepsie: IBM; 1964. p. 463–85.
19. Blum BI, Lenhard RE J, McColligan EE. An integrated data model for patient care. IEEE Trans Biomed Eng. 1985;32:277–88.
20. Blum B, Lenhard Jr R. A clinical information display system. Proc SCAMC. 1977;131–8.
21. Blum BI, Orthner HE. The MUMPS programming language. In: Helmuth HF, Blum BI, editors. Implementing health care information systems. New York: Springer; 1989. p. 396–420.
22. Blum BI. Clinical information systems. New York: Springer-Verlag; 1986.
23. Blum BI. An information system for developing information systems. AFIPS Natl Comput Conf Proc. 1983;52:743–52.
24. Blum RL. Automating the study of clinical hypotheses on a time-oriented clinical database: The Rx Project. Proc MEDINFO. 1980:456–60.

25. Blum RL. Automating the study of clinical hypotheses on a time-oriented data base: the RX project. Proc MEDINFO. 1979;456–60.
26. Brame RG, Hammond WE, Stead WW. The computerized obstetrical record of Duke University. J Clin Comput. 1974;4:107–20.
27. Brown A. A computer generated aid for scheduling operating rooms. Proc AAMSI Congress. 1984;259–99.
28. Budd JR, Warwick WJ, Wielinski CL, Finkelstein SM. A medical information relational database system (MIRDS). Comp Biomed Res. 1988;21:419–33.
29. Budetti P, Barrand N, McManus P, Heinen LA. The costs and effectiveness of neonatal intensive care. Darby: Diane Publishing; 1981.
30. Burgess CJ, Swigger KM. A data collection system for use by psychiatric patients. Proc SCAMC. 1984;286–9.
31. Burstein E. Use of a microcomputer system for administration and evaluation of psychological testing: the Minnesota Multiphasic Personality Inventory (MMPI). Proc SCAMC. 1980;1872–80.
32. Chodoff P, Gianaris II C. A nurse-computer assisted preoperative anesthesia management system. Comp Biomed Res. 1973;6:371–92.
33. Clark JS, Veasy LG, Jung AL, Jenkins JL. Automated PO2, PCO2, AND PH monitoring of infants. Comp Biomed Res. 1971;4:262–74.
34. Clayton PD, Urie PM, Marshall HW, Warner HR. A computerized system for the cardiovascular laboratory. In: Cox JR, Hugenholt, editors. Computers in cardiology. Long Beach: IEEE Computing Society; 1974. p. 89–93.
35. Coffman GA, Mezzich JE. Research use of a general psychiatric data base. Proc SCAMC. 1983;721–3.
36. Collen MF. A history of medical informatics in the United States, 1950 to 1990. Indianapolis: American Medical Informatics Association; 1995.
37. Collen MF. General requirements for clinical departmental systems. Proc MEDINFO. 1983;83–9.
38. Collen MF. General requirements of a medical information (MIS). Comput Biomed Res. 1970;3:393–406.
39. Colligan RC, Offord KP. Revitalizing the MMPI: the development of contemporary norms. Psychiatr Ann. 1985;15:558–68.
40. Congleton MW, Glogower FD, Ramsey-Klee D, Roberts AS. Navy Mental Health Information System (NAMHIS): a psychiatric application of COSTAR. Proc SCAMC. 1984;437–40.
41. Connelly D, Dean DW, Hultman BK. Physician-oriented result reporting in an intensive care environment. Proc MEDINFO 1986;810–2.
42. Cox Jr J, Kimura TD, Moore P, Gillett W, Stucki MJ. Design studies suggested by an abstract model for a medical information system. Proc SCAMC. 1980;3:1485–94.
43. Cozen HJ. Computer generated anesthesia record. Proc SCAMC. 1979;615–7.
44. Crouse L, Wiederhold G. An advanced computer for real-time medical applications. Comp Biomed Res. 1969;2:582–98.
45. Davis RS, Jack DB. A surgical cut into computers. MD Comput. 1985;3:21–8.
46. Dayhoff RE, Ledley RS, Rotolo LS. Newborn screening information system (NBSIS). Proc SCAMC. 1984;253–6.
47. Diehl M. Strategy for large-scale dental automation. Dent Clin N Am. 1986;30:745–53.
48. Diehl MC, Neiburger EJ. A history of computer applications in dental practice. Proc AAMSI. 1987;362–6.
49. ECRI. Clinical information systems improve with new standard. Health Tech Trends. 1989;1:3–6.
50. Elshtain EL, Haessler HA, Harden CM, Holland T. Field study of an automated pediatric data base history. Proc Symp Medical Data Processing. Toulouse: IRIA; 1973. p. 47–53.
51. Engelke SC, Paulette EW, Kopelman AE. Neonatal information system using an interactive microcomputer data base management program. Proc SCAMC. 1981;284–5.
52. Enterline JP, Lenhard RE, Blum BI. The oncology clinical information system. In: Enterline JP, Lenhard RE, Blum BI, editors. A Clinical Information System for Oncology. New York: Springer; 1989. p. 1–21.

53. Ertel PY, Pritchett EL, Chase RC, Ambuel JP. An outpatient data system. New techniques to meet new demands. JAMA. 1970;211:964–72.
54. Farr FL, Clark JS, Gardner RM, Veasy LG. Using a dedicated small computer in conjunction with a time-shared system in a hospital intensive care unit. Comp Biomed Res. 1972;5:535–9.
55. Finney JC. Programmed interpretation of MMPI and CPI. Arch Gen Psychiatry. 1966;15:75–81.
56. Fowler RD. The current status of computer interpretation of psychological tests. Am J Psychiatry. 1969;125:21–7.
57. Friedman C, Hripcsak G, Johnson SB, Cimino JJ, Clayton PD. A generalized relational schema for an integrated clinical patient database. Proc SCAMC. 1990;335–9.
58. Friedman RH, Krikorian JG, Horwitz JH, Concannon TI. An information system for clinical research: the cancer data management system. Proc MEDINFO. 1980;876–80.
59. Fries JF, McShane DJ. ARAMIS: a prototypical national chronic-disease data bank. West J Med. 1986;145:798–804.
60. Fries JF, McShane D. ARAMIS: a national chronic disease data bank system. Proc SCAMC. 1979;798–801.
61. Gabrieli ER. Standardization of medical informatics (special issue). J Clin Comput. 1985;14:62–104.
62. Garrett Jr L, Stead WW, Hammond WE. Conversion of manual to total computerized medical records. J Med Syst. 1983;7:301–5.
63. Gardner DW, Klatchko DM. A microcomputer based diabetic patient registry for patient management and clinical research. Proc SCAMC. 1985;87–9.
64. Giebink GA, Hurst LL. Computer projects in health care. Ann Arbor: Health Administration Press; 1975.
65. Gildea TJ, Bell CW. Advanced techniques in pulmonary function test analysis interpretation and diagnosis. Proc SCAMC. 1980;1:258–65.
66. Goldsmith MF. Computers star in new communication concepts for physically disabled people. JAMA. 1989;261:1256–9.
67. Gonzalez F, Fox H. The development and implementation of a computerized on-line obstetric record. BJOG Int J Obstet Gynaecol. 1989;96:1323–7.
68. Gotcher SB, Carrick J, Vallbona C, Spencer WA, Carter RE, Cornell S. Daily treatment planning with an on-line shared computer system. Methods Inf Med. 1969;8:200–5.
69. Greist JH, Klein MH, Erdman HP, Jefferson JW. Clinical computer applications in mental health. J Med Syst. 1983;7:175–85.
70. Grover J, Spellacy W, Winegar A. Utilization of the University of Illinois regional perinatal database in three areas. Proc AAMSI. 1983;144–7.
71. Hammer JS, Lyons JS, Strain JJ. Micro-cares: an information management system for psychosocial services in hospital settings. Proc SCAMC. 1984; 234–7.
72. Hammond KW, Munnecke TH. A computerized psychiatric treatment planning system. Psychiat Serv. 1984;35:160–3.
73. Hammond WE, Stead WW. Bedside terminals: an editorial. MD Comput. 1988;5(1):5–6.
74. Hancock WM, Walter PF, More RA, Glick ND. Operating room scheduling data base analysis for scheduling. J Med Syst. 1988;12:397–409.
75. Harbort RA, Paulsen AW, Frazier WT. Computer generated anesthesia records. Proc SCAMC. 1980;3:1603–10.
76. Harris TR, Bahr JP, editors. The use of computers in perinatal medicine. New York: Praeger Publishing; 1982.
77. Henley RR, Wiederhold G. An analysis of automated ambulatory medical record systems. San Francisco: Office of Medical Information Systems, University of California, San Francisco Medical Center; 1975.
78. Herner & Co. The use of computers in hospitals: report III-survey analysis; report IV- descriptions of computer applications. Bethesda: National Center for Health Services Research; 1968.

79. Hilberman M, Kamm B, Lamy M, Dietrich HP, Martz K, Osborn JJ. Prediction of respiratory adequacy following cardiac surgery. In: Cox JR, Hugenholtz PG, editors. Computers in Cardiology. Long Beach: IEEE Computer Society. 1974;2–4.

80. Hogan MJ, Wallin JD, Kelly MR, Baer R, Barzyk P, Sparks HA. A computerized paramedical approach to the outpatient management of essential hypertension. Mil Med. 1978;143:771–5.

81. Hon EH. Computer aids in evaluating fetal distress. In: Stacy RW, Waxman BD, editors. Computers in biomedical research. New York: Academic; 1965. p. 409–37.

82. Hoppenbrouwers T, Jilek J, Arakawa K. A system for monitoring cardiorespiratory variables and transcutaneous blood gases during sleep in the newborn and young infant. Proc MEDINFO. 1983;644–7.

83. Horwitz J, Thompson H, Concannon T, Friedman RH, Krikorian J, Gertman PM. Computer-assisted patient care management in medical oncology. Proc SCAMC. 1980;2:771–8.

84. Hubbard SM, Martin NB, Blankenbaker LW, Esterhay RJ, Masys DR, et al. The physician data query (PDQ) cancer information system. J Cancer Educ. 1986;1:79–87.

85. Jacobs I. Computers in ophthalmology. MD Comput. 1985;2:28–34.

86. Jacobsen TJ, Lockee C, Sands C. Development of an operating room management information system using multi-user microcomputer technology. Proc SCAMC. 1984;646–8.

87. Janik DS, Swarner OW, Henriksen KM, Wyman ML. A computerized single entry system for recording and reporting data on high-risk newborn infants. J Pediatr. 1978;93:519–23.

88. Jelovsek FR. Computers in the examining room, the delivery room, and the nursery. MD Comput. 1984;1:52–8.

89. Jelovsek F, Hammond WE. Experience in computerization of perinatal medical records. Univ Mich Med Cent J. 1977;43:5–8.

90. Jelovsek FR. Computers in the examining room, the delivery room, and the nursery. MD Comput. 1987;1:153–9.

91. Jelovsek FR, Deason BP, Richard H. Impact of an on-line information system on patients and personnel in the medical office. Proc SCAMC. 1982;85–8.

92. Jenkin MA. Clinical specialty systems as an introduction to clinical informatics. Proc AAMSI. 1983;223–7.

93. Jennett RJ, Gall D, Waterkotte GW, Warford HS. A computerized perinatal data system for a region. Am J Obstet Gynecol. 1978;131:157–61.

94. Johns RJ, Blum BI. The use of clinical information systems to control cost as well as to improve care. Trans Am Clin Climatol Assoc. 1978;80:140–51.

95. Johnson ME. Pulmonary testing laboratory computer application. Proc SCAMC. 1980;1:253–7.

96. Kahane SN, Goldberg HR, Roth HP, Lenhard RE, Johannes RS. A multimodal communications interface for endoscopy data collection with automated text report generation. Proc MEDINFO. 1986;26–30.

97. Kassirer JP, Brand DH, Schwartz WB. An automated system for data processing in the metabolic balance laboratory. Comp Biomed Res. 1971;4:181–96.

98. Keating III H.J., Sims SC, Balk MA. Computer assisted pre-operative evaluation (CAPE): a system description. Proc SCAMC. 1984;269.

99. Kessler RR. A comprehensive computer package for ambulatory surgical facilities. Proc SCAMC. 1980;3:1436–40.

100. Kilpatrick KE, Mackenzie RS, Delaney AG. Expanded-function auxiliaries in general dentistry: a computer simulation. Health Serv Res. 1972;7:288–300.

101. Knesper DJ, Quarton GC, Gorodezky MJ, Murray CW. A survey of the users of a working state mental health information system: implications for the development of improved systems. Proc SCAMC. 1978; 160–5.

102. Laboratories – Berekeley Scientific. A study of automated clinical laboratory systems. U.S. health services and mental health administration. Springfield: National Technical Information Service; 1971.

103. Larks SD. Present status of fetal electrocardiography. Bio-Med Electron IRE Trans. 1962;9:176–80.

104. Laurent D, Mashruwala MD, Lucas CP. A computerized data-handling system in hypertension management. Arch Intern Med. 1980;140:345–50.
105. Lederman M, Weil JP. ORIS (operating room information system): a solution whose time has come. US Healthc. 1989;6:32–3.
106. Lenhard RE, Blum BI, McColligan EE. An information system for oncology. In: Blum BI, editor. An Information System for Patient Care. New York: Springer-Verlag;1984;385–403.
107. Lenhard RE, Waalkes TP, Herring D. Evaluation of the clinical management of cancer patients: a pilot study. JAMA. 1983;250:3310–6.
108. Lenhard RE, Blum BI, Sunderland JM, Braine HG, Saral R. The Johns Hopkins oncology clinical information system. J Med Syst. 1983;7:147–74.
109. Levy N, Say BA. Henry Ford Hospital nephrology information system. Proc MEDINFO. 1983;801–3.
110. Lewis HM, Wheeler JR, Gregory RT. Clinical data base management by microcomputer. J Med Syst. 1982;6:255–8.
111. Lindberg DAB. The computer and medical care. Springfield: Charles C. Thomas; 1968.
112. Lomatch D, Truax T, Savage P. Use of a relational database to support clinical research: application in a diabetes Program. Proc SCAMC. 1981;291–5.
113. Lowensohn RI, Moawad AH, Pishotta FT, Gibbons PS. The computer-based OBFILE perinatal reporting system. Proc SCAMC. 1980;2:1192–5.
114. Lyman M, Chi E, Sager N. Automated case review of acute bacterial meningitis of childhood. Proc MEDINFO. 1983;790–3.
115. Malerstein AJ, Strotz CR, Starkweather JA. A practical approach to automation of psychiatric hospital records. J Biomed Syst. 1971;2:19–29.
116. Marciniak TA, Leahey CF, Zufall E. Information systems in oncology. Proc MEDINFO. 1986;508–12.
117. Maurer Jr M, Moore P, Mead CN, Johnson JA, Marshall RE, Thomas Jr L. Data management for rapid access to newborn intensive care information. Proc SCAMC. 1980;3:1621–9.
118. McColligan EE. Implementing OCIS at Ohio State University. In: Enterline JP, Lenhard RE, Blum BI, editors. A clinical information systems for oncology. New York: Springer; 1989. p. 241–59.
119. McColligan E, Blum B, Brunn C. An automated care medical record system for ambulatory care. In: Kaplan B, Jelovsek FR, editors. Proc SCM/SAMS Joint Conf on Ambulatory Care. 1981;72–6.
120. McColligan EE, Jones CE, Lindberg D. An automated operating room scheduling and management information system. AAMSI Congress. 1983;83:517–22.
121. McColligan EE, Blum BI, Lenhard RE, Johnson MB. The human element in computer-generated patient management plans. J Med Syst. 1982;6:265–76.
122. McColligan EE, Gordon TA, Jones CE, Stiff JL, Donham RT, Rogers MC. Automated utilization analysis as a foundation for effective operating room management. Proc SCAMC. 1984;227–30.
123. McDonald CJ, Tierney W, Blevins L. The benefits of automated medical record systems for ambulatory care. In: Orthner HE, Blum BI, editors. Implementing health care information systems. New York: Springer; 1989. p. 67–84.
124. McDonald C, Blevins L, Glazener T, Haas J, Lemmon L, Meeks-Johnson J. Data base management, feedback control, and the regenstrief medical record. J Med Syst. 1983;7:111–25.
125. McDonald CJ, Wilson G, Blevins L, Seeger J, Chamness D, Smith D, et al. The Regenstrief medical record system. Proc SCAMC. 1977;168.
126. Meldman MJ. Microprocessor technology for psychiatrists. Proc SCAMC. 1978;216–20.
127. Meldman MJ. Clinical computing in psychiatry: an integrated patient data base approach. Comput Med. 1975;4:1–2.
128. Menn SJ, Barnett GO, Schmechel D, Owens WD, Pontoppidan H. A computer program to assist in the care of acute respiratory failure. JAMA. 1973;223:308–12.
129. Mezzich JE, Coffman GA. A computerized alerting system regarding special-concern psychiatric patients. Proc SCAMC. 1984;449–52.

130. Michas CA, Wilcox JC, Walters RF. A computer-based surgery reporting system: an entry point to clinical information systems. West J Med. 1976;124:151–8.
131. Michenfelder JD, Terry HR, Anderholm FR, Shaw DG. The application of a new system for monitoring the surgical patient. Proc 18th Annual Conf Eng Med Biol. 1965;7: 233.
132. Miller PL. ATTENDING: a system which critiques an anesthetic management plan. Proc AMIA. 1982;36–40.
133. Miller RA, Kapoor WN, Peterson J. The use of relational databases as a tool for conducting clinical studies. Proc SCAMC. 1983;705–8.
134. Moffatt PH, Heisler BD, Mela WD, Alpert JJ, Goldstein HM. MARCO (Medical Record Communications): system concept, design and evaluation. Proc SCAMC. 1978;451–68.
135. Muller JH, Kerner ER, Fitzgerald MA. Spirometry for office-based physicians. Med Electron. 1986;70–6.
136. Nagey DA, Wright JN, Mulligan K, Crenshaw Jr C. A convertible perinatal database. MD Comput Comp Med Pract. 1988;6:28–36.
137. Nault FG, Hanson RJ, L'Heureux D, Mermelstein PD. Evaluation of operating room facilities and personnel utilization. In: Emlet HE, editor. Challenges and prospects for advanced medical systems. Miami: Symposia Specialists; 1978. p. 61–8.
138. Overall JE, Hollister LE. Computer program for recommendation of treatment for psychiatry patients. Proc 16th Annual Conf Eng Biol. 1963;5:126–7.
139. Pearlman MH, Hammond E, Thompson HK. An automated "well-baby" questionnaire. Pediatrics. 1973;51:972–9.
140. Pearson JS, Swenson WM, Rome HP, Mataya P, Brannick TL. Further experience with the automated Minnesota multiphasic personality inventory. Mayo Clin Proc. 1964;39:823–9.
141. Piotrowski ZA. Digital-computer interpretation of inkblot test data. Psychiatr Q. 1964;38:1–26.
142. Pollak VE, Buncher CR, Donovan ER. On-line computerized data handling system for treating patients with renal disease. Arch Intern Med. 1977;137:446–56.
143. Porter D. Patient responses to computer counseling. Proc SCAMC. 1978;233–7.
144. Post EM, Bolitsky BA. Integration of computer utilization for medical office practice. Proc SCAMC. 1987;631–5.
145. Pryor DB, Stead WW, Hammond WE, Califf RM, Rosati RA. Features of TMR for a successful clinical and research database. Proc SCAMC. 1982;79–83.
146. Pryor DB, Califf RM, Harrell FE, Hlatky MA, Lee KL, Mark DB, et al. Clinical data bases: accomplishments and unrealized potential. Med Care. 1985;23:623–47.
147. Pryor TA, Ho SJ, Stephen RL. Computer systems for management and research in end-stage renal disease. In: Shoemaker WC, Tavares BM, editors. Current topics in critical care medicine, vol. 3. Basel: S. Karger; 1977. p. 93–111.
148. Reisman A, Emmons H, Morito S, Rivaud J, Green EJ. Planning a dental practice with a management game. J Med Syst. 1978;2:71–83.
149. Robson J, Braunstein HM. Computerized growth record for clinic use. Pediatrics. 1977;60:643–6.
150. Rome HP. Automation techniques in personality assessment: the problem and procedure. JAMA. 1962;182:1069–72.
151. Rosen MG, Sokol RJ, Chik L. Use of computers in the labor and delivery suite: an overview. Obstet Gynecol. 1978;132:589–94.
152. Rosner SW, Palmer A, Caceres CA. A computer program for computation and interpretation of pulmonary function data. Comp Biomed Res. 1971;4:141–56.
153. Rothrock JJ. ASTM: the standards make the pieces fit. Proc AAMSI Congr. 1989;327–35.
154. Rutt TE. Work of IEEE P1157 medical data interchange committee. Int J Clin Monit Comput. 1989;6:45–57.
155. Sadler Jr C. Orthopedic computing: bone and joint computer connection. MD Comput. 1984;1:39–47.
156. Safran C, Porter D, Lightfoot J, Rury CD, Underhill LH, Bleich HL, et al. ClinQuery: a system for online searching of data in a teaching hospital. Ann Intern Med. 1989;111:751–6.
157. Sanders SJ, Sheppard AP, Spurlock JM. Micro-computer controlled care system for the severely physically impaired. Proc SCAMC. 1984;886–91.

158. Schenthal JE. Clinical concepts in the application of large scale electronic data processing. Proc 2nd IBM Medical Symp. Endicott, NY: IBM.1960;391–9.

159. Schenthal JE. Development aspects of a biomedical data processing systems. Proc 3rd IBM medical symposium. Endicott: IBM; pp 167–74.

160. Schmidt NM, Brown ACD. The prediction of surgeon-specific operating room time. Proc SCAMC. 1984;800–4.

161. Seime RJ, Rine DC. The behavioral medicine data retrieval and analysis program at West Virginia University Medical Center. Proc SCAMC. 1978;125–36.

162. Serber MJ, Mackey R, Young CW. The Sloan-Kettering information system for clinical oncology. Proc SCAMC. 1980;2:728–32.

163. Shaffer MJ, Kaiser PR, Klingenmaier CH, Gordon MR. Manual record-keeping and statistical records for the operating room. Med Instrum. 1978;12:192–7.

164. Shonfeld EM, Kerekes J, Rademacher CA, Weihrer AL, Abraham S, Silver H, et al. Methodology for computer measurement of pulmonary function curves. CHEST J. 1964;46:427–34.

165. Simborg DW. An emerging standard for health communications: the HL7 standard. Healthc Comput Commun. 1987;4:58. 60.

166. Slack WV. Patient counseling by computer. Proc SCAMC. 1978;222–6.

167. Slack WV, Slack CW. Talking to a computer about emotional problems: a comparative study. Psychother Theory Res Pract. 1977;14:156–63.

168. Slack WV, Slack CW. Patient-computer dialogue. N Engl J Med. 1972;286:1304–9.

169. Slosarik W, Luger G, Kirkpatrick J, Koffler H, Burstein R. The UNMH intensive care information system. Proc SCAMC. 1980;1576–80.

170. Southard TE, Rails SA. A computerized dental examination record system. Comput Bio Med. 1986;16:59–67.

171. Spencer WA, Vallbona C. Digitation of clinical and research data in serial evaluation of disease processes. IRE Trans Med Electron. 1960;ME-7:296–308.

172. Spencer WA. An opinion survey of computer applications in 149 hospitals in the USA, Europe and Japan. Inform Health Soc Care. 1976;1:215–34.

173. Spencer WA, Vallbona C. A preliminary report on the use of electronic data processing technics in the description and evaluation of disability. Arch Phys Med Rehabil. 1962;43:22–35.

174. Starkweather JA. Computer simulation of psychiatric interviewing. In: Kline N, Laska EM, editors. Computers and electronic devices in psychiatry. New York: Grune & Stratton; 1968. p. 12–9.

175. Starkweather JA. Computer methods for the study of psychiatric interviews. Compr Psychiatry. 1967;8:509–20.

176. Starkweather JA. Computest: a computer language for individual testing, instruction, and interviewing. Psychol Rep. 1965;17:227–37.

177. Starkweather JA, Decker JB. Computer analysis of interview content. Psychol Rep. 1964;15:875–82.

178. Stead WW, Brame RG, Hammond WE, Jelovser FR, Estes EH, Parker RT. A computerized obstetric medical record. Obstet Gynecol. 1977;49:502–9.

179. Stead WW, Hammond WE. How to realize savings with a computerized medical record. Proc SCAMC. 1980;2:1200–5.

180. Stead WW, Hammond WE, Straube MJ. A chartless record: is it adequate? Proc SCAMC. 1982;89–94.

181. Stead WW, Hammond WE. Functions required to allow TMR to support the information requirements of a hospital. Proc SCAMC. 1983;106–9.

182. Stead WW, Hammond WE, Winfree RG. Beyond a basic HIS: work stations for department management. Proc SCAMC. 1984;197–9.

183. Stead WW, Hammond WE, Straube MJ. A chartless record: is it adequate? J Med Syst. 1983;7:103–9.

184. Stillman R, Roth WT, Colby KM, Rosenbaum CP. An on-line computer system for initial psychiatric inventory. Am J Psychiatry. 1969;125:8–11.

185. Stodolsky D. The computer as a psychotherapist. Int J Man-Mach Stud. 1970;2:327–50.

186. Strotz CR, Malerstein AJ, Starkweather JA. SEARCH: a physician-oriented, computer-based information retrieval system. J Biomed Syst. 1970;1:41–8.
187. Swenson WM. An aging psychologist assesses the impact of age on MMPI profiles. Psychiatr Ann. 1985;15:554–7.
188. Swenson WM. Symposium on automation technics in personality testing: the test. Mayo Clinic Proc. 1962;37:65–72.
189. Swenson WM, Pearson JS. Psychiatry: psychiatric screening. J Chronic Dis. 1966;19:497–507.
190. Tepas DI. Computer use in the psychology laboratory: a survey. Comput Programs Biomed. 1974;4:53–8.
191. Thomas JC, Moore AC. Content of an automated ambulatory record system for clinical decisions. In: Hinman EJ, editor. Advanced medical systems: the 3rd century. Miami: Symposia Specialists; 1977. p. 153–60.
192. Thompson DA. Monitoring total parenteral nutrition with the pocket computer. Comput Nurs. 1984;2:183–8.
193. Tira DE, Tharp LB, Lipson LF. Computers in dental education. Promise of the past versus reality of the present. Dent Clin N Am. 1986;30:681–94.
194. Tolchin SG, Barta W. Local network and distributed processing issues in the Johns Hopkins Hospital. J Med Syst. 1986;10:339–53.
195. Truax T, Savage P, Lomatch D. Microcomputer assisted data management in a diabetes clinic. Proc SCAMC. 1980;2:1183–91.
196. Vallbona C. The usefulness of computers in the management of the chronically ill and disabled. So Med Bull. 1969;57:25–8.
197. Vallbona C, Spencer WA. Texas institute for research and rehabilitation hospital computer system (Houston). In: Collen MF, editor. Hospital computer systems. New York: Wiley; 1974. p. 662–700.
198. Vallbona C, Spencer WA, Moffet CL. The patient care centered information system of the Texas Institute for Rehabilitation and Research. In: Collen MF, editor. Proc Int Conf on Health Technol Syst. ORSA. 1973;232–60.
199. Vallbona C, Spencer WA, Geddes LA, Blose WF, Canzoneri J. Experience with on-line monitoring in critical illness. Spectr IEEE. 1966;3:136–40.
200. Vallbona C, Pevny E, McMath F. Computer analysis of blood gases and of acid-base status. Comput Biomed Res. 1971;4:623–33.
201. Warner HR. Experiences with computer-based patient monitoring. Anesth Analg. 1968;47:453–62.
202. Wasserman AI, Stinson SK. A specification method for interactive medical information systems. Proc SCAMC. 1980;3:1471–8.
203. Wheeler PS, Simborg DW, Gitlin JN. The Johns Hopkins radiology reporting system. Radiology. 1976;119:315–9.
204. Wilson DH. A private practice medical computing system: an evolutionary approach. Comput Med. 1974;3:1–2.
205. Wirtschafter DD, Blackwell WC, Goldenberg RL, et al. A county-wide obstetrical automated medical record system. J Med Syst. 1982;6:277–90.
206. Witten M. PEDS: an expert pediatric evaluation and diagnostic system. Proc SCAMC. 1987;507–13.
207. Yeh S, Lincoln T. From micro to mainframe. Am J Perinatol. 1985;2:158–60.
208. Yeh S, Teberg AJ, Phelan JR. A practical approach to perinatal data processing in a large obsteric population. Proc MEDINFO. 1983;656–8.
209. Young B. Anesthesiologists breathe easier with computer assistance. Comput Med. 1981;10:1.
210. Zajac TH. A microcomputer based management control system in the operating suite. Proc SCAMC. 1984;242–5.
211. Zimmerman JL. Computer applications in dentistry. Philadelphia: WB Saunders Co; 1986.
212. Zviran M, Blow R. DMSS: a computer-based diabetes monitoring system. J Med Syst. 1989;13:293–308.

Chapter 10
Multi-Hospital Information Systems (MHISs)

Morris F. Collen and Don Eugene Detmer

Abstract Changing economics gave rise to the development of Multi-Hospital Information Systems (MHISs) serving systems of three or more hospitals and their associated services. Functional and technical capabilities, including translational databases, were developed to support the exchange and integration of multiple forms of information within and among facilities. Early examples in the private sector included MHISs at The Sisters of the Third Order of St. Francis (1960s) and Intermountain Health Care (1970s), and in mental health hospitals (1960s–1970s). In the federal sector, the U.S. Public Health Service and Indian Health Services began to develop MHISs in the 1970s. Efforts to use automation to support services started in the 1960s at the Department of Defense, which used a top down approach, and Veterans Administration, which worked bottom up; the complicated histories of these developments spanned decades. Also in the MHIS marketplace were commercial entities, such as IBM, McDonnell Douglas (later Technicon), and many others. By the end of the 1980s the Institute of Medicine deemed that MHISs had reached sufficient maturity to warrant study, published as *The Computer-based Patient Record: An Essential Technology for Patient Care* in 1991. The development of functioning information technology for health systems had hit a plateau with the focus now shifting sharply toward informatics, e.g., the *use* of information and communications technology to produce safer, higher quality care for individuals and populations.

Keywords Multi hospital information systems • Functional capabilities • Early installations • Commercial systems • Translational databases • Federal sector systems • VA DHCP • DoD CHCS

Multi-hospital information systems (MHISs) are medical information systems (MISs) that service three or more hospitals with their associated medical offices,

---

Author was deceased at the time of publication.

M.F. Collen (deceased)

D.E. Detmer, M.D., M.A. (✉)
Department of Public Health Sciences, University of Virginia, Charlottesville, VA, USA
e-mail: detmer@virginia.edu

© Springer-Verlag London 2015   459
M.F. Collen, M.J. Ball (eds.), *The History of Medical Informatics in the United States*, Health Informatics, DOI 10.1007/978-1-4471-6732-7_10

clinics, and clinical support services. The important effect of economics on the development of MHISs was emphasized by Ermann and Gabel [39], who observed that at the time of the enactment of Medicare and Medicaid legislation in 1965, there were no investor-owned hospital information systems in the United States. By 1970 there were 29 investor-owned MHISs that owned 207 hospitals. In 1975 about 25 % of community hospitals belonged to a MHIS. In 1983 one in every seven hospitals, with nearly 19 % of the nation's hospital beds, was part of an investor-owned MHIS. In September 1984 there were 53 investor-owned systems in operation; the four largest, Hospital Corporation of America (HCA), Humana, Inc., National Medical Enterprises, Inc. (NMR), and American Medical International, Inc. (AMI), owned or managed 53 % of investor-owned systems of hospitals and 75 % of the hospital beds [39]. By the mid-1980s, 44 % of hospitals were part of some MHIS [102]. Ermann and Gabel [39] further explained that the increasing financial pressure on hospitals to remain solvent stimulated the growth of MHISs. Hospitals required large sums of capital to replace, renovate, modernize, and expand, resulting in an increased use of cost-based reimbursement by Medicare, Medicaid, and Blue Cross. It also reduced the hospital's incentive to control expenditures of finance capital in the least expensive manner, further fostering debt financing.

It was soon recognized that very complex information systems were essential if the perceived advantages of multi-hospital information systems (MHISs) over independent single hospital information systems (HISs) were to be fully realized. The expected advantages of MHISs included (1) economic benefits, including improved access to capital, increased efficiency, economies of scale, and ability to diversify; (2) personnel and management benefits, such as improved recruiting, and ability to develop and retain high caliber staff; and (3) planning, program, and organizational benefits with a regional rather than a local perspective on health needs; and greater power to control environmental factors [40].

When health care systems merged and evolved into a higher level of organization, such as was required in a MHIS, the amount of information that was processed at this new level was more than that at the lower levels owing to the greater diversity of the components. MHISs required more complex information systems with sophisticated communications and networks between facilities, and thus they evolved. The added information needs of a MHIS resulted from the associated responsibility for continuing, long-term patient care, such as under governmental sponsorship as in the Department of Defense and the Veterans Administration, or under private ownership such as health insurance agencies and health maintenance organizations. The need developed for MHISs to link and integrate all information from all affiliated facilities for each patient into one medical record for the full period of time that the health care program was responsible for the patient's care. In such large health care programs, patients moved continually between hospitals and clinics and physicians' offices; and sometimes these facilities were located some distances from each other. In such instances, the traditional separation of the patient's medical record in each facility could be a serious impediment to a good quality of continuing care. For example, a physician might be unaware of a prior treatment for a chronic or recurring ailment because the medical record had not arrived from another treatment facility. As a result, by the 1980s, larger health care systems in the United States were becoming more vertically integrated for all inpatient, outpatient, and ancillary services. In addition, they were acquiring multiple facilities and becoming more horizontally integrated to provide a broader range of acute, specialized, chronic, and extended care services.

10.1   MHIS Added Requirements

The functional and technical requirements for MHISs were basically similar to those described in Chaps. 5 and 6 for outpatient information systems (OISs) and hospital information systems (HISs). The primary differences in their requirements were in scale for an increased workload and broader communications and interoperability. Because a patient's data was collected in multiple facilities, MHISs had to link, communicate, and integrate this data among all these facilities, as well as between their multiple departments and subsystems. A completely integrated MHIS often had difficulty in meeting all the different objectives of its individual components. As a result, they usually exercised central coordination of their information services, supervised the security and confidentiality of computer-based patient data, and controlled the central databases for patients, personnel, services, and resources. Yet they generally supported decentralized computing applications to allow for differences in local business, administrative, and clinical requirements. In time, the MHISs usually provided centralized patient identification and eligibility files; scheduling, order entry, and results reporting for centralized services such as a regional laboratory; and tracking of pharmacy drug usage prescribed for patients by different physicians within multiple facilities. In the 1980s and into the 1990s users needed not only to exchange data between facilities, but also to exchange images and documents; they required electronic mail for interfacility consultations; they needed word processing and facsimile exchange; and they wanted online access to the National Library of Medicine's MEDLINE and its factual databases. For planning purposes, management sought patient demographic, broad environmental, and community social data.

Prior to the advent of open architecture systems in the 1980s, the technical specifications for a MHIS required uniform computer and communication standards for all hospitals and clinics in the system, so as to permit the integration of data from its various subsystem databases. Because MHISs required a high level of data integration, a single vendor was often mandated to support more consistent, interoperable, and compatible data handling procedures, file management, database organization, patient data security, computer hardware and software. In the 1980s and into the 1990s local area network (LAN) links were being used within most large hospitals between computers, between computers and workstations, and between workstations. Wide area networks (WAN) and satellite links were being used for communication between distant hospitals' computers. The new integrated services digital network (ISDN) began to allow integration of voice, text, and images on one physical line. The ability of ISDN to use twisted-pair cables within a hospital offered an alternative to other network technologies and permitted transmission of high quality images between hospitals.

10.1.1 Translational Databases

Frey [42] and associates at Stanford Medical Center described the Advanced Computer for Medical Research (ACME) system that was developed as a research database able to (1) handle many data sets of many varieties and sizes, some that had to be held for long periods of time and some that required frequent updating; (2) minimize inadvertent loss of data; and (3) serve a group of medical researchers who often were inexperienced in computer technology. A typewriter terminal-driven, time-sharing system, ACME was designed to acquire, analyze, store, and retrieve medical research data, and to control laboratory instruments; it was served by an IBM 360-50 computer, with access to 2,741 typewriter terminals, and a variety of laboratory instruments that were interfaced through an IBM 1800 analog-digital computer with disc drives for storage and magnetic tape storage for backup and archival storage.

Translational databases evolved in the 1990s with the development of federated databases and more advanced designs of database management systems to (1) optimize the translation, transformation, linkage, exchange, and integration of the increasingly voluminous medical information that was becoming accessible from many large databases in multiple institutions that were widely located, by using wide area networks, the Internet, and the World Wide Web; (2) provide access to high-performance, super-computing resources; (3) facilitate the concurrent query, analyses, and applications of large amounts of data by multidisciplinary teams; (4) encourage knowledge discovery and data mining, and support the transfer of new evidence-based knowledge into direct patient care; and (5) advance the use of biomedical computational methods. Since most data warehouses had been developed with database management systems that employed their own legacy and data-encoding standards, their source data usually required some reorganization and modification in order to be compatible and interoperable with data transferred from other data warehouses, and then be merged into a single database schema. Thus the development of translational database software became necessary.

Translational informatics was developed in the 2000s to support querying diverse information resources located in multiple institutions. The National Center of Biomedical Computing (NCBC) developed technologies to address locating, querying, composing, combining, and mining biomedical resources; each site that intended to contribute to the inventory needed to transfer a biosite-map that conformed to a defined schema and a standard set of metadata. Mirel and associates [94] at the University of Michigan described using their Clinical and Translational Research Explorer project with its Web-based browser to facilitate searching and finding relevant biomedical resources for biomedical research. They were able to query more than 800 data resources from 38 institutions with Clinical and Translational Science Awards (CTSA) funding. Funded by the National Centers for Biomedical Computing (NCBC), they collaborated with ten institutions and 40 cross-disciplinary specialists in defining task-based objectives and user requirements to support users of their project.

Denny and associates [31] at Vanderbilt University developed an algorithm for phenome-wide association scans (PheWAS) when identifying genetic associations in electronic patient records (EPRs). Using the International Classification of Diseases (ICD9) codes, they developed a code translation table and automatically defined 776 different disease population groups derived from their EPR data. They genotyped a group of 6005 patients in their Vanderbilt DNA biobank, at five single nucleotide polymorphisms (SNPs), who also had ICD9 codes for seven selected medical diagnoses (atrial fibrillation, coronary artery disease, carotid artery disease, Crohn's disease, multiple sclerosis, rheumatoid arthritis, and systemic lupus erythematosis) to investigate SNP-disease associations. They reported that using the PheWAS algorithm, four of seven known SNP-disease associations were replicated, and also identified 19 previously unknown statistical associations between these SNPs and diseases at $P < 0.01$.

10.2 Examples of Early Multi-Hospital Information Systems (MHISs)

In the 1960s The Sisters of the Third Order of St. Francis had a centralized administration for their multi-hospital information system (MHIS) that comprised 12 health care institutions; which included ten general hospitals, a continuing care center, and a geriatric care unit, all located in Illinois, Michigan, and Iowa. In 1961 a group headed by Huff [68] initiated time-shared services in their hospital in Peoria, Illinois; over the next few years they expanded the services to all their facilities. By the end of 1963, their MHIS provided centralized payroll, accounts payable, general ledger, financial reporting, accounts receivable, and inpatient billing. In 1970 they were acquired by the McDonnell-Douglas Automation Company (MCAUTO) of St. Louis, and became the Health Services Division of MCAUTO. In 1979 McDonnell-Douglas introduced its Patient Care System (PCS), after having acquired additional modules to provide a fairly comprehensive MHIS. In the mid-1980s it responded with its PCS to requests for proposals from the Veterans Administration (VA) and the Department of Defense (DoD). Lindberg [85] at the University of Missouri-Columbia, was already operating a MHIS for a statewide network in Missouri and using standard telephone lines. Lindberg found that the costs for transmission of data via telephone lines over a network were about equal to the costs for computer rental, but likely exceeded the computer problems in complexity and importance; and concluded that the issue of backup systems, ready access to distant medical communities, interactive inquiry for users, integrity of systems against unauthorized invasion of privacy, all depended primarily upon the capacity, adequacy, and cost of the data transmission services.

In 1975 when the Church of Jesus Christ of Latter Day Saints (LDS) divested itself of its LDS hospital holdings, Intermountain Health Care (IHC) was formed as a nonprofit multi-hospital corporation of 15 hospitals located in Utah, Idaho, and Wyoming. By 1982 IHC was servicing 22 hospitals with central services for applications such as payroll, general ledger, and productivity monitoring, designed for multi-hospital reporting and control; but the software had been developed permitting the sharing of a single S/38 IBM computer among multiple smaller institutions for decentralized data processing operations [53]. In the 1990s the IHC system expanded to provide comprehensive clinical support services in nine affiliated Intermountain Health Care Hospitals in Utah [46].

In 1973 the Health Maintenance Organization (HMO) Act was passed; by 1977 more than 150 HMOs were operational. Larger HMOs used multiple hospitals and office facilities and required the information processing capabilities of a multiple hospital information system (MHIS). In addition, to plan to meet their service requirements and an increasing competition, HMOs were dependent on an adequate, integrated database of their health plan members' demographic attributes, their members' utilization of services, the mix of health professionals needed to provide these services, the operational direct and indirect costs of all services provided, the facilities and equipment used and their capital costs, and the predicted changes of their competition and changes in their community [25, 132].

In 1994 Brigham and Women's Hospital joined with Massachusetts General Hospital to form Partners Healthcare System that included ten hospitals and more than 250 medical practice sites [125]. In 1994 the Harvard Community Health Plan merged with Pilgrim Health Care and in 1998 joined with the Harvard Vanguard Medical Group. The largest inpatient facility for their hospitalized patients was Brigham and Women's Hospital in Boston, with 720 beds; there an internally developed hospital information system, the Brigham Integrated Computing System built using Datatree MUMPS [118], had a patient database that already contained medical records for more than one million people and a PHARM system that contained some pharmacy data since 1981 [74]. By 1998, as a result of these mergers, automated pharmacy data for ambulatory patients with Harvard Community Health Plan could have their outpatient pharmacy data linked with their inpatient pharmacy data from their records with the Brigham and Women's Hospital [21].

10.2.1   Federal MHISs

The U.S. Public Health Service (PHS) began in 1976 to develop for its PHS hospitals its own multi-hospital information system (MHIS), called the Public Health Automated Medical Information System (PHAMIS). PHAMIS was designed to meet the clinical data processing requirements of nine hospitals and of 26 freestanding PHS clinics. The primary beneficiaries of the PHS hospitals and clinics were American seamen, active duty and retired uniformed members of the Coast Guard, members of the National Oceanic and Atmospheric Administration, and PHS officers. In his comments on the PHAMIS concept at the 1979 Symposium for Computer Applications in Medical Care (SCAMC), Glaser reported that in 1976 approximately 540,000 individuals received care in PHS facilities. The ultimate objective of PHAMIS was to replace the handwritten medical record with a computer-based health information system which would support patient care, hospital management, and clinical research activities.

In 1979 PHAMIS was still in a developmental stage. Its patient registration module gave patients a unique identification number and included demographic information. An admission, discharge, transfer (ADT) and bed-control system recorded the admission of patients to the facility and kept track of bed occupancy. At the PHS facility in Seattle, there was an appointment scheduling system in one clinic. An outpatient pharmacy module maintained a complete medication history, which included known allergies, as part of the patient's medical database. In 1979 an automated laboratory information system was in the procurement phase, to be interfaced with PHAMIS. Problem lists for outpatients were maintained in one clinic. The patient database stored all patient information in a single central file. With the same patient identification number used in all facilities, it was possible to integrate a patient record from different facilities by storing the information in a central database common to all facilities and also in local databases that were queried as required. For example, a request for a medication profile retrieved all the recent medications received, regardless of the dispensing facility. The PHS hospitals were closed in the 1980s. In 1981 Glaser founded PHAMIS, Inc., as a private vendor; and further development and marketing was continued commercially. By the end of the 1980s Seattle-based PHAMIS was installing its own MHIS, now called LASTWORD, with a long-term integrated relational database and modules for inpatient and outpatient care, in the Humana Hospitals system [89].

The U.S. Indian Health Service (IHS) had unique requirements for providing health services to its patients. In 1955 responsibility for the health care of Native Americans and Native Alaskans was transferred to the PHS from the Bureau of Indian Affairs. The Surgeon General established the Division of Indian Health to administer the program. In the 1960s there were 380,000 Native American and Alaskan people living in 23 states on federal Indian reservations and in Alaska [108]. In the 1970s the IHS took care of about 750,000 people and operated 52 hospitals, 99 full-time health centers, and several hundred health stations. Garratt [47] described the status of the MHIS being developed by the IHS in 1979 as being a widely dispersed, multi-facility, multi-disciplinary, multi-organizational, multi-level Patient Care Information System (PCIS) designed to operate in this environment. Prototype versions of PCIS became operational in southern Arizona in 1969 and in central Alaska in 1974. A pilot test of the PCIS was implemented in all IHS facilities in the states of Montana and Wyoming, and it became operational in December 1978. A second pilot test including all IHS facilities in Alaska became operational in April 1979.

A third large-scale project was initiated in 1979 on the Navajo Reservation. The PCIS maintained a computer-stored single record for each patient; and the record contained relevant health data from each encounter with all providers of care at all facilities. This required the linkage of health data from all sources of care. Multipart encounter forms were used by all health professionals to document all visits. The original copy of the encounter form provided the legal record of the patient visit and included prescription blanks for ordering medications, consultation and referral requests, appointment slips, and instructions to patients. Copies of all PCIS forms were mailed to a central data processing center in Tucson, Arizona, where ICD-9-CM codes were added for all diagnoses and to any narrative free text. The data were then entered by keyboard, and stored on magnetic tape. The tape files of data were then sent to the computer center in Albuquerque, New Mexico, where a master tape file was created from which all reports were generated. Computer output to microfiche was used to provide patient health summaries that contained significant medical data from all services. The health summaries were updated every 2 weeks and were distributed to all appropriate PCIS users. The average turnaround time from the date of encounter to the receipt and availability of health summaries back in Alaska was approximately 4–6 weeks [18]. The data available to a clinician at a facility included the facility's medical record, which contained the original copies of past input forms completed at that facility, together with paper copies of the computer-generated microfiche health summaries with essential medical information from all inpatient and outpatient facilities [131].

In 1983 the IHS implemented its Resource and Patient Management System (RPMS). This replaced the centralized PCIS, which had been programmed in COBOL language, and operated in a mainframe environment. RPMS used the VA Decentralized Hospital Computer Program (DHCP), which was programmed in the MUMPS language, used the DHCP File Manager database management system, and operated in a distributed minicomputer setting [30]. At the end of the 1980s, a typical RPMS configuration in a health facility included patient registration, pharmacy, dental, maternal and child health, contract health services, and laboratory, together with its Patient Care Component (PCC) [69]. The PCC of the RPMS used the File Manager database and provided a computer-based patient record for the collection, storage, and retrieval of the patient health data from all sites. Ultimately, the patient's health information from multiple facilities was integrated in the PCC database at each site where the patient had an active medical record. Revised multi-purpose forms were still used for collecting patient data, and the originals were filed in the patients' paper charts. A data entry module featured English language textual data entered from PCC encounter forms, with automated coding of the data where necessary. At that date the health summary report was the principal output of the PCC. A structured report extracted from the PCC database, it was displayed in a standardized format, printed routinely whenever a patient was seen, and updated by the entry of new data from the encounter forms. The health summary included an integrated report of the patient's demographic data, an overview of the medical history, a list of active medical problems, inpatient and outpatient visits, recent medications, laboratory test reports, allergies and immunizations, and health reminders. The facility's visual display terminals permitted users to retrieve a variety of other reports from a displayed menu. In 1989 the IHS had the PCC operational in 53 sites.

10.2.2   *Veterans Administration Decentralized Hospital Computer Program (DHCP)*

In the 1980s the Veterans Administration (VA), an agency of the federal government, operated 172 hospitals and 229 outpatient clinics. There were about 26 million veterans in the United States; the VA provided care to 1.5 million inpatients and furnished almost 20 million outpatient visits per year to these veterans. The VA was the largest centrally coordinated civilian health care system in the United States.

Since the 1950s the VA had maintained, in Chicago, a national centralized computer-based file of all VA patients that included their identification data, claims, and Social Security numbers. A Patient Treatment File contained inpatient admission and discharge data including diagnoses, surgical procedures, and patient disposition data. Initially, each month every VA hospital submitted a deck of punched cards to the processing center. Each card represented data covering a completed hospital episode for an individual patient [23]. They soon extended the Patient Treatment File to include outpatient visits and used this central database as their Automated Management Information System (AMIS) at the Veterans Administration Central Office [110]. Data from clinical records in all VA treatment facilities were coded locally onto standardized forms, and these coded data forms were sent to the computer center for editing and entry into the computer. These data were used primarily for statistical analyses by the VA Administration [28].

In 1960 the VA began to explore the use of computers in its medical program when it reached an agreement with the Systems Development Corporation in Santa Monica, California, to use the Los Angeles VA Center and the Wadsworth General Medical and Surgical Hospital to prepare a comprehensive HIS functional requirements description. Successful implementation of the total simulated hospital operations was started the last week of March 1962 [133]. In 1965 the VA installed a pilot Automated Hospital Information System (AHIS) in its 710-bed hospital in Washington, DC. They used an IBM 360/40 computer with 40 input-output terminal devices consisting of IBM 1052 typewriters and IBM 1092 keyboards with variable-overlay plastic key mats. Plans were to develop subsystems corresponding to the organizational divisions of the hospital: admissions and dispositions, medications, laboratory, radiology, dietetics, surgery, central services, clinic and ward care, patient information, and medical administration [111]. A regional data processing center was to collect and store the current patient-treatment data while the patient was in the hospital. Any permanently required data would be transferred into a Patient Treatment File in a central database, which would serve as the historical record of all treatment episodes for each person served by a VA medical installation. Budd [19], then chief data manager of the VA, reported that they expected the date for completion of the pilot AHIS project in September 1967. In 1968 and 1969, several modules were reported as being operational in the VA hospital in Washington, DC [24]. However, this pilot system was soon found to be an inadequate solution for the VA's requirements for an MHIS, and the pilot project was terminated. During the 1970s a variety of clinical computer applications were developed independently in several different VA hospitals, mostly using MUMPS software for applications programming and File Manager as the database management system [71].

The File Manager had its origin in the early 1970s at the Beth Israel Hospital in Boston as the MISAR application package [73]. MISAR (Miniature Information Storage and Retrieval System) was developed by Karpinski and Bleich [75] as a general-purpose, time-sharing, information storing and retrieval system that facilitated the rapid creation, maintenance, and searching of small data files. In 1978 the rewriting of the MISAR II program from a dialect of MUMPS into the Standard MUMPS language, while adding a substantial number of desired enhancements, was undertaken by a San Francisco VA hospital staff member [73]. The VA File Manager allowed the user to define new files; add new attributes to existing files; enter, edit, and delete data within those files; and then list or search the files for any combination of data elements [126]. Hauser [57] extolled the importance of the advocates of the MUMPS language in the development of the DHCP by noting that there were two non-VA organizations which had significant roles in the success of the DHCP, namely the MUMPS Users Group (MUG) and the MUMPS Development Committee (MDC), custodian of the MUMPS ANSI standard. Many VA medical professionals employed professional networks and used MUMPS to create small prototype applications in the clinic setting; this grass roots effort was dubbed the MUMPS "Underground Railroad."

In February 1982, to provide some central management, the VA Administrator developed a policy of support for the decentralized computer operations in the VA medical centers, and directed the establishment of six regional Verification and Development Centers (VDCs) to assist with the implementation of computer-based medical applications at the medical centers. In addition, a VA Project Management Task Force was formed to compile an inventory of computer capabilities in the field and to develop plans for implementing existing in-house developed software on available computers. In June 1982 the Medical Information Resources Management Office (MIRMO) was established to further the task force's objectives by assisting with the creation of the regional VDCs, developing a complete Department of Medicine and Surgery (DM&S) Automated Data Processing (ADP) Plan, and formulating procurement and budget strategies in support of field ADP needs [34]. Originally MIRMO had been given the responsibility for the planning, direction, and control of the DM&S information-system development program, but its overall responsibilities were re-delegated to the VA's regional directors and the VDCs. In April 1983 DM&S published its first ADP Plan that identified the major objectives of the Veterans Administration Decentralized Hospital Computer Program (DHCP): (1) Provide adequate ADP support for key functions in all VA medical centers; (2) Implement an integrated DM&S management information system; (3) Decentralize to the field the responsibilities for ADP planning, budgeting, and operations to the maximum extent possible; and (4) Improve the management of information resources [34].

In 1983 Special Interest User Groups (SIUGs) composed of field- and central-office program-area experts were established, and they initiated a department-wide computer literacy effort. The high degree of decentralization in the VA Decentralized Hospital Computer Program (DHCP) was demonstrated by the great responsibilities delegated to the SIUGs for system development. The SIUG's many responsibilities were to: (1) Recommend development, enhancement, and modification of a data processing system, and work closely with the Verification and Development Centers (VDCs) which were assigned the primary responsibility for the software development. (2) Establish priorities for system development. (3) Develop and maintain functional requirements for DM&S automated systems. (4) Provide professional assistance to the VDCs in the specialty area. (5) Assist VDCs in system validation and certification. (6) Recommend means for resolving conflicts between automated systems and the current modes of operation. (7) Participate in implementation planning and execution. (8) Monitor the status of system development in the specialty areas. (9) Represent the program area in DHCP/CORE activities. (10) Serve as an advocate for program-area interests in the competition for system resources (DM&S [35]).

Great authority was granted to the six Verification and Development Centers (VDCs), one for each VA medical region and to their Council, to ensure uniform and compatible systems throughout the VA. This arrangement essentially delegated oversight, direction, and control of the DHCP to the VDC Council. Each VDC provided a central point of technical expertise and support for its region and was responsible for installation, implementation, support, and maintenance of the DHCP CORE and all CORE applications in each VA medical center (VAMC) within the region. It was responsible for dissemination of standard programs, for new releases of existing programs and locally developed software, and for maintenance of an inventory of all software. The VDC assisted in the preparation, review, and approval of facility data processing plans. Some VDCs were also responsible for the development and maintenance of CORE software modules. The VDC Council was composed of six VDC directors, and was responsible for recommending software development and verification, and for providing guidance to the VA in the implementation of the DHCP. Coordination of activities at a national level was established to prevent duplication of effort, to assure exportability of systems, and to assure the rapid development of a complete VA Management Information System made possible by VA Standardized Data Dictionaries in use at every VAMC. To carry out the continuing decentralized effort, the DHCP was initiated and administered by the DM&S. Within the DHCP a DHCP Kernel and a DHCP CORE system were developed, both written in the MUMPS programming language and sharing a common patient database.

A set of software tools for database management, electronic communications, security, and software management, the Kernel provided the basic tools that held the system together and provided the means for individual sites to adapt to their unique user, database, and security needs. The Kernel allowed both centrally developed and locally adapted software to coexist [99]. Composed of routines that interfaced DHCP application packages with the MUMPS operating system, the Kernel insulated applications from operating system-specific concerns, and allowed the writing of applications that would run on any MUMPS operating system. The Kernel included the VA FileMan (File Manager), which was the database for the DHCP. Initially the CORE system of applications included patient identification and registration, admission/discharge/transfer, ward census, clinic scheduling, and outpatient pharmacy. The Full VA CORE system added inpatient pharmacy, clinical laboratory, and radiology [71]. The Full CORE system was planned for all VAMCs, with terminals located on wards for order entry and ward reporting.

Developers of the DHCPs recognized the importance of system and data standardization, and the difficulty of achieving standardization in a decentralized operation. Before any program was put into operational use at more than one location, it was verified by one of the Verification and Development Centers (VDCs). The Kernel database approach allowed system users to modify the CORE system at its local level; for example, by appending extra fields to the standard data elements of the CORE database, without foregoing standardization. The format, definition, names, and range of values of the CORE data elements were mandatory and could not be changed by an individual VAMC. The Department of Medicine and Surgery (DM&S) established a VA Hospital Information Systems Data Dictionary to mandate a common data structure for use in the various field-developed systems, and to insure standardization throughout the hospital network. By December 1987 the DHCP Data Dictionary comprised several volumes. For example, the second volume contained for each data element, a file location, label, type, and description. It had a glossary of specific terms used by the inpatient pharmacy and clinical laboratory. VA Medical Center (VAMC) directors had the authority to add optional application programs; they produced an Enhanced DHCP Software that was developed in the standard MUMPS programming language in various VAMCs, and was made available to other VAMCs that had a need for such support. Although not considered part of CORE, the Enhanced DHCP software was used in conjunction with the CORE system, sharing the same patient database. Enhanced DHCP software included the medical service, surgical service, radiology, dietetics, patient records tracking, nursing, mental health, social work, dentistry, and engineering. In 1982, so that they would conform to generally used community hospital standards, the computer programs were modified to permit the Patient Treatment File to calculate patients' length of stay, average daily census, projected annual hospital days, and required hospital beds. Later, an algorithm was added to adjust for diagnostic related group (DRG) classification for claims reimbursement [76]. In December 1982 legislation was passed that supported the VA program and directed the agency to concentrate its resources on DHCP implementation and to provide a single VA patient database that could be accessed by all users.

In 1983 the U.S. Congress, which controlled the VA's budget and had repeatedly directed the VA to examine commercially available vendor HISs, mandated (as it also did for the DoD TRIMIS program) that the VA procure, install, and assess three competing commercial HISs and compare their effectiveness for the VA DHCP. In

April 1986 the Congress's House Appropriations Committee requested an investigation be made into the progress of the medical computer program of the VA. The committee reported that VA DHCP contracts were awarded in 1984 to Shared Medical Systems for the Philadelphia VAMC; to McDonnell-Douglas Health Systems for the Saginaw, Michigan, VAMC; and to Electronic Data Systems for the Big Spring, Texas, VAMC. They were designated by the VA as the VA Integrated Hospital Systems (IHS) Program and were scheduled to end in 1987. The Medical Information Resources Management Office (MIRMO) awarded a \$2.9 million contract to A. Andersen to perform an objective evaluation of the three IHS test sites and to compare them to the VA DHCP. The House Appropriations Committee Report pointed out that the DHCP was not required to document performance, objectives, schedules, or fixed and operational costs, whereas the vendor Integrated Hospital Systems (IHS) sites were required to do so; thus comparable evaluations were not possible. The VA provided little management or staff support to carry out the IHS program, and it was generally acknowledged that the VA DHCP in the mid-1980s could not equal the capabilities of the commercial systems [26]. The 1984 DM&S ADP Plan reported that 429 DEC PDP 11/44 computers had been procured at a cost of \$48 million. Implementation of the DHCP Full CORE system began in 1985; in that year, the VA Decentralized Hospital Computer Program (DHCP) installed computer systems in 169 medical centers with the basic software package called the Kernel.

The Kernel was now written entirely in American Standard National MUMPS and included: FileMan (a database management system, data-entry editor, report writer, and data dictionary); MailMan (a computer-based messaging, teleprocessing, and networking system); a log-on security system; and a set of programs and tables to allow applications programs to be written in a manner independent of device; operating systems, communications protocols, and vendors [100]. A VA Integrated Planning Model was also developed in 1987 that ran on minicomputers and was programmed in the Pascal language [76]. A strong training program for users of DHCP contributed to the successful implementation of various modules. Computer overview classes were mandatory for all users and were held at least once a week. Attempts were made to teach physicians, nurses, etc., in professional groups, thus allowing user-specific issues to be addressed in the class; training manuals were developed as an important adjunct [20].

An independent review of the VA's DHCP conducted by the Office of Technology Assessment (OTA) of the U.S. Congress in 1987 produced an OTA VA report recommending that, if the VA was to implement at least a minimum level of automation in all its hospitals within the next year or two, the OTA found no reasonable alternative to the VA DHCP since DHCP modules offered reasonable features and functions to meet the VA's near-term needs for hospital information. In the long term DHCP might have limitations that could make it an unsuitable platform for the transition to the information system VA would need in the 1990s [105]. The OTA report included an analysis of the VA DHCP's costs: VA historical cost data and projections for the period 1983 through 1987 indicated that the total costs for Core Plus 8 would be about \$1.1 billion. VA's 10-year (fiscal years 1987–1996) lifecycle costs were estimated at about $930 million for six Core modules plus eight Enhanced Modules [105]. Since the VA Decentralized Hospital Computer Program was not yet an integrated system, but was rather a series of interfaced applications, the OTA report addressed its capability to integrate patient data entered and retrieved from the various system modules, a critical requirement of any MIS. A shortcoming observed in DHCP was the order entry/result reporting function that was inherently difficult to operate due to the separate development of the pharmacy, laboratory, and dietetics modules used on the nursing wards [105]. Andrews and Beauchamp [3] described the development of a pilot integrated uniform database (UDB) to extract patient data from the separate laboratory, pharmacy, and radiology databases installed at the Sioux Falls, South Dakota, VAMC. They found it difficult to integrate information across the modules, so they wrote a new set of programs, the clinical database management system (CDMS) that supported the UDB; and was used to assist most clinical functions. While the file structures were created and maintained with FileMan, the CDMS provided utilities for queries, reporting, entry, and translation of data from ancillary packages into the UDB, and provided some decision support. By the end of 1989 the DHCP contained clinical management packages for inpatient and outpatient pharmacy, clinical laboratory, radiology, anatomic pathology, blood bank, dietetics, medicine, surgery, oncology, nursing, mental health, dentistry, social work, quality assurance and utilization review, order entry, and results reporting. A health summary served as the beginning of a computer-based patient record that integrated clinical data from ancillary support packages into patient health summaries for viewing by clinicians on display terminals or as printed reports. VA admission, discharge, and transfer (ADT) module functioned as the focal point in the collection of patient information for DHCP to encompass demographic, employment, insurance, and medical history data; and was used by other DHCP subsystems including laboratory, pharmacy, radiology, and dietetics [35]. The decentralized nature of the VA DHCP program was clearly shown in its November 1989 report, which detailed the responsibilities of each of the VDCs, now called Information Systems Centers (ISCs): (1) The Albany ISC was responsible for the radiology, ADT, medical administration, and outpatient-scheduling and record-tracking packages; (2) Birmingham ISC for pharmacy, surgery, and social work; (3) Hines ISC for dietetics, nursing, and quality-assurance; (4) Salt Lake City ISC for laboratory, pathology, mental health, order entry and results reporting, and health summary; (5) San Francisco ISC for the Kernel FileMan; and (6) Washington, DC, for oncology, medicine, dentistry, library, and MailMan, in addition to Integrated-Funds Control, Accounting, and Procurement (IFCAP) [35].

In 1988 DoD awarded a contract to Science Applications International Corporation (SAIC) of San Diego, California, to implement DoD's Composite Health Care System (CHCS) with a MUMPS-based system derived from the VA DHCP experience [98]. At the end of 1989, the VA decided to award a contract for $52 million to SAIC to install health information systems at three of its medical centers [97].

10.2.3 Department of Defense Composite Health Care System (CHCS)

The Department of Defense (DoD) oversees a large health care delivery system with many and varied facilities that are managed and operated by the three armed services: the Army, Navy, and the Air Force. DoD provides a full spectrum of clinical and hospital services throughout the world to active-duty and retired military members and their eligible dependents, while it maintains a constant state of readiness to support the national defense. In the 1970s within the continental United States, there were nearly one million hospital admissions and about 35 million outpatient visits annually. Military medical facilities within the continental United States then numbered 126 hospitals; the 4 largest had up to 1,000 beds. All medical facilities had extensive outpatient services, with the largest having two million patient visits per year; and there also were several hundred free-standing clinics.

In 1959 the U.S. Air Force Research and Development Command at Andrews Air Force Base undertook with the Lovelace Foundation the development of a database on punched cards for the Air Force's Man in Space program. Data from a fairly comprehensive medical examination were recorded on mark-sense cards. The decks of cards were transferred to an IBM facility at Kirtland Air Force Base, where the data were assembled and were used to select candidates for the National Aeronautics and Space Administration (NASA) program [115]. In 1968 the Secretary of Defense directed that studies be made to determine the feasibility of improving health care delivery within DoD through the use of automated data processing. The period during the late 1960s and early 1970s also saw independent development efforts within each of the three armed services. In the late 1960s, with the Air Force as lead service, DoD undertook a project with A.D. Little, Inc. that resulted in a nine-volume, Systems Analysis for a New Generation of Military Hospitals [86]. Its aim was to use computers to improve patient care and to help to control resource consumption with a prototype hospital; but this hospital was never built [4]. In 1971 Craemer initiated service with an outpatient information system (OIS) at the U.S. Naval Air Station Dispensary in Brunswick, Maine, a primary care clinic that served about 15,000 active-duty and retired Navy personnel and their dependents (about 20,000 visits a year). Physicians dictated their patient care notes, and the full text was entered by transcriptionists using display terminal keyboards. The patients' medical complaints and diagnoses were coded, and then were stored by keyboard entry. Laboratory findings were entered by the clinical laboratory. Computer services were provided by a commercial vendor located about 130 miles away. The medical record available during a patient's visit was a computer-generated abstract that contained a limited amount of essential medical data. During the visit, more medical record data could be obtained, if needed, within a few seconds from the terminal on an online basis [64].

In 1973 the Defense Systems Acquisition Review Council (DSARC), with the concurrence of the three Surgeons General, recommended that the automated information systems development efforts of the three military departments be combined into a single tri-service program. In July 1974 the Deputy Secretary of Defense established the Tri-Service Medical Information Systems (TRIMIS) Program [15]. The mission of TRIMIS was defined as to: (1) Improve the effectiveness and economy of health care delivery administered by the Military Departments, through the application of standardized automatic data processing (ADP) techniques to health care information systems; (2) Centralize and coordinate the application of existing technology and the development of standardized automated systems to meet the Tri-Service functional requirements in the medical area; (3) Adapt advanced data automation technology to health care delivery, and streamline, modernize, and standardize DoD medical information systems [127]. Initially the TRIMIS requirements and direction were provided by the three Surgeons General. However, in June 1976 the TRIMIS Program Office (TPO) was formed, and its direct management was taken over by the Assistant Secretary of Defense for Health Affairs. Responsible for planning, budgeting, and managing program activities, the TPO focused its activities on achieving three related objectives: functional (work-center) applications to improve patient care; resources to improve management applications; and integration of functional and management applications into an overall replicable system to be applied first for a single hospital, and then for successively larger entities. The TPO centrally funded all tri-service systems and provided coordination and direction for the program. The Assistant Secretary of Defense for Health Affairs managed the TRIMIS program with the advice and guidance of the *TRIMIS Steering Group*. In addition to the three Surgeons General, this group included the Principal Deputy Assistant Secretary of Defense for Health Affairs as Chair, the President of the Uniformed Services University of Health Sciences, and representatives of the VA and HEW. In addition, three defined critical milestones in the procurement and diffusion of TRIMIS systems had to be reviewed and approved by the Major Automated Information Systems Review Council (MAISRC), which consisted of the Assistant Secretary of Defense Comptroller as Chair, the Assistant Secretary of Defense for Manpower, the Assistant Secretary of Defense for Health Affairs, and the Assistant Secretary of Defense for Command, Control, Communications, and Intelligence.

A TRIMIS Peer Review Group was assembled in 1978. An interdisciplinary body of nationally known experts from outside the Government, the group reviewed various aspects of the TRIMIS Program several times a year and provided their assessment of the Program's progress and activities to the Assistant Secretary of Defense for Health Affairs [14]. Managed in the late 1970s by Roberts of Medical Systems Technical Services, Inc., under contract with the National Bureau of Standards, throughout the 1980s, the group was managed by Simpkins of Battelle Laboratories through a contract with the TPO. Collen (Director, Division of Research, Northern California Kaiser Permanente), Cunningham (formerly Chief, ADP Management Branch, ODP), Dammkoehler (Department of Computer Sciences, Washington University), and McDonald (Chief Scientist, Missile System Division, Rockwell International Corporation) were continuing members of this Peer Review Group from 1978 to 1989. Other members who participated in the Peer Review Group in the later 1970s, included Cox (Washington University), Lindberg

(University of Missouri-Columbia), Reals (University of Kansas-Wichita), and Sorensen (Southern California Permanente Medical Group). In the later 1980s, they included Ball (University of Maryland Baltimore) and McDonald (Indiana University).

The basic planning document that guided TRIMIS decision-making within this rather complicated environment was known as the TRIMIS Master Plan (TPM) produced in the TPO in February 1977 [14]. The TMP was an overall technical approach to address its objectives through three levels of automated data processing capabilities, namely, the work center, the medical treatment facility (MTF), and DoD higher command; all were to be implemented through a four-phase time schedule. In phase I, Initial Operational Capabilities (IOCs) pilot systems were to be acquired by competitive procurements of commercially available applications modules to support selected high-volume work centers. Other than to accommodate such features as unique military data elements, there was to be no major modification to these systems. The strategy was for these IOC subsystems to achieve a significant level of standardization of their functional and operational characteristics within the work centers so that the experience gained from using these systems would lead directly to the determination of the functional specifications for the next phase. In phase II, Standardized TRIMIS Systems would evolve to permit some expanded functional support of additional work centers; to develop applicable TRIMIS standards necessary for integration of the initial modules; and to design a network-integrating system. In phase III, a Composite Hospital System (CHS) would be designed from the experience gained in the first two phases and culminate in specifications by which the Standardized Systems would be integrated within the medical treatment facilities (MTFs). In phase IV, a DoD Health Care Information System (HCIS) was to be implemented to manage both resource and patient-centered data on a system-wide basis; collect transaction data from a CHS or from Standardized Systems; provide patient record data and resource management data to multiple MTFs; and provide data to facilitate reporting requirements above the MTF level [127].

The initial DoD Master Plan was for the TPO to acquire the major automated support for the military treatment facilities in three procurement steps. First, a limited number of systems were to be procured to satisfy the immediate support requirements of the three armed services in four functional work centers: laboratory (LAB), pharmacy (PHARM), radiology (RAD), and patient appointment and scheduling (PAS). Next the principal thrust would be to interface these four modules in an operational environment through the development of a DoD Network Interface System. Finally, integratable systems to fulfill the CHS requirements were to be acquired in sufficient quantity to support all treatment facilities justified by the armed services. In advance of the development of the TRIMIS modules in the mid-1970s, each of the three services was allowed to proceed with some pilot automation projects in their larger hospitals. A clinical laboratory system was installed at Wilford Hall Air Force Medical Center; a pharmacy system at Charleston Naval Hospital; a radiology system at San Diego Naval Hospital; food service and hospital logistics systems at Walter Reed Army Medical Center.

One of the earliest TPO cost-benefit analyses was reported in 1978 for a Tri-Service Wards and Clinics Support module implemented as a part of the early CHS. It compared the automated system's costs and benefits to the traditional manual alternative in three medical treatment facility sites: the Naval Regional Medical Center, Jacksonville, Florida; the U.S. Air Force Regional Hospital, Eglin AFB, Florida; and the Dwight David Eisenhower Army Medical Center, Ft. Gordon, Georgia. Based on actual 1977 data from these three sites viewed as a single regional system, the total (11 years, discounted) cost for the TRIMIS system was 0.5 % less than for the manual system. The following were identified as quantified advantages of implementing the TRIMIS system in the hospital and clinics: reduction in the cost of patient services, notably of redundant or unnecessary services delivered to the wrong location or after the patient had left; reduction of clerical support required; improvement of outpatient pharmacy management and control; reduction in administrative supplies costs; and relief from an excessive clerical workload burden on military health care providers in reduction in patient non-effective time and time away from active duty. Unquantifiable benefits attributed to TRIMIS were improvements in the quality of information associated with patient care through more thorough accumulation, systematic organization, and accurate transmission. TRIMIS reduced the interval required to transmit information on admission, patient status, physicians' orders, diagnostic results, and supportive services throughout the medical treatment facility; and improved the accuracy of information by providing system edits that reduced the number of opportunities for error and the automatic transmission of multiple errors. By capturing data at their source, TRIMIS improved resource utilization, collected data for research and peer review activities, and supported consistent and reliable patient care planning and its documentation for the medical record [127].

By 1979 TRIMIS had made considerable progress with the procurement and installation of its phase I nonintegrated modules. In that year, the program provided full funding and management-support coordination for a number of existing operational, interim, and pilot systems. These included the following:

- Clinical Laboratory (AFCLAS/TRILAB and LABIS) systems at USAF Medical Center, Wright-Patterson AFB, Ohio; Malcolm Grow USAF Medical Center, Andrews AFB, Maryland; and the National Naval Medical Center, Bethesda, Maryland.
- Pharmacy (PROHECA/Data Stat) pilot systems at the Naval Regional Center, Charleston, South Carolina; Naval Hospital, Beaufort, South Carolina; USAF Clinic, Charleston AFB, South Carolina; Naval Weapons Station Clinic, Charleston, South Carolina; Outpatient Clinic, Charleston Naval Base, South Carolina; USAF Regional Hospital Shaw, Shaw AFB, South Carolina; and Dwight David Eisenhower Medical Center, Augusta, Georgia.
- A Tri-Service Formulary at Health Services Command, San Antonio, Texas, that supported 77 health care facilities.
- A Medical Administrative Management System at USAF Regional Hospital, McDill AFB, Florida; USAF Medical Center, Wright-Patterson AFB, Ohio; Wilford Hall USAF Medical Center and Lackland AFB, Texas.

- A Patient Registration System at Walter Reed Army Medical Center, Washington, DC.
- An Interim Hospital Logistics System and an Interim Food Service System at Walter Reed Army Medical Center, Washington, DC.
- An Automated Multiphasic Health Testing system at National Naval Medical Center, Bethesda, Maryland.
- A Clinical Decision Support system for hypertension and diabetes at the Naval Regional Medical Center, Oakland, California [14].

At that time TRIMIS also installed a Computer Assisted Practice of Cardiology (CAPOC) system at the Naval Regional Medical Center, San Diego, California, to provide electrocardiogram analysis to military facilities in southern California and portions of Nevada. They were also procuring an Automated Cardiac Catheterization Laboratory System (ACCLS) to provide 12 existing manual cardiac catheterization laboratories with a computer processing capability [14]. In 1979 the TPO had satisfied its phase I requirements. It had acquired an adequate number of commercial stand-alone Initial Operational Capabilities (IOCs) work-center systems and had installed them in military treatment facilities for pharmacy, laboratory, radiology, patient administration, and patient appointment and scheduling. The implementation of the IOCs created some user problems, since each was a separate operating unit, and without an integrating system, the professional users had to access each module individually to retrieve data from their respective databases. In February 1979 the Major Automated Information Systems Review Council (MAISRC) approved the installed IOCs as having achieved Milestone 0 for the TRIMIS program and authorized their further implementation to provide interim support in the larger DoD hospitals until replaced by the soon-to-be-initiated Composite Health Care System (CHCS). December 1984 became the target date for Milestone I to obtain the approval of the functional requirements, developed from the experiences of using the IOCs by the three armed services, for the core modules to be included in its phase II Network Interface System. These core modules included patient administration, patient appointment and scheduling, nursing, clinical laboratory, radiology, pharmacy, and clinical dietetics [129].

In March 1979 the TRIMIS Program Office received a critical report from Congressman Brooks, Chair of the House Committee on Government Operations, which stated that the TPO had spent or obligated approximately $70 million on TRIMIS since DoD assumed responsibility in 1974; that this money, for all intents and purposes, had been wasted; and after 5 years of operations few concrete results could be found. The Brooks report included a strong recommendation to terminate the outside contractor, a major reorganization of the TPO structure should be undertaken if the TRIMIS concept was to be saved; and systems to be procured, at least initially, should be commercial off-the-shelf items [17]. It was apparent to TPO and to the Peer Review Group that the Congressman had not fully appreciated the substantive accomplishments of TRIMIS under its many difficult constraints. Following the Brooks report, the TPO decided to skip phase II and to move directly into phase III, and to develop the requirements and plans for the acquisition of a comprehensive, fully integrated system, now called the Composite Health Care System (CHCS).

In 1980 the U.S. Congress directed the DoD to install and assess two or three competing commercial HISs, as it had for the VA. As a result, in 1982 DoD awarded three separate contracts to two vendors: Technicon Data Systems to install its system in the William Beaumont Army Medical Center at Fort Bliss, Texas, and Martin Marietta Data Systems to install its system in the Naval Regional Medical Center at Jacksonville, Florida, and in the U.S. Air Force Regional Hospital at Eglin Air Force Base in Fort Walton Beach, Florida. Using a phased approach, the plans selected by the Air Force and the Naval facilities consisted of initially bringing the registration, admission, disposition, and transfer module online [67]. This was to be followed by outpatient appointment scheduling and order entry and results reporting for pharmacy, laboratory, and radiology, with inpatient applications to be implemented last.

In 1981 A.D. Little, Inc. was awarded a contract to evaluate the TRIMIS IOC systems and to provide information needed for the decision regarding further system proliferation. Based on evaluations already completed, A.D. Little's project director, Drazen, estimated that the annual benefits of automated information systems in DoD medical treatment facilities would be derived from the following: 31 % from increased service capacity resulting from more effective utilization of the DoD health care system due to fewer repeat clinic visits because of missing laboratory tests, and a reduced length of hospital stay from more timely test reporting and earlier initiation of treatment; 28 % from increased availability of time on the part of the health care provider from less time spent in searching for charts and test results; 15 % increased availability in staff time due to less clerical time spent in scheduling, registering, and maintaining records; 15 % from improved patient health status from better review of care plans and treatments and automated monitoring of adverse drug reactions; 7 % increase in availability of effective time of military personnel due to less of their time being spent in obtaining needed office visits; and 4 % in other savings [37].

Because of its concerns about the possible duplication of effort between the DoD and the VA, Congress directed DoD to test the feasibility of using the VA Decentralized Hospital Computer Program (DHCP) software [26]. The MITRE Corporation had in 1984 completed an assessment of the VA DHCP's ability at that date to satisfy the functional requirements of the DoD's CHCS; and it reported that the TRIMIS functionality demonstrated by the VA system was adequate for the CHCS [96]. Tests were carried out using the VA DHCP software at March Air Force Base in Riverside, California, and at Fitzsimmons Army Medical center in Aurora, Colorado, to test the feasibility and cost-effectiveness of the VA DHCP in DoD MTFs. To determine the cost and level of effort required to meet the Composite Health Care System (CHCS) requirements using DHCP as a baseline [93]. Some evaluation results were reported, such as the early findings from A. D. Little on the VA Patient Appointment and Scheduling (PAS) module of the DHCP at March Air Force Base that had been chosen because of the high priority placed on this application by its hospital commander. The VA PAS was readily modified to meet the requirements of March Air Force Base; its users were generally pleased with the system [50].

In 1984 to accomplish a more complete integration of all the military MISs, the Assistant Secretary of Defense for Health Affairs established the Defense Medical Systems Support Center (DMSSC) composed of six program offices: TRIMIS and Hospital Systems; Defense Enrollment Eligibility Reporting System (DEERS); Medical Readiness and Theater Systems; Management Information Systems; Architecture, Communications and Technology; and Quality Engineering. Mestrovich, who had headed DEERS, was appointed the first director of DMSCC. In 1984 the experience gained from these assessments became the basis for the specific requirements developed for the Composite Health Care System (CHCS). In May 1985 the TPO released to commercial vendors a Request for Proposals (RFP) for the design, development, deployment, and maintenance of the CHCS. Detailed and comprehensive as to functional and operational requirements, the RFP kept technical specifications to a minimum to encourage competing vendors to use products they had already developed. The RFP specified that CHCS should support the full set of CHCS system capabilities for eight functional areas: patient administration (PAD), patient appointment and scheduling (PAS), laboratory, radiology, pharmacy, nursing support, clinical dietetics, and health care provider support. Detailed functional requirements for each of these areas were presented as appendices. The RFP further specified that the CHCS contractor should provide a Data Base Management System (DBMS) as the primary vehicle through which the CHCS database would be constructed, accessed, and maintained. The DBMS requirements for CHCS fell into seven major functional areas: general DBMS requirements, integrated data dictionary, data base management, data query and data transactions, report generator, DBMS backup and recovery, and data base utilities. TPO recognized the need for requiring a capability for maintaining the logical integrity of the data base [130]. It was also required that users of the DBMS had online access to their Integrated Data Dictionary, which was to have a set of basic characteristics that included unique identifiers, physical characteristics, and textual information for each data element; showed the relationships between elements; contained the official external name and acceptable synonyms for each data element, the type of units to be used for the data items (for example, degrees Celsius, milligrams); and the rules or algorithms to be used by the DBMS for data elements which were computed from the values of other data elements (for example, body surface area). An English-like query language was to be a highly supportive interactive display of the data dictionary, with prompts, HELP messages, query and modification status displays. The Report Generator was to have the capability of generating low-resolution simple graphic outputs such as scatter plots, histograms and pie charts; for data security, it required the capability to record the name of the user, the identification of the actual device used, and the dates and times of log-in and subsequent log-off. The CHCS System Manager was to have the capability to prevent dial-in access to CHCS without the System Manager's approval for each dial-in session. The RFP required that CHCS have the ability to communicate with other external support services, including the Tri-Service Food and Tri-Service Logistics systems; and it specified that the CHCS Contractor should utilize the Reference Model for Open Systems Interconnections (OSI) developed by the International Standards Organization for these interfaces. It also required an interface with DEERS that provided the basic eligibility information on all DoD personnel. The RFP furthermore specified that the contractor should provide initial and follow-up training programs specific to military treatment facility users that included supervisors, professionals, and clerks and administrative personnel [130].

Earlier the TRIMIS Program Office had developed a statement that described the requirements for a Computerized Medical Record Information System (CMRIS) for both hospital and outpatient care, since the TPO had expressed the need that readily accessible patient medical information was necessary to provide the military health care provider with accurate, timely, legible, and well-organized medical information to support the patient's treatment and follow-up care. Thus the CMRIS RFP required that the automated comprehensive medical record (inpatient and outpatient data) would be a component part of the Composite Health Care System (CHCS) database so that required data could be transmitted automatically [129, 130]. As a part of the CMRIS project and to obtain some experience with other computer-based patient records, the Computer-Stored Ambulatory Record (COSTAR) was installed in 1981 in the Family Practice Clinic in the Silas B. Hays Army Community Hospital at Ford Ord, California, [103] and also in the Family Practice and Primary Care clinics at the USAF Hospital Pease at Pease Air Force Base, New Hampshire, that used the time-sharing capabilities from G. Barnett's Laboratory of Computer Science at the Massachusetts General Hospital [38]. Because the Brooks Congressional Committee considered the computer-based patient record and the health care provider functional requirements as "gold-plated" enhancements of CHCS, both of these requirements were removed from the 1984 RFP; and a second RFP for CHCS was released in March 1987. Even at the end of the 1980s, however, CHCS had not yet planned to provide an integrated, computer-based medical record, nor did it satisfy such functional requirements of the health care professional as the inclusion of patients' medical histories, physicians' physical examination findings, or consultation reports. These functions were to await a later phase of CHCS enhancements in the 1990s.

In September 1986 a stage I, cost-plus-fixed-fee contract was awarded to four contractors: TDS Healthcare Systems Corporation (formerly Technicon Data Systems), McDonnell-Douglas Health Information Systems, Science Applications International Corporation (SAIC), and Baxter International, Inc. The contracts specified that each was to develop a proposal to meet the functional and technical requirements of CHCS. Since a system design was not specified in the contract, the vendors were allowed considerable flexibility in this regard, but TDS Healthcare Systems soon withdrew from this contest. Following extensive tests, demonstrations, and evaluations, DoD conducted a complex, competitive bidding process among the remaining vendors. In March 1988 the Milestone II review was completed that authorized proceeding with the installation of CHCS in selected sites; and DoD awarded a stage II fixed-price contract in the amount of about $1.1 billion to SAIC for the development and deployment of CHCS. The report of the Source Selection Evaluation Board concluded that SAIC was clearly superior to its competitors: it developed more health care functionality, offered the only completely integrated system, received slightly better ratings than its nearest competitor in management, and slightly lower ratings than the highest-rated competitor in deployment. In addition its system cost was significantly less than the nearest competitor's system. The U.S. General Accounting Office (GAO) published a report that called the selection process results fair and reasonable [48].

An employee-owned company in San Diego, Science Applications International Corporation (SAIC) used a major software contractor, Di-Star, whose founders had helped develop the MUMPS-based VA DHCP [70]. MUMPS users were delighted with the selection of SAIC and its proposed MUMPS-based CHCS, and published an announcement that DOD had awarded to SAIC a $1 billion, 8-year contract for a MUMPS-based integrated hospital information system. SAIC's major subcontractor for most of the CHCS hardware components was Digital Equipment Corporation (DEC). The selected CHCS architecture was to be decentralized at the hospital level, with a mainframe computer in each hospital linked to its associated clinics with a communications network. Independent clinics that were separate from hospitals were to receive their own mainframe computer. All software was to be written in ANSI-standard MUMPS. The database manager was FILEMAN, an updated version of the VA's FileMan. A comprehensive data dictionary, SCREENMAN, provided a standard terminal-display presentation and editing tool. TASKMAN allowed control over the timing and priority of both interactive and batch processes. MAILMAN provided electronic mail to all users.

Mestrovich [93] described the planned operational features of CHCS in 1988. The CHCS would provide the health care providers with patient care data through integration with the functional work centers of clinical dietetics, laboratory, nursing, patient administration, patient appointment and scheduling, pharmacy, and radiology. It would assist health care professionals by providing support to the entry of orders and the reporting of results, and support administration in quality assurance, management of resources, mobilization, and mass casualty operations. CHCS would also provide interfaces to other TRIMIS and DoD activities such as the Medical Expense and Performance Reporting System (MEPRS), DEERS, food service, medical logistics, service-specific administrative systems, tactical automation systems, national disaster medical system, and the VA systems. CHCS would provide support to military hospitals, clinics, dental clinics, and Service schools throughout the world. Eventually 14 sites were selected for Stage II CHCS beta testing: the Bethesda, Camp Lejuene, Charleston, and Jacksonville Naval hospitals; the Carswell, Eglin, Keesler, Shaw, and Shepard Air Force hospitals; and the Eisenhower, Ireland, Nuernberg, Tripler, and Walter Reed Army hospitals. By the end of 1989 DoD had ten operational CHCS beta test sites; and deployment activities were under way at four additional sites for operational testing and evaluation [2]. Most of the stand-alone IOC modules were expected to be replaced in the early 1990s by CHCS installations.

Following full deployment, the annual operating cost of CHCS in 167 military hospitals and 583 clinics worldwide was estimated at $108 million [93]. This level of expenditure obviously called for appropriate cost-benefit evaluations. The TPO prepared a two-stage Test and Evaluation Master Plan (TEMP) to review and monitor in selected sites the extent to which the installed CHCS fulfilled its specified functional and technical requirements. The first stage included pre-installation and acceptance testing to see whether the contractor's system met the functional and technical requirements prior to the system deployment. The initial alpha testing of CHCS software was conducted at Ireland Army Community Hospital in Fort Knox, Kentucky, and at Tripler Army Medical Center in Hawaii, after which the approved software was released to beta test sites. The second stage included installation and acceptance testing of the CHCS at each beta site. Data collection at the beta sites began at the end of 1988, and analysis and reporting of evaluation results of CHCS to be completed by Milestone III in the early 1990s, at which time worldwide deployment would be authorized. The A. D. Little group obtained a contract to provide a CHCS benefits assessment that used a list of 168 pre-specified measures and indicators as evidence of obtained benefits. Data that measured these indicators of potential benefits were to be collected at the beta sites (and also at matched non-automated control sites) prior to the implementation of CHCS (so-called "period X") and scheduled for release in 1990. These period X data then would be compared to data collected for these same indicators after each CHCS site became operational (in "period Y") in the 1990s [87]. The TPO was especially interested in the determination of any significant changes in the quality of health care services following the introduction of CHCS. The system would be assessed in regard to whether it effectively performed all the required functions in typical DoD medical treatment facilities; whether the process of delivering health care services became more efficient after the CHCS was introduced; whether the system was easy to use; whether it was flexible enough to handle future workload expansion and technological developments; whether the training procedures were adequate; whether the system provided the required security, confidentiality and data integrity without constraining legitimate authorized access; and whether the system exhibited in the operational environment, the desired reliability, availability, restorability and safety characteristics [128].

In the 1970s and 1980s the TRIMIS Program Office provided an instructive model for the development of a very large MHIS. The TPO first developed detailed functional requirements by user committees. It then procured, tested, and evaluated vendor-supplied, prototype, stand-alone modules for all major functional departments. Following this, it revised its functional requirements and technical specifications for integrating all modules into one CHCS. Finally, after competitive bidding, it contracted for a phased-in procurement and installation of CHCS in all of DoD's worldwide military medical facilities. DoD also contracted for and completed an independent cost-benefit evaluation of CHCS. Despite its shortcomings, by the end of the 1980s, DoD's CHCS represented the largest and most comprehensive MHIS in the world.

10.3   Mental Health Information Systems

Mental health information systems was the term used by Hedlund [61] at the University of Missouri-Columbia in a review of computers in mental health hospitals. Such systems attempted to integrate information about mental health care from a number of different sources in order to satisfy a variety of administrative and clinical needs. Laska [80] noted that the magnitude of the economic costs to society of mental illness was already immense. In the United States almost half of the hospital beds in the 1970s were set aside for the treatment of the mentally ill.

Glueck [51] described the operation of a psychiatry information system using an IBM 1440 computer, partially funded by NIMH, at the Institute of Living, a 400-bed private mental hospital in Hartford, Connecticut. Their first data reporting process used descriptive statements of patient's behavior that were listed on punch cards. Numbers corresponding to the appropriate statements were circled, key-punched, and processed to produce a set of narrative statements corresponding to the patient's behavioral index [51]. The primary objective of the computer project was the application of automated techniques to the clinical aspects of hospital care [13]. It was this system's emphasis on clinical applications directed to individual patient care that served as an operational model for other mental health information systems [61]. By 1980 Glueck's staff had developed programs in such areas as mental status, behavioral assessment, biofeedback monitoring, automated nursing notes, computerized education, and psychophysiological monitoring [27]. The need for adequate information about the mentally ill was so basic that the National Institute of Mental Health (NIMH) and many state departments of mental health shared in the financial support of many of the early mental hospital information systems. However, governmental support sometimes emphasized administrative needs over clinical needs of mental health institutions. This led Lindberg [84] to ask whether computer applications and systems in mental health were being shaped by exterior mandates such as the production of mental health statistical reports, and to advise that computers should be primarily used to help in patient care, to help to improve the lot of the patients, and increase our understanding of mental illness. Consistent with Lindberg's advice, clinically oriented mental health information systems soon became more common.

Hedlund [61] credited the National Institute of Mental Health (NIMH) with funding the earliest mental health information systems, and reported that in the mid-1970s there were five multi-state mental health information systems in the United States. The Fort Logan Mental Health Center was one of the first to automate a relatively comprehensive psychiatric patient record system that became operational in 1961. In 1962 the Camarillo State Hospital in California, with NIMH funding, became what is generally considered to be the first large inpatient facility to attempt to computer- process comprehensive psychiatric case- record data in a time frame prompt enough to be of day-to-day clinical use. In 1966 the Missouri Division of Mental Health initiated a statewide information system. Begun as a joint project with the Missouri Institute of Psychiatry, a branch of the University of Missouri [119], the Missouri Mental Health Information System provided support to five large mental hospitals, three large community mental health centers, three state schools and hospitals for the mentally retarded, and nine smaller regional centers for the developmentally disabled.

Also in the 1960s a multi-state mental health information system was developed at the Rockland Research Institute in Orangeburg, New York, a state mental institution with a capacity of 5,200 beds, in a program that grew to involve seven states in developing a common computer-based patient record system designed to follow the patient through all phases of psychiatric service [79]. In 1966 Laska had used an IBM 360/30 computer for its computer-based electronic patient record (EPR) system at the Rockland State Hospital. In 1967, funded in part by a 5-year demonstration grant from the NIMH, the system was expanded to support five large mental hospitals, three large community mental health centers, three state schools and hospitals for the mentally retarded, and ten regional centers for mental retardation and developmental disabilities. Its software was compatible with IBM 360/370 model computers. In 1968 the IBM 360/30 computer was replaced by a 360/50 model and an IBM 360/44 computer was added for backup; each had direct-access disk drives and optical mark page readers. Remote terminals included an optical mark page reader and a keypunch machine linked to the central computer by telephone lines. In 1970 the files at Rockland contained more than 20,000 patient records from 13 facilities in seven states (Connecticut, Maine, Massachusetts, New Hampshire, New York, Rhode Island, and Vermont); and had about 300,000 patient records in its database.

Using a central IBM 370/155 computer in its Institute of Psychiatry, with remote terminals in each facility, it provided a computer-stored database for clinical and administrative information. Computer-generated reports provided clinicians, supervisors, and auditors with information about which patients had been treated, which patients were receiving what types of treatment for what types of problems, and which patients were receiving multiple or even incompatible medications [59, 61]. The electronic patient record included identifying data, examination and treatment data, medical problems, mental status examinations, medical and neurological examinations, medications, laboratory reports, and follow-up information after discharge. Users recorded the data by placing marks on forms that either were read directly by an optical mark reader to a card-punch machine or were keypunched. The forms were generally designed as multiple-choice checklists to reflect the clinical information from all health professionals who came in contact with the patient. The records included both hospital inpatients and patients seen in other psychiatric settings, such as clinics and community health centers. Data were transmitted in batches to the central computer over telephone lines from card-reader terminals located in each participating facility. The computer updated the patient's record as indicated, and sent back a series of reports reflecting the information received. These reports included daily patient census, narratives based on mental status examinations, progress notes, and admission-record face sheets. The psychiatric services rendered to a patient could be identified in their continuity through different services in various types of facilities, for example, inpatient service in a state hospital or day care in a clinic. The same computer record followed as a patient moved from facility to facility.

In 1972 all participating states began contributing to its operating costs [29], and in 1974 this Multi-State Information System began to operate as a nonprofit, user-supported system. By 1975 they had added to their system the states of Hawaii, South Carolina, and Tennessee, as well as the District of Columbia [80]. In 1975 they replaced the IBM 360/50 computer with an IBM 360/67 model [131]. Their database contained all their accumulated patient records, in addition to information needed for generation and transmission of reports and reference tables. Each facility was allocated a storage area to contain its files. Since these computer-based storage areas were physically distinct, each facility's data were protected from unwarranted access and accidental damage while the computer system processed another facility's files. Provision was made within the database to link separate episodes within the patient records. In some facilities, the records for many episodes were linked together by the same case number. Other facilities allocated a new case number for each episode, including multiple episodes occurring within the same facility; these facilities, in most cases, used the patient's Social Security number for linking episodes. The master patient record file and case index were stored on direct-access devices. Magnetic tapes were used to store historical copies of the patient files. In 1973 the files had grown to include approximately 165,000 patient records.

Using the central IBM computer in its Institute of Psychiatry, with remote terminals in each facility, it provided a computer-stored database for clinical and administrative information. Computer-generated reports provided clinicians, supervisors, and auditors with information about which patients had been treated, which patients were receiving what types of treatment for what types of problems, which patients were receiving multiple or even incompatible medications [60, 61]. In 1980 visual display terminals with keyboards for data entry replaced the optically scanned forms [78]. The team developed a Patient Narrative Document Display Program in which they entered the information that had been filled out on their periodic evaluation record document. This information was then processed to produce a narrative equivalent to the data just entered. The narrative was then displayed to the user, who could make changes, if necessary, to the original input. The system permitted the user to request a complete record or selected areas of specific interest. More than one user with a display terminal could access the database simultaneously. The group also developed a psychotropic-drug monitoring system that provided prescribing rules for medications as they were ordered. Lists of exceptions to approved rules provided alert to clinicians and supervisors to the occurrence of possibly inappropriate prescribing practices [114].

To satisfy the strict legal requirements for maintaining the confidentiality of psychiatric patient data, the group set up the system in a way that each terminal had access to only its own data files and could not access those of any other terminal. Personnel at each terminal dialed the computer when data were ready to be transmitted. A password was required to identify the individual. Failure to provide the correct password resulted in the immediate termination of the call. Passwords were changed periodically and as needed. At the headquarters, guards were posted 24 h a day to prevent unauthorized personnel from entering the computer room [29]. After visiting the Rockland Center, Wiederhold [131] reported that data were protected by limiting physical access to the terminal sites and by using passwords, and this protection was considered adequate.

Community mental health centers (CMHC) were usually understaffed and underfunded, but were well suited to use computer-based interviews. Harman and Meinhardt [56] explored the use of automated multi-test evaluations that eliminated the need for human raters, and provided a comprehensive and reliable method for acquiring data directly from patients. He proposed that for a community mental health center, an independent automated data-acquisition and follow-up system could be operated by community volunteers or other nonprofessionals. Such a system could produce printouts of comprehensive intake and follow-up evaluations, and provide a coordinated identification and tracking system utilizing a uniform data-acquisition and follow-up system for all county agencies. The results of a 1978 survey of the directors of 149 community mental health centers indicated that there was then a moderate use of computers, primarily in administrative areas; three-fourths of the centers had computer applications for financial procedures and for external reporting to accountability sources; and some automation had been applied to client monitoring and to program evaluation [49].

As a centralized approach to support computer applications in community mental health centers, the NIMH designed a prototype minicomputer-based management information system for such centers. The NIMH system comprised seven subsystems. The first was the Service/Activity Event Monitoring Subsystem which collected, organized, and reported data related to the services provided and the activities performed by community mental health center personnel [134]. The second subsystem provided patient demographics and case-manager caseloads. The remaining subsystems were for accounts receivable and billing, cost finding, general accounting, payroll/personnel reporting, and statistical analysis. Hedlund expressed hope that community mental health centers had the potential of improving direct patient care [58, 62].

10.4 Commercial Vendors' MHIS

In the 1950s users of commercial mainframe computers began to explore the capabilities of vendors' time-sharing computers for data processing in hospitals; and in the 1960s some hospitals began to use commercial time-sharing computer systems. In 1961 the Sisters of the Third Order of St. Francis established a centralized administration for their 12 health care institutions that included ten general hospitals, a continuing care center, and a geriatric care unit, located in Illinois, Michigan, and Iowa. In 1961 a group headed by Huff [68] initiated time-shared services in their hospital in Peoria, Illinois; and over the next few years expanded the computing services to all their facilities. By the end of 1963 their multi-hospital information system provided centralized payroll services, accounts payable, general ledger, financial reporting, accounts receivable, and inpatient billing. In 1970 they were acquired by the McDonnell-Douglas Automation Company (MCAUTO) of St. Louis, and became the Health Services Division of MCAUTO.

In 1964 the Information Systems Division of the Lockheed Missiles and Space Company in Sunnyvale, California, began to apply their aerospace expertise to develop a Lockheed Hospital Information System. In 1969 the Lockheed management decided to develop its Lockheed HIS in the El Camino Hospital in Mountain

View, California, a 464 bed, general community hospital with a medical staff of 340 physicians [44, 45]. In 1971 Lockheed sold its system to the Technicon Corporation, which had come to dominate automation in the clinical laboratory; its new owner, Whitehead, saw an opportunity to extend computer automation from the clinical laboratory into the entire hospital information system by developing its Technicon Medical Information System (MIS). In March 1971 the El Camino Hospital signed a contract for the installation of the Technicon MIS, that operated on an IBM 370/155 time-shared computer located in Technicon's Mountain View offices [116]. In 1972 the Technicon MIS was installed at the Ralph E. Davies Medical Center in San Francisco that operated off of the Technicon regional time-sharing computer center. In 1973 the first in-hospital computer installation was implemented at the Nebraska Methodist Hospital in Omaha. The next two systems Technicon installed ran from the company's second regional center in Fairfield, New Jersey; one was at St. Barnabas Hospital in Livingston, New Jersey, the other at the Maine Medical Center in Portland. In 1975 Technicon installed its system at the Clinical Center of the National Institutes of Health. Initially operated from a time-shared computer at the Technicon Fairfield Center, it was later transferred to the NIH computer facility in Bethesda, Maryland. The El Camino Hospital continued through the 1980s to operate with a time-shared computer.

In 1980 the Technicon Data Systems Corporation (TDS) was acquired by Revlon, Inc. In 1986 it was repurchased by a new company called TDS Healthcare Systems Co., headed by the son of the founder of Technicon; its enhanced TDS 4000 system was announced in 1987 [22]. By 1986 the Technicon Data Systems (TDS) MIS had been installed in about 40 hospitals [16]; by the end of the 1980s, 85 TDS systems had been installed in the United States, Canada, and the United Kingdom. These installations included the Clinical Center in the NIH and sites in major teaching institutions such as New York University, Temple University, Medical College of Virginia, University of Illinois, Loyola, University of Chicago, Baylor University, and University of California at Irvine [66]. The Lockheed HIS that was initiated in 1966 became the Technicon MIS in 1971, and then the TDS. It was probably one of the best commercially developed HIS in the United States throughout the 1970s and 1980s, although it had deficiencies, such as a discontinuous patient record that did not integrate patient data collected over multiple admissions, and it did not allow for an office information system. By the end of the 1980s enhancements had been added to the TDS 4000 system that partially corrected these deficiencies by an expanded electronic patient record (EPR) with linkages of the hospital system and to attending physicians' offices. In 1986 Technicon TDS was sold to Revlon; and it became Allscripts. In 2008 Allscripts acquired several health care information system vendors and became a major vendor for electronic health record (EHR) systems.

In 1965 a survey of computer-based information systems in medicine by Summerfield and Empey [124] at Systems Development Corporation (SDC) in Santa Monica, California, listed 73 ongoing projects developing hospital information systems or subsystems. In a review of commercial HIS vendors in the 1960s, Jacobs [72] noted that it was not until the mid-1960s that vendors began to take notice of the potential of the hospital data processing market. In 1966 Honeywell announced the availability of a business and financial package, acquired from Blue Cross of Minnesota, for a shared hospital data processing center. International Business Machines (IBM) followed in the next year with Shared Hospital Accounting System (SHAS). Lockheed and National Data Communications, Inc. (then known as REACH, Inc.) began the development of HISs to be offered to hospitals on a turnkey basis. In the late 1960s MEDELCO, Inc. brought a simplified HIS to the market that met with some success.

In 1968 Thompson in the Department of Health Services in Los Angeles County, California, operated a large countywide system with terminals at 48 different sites that provided patient identification data, clinic registration and appointment scheduling with a limited amount of clinical information for about 550,000 patient visits a year. Thompson also operated at the East Los Angeles Child and Youth Clinic, California, a Los Angeles County-supported clinic that collected patient data on paper forms, coded the data by a medical technician, and entered the data by keypunch off-line batch processing to provide a supplement to the paper-based medical record for about 10,000 patients [64]. In 1969 a centralized information system for nine Los Angeles County Hospitals was initiated using an IBM 360/40 computer connected by telephone cable to remote display terminals and printers, located initially in the admitting offices and pharmacies, and then to a centralized patient records database, it soon added order entry of medications, diets, and laboratory tests [113].

In 1968 a survey conducted for the National Center for Health Services Research and Development (NCHSR&D) reported that in the United States about half of the 1,200 hospitals with more than 200 beds used computers for some business functions, but only about 15 % of these had some operational medical or medical research computing applications. For 248 respondents who used computer manufacturers for advice or assistance in the development of their hospital computer activity, the following vendors and the number of systems they had installed were listed as IBM 168, National Cash Register 37, Honeywell 19, Burroughs 10, UNIVAC 10, General Electric two, RCA one, and unspecified one [65]. An Arthur Young & Co. report identified four well-known, large, time-sharing HISs capable of servicing several hospitals in the 1960s [117]. The Medi-Data system, formed by a group of four hospitals in North and South Carolina, shared a common data processing center using Burroughs computers [6]. In an attempt to maintain low operational costs, Medi-Data avoided the use of real-time processing and provided all output reports on a regularly scheduled basis; its terminals were designed for use by clerks rather than by health professionals. The Medinet system, based on General Electric (GE) equipment, was used in a number of hospitals in the New England area. The MISs Program (MISP) used a number of programs developed at teaching hospitals supported by research grants, and was designed for the IBM 360 series of computers. Fourth was the Technicon HIS which also used IBM equipment. By the end of the 1960s a number of commercial HISs were competing for what was heralded as a potentially great market.

In the early 1970s a series of reviews [6, 8, 9] reported on the status of vendor HISs and added the following as offering systems that attempted to meet the needs for comprehensive services: Biomedical Computer Services, which focused on the medical record, and used a variety of computers linked to touch-screen terminals; Control Data Corporation (CDC); MEDICOM, which used CDC computers connected to CDC touch-screen terminals; Medelco's Total HIS (T.H.I.S.), which used prepunched cards for each order, service, or product available in the hospital and read into a hard-wired, pre-programmed machine; McDonnell-Douglas Automation Company (MCAUTO), which in 1970 acquired the HIS of the Sisters of the Third Order of St. Francis; Medical Information Technology, Inc. (Meditech), which originated with the MUMPS founder Pappalardo, and initially used DEC or Data General minicomputers with display terminals and their own software developed for a relatively comprehensive integrated HIS; National Data Communications, whose Real-Time Electronic Access Communications for Hospitals (REACH) System used Honeywell and other computers connected to Raytheon cathode ray tube (CRT) display terminals with 20 selector push buttons located along the left side of the display for order entry and routine tasks; and a keyboard for entering textual data; Searle's Medidata System, with touch terminals that used sets of overlays (for example, one for laboratory, another for pharmacy, and so on), each of which presented 320 order choices in addition to display terminals with keyboards for entry of text. However, Searle offered Medidata for only a few years when it was taken over by Mediquip, a subsidiary of Quanta System Corporation and Spectra Medical Systems, which used a Data General Nova minicomputer connected to color display terminals with keyboards and light-pen selectors designed for data entry by physicians. In 1974 Huff and associates, who had developed the system at the Sisters of the Third Order of St. Francis Hospital acquired by MCAUTO, left MCAUTO and formed HBO and Co. [73]. In 1975 the company unveiled a new second-generation level-1 system, MEDPRO, which used modern cathode ray tube (CRT) order-entry terminals [7].

Until the mid-1970s the majority of hospitals subscribed to out-of-hospital, shared computing services [11]. In the mid-1970s lower-cost minicomputers introduced the capabilities of locating small, special purpose computers in various departments, all linked to one or more central, large mainframe computers. Ball [10] considered this distributed approach to functionally oriented HISs a major change in their development. The use of minicomputers in subsystems such as laboratory and pharmacy expanded the concept of a HIS into a network of interrelated, modular, functional processing systems. In the mid-1970s a survey of computer applications in approximately 100 hospitals in the United States reported that only about one-third had clinical laboratory or other patient care applications [120]. In 1976 a Spectra 2000 system for 800 beds was installed at Rush-Presbyterian-St. Luke's Medical Center in Chicago; in 1980 it was replaced by a Spectra 3000 system that was linked to minicomputers and used visual display terminals with light-pen selectors for users to select items from displayed, predefined data sets. Physicians entered their orders directly, and a nursing module was well accepted [109]. In 1976 Bleich, Slack and associates at Beth Israel Hospital in Boston initiated their HIS. In 1982 they expanded it into the Brigham and Women's Hospital. By 1984 it ran on a network of Data General Eclipse minicomputers that supported 300 video-display terminals located throughout the hospital. In 1994 Brigham and Women's Hospital joined with Massachusetts General Hospital to form Partners Health Care *System* including 10 hospitals and more than 250 practice sites [125].

After reviewing the history of the diffusion of HISs through the early 1970s, Jacobs [72] concluded that there had been a rapid growth that decade in the number of hospitals with on-site computers, especially in the larger, general, not-for-profit, non-governmental hospitals. In a smaller survey of computer applications in approximately 100 responding U.S. hospitals [120], three-fourths indicated they had some computer applications for administrative functions, and about one-third reported clinical laboratory or other patient care applications. Ball [12] and Jacobs reported that although level-1 HISs, which provided primarily administrative, business, and communication applications had begun to be accepted in the second half of the 1960s, a 1974 survey showed that the majority of hospitals still subscribed to out-of-hospital shared computing services. However, the percentage of short-term general hospitals with in-hospital computers had increased from 30 % for small hospitals to 75 % for hospitals with 500 or more beds. Other surveys of U.S. hospitals found that 80 % in 1975 and 90 % in 1976 used some sort of data processing for business applications [1].

In 1976 a prototype of IBM's Patient Care System (PCS) began to be implemented as a joint project with Stead and Hammond's group at Duke University Medical Center in Durham, North Carolina. The Duke HIS used an IBM 3033 computer with IBM's IMS database management system and its terminal handlers [55]. It used IBM 3278 visual displays with light-pen selectors; and its terminals were available at each nursing station and in each service department. It stored all clinical information in its database and was interfaced with Duke's outpatient information system (OIS) and system known as The Medical Record (TMR). The initial Duke HIS transmitted its OIS prenatal records to the inpatient obstetrics department when a woman in labor was admitted [55].

By 1984 the Duke HIS serviced 52 nursing stations containing an aggregate of 1,008 beds, and was linked to 18 service departments and 64 specimen laboratories [121]. Microcomputers were used as departmental workstations linked to the central computer. In 1987 the Duke HIS central computer was upgraded to an IBM 3090–200 computer that serviced 550 display terminals. It used an application generator program called the Application Development System (ADS), also marketed by IBM. IBM's Patient Care System (PCS) was also developed to run under ADS [77]. IBM's PCS/ADS provided the development-modification tools for any desired modifications after the delivered applications had been installed and thus served as an application-enabling system for large mainframe HISs. In 1987 IBM announced its Patient Care System/ Application Development System (PCS/ADS) was available as a licensed product for ADS-based application development [63]. Through the 1980s IBM continued to provide most of the mainframe HISs in the United States. In parallel with the development of the Duke HIS, IBM also began in 1976 to install its PCS using an IBM 370 computer at Parkland Memorial Hospital in Dallas, Texas, where it was called the Parkland Online Information System (POIS), and was under the direction of Mishelevich and associates; by 1978 a relatively comprehensive HIS was operational with terminals at all 40 nursing stations [95].

In 1979 McDonnell-Douglas introduced its Patient Care System (PCS), after having acquired additional modules to provide a fairly comprehensive HIS. In the mid-1980s it responded with its *MCAUTO PCS* to requests for proposals from the Veterans Administration (VA) and the Department of Defense (DoD). In 1979 Fetter [41] described a Yale University microcomputer-based MIS (medical information system) using a Digital Equipment Corporation (DEC) 16-bit LSI-11 processor, with computer terminals installed in Yale's radiology department and clinical laboratory.

At the end of the 1970s Maturi and DuBois [90] conducted a survey for the National Center for Health Services Research (NCHSR) of the state of commercially available hospital department information systems (HISs), including their relationship to hospital-wide communication systems. The department-specific applications that they reviewed were medical record room functions (tracking charts, coding diseases, and similar record librarian activities); and also laboratory, radiology, and pharmacy systems; but they did not include computer-based patient records or general clinical applications. They reported that the department specific subsystems were usually acquired by the hospital before a hospital-wide communication system was in place. However, many department-specific systems soon became part of a communication network as industry provided expanded interfacing capabilities, a trend which encouraged distributed systems involving department-specific and hospital-wide systems. They reported that the major clinical laboratory vendors at that time were Becton Dickenson, Technicon, Medlab, and Community Health Computing. The major vendors of radiology systems were Siemens and General Electric; and of pharmacy systems were Becton Dickenson, International Business Machines, and Shared Medical Systems.

At the end of the 1970s, Young [137] and associates at the University of Southern California also conducted a survey of minicomputer-based HISs in medium-sized hospitals with 100–300 beds. They identified 75 different applications that they grouped into five levels or steps of difficulty in a modular implementation of an HIS. They found that essentially all had level-1 hospital applications (primarily by batch processing), which included billing and accounting, payroll, and inpatient census. Some also had level-2 hospital applications (with limited online data entry), which included admission-discharge-transfer (ADT), patient record data collection, patient identification number assignment, general ledger interface, and credit and collections. Only about one-half of the hospitals had level-3 hospital applications (using online data entry terminals), which included order entry transmission, message communication, patient number retrieval, discharge abstract preparation, and various inventory applications. Less than one-fourth had level-4 hospital applications (with most functions automated), which included patient identification number (ID) assignment, discharge analysis and reports, laboratory worksheets and schedules, budget preparation and expense reports, and labor time collection. Few hospitals in this survey had level-5 hospital applications (with two-way data transmission and clinical functions), which included test results reporting, medical chart reports, personnel history, and utilization review. Young [137] concluded that smaller HISs with minicomputers fell short of the more sophisticated HISs in larger hospitals with mainframe computers supporting a variety of patient care applications.

In the late 1970s and early 1980s constant changes occurred in the vendors providing HISs as increasing competition resulted from the new hardware and software that evolved in this time period. Among some of the more notable changes were the following: HBO expanded and acquired new subsystems; Whittaker Corporation's MEDICUS, initially organized in 1969, acquired Spectra Medical Systems; Perot's Electronic Data Systems (EDS) expanded into the HIS market in 1980; and IBM offered its new PCS with some applications developed at Duke University Medical Center and Parkland Memorial Hospital [72]. In the early 1980s federal legislation gave a major impetus to HISs when Medicare reimbursement policies changed to require the payments for hospital services to Medicare patients be made on the basis of classifying patients' conditions into Diagnostic Related Groups (DRGs). As a result, every hospital in the United States providing care to Medicare patients required major changes in its HIS to accommodate these DRG requirements.

In the early 1980s strategies for designing an HIS were sufficiently advanced that a hospital administrator could select the HIS functional components desired and refer to the Automated Hospital Information System (AHIS) Component Catalog developed at the Health Services Research Center of the University of Columbia-Missouri by Leonard, Goldman, and associates. This document described 112 commercially available components that might be used to design an HIS, and it provided standardized descriptions of cost and performance of each component [82, 83]. Young [136] published an *Automated Hospital Information Systems Workbook* in two volumes: the first was designed to guide the planning, selecting, acquiring, implementing, and managing a HIS; and the second described 180 available HIS applications, and the characteristics of 24 HISs available from 22 vendors. In 1980 a survey by Ball and Jacobs [7] found that 18 HIS vendors provided some nursing, pharmacy, laboratory, and radiology functions. Another survey by Ball and Jacobs [12] found that 18 vendors offered second-generation, Level-1 HISs (which provided some nursing, pharmacy, laboratory, x-ray, and medical record-room functions, in addition to business and administrative applications); more than 500 such systems had been sold as of the spring of 1980. As of that time, eight vendors also offered Level-2 HISs which also provided a computer-based patient record (CPR) and supported nursing and clinical applications. In the 1980s local area networks (LANs) permitted their users with inexpensive microcomputers to integrate their various individual databases into large, centrally shared databases. Multiple computers in affiliated hospitals began to use communication networks to link their hospital databases.

In 1981 Grams [52] at the University of Florida initiated a series of annual surveys of HISs in the United States, offering the data collected in 1982 prior to the imposition of DRGs and the new federal requirements for prepaid medical care as a reference point for analyzing any new changes or trends in HISs. In the 1982 survey, 37 % of 1,430 responding hospitals reported that they used their own in-house developed financial computer system (of these, 55 % used *IBM* computers, 14 % used *NCR*, 13 % used Burroughs, and 4 % used DEC computers); 42 % of the respondent hospitals used a vendor-maintained turnkey financial system (of these, 26 % used Shared Medical Systems (SMS), 25 % used McDonnell-Douglas Automation Company (MCAUTO), 5 % used Systems Associates, Inc. (SAI), and 2 % used HBO systems). In 1984, only 30 % of 1,263 respondents used an in-house developed financial system (with approximately the same distribution of computer vendors as in 1982); 44 % used vendor turnkey systems (of these, 24 % used SMS, 19 % used MCAUTO, 8 % used SAI, 5 % used HBO, and 2 % used Dynamic Control Co (DCC) financial systems. The success of vendor time-shared systems such as SMS and MCAUTO for hospital business and financial applications was highly apparent.

The responding hospitals also reported on hospital nursing-station and order-entry systems. In the 1982 survey, 7% used an in-house developed system (of these, 64 % used IBM computers, 9 % NCR, 7 % Burroughs, 7 % DEC computers); 14 % used vendor turnkey systems (40 % used HBO, 23 % SMS, 14 % MCAUTO, 4 % Technicon, and 3 % used EDS systems). In the 1984 survey, 8 % used in-house developed nursing-station and order-entry systems (of these, 56 % used IBM, 16 % DEC, 7 % Burroughs, 6 % NCR, 1 % Data General computers); 16 % used vendor turnkey nursing systems (34 % HBO, 21 % SMS, 11 % MCAUTO, 5 % Technicon, 5 % DCC, 4 % EDS, 4% Meditech, and 3% SAI systems [52].

Rozner [112] noted that competition was intense with over 150 companies providing products and services to support hospital computerization, with IBM, SMS, and MCAUTO accounting for 45 % of the total market in 1982. In the 1984 and 1985 market, after several acquisitions and mergers, eight vendors accounted for almost one-half of the total market revenues: IBM for 19 %, SMS 10 %, McDonnell-Douglas (formerly MCAUTO) 7 %, Baxter Travenol (who acquired Dynamic Control Co.) 4 %, Meditech 1 %, and SAI 1 % [106].

In the 1980s Leberto [81] ranked the top vendors of HISs with patient care systems by their 1986 sales (in millions of dollars), as follows: IBM $925; SMS $350; McDonnell-Douglas $185; DEC $175; Data General Corp. $140; Unisys Corp. $125; Baxter Management Services $115; NCR Corp. $75; Hewlett Packard $50; Technicon Data Corp $40; Professional Healthcare Systems, Inc. $30; Systems Associates, Inc. $30; Meditech $28; Tandem Computers $25; Ferranti Healthcare Systems Corp. $20; Motorola Computer Systems $15; Electronic Data Systems $15; 3 M Health Information Systems $12; and Gerber Alley $12.

Through the 1980s *IBM* continued to provide most of the mainframe HISs in the United States. Ball [5] observed that despite the diversity of the marketplace with more than 400 vendors, *IBM* still comprised the largest one-vendor commitment to HISs, with 34 % of HISs using IBM computers. Over half of these used IBM mainframes, while the remainder used mini- and/or microcomputers; about half of the IBM mainframe users relied on in-house development rather than on turnkey systems; and over 70 % used IBM Patient Care System (PCS).

Stoneburner [123] listed 73 vendors of outpatient information systems (OISs) in the United States. Friedman and MacDonald [43] reported that more than 100 different varieties of personal computers were available for use by physicians, most of them based on 8-bit microcomputer chips; but 16-bit microprocessors were beginning to appear in 1983. Lund and associates [88] at the Henry Ford Hospital in Detroit, Michigan, reported the installation of a broadband, cable-television LAN that connected by cable a variety of computers located in seven buildings. The system was capable of transmitting digital computer data, as well as analog video information. In 1985 the Health Data Sciences (HDS) Corporation in San Bernardino, California installed a pilot system of its Ulticare HIS, a bedside terminal system that used keyboard data entry, in the 1,120-bed William Beaumont Hospital in Royal Oaks and Troy, Michigan. This system used distributed Data General minicomputers for its applications, and one archival computer that stored a duplicate copy of all information. By 1989 the Ulticare HIS with a MUMPS-based operating system had 15 operational applications, including a computer-based patient record, order entry and results reporting, patient assessment, care planning, patient scheduling, nurse charting, and medication programs. Humana, Inc., Louisville, Kentucky, that operated 88 hospitals nationwide, also began using the Ulticare system [101].

By the second half of the 1980s, a large HIS generally used a mix of large, mini- and microcomputers linked by a LAN. More advanced HISs linked clinical data to the financial database and permitted association of quality-assurance measures with cost data, so as to provide guidelines for more cost-effective procedures [135]. By 1987 almost all hospitals with more than 100 beds had a HIS financial system, and 44 % had a nursing station order entry system [122]. About 20 % of U.S. hospitals had computer links between their HISs and affiliated physicians' offices. Some had workstation terminals that enabled data to be exchanged, copied, and modified; some permitted direct access to laboratory and radiology reports from an office information system [104]. Such linkage required additional security procedures to protect patient confidentiality and to prevent unauthorized access to patient data. Linkage of a HIS to staff physicians' offices was encouraged because it facilitated the transfer of results of diagnostic tests to the physicians [91]. In 1987 a Medical Software Buyer's Guide listed more than 900 products that included software for laboratory, pharmacy, and radiology systems [107]. Leberto [81] ranked the top vendors of HISs with patient care systems by their 1986 sales (in millions of dollars), as follows: IBM 925; SMS 350; McDonnell-Douglas 185; DEC 175; HBO & Co. 145; Data General Corp. 140; Unisys Corp. 125; Baxter Management Services 115; NCR Corp. 75; Hewlett Packard 50; TDS Corp. 40; Professional Healthcare Systems, Inc. 30; Systems Associates, Inc. 30; Meditech 28; Tandem Computers 25; Ferranti Healthcare Systems Corp. 20; Motorola Computer Systems 15; Electronic Data Systems 15; 3 M Health Information Systems 12; and Gerber Alley 12.

The fifth annual edition of the *Computers in Healthcare* (1988) market directory listed 750 vendors of computer systems and supplies available to the health care industry. Hammon [54] noted that average hospital data processing costs, as a percentage of the hospital budget, had increased from 2.85 % in 1985 to 3.73 % in

1987, an increase of 30 % in 2 years; and that the use of computers in hospitals was moving from the financial applications to the clinical applications. Dorenfest [36] also reported that the number of hospitals using computers for other than finance had risen dramatically as computers moved into patient registration, pharmacy, nursing, and laboratory; when the manual systems that supported patient care processes in the 1960s proved inadequate in the 1980s, there was a huge opportunity to improve hospital operations through better automation in the 1990s.

By the 1990s most hospitals had a variety of integrated or linked clinical subsystems. In 2010 commercial vendors of the systems reported that Meditech had 1,212 EHR installations, Cerner Corporations 606; McKesson Provider Technologies 573, Epic Systems 413, Siemens Healthcare 397. In 2014 Epic Systems Corp. was reported to be the top vendor of complete EHR systems used by physicians and other professionals who earned Medicare incentive payments for using the technology, according to federal data; and Cerner Corp. led among the smaller number of physicians who used modular EHR systems.

10.5 Summary and Commentary

Up to the 1980s, the two largest multi-hospital information systems (MHISs) in the United States were independently developed: one by the Veterans Administration (VA) for its hospitals, and the other by the Department of Defense (DoD) for its hospitals. Both systems were similar in their requirements in that each served more than 100 hospitals with associated clinics in the continental United States, and both began to develop their systems in the 1960s. Both ended up with MUMPS-based software systems; each was operated by a different national governmental agency, but the multimillion-dollar annual budgets of both were controlled by the U.S. Congress. There was a difference in design and development taken by these two systems, in that DoD took a centralized "top-down approach" in which a central office for the three armed services, the TRIMIS Program Office (TPO), did all the planning, developed the functional and technical requirements, budgeted for and procured its hardware and software, and installed and maintained all of its medical treatment facilities. The VA, on the other hand, took a decentralized "bottom-up approach," in that the development of functional and technical requirements, all software development, installation, and maintenance of all systems were done in the various VA Medical Centers (VAMCs). The DoD implemented its stages of system evolution by purchasing vendor turnkey systems, whereas the VA DHCP was predominately an in-house development. Costs for the DoD system were closely monitored each year. In the VA system, only VA budgeting and hardware procurement were done centrally; therefore, only the costs for procurement of hardware were monitored, since most other systems and software costs were absorbed by the local VAMCs and these costs were not always identified. DoD contracted for independent evaluation of the effectiveness of achieving its system objectives and of the cost-effectiveness of system modules, whereas the VA evaluated the effectiveness of system modules by its own regional Verification and Development Centers (VDCs), and it did so primarily for purposes of standardization and transportability. User satisfaction was variable in the DoD systems, whereas in the VA systems user satisfaction was generally high wherever the software had been locally developed. These two examples of MHISs sponsored by the U.S. government were of special interest, since they demonstrated that, with relatively unlimited resources, huge MHISs could be implemented successfully using different approaches. Since the SAIC's DoD's CHCS that was installed in all DoD medical centers had some features of the VA's DHCP, and since both systems were using similar computers and MUMPS-based software, some potential benefits were possible if the DoD and VA information systems would eventually become interoperable.

By the end of the 1980s, the multi-system information systems had matured such that the Institute of Medicine decided that a committee should be formed to examine the impact of this maturing technology on the future of medical care. The report from this group, *The Computer-Based Patient Record: An Essential Technology for Patient Care*, was released in 1991 and re-released in 1997 with an update [32, 33]. Morris Collen was a member of the study and was responsible for the choice of its title, the computer-based patient record. With the exception of the challenge of managing personal authentication since the use of a unique national personal health identifier was banned from the USA in the mid-1990s and interoperability among EHRs, the era of health information technology (HIT) research and development had largely ended, that is in the context that practical systems for the mass market were now available and being used in a variety of clinical care settings. Looking forward, the challenging work that remains relates to informatics versus information technology (IT) per se, e.g., the science of the *use* of information and communications. Improving user interfaces as well as better natural language processing remain with us and these are not to be trivialized but some consider these to be informatics rather than IT challenges. Informatics challenges in terms of better decision support, system improvements through the use of "big data" analytics, etc., gain ever more attention as healthcare budget pressures rise.

As noted earlier, the next two decades saw continued expansion of a few large MSIS into broader commercial use. Following the federal investment in EHRs through the HITECH provisions of the Recovery and Reinvestment Act of 2009, a few vendors, especially Epic, separated from the pack as industry consolidation occurred [58].

One could argue that from 2000 through today much of the excitement and continued development in MSIS have related to communications rather than information technology and its impact on care. From the personal digital assistants of the period from 1999 to the emergence of the iPhone in 2007, linking providers and other users to EHRs data, especially via secure websites referred to as "patient portals," has represented the most dramatic leap of technology. Telemedicine that had required large investments of personnel and equipment by MSISs for image transfers and assured connectivity suddenly began to merge into a routine care dimension furthered by the arrival of the iPad and other tablets.

The HITECH provisions also placed a premium on Health Information Exchanges (HIEs) to deal with the continued angst especially among care providers over the lack of interoperability and limits to secure data exchange. HIEs had been around using different terminology, e.g., community health information networks (CHINs) among other titles, for a few decades as efforts were made to improve interoperability across MSIS.

Alas, their major limitation was not technology per se but rather the absence of a sustainable value proposition to underwrite the costs relating to assuring that the system remained live. While HIEs hold great value to the overall system, their function as a utility failed since no single player seemed willing to come forward to pick up the costs over time. Further, few innovators have figured out an acceptable way for all users of the commons to support the service. Even today there are too few working examples akin to the Indiana Network for Patient Care that imports data from 103 of Indiana's 120-some hospitals and their hospital-based outpatient practices as well as four small ones that are mostly based in surrounding states (Michigan, Ohio) and include some of the border hospital systems It is managed by the Indiana Health Information Exchange, a non-profit organization [92]. The HIEs remain as arguably the dominant challenge for HIT and MSISs in this nation today.

References

1. Abdelhak M, Firouzan PA, Ullman L. Hospital information systems applications and potential: a literature review revisited, 1982–1992. Top Health Inf Manag. 1993;13:1–14.
2. Andreoni AJ. From the DMSCC directors desk. CHCS Parameters. 1990;1:1.
3. Andrews RD, Beauchamp C. A clinical database management system for improved integration of the Veterans Affairs Hospital Information System. J Med Syst. 1989;13:309–20.
4. Baker BR. The Tri-Service Medical Information System (TRIMIS) Program: an overview. In: Emlet HE, editor. Challenges and prospects for advanced medical systems. Miami: Symposia Specialists; 1978. p. 171–4.
5. Ball M. Integrating information systems in health care. In: Bakker AR et al., editors. Towards new hospital information systems. Amsterdam: North-Holland; 1988. p. 39–44.
6. Ball MJ. An overview of total medical information systems. Methods Inf Med. 1971;10:73–82.
7. Ball MJ, Jacobs SE. Information systems: the status of level 1. Hospitals. 1980;54:179–86.
8. Ball MJ, Hammon GL. Overview of computer applications in a variety of health care areas. CRC Crit Rev Bioeng. 1975;2:183.
9. Ball MJ, Jacobs SE, Colavecchio FR, Potters JR. HIS: a status report. Hosp JAHA. 1972;46:48–52.
10. Ball MJ. Computers-prescription for hospital ills. Datamation. 1975;21:50–1.
11. Ball MJ. Available computer systems. In: Ball MJ, editor. Selecting a computer system for the clinical laboratory. Springfield: Thomas; 1971. p. 54–73.
12. Ball MJ, Jacobs SE. Hospital information systems as we enter the decade of the 80's. Proc SCAMC. 1980;1:646–50.
13. Bennett WL. A viable computer-based hospital information system. Hosp Manag. 1967;103:43–7.
14. Bickel RG. The TRIMIS concept. Proc SCAMC. 1979;839–42.

15. Bickel RG. In: Emlet HE, editor. The TRIMIS planning process: decisions, decisions, decisions. Miami: Symposia Specialists; 1978. p. 175–81.
16. Blum BI. Clinical information systems. New York: Springer-Verlag; 1986.
17. Brooks J. Congressional memorandum re: Investigation of the TRIMIS Project. Washington, DC: U.S. Congress; 1979.
18. Brown GA. Patient care information system: a description of its utilization in Alaska. Proc SCAMC. 1980;2:873–81.
19. Budd PJ. Planning a comprehensive hospital information system. International advanced symposium on data processing in medicine elsinore, Denmark; 1966.
20. Catellier J, Benway PK, Perez K. Meeting the DHCP challenge: a model for implementing a Decentralized Hospital Computer Program. Proc SCAMC. 1987:595–8.
21. Chan KA, Platt R. Harvard pilgrim health care/Harvard vanguard medical associates. In: Strom BL, editor. Pharmacoepidemiology. 3rd ed. New York: Wiley; 2000. p. 285–93.
22. Childs BW. TDS is changing to meet the challenges of the future. Healthc Comput Commun. 1987;4:12–3.
23. Christianson LG. Medical data automation in VA. Mil Med. 1964;129:614–7.
24. Christianson LG. Toward an automated hospital information system. Ann N Y Acad Sci. 1969;161:694–706.
25. Coleman JR, Kaminsky FC. A computerized financial planning model for HMOs. In: Hinman EJ, editor. Advanced medical systems: the 3rd century. Miami: Symposia Specialists; 1977. p. 187–95.
26. Congress. House Appropriations Committee Report 1986. Washington, DC: U. S. Congress, 1986.
27. Conklin TJ. A data support system for clinicians. Proc SCAMC. 1980;2:913–22.
28. Cope CB. A centralized nation-wide patient data system. In: Acheson ED, editor. Record linkage in medicine. Edinburgh: E & S Livingstone; 1968. p. 34–8.
29. Curran WJ, Kaplan H, Laska EM, Bank R. Protection of privacy and confidentiality: unique law protects patient records in a multistate psychiatric information system. Science. 1973;182:797–802.
30. Curtis AC. Portability of large-scale medical information systems: the IHS-VA experience. Proc MEDINFO. 1986;86:371–3.
31. Denny JC, Ritchie MD, Basford MA, Pulley JM, Bastarache L, et al. PheWAS: demonstrating the feasibility of a phenome-wide scan to discover gene-disease associations. Bioinformatics. 2010;26:1205–10.
32. Dick RS, Steen EB, Detmer DE. The computer-based patient record: an essential technology for health care. Washington, DC: National Academy Press; 1997. Revised Edition.
33. Dick RS, Steen EB, Detmer DE. The computer-based patient record: an essential technology for health care. Washington, DC: National Academy Press; 1991.
34. DM&S Automated Data Processing (ADP) Plan, Fiscal Years 1984–1989. Washington, DC: Veterans Administration, Medical Information Services Management Office (MIRMO); February 1984.
35. DM&S. Decentralized Hospital Computer Program (DHCP). Washington, DC: Veterans Administration, Medical Information Resources Management Office (MIRMO); 1988.
36. Dorenfest SI. The decade of the 1980's: large expenditures produce limited progress in hospital automation. US Healthc. 1989;6:20–2.
37. Drazen E, Metzger J, Koran R, Nadell A. Benefits of automation within DoD Hospitals. Proc SCAMC. 1982;441–4.
38. Ehemann LJ. Computerized medical record information system (CMRIS): COSTAR experience in USAF Hospital Pease, Pease AFB, New Hampshire. 1st annual TRIMIS program conference. Bethesda, MD: Uniformed Services University of the Health Sciences; 1982. p. 55–6.
39. Ermann D, Gabel J. Investor-owned multihospital systems: a synthesis of research findings. In: BH Gray, For-Profit Enterprise in Health Care. Washington, DC: National Academy Press; 1986. p. 474–91.

40. Ermann D, Gabel J. Multihospital systems: issues and empirical findings. Health Aff. 1984;3:50–64.
41. Fetter RR, Mills RE. A micro computer based medical information system. Proceedings of the 2nd annual WAMI meeting. Paris: World Association for Medical Informatics; 1979. p. 388–91.
42. Frey R, Girardi S, Wiederhold G. A filing system for medical research. Int J Biomed Comput. 1971;2(1):1–26.
43. Friedman RB, MacDonald CJ. A buyer's guide to microcomputers for the home or the office. Medcomp. 1983;1:60–71.
44. Gall J. Computerized hospital information system cost-effectiveness: a case study. In: Van Egmond J, de Vries Robbe PF, Levy AH, editors. Information systems for patient care. Amsterdam: North Holland; 1976. p. 281–93.
45. Gall J. Cost-benefit analysis: total hospital information systems. In: Koza, editor. Health information system evaluation. Boulder: Colorado Associated University Press; 1974. p. 299–327.
46. Gardner RM, Pryor TA, Warner HR. The HELP hospital information system: update 1998. Int J Med Inf. 1999;54:169–82.
47. Garratt AE. An information system for ambulatory care. Proc SCAMC. 1979;856–8.
48. General Accounting Office. GAO report: medical ADP systems: composite health care systems acquisition-fair, reasonable, supported. Gaithersburg, MD: General Accounting Office; 1988.
49. Giannetti RA, Johnson JH, Williams TA. Computer technology in community mental health centers: current status and future prospects. Proc SCAMC 1978;117–21.
50. Glaser JP, Coburn MJ. Evaluation of the VA decentralized hospital computer program in a military hospital. Proc MEDINFO. 1986;430–4.
51. Gluek BC. A psychiatric patient observation system. Proceedings of the 7th IBM medical symposium; 1965. p. 317–22.
52. Grams RR, Peck GC, Massey JK, Austin JJ. Review of hospital data processing in the United States (1982–1984). J Med Syst. 1985;9:175–269.
53. Grandia LD, Rosqvist WV. Decentralized information system in a multihospital environment. Proc SCAMC. 1984;193–6.
54. Hammon GL. Cost allocation and forecasting. In: Bakker AR et al., editors. Towards new hospital information systems. Amsterdam: North-Holland; 1988. p. 315–9.
55. Hammond WE, Stead WW, Straube MJ. An interface between a hospital information system and a computerized medical record. Proc SCAMC. 1980;1537–40.
56. Harman CE, Meinhardt K. A computer system for treatment evaluation at the community mental health center. Am J Public Health. 1972;62:1596–601.
57. Hauser WR. Using the VA's public domain medical software to meet the needs of health care providers. MUG Q. 1985;XIV:3–18.
58. Health Information Technology for Economic and Clinical Health (HITECH) Act. American Recovery and Reinvestment Act of 2009 (ARRA) Pub. L. No. 111-5. 2009.
59. Healy JC, Spackman KA, Beck JR. Small expert systems in clinical pathology: are they useful? Arch Pathol Lab Med. 1989;113:981–3.
60. Hedlund JL, Vieweg BW, Cho D. Mental health information systems. Columbia, MO: University of Missouri-Columbia: Health Services Research Center; 1979.
61. Hedlund JL. Mental health information systems: some national trends. Proc SCAMC. 1978; 109–16.
62. Hedlund JL, Gorodezky MJ. Recent developments in computer applications in mental health: discussion and perspective. Proc SCAMC. 1980;2:885–95.
63. Helppie R. Superior insight. Comput Healthc. 1987 (March);20.
64. Henley RR, Wiederhold G. An Analysis of Automated Ambulatory Medical Record Systems. Office of Medical Information Systems, University of California, San Francisco Medical Center. 1975.

65. Herner & Co. The use of computers in hospitals. Report III-Survey analysis; report IV-descriptions of computer applications. Bethesda: National Center for Health Services Research; 1968.
66. Hodge MH. History of the TDS medical information system. In: Blum BI, Duncan KA, editors. A history of medical informatics. New York: Addison-Wesley; 1990. p. 328–44.
67. Houser ML, Barlow JL, Tedeschi RJ, Spicer M, Shields D, Diamond L. The implementation of hospital information systems: change, challenge, and commitment. Proc SCAMC. 1984;221–4.
68. Huff Jr WS. Automatic data processing in hospitals: computer handles total financial workload for 12-unit hospital system. Hospitals. 1964;38:81.
69. IHS Patient care component health summary. Tuscon, AZ: Indian Health Service; 1990.
70. Ivers MT, Timson GF. The applicability of the CA integrated clinical CORE information system to the needs of other health care providers. MUG Q. 1985;14:19–22.
71. Ivers MT, Timson GF, Hv B, Whitfield G, Keltz PD, Pfeil CN. Large scale implementation of compatible hospital computer systems within the Veterans Administration. Proc SCAMC 1983;53–6.
72. Jacobs SE. Hospital-wide computer systems: the market and the vendors. MUG Q. 1982;7:25–6.
73. Johnson ME. Pulmonary testing laboratory computer application. Proc SCAMC. 1980;1:253–7.
74. Jones JK. Inpatient databases. In: Strom BL, editor. Pharmacolepidemiology. 2nd ed. New York: Wiley; 1994. p. 257–76.
75. Karpinski RHS, Bleich HL. MISAR: a miniature information storage and retrieval system. Comput Biomed Res. 1971;4:655–60.
76. Kilpatrick KE, Vogel WB, Carswell JL. Evolution of a computerized support system for health care capacity planning. J Med Syst. 1988;12:305–17.
77. Kirby JD, Pickett MP, Boyarsky MW, Stead WW. Distributed processing with a mainframe-based hospital information system: a generalized solution. Proc SCAMC. 1987;764–70.
78. Kuhn IM, Wiederhold G, Rodnick JE, Ransey-Klee D, Benett S, Beck DD. Automated ambulatory record systems in the US. NTIS Publication; 1982. p. 178–89.
79. Laska E, Logemann G. Computing at the information sciences division, Rockland State Hospital. Proc Annual Conf ACM;1971. p. 672–83.
80. Laska E, Siegel C, Meisner M. Data systems in mental health. Methods Inf Med. 1975;14:1–6.
81. Leberto T. Top 25 hospital management information vendors. HealthWeek Insight. 1988;25.
82. Leonard MS, Goldman J. A strategy for the implementation of automated information systems. Inform Health Soc Care. 1985;10:13–8.
83. Leonard MS, Ashton WB, Blackwell PW. Automated Hospital Information System: AHIS component catalog. Columbia, MO: University of Missouri-Columbia; 1980.
84. Lindberg D. Computers in mental health care. In: Crawford JL, Morgan DW, Gianturco DT, editors. Progress in mental health information system computer applications. Cambridge, MA: Ballinger Pub. Co; 1973. p. 333–8.
85. Lindberg DAB. A statewide medical information system. Comput Biomed Res. 1970;3:453–63.
86. Little AD. Systems analysis for a new generation of military hospitals. Summary. Cambridge, MA: Arthur D. Little NTIS AD 722 980;1971.
87. Little AD. Benefits assessment of CHCS: peer review of work in progress. Cambridge, MA: Arthur D. Little;1988.
88. Lund SR, Ackerman LV, Martin JB, Somand ME. Distributed processing with a local area network. Proc AAMSI. 1984;52–6.
89. Marlowe K. The key to supporting comprehensive healthcare, research and planning. Healthc Inform. 1990;7:22–4.
90. Maturi VF, DuBois RM. Recent trends in computerized medical information systems for hospital departments. Proc SCAMC. 1980;3:1541–9.

91. McDonald CJ, Blevins L, Tierney WM, Martin DK. The Regenstrief medical records. MD Comput. 1987;5:34–47.
92. McDonald CJ, Overhage JM, Barnes M, Schadow G, Blevins L, Dexter PR, et al. The Indiana network for patient care: a working local health information infrastructure. Health Aff. 2005;24:1214–20.
93. Mestrovich MJ. Defense medical systems support center factbook. Falls Church: DMSSC; 1988.
94. Mirel BR, Wright Z, Tenenbaum JD, Saxman P, Smith KA. User requirements for exploring a resource inventory for clinical research. AMIA SummitsTrans Sci Proc. 2010;2010:31.
95. Mishelevich DJ, Kesinger G, Jasper M. Medical record control and the computer. Topics in health record management. 1981;2(2):47–55.
96. MITRE: Utilization of the Veterans Administration Software in the TRIMIS Program: Presentation of the MITRE Final Report. The MITRE Corp. Jul 17, 1984.
97. MUMPS News. SAIC, PRC wins VA HIS contract, MUMPS News 1990;7:1.
98. MUMPS News. MUMPS users group. MUMPS News 1988;5:2.
99. Munnecke TH, Kuhn IM. Large scale portability of hospital information system software. Proc SCAMC. 1986;133–40.
100. Munnecke TH, Davis RG, Timson GF. The Veterans' administration kernel programming environment. Proc SCAMC. 1985;523.
101. Myers E. Shot in the arm. Datamation. 1985;31:75–83.
102. NCHSR. The role of market forces in the delivery of health care: issues for research. Washington, DC: National Center for Health Services Research; 1988.
103. Nevarez L. Computerized medical record system. Proc 1st Annual TRIMIS Program Conf. Bethesda, MD: Uniformed Services University of Health Sciences. 1982;53–4.
104. Newald J. Hospitals look to computerization of physician office linkage. Hospitals. 1987;61:92–4.
105. OTA. OTA special report: hospital information systems at the Veterans Administration. 1987.
106. Packer CL. Changing environment spurs new HIS demand. Hospitals. 1985;59:99.
107. Polacsek RA. The fourth annual medical software buyer's guide. MD Comput. 1987;4:23–136.
108. Rabeau ES. Applied research in health program management. Proceedings of the first Operation SAM orientation conference. 1966.
109. Reynolds RE, Heller Jr EE. An academic medical center experience with a computerized hospital information system: the first four years. Proc SCAMC. 1980;1:13–6.
110. Rosen D. Medical care information system of the Veterans Administration. Public Health Rep. 1968;83:363–71.
111. Rosenthal M. The new VA's new automated hospital. Hosp JAHA. 1966;40:40–6.
112. Rozner E. HIS Market review (Part II): competitive forces are reshaping the industry. HC&C. 1984;4:38–40.
113. Runck HM. Computer planning for hospitals: large-scale education and involvement of employees. Comput Autom. 1969;18:33–6.
114. Schwartz SR, Stinson C, Berlant J. Computers in psychiatry. MD Comput. 1985;2:42–50.
115. Schwichtenberg AH, Flickinger DD, Lovelace I, Randolph W. Development and use of medical machine record cards in astronaut selection. US Armed Forces Med J. 1959;10:1324–51.
116. Shieman BM. Medical information system, El Camino Hospital. IMS Ind Med Surg. 1971;40:25–6.
117. Singer JP. Computer-based hospital information systems. Datamation. 1969;15:38.
118. Sittig DF, Franklin M, Turetsky M, Sussman AJ, Bates DW, Komaroff AL, et al. Design and development of a computer-based clinical referral system for use within a physician hospital organization. Stud Health Technol Inform. 1998;52(Pt 1):98–102.
119. Sletten IW. The Missouri statewide automated standard system of psychiatry problems and partial solutions. Proceedings of the ACM annual conference. 1973, p. 5–6.
120. Spencer WA. An opinion survey of computer applications in 149 hospitals in the USA, Europe and Japan. Inf Health Soc Care. 1976;1:215–34.

121. Stead WW, Hammond WE, Winfree RG. Beyond a basic HIS: work stations for department management. Proc SCAMC. 1984;197–9.
122. Stefanchik MF. Point-of-care information systems: improving patient care. Comput Healthc. 1987;8:78.
123. Stoneburner LL. Survey of computer systems for the physician's office: current systems. Proc MEDINFO. 1983;164–9.
124. Summerfield AB, Empey S. Computer-based information systems for medicine: a survey and brief discussion of current projects. Santa Monica: System Development Corporation; 1965.
125. Teich JM, Glaser JP, Beckley RF, Aranow M, Bates DW, Kuperman GJ, et al. The Brigham integrated computing system (BICS): advanced clinical systems in an academic hospital environment. Int J Med Inf. 1999;54:197–208.
126. Timson G. The file manager system. Proc SCAMC. 1980;1645–9.
127. TRIMIS. Master plan. Bethesda: TRIMIS Program Office; 1978.
128. TRIMIS Program Office. TRIMIS, composite health care systems: test and evaluation plan. Bethesda: TRIMIS Program Office; 1988.
129. TRIMIS Program Office. TPO fact sheet: Computerized Medical Record Information System (CMRIS). Bethesda: TRIMIS Program Office; 1981.
130. TRIMIS RFP. Request for proposals for composite health care systems (CHCS) and small composite health care systems (SMCHCS). Bethesda: TRIMIS; 1984.
131. Wiederhold G, Fries JF, Weyl S. Structured organization of clinical data bases. Proc AFIPS Conf. 1975;479–85.
132. Wilkins M, Eberhardy J, Plotnik D, Rock A. Information requirements for health maintenance organizations. Proc SCAMC. 1984;417–9.
133. Wilson HH. Automated data processing for a modern hospital. Santa Monica: System Development Corporation; 1962.
134. Wurster CR, Goodman JD. NIMH prototype management information system for community mental health centers. Proc SCAMC. 1980;2:907–12.
135. Yeh S, Lincoln T. From micro to mainframe. Am J Perinatol. 1985;2:158–60.
136. Young EM, Brian EW, Hardy DR. Automated hospital information systems workbook. Los Angeles: USC Center for Health Services Publications; 1981.
137. Young EM, Brian EW, Hardy DR, et al. Evaluation of automated hospital data management systems (AHDMS). Proc SCAMC. 1980;651–7.

Part III
Support Systems

Chapter 11
Clinical Support Information Systems (CSISs)

Morris F. Collen and John S. Silva

Abstract Operating within a larger medical information system (MIS), clinical support information systems (CSISs) process the specialized subsystem information used in support of the direct care of patients. Most of these CSISs were developed as stand-alone systems. This chapter highlights the early efforts to combine data from disparate departmental data systems into more "integrated ones" that support the full spectrum of data management needs of multi-hospital and ambulatory health systems. In the 1960s and 1970s, institutions incorporated clinical laboratory and medication subsystems into their MISs; more subsystems were added (pathology, imaging, etc.); and systems with integrated CSIS were developed for ambulatory care settings. Despite all the progress made over the past 40 years, two key challenges remain unsolved: first is the lack of data interoperability among myriad systems; second is the lack of a useful point of care system. Both threaten to make the clinician's work harder; overcoming them is key to transforming the health care system.

Keywords Clinical support information systems • Integrated CSIS • Interoperability • Point of care systems • Clinical subsystems • Dietary information systems

Taking care of a patient in 1950 or 2010 usually involved a physician seeing the patient in a medical office or in a hospital. To evaluate the patient's health status, the physician took a history of the patient's medical problems (symptoms), performed a physical examination to discover any physical abnormalities (signs), and combined the symptoms and signs to see if they fitted any syndrome. He then recorded the patient's history and examination findings and any preliminary impressions of any syndromes in the patient's medical record, which was usually a paper-based chart. The physician often referred the patient for tests and procedures that involved clinical laboratory, radiology, and other clinical support services. Upon reviewing the results from these services, the physician could make a preliminary diagnosis

Author Collen was deceased at the time of publication.

M.F. Collen (deceased)

J.S. Silva, M.D., F.A.C.M.I. (✉)
Silva Consulting Services, LLC, Eldersburg, MD, USA
e-mail: Jc-silva-md@att.net

© Springer-Verlag London 2016
M.F. Collen, M.J. Ball (eds.), *The History of Medical Informatics in the United States*, Health Informatics, DOI 10.1007/978-1-4471-6732-7_11

505

and send the patient to the pharmacy for any needed medications. In some instances, patients had to undergo one or more surgical procedures to take tissue specimens to send to pathology for analysis and interpretation. Using all the information received from these clinical support services, the physician usually arrived at a final diagnosis. To prescribe the most appropriate therapy, the physician might consult one or more colleagues and/or computer databases. In summary, most patients who were cared for by physicians in hospitals or in medical offices were referred to one or more clinical support services to receive procedures that could aid in the processes of diagnosis and/or treatment.

Specialized departmental clinical support information systems (CSISs) have evolved for the clinical laboratory, pathology, pharmacy, and imaging, each covered in a separate chapter following this overview. This chapter details the requirements for a CSIS and provides a summary of early examples of the integration of CSISs within clinical practice, describes the unique features of dietary information systems, and concludes with a summary and commentary regarding the future of CSIS.

11.1 Requirements of a CSIS

The primary objective of clinical support information systems (CSISs) is to process the specialized subsystem information used in support of the direct care of patients. As for any module in a medical information system (MIS), the users of a CSIS had to first define exactly what they wanted the CSIS to do. Since a CSIS usually operated within a larger MIS, the functional requirements of the CSIS had to be compatible with those of the MIS of which it was a part. Thus, a CSIS usually had the general requirements to: (1) Identify and register the patient, identify the procedures requested, and the specific technical unit where the procedures were to be performed. (2) Record the date, the time, and the location of every patient care transaction. (3) Collect and store all data about the patient and the procedures performed; and also store all internal processing information, such as that collected for process quality control. (4) Fulfill billing and accounting procedures for all services provided to each patient. (5) Satisfy economic requirements. (6) Communicate and provide capabilities for data linkages to other medical sites when necessary for the transfer of patient data [28].

Prior to the advent of the CSIS, physicians' orders for procedures were handwritten and transmitted to the clinical support service. The clinical support service then communicated test results to physicians verbally or via printed forms, documents, or typed reports. To replace these error-prone methods, a CSIS needed a computer-based physician order entry (CPOE) and a results reporting (RR) module capable of receiving requests for the procedures to be performed and of reporting back the results after the procedures were completed. Until the 1970s each CSIS provided its own OE-RR application, so that when a hospital implemented its laboratory, radiology, or pharmacy subsystems, each had its own separate order entry (OE) terminal. It was frustrating for hospital personnel, when entering new orders, or changing old orders for a patient, to have to repeatedly enter the patient's identification into separate terminals for laboratory, pharmacy, radiology, and/or patient bed transfer, or discharge orders. Furthermore, many orders were of such a nature that they required associated secondary orders that involved communications to another department, such as to dietetics. For example, an order for an upper-gastrointestinal x-ray examination to be done on a specified day, required that the procedure be scheduled in the radiology department, that nursing and dietetics departments be notified that food and fluids should be withheld from the patient prior to the procedure, that the patient should be transported to the radiology department at the time of the scheduled examination, and that appropriate instructions be given as to feeding on the patient's return.

An entirely new set of requirements were necessary when the CSIS functioned within or was linked to the MIS: (1) Interface to an available order entry (O/E) module that communicated to the CSIS all requisitions for procedures that the patient was to receive, provide any special instructions to the patient and to relevant personnel that included the time the procedure was to be done, and noted any restrictions as to the patient's physical activity and food intake prior to the procedure. (2) Interface to a results reporting module and be able to communicate to one or more desired locations the dates and times of completing the procedure; and the results of the procedure including any interpretive comments. (3) Transmit the data into a computer-based patient record, if available. (4) Support the decision-making processes involved in patient care.

As the CSIS technology and systems evolved, a whole new set of technical requirements and design specifications were needed. The CSIS had to be designed to: (1) Have acceptable computer terminals for entering patient and procedure data; and for reporting the results of the completed procedures. (2) Provide appropriate interfaces between specialized instruments, data-acquisition equipment, and the CSIS computer. (3) Include computer programs for processing order entry requisitions for services, for providing quality control measures, and for processing and reporting procedure and/or test results. (4) Provide for a CSIS computer database adequate in capacity to store all of the patients' data, and the information associated with and resulting from all procedures, while ensuring 24×7 access to the CSIS. (5) Have a computer-stored data dictionary (metadatabase) that described all tests and procedures performed with any special instructions for conducting them; and their normal and alert boundary limits. (6) Provide communication links to the information systems in affiliated medical offices and hospitals from which the patients came; and also provide links to any needed external databases. (7) Provide reliable and rapid turn-around services for urgent and emergency medical conditions. (8) Have a flexible information system design and implementation that could adapt to changes in medical technology and knowledge. (9) Accommodate an increasing volume and variety of procedures technical and medical innovations. (10) Employ a vocabulary of standard terms to facilitate exchange of information with other information systems.

Since the exchange of clinical data between different CSIS databases required the use of standard terms, in 1983 standards for the transmission of clinical data between computers began to be developed [65]. The proposed standards addressed what items of information should be included in defining and recording an observation, how individual items should be encoded and formatted, and what transmission media should be employed. Formal attempts to improve the standardization of medical information were carried out by collaborating committees, such as the subcommittees on Computerized Systems of the American Standards for Testing Materials (ASTM), the oldest of the nonprofit standard setting societies and a standards-producing member of the American National Standards Institute [76]. The ASTM technical subcommittee E31.12 on Medical Informatics considered nomenclatures and medical records [38]. In 1988 ASTM's subcommittee E31.11 on Data Exchange Standards for Clinical Laboratory Results published its specifications E1238 for clinical data interchange, and set standards for the two-way digital transmission of clinical data between different computers for laboratory, office and hospital systems; so that, as a simple example, all dates would be recorded as an eight-character string, YYYYMMDD. Thus the date January 12, 1988 would always be transmitted as 19880112 [3–5].

Health Level Seven (HL7), an organization made up of vendors, hospitals, and consultants, was formed in 1987 to develop interface standards for transmitting data between applications that used different CSIS' within hospital information systems [85]. The message content for HL7 was to conform to the International Standards Organization (ISO) standards for the applications level 7 of the Open Systems Interconnection (OSI) model. The HL7 standards used the same message syntax, the same data types, and some of the same segment definitions as ASTM 1238 [64]. The Medical Data Interchange (MEDIX) P1157 committee of the Institute of Electrical and Electronics Engineers (IEEE), formed at the Symposium on Computer Applications in Medical Care (SCAMC) in 1987, was also developing a set of standards, based on the ISO application-level standards, for the transferring of clinical data over large networks from mixed sources, such as from a clinical laboratory and a pharmacy, for both intra- and inter-hospital communications [78].

11.2   Examples of Early CSIS and Integration with MIS

In 1959 the evolution of clinical support information systems (CSISs) began when Schenthal [79, 80] and Sweeney at Tulane Medical School, used an IBM 650 computer equipped with magnetic tape storage to process medical record data that included laboratory test results for clinic patients. They used a mark-sense card reader that sensed marks made with high-carbon content pencils on special formatted cards. The marks were converted into punched holes in standard punch cards. They read these punched cards into the computer, which then processed and stored the data for the clinic's physicians. At about the same time, Spencer and Vallbona, at the Texas Institute for Rehabilitation and Research (TIRR), began to develop a fairly comprehensive MIS with several clinical support subsystems. TIRR was a private, non-profit, special-purpose hospital in the Texas Medical Center at Houston that delivered comprehensive rehabilitation services to patients having a wide variety of physical disabilities. In February 1959 laboratory reports and physiological test data were manually recorded on specially designed source documents. The data were then coded, keypunched, and then processed on a batch basis with unit-record equipment. The software consisted of diagrams of complex patch boards. In 1961 the acquisition of IBM 1401 and 1620 computers with magnetic tape storage provided for data processing, storage, and data retrieval capabilities [20]. In 1965 the problem of errors in data entry associated with the use of punched paper tape and cards required TIRR to advance to online computing with an IBM 1410 computer. Data entries were made by a clerk at TIRR via a remote typewriter terminal. With the establishment of a conversational mode between the terminal and the computer, error detection and correction by staff personnel became feasible. In 1967 the system was enhanced by the acquisition of an IBM 360/50 computer [91].

In 1968 physicians' orders began to be entered into their medical information system; and appropriate displays were accessed on IBM 2260 cathode-ray-tube terminals located in various clinical departments [18]. In 1969 using these display terminals connected to the Baylor University IBM/360 computer, updated reports were batch processed daily for each patient [43]. In 1970 they initiated their pharmacy information system; and in 1971 TIRR added a Four-Phase Systems minicomputer that supported the clinical laboratory. By the mid-1970s TIRR had an information system with several operational modules, including the provision of results of all patients' laboratory and functional capacity tests [91].

In 1962 Children's Hospital in Akron, Ohio, installed an IBM 1401 computer that processed doctors' orders. After physicians had written their orders for medications, laboratory tests, and x-ray examinations, the orders were numerically coded and keypunched into cards for data processing [33]. In 1964 they discontinued using punched cards and installed at every hospital nursing station a terminal unit with a matrix of 120 buttons to be used for data entry, and an electric typewriter that served as an output printer, each connected to the central computer. A scroll on the data-entry unit was turned to show the type of entry to be made. The first two columns of buttons were used to enter the type of order, the next three columns of buttons were to enter the patient's identification number, the next four columns designated the order number, and the remaining three columns of buttons were used to enter modifiers such as the type of order and its frequency. The printer then provided the printouts for use as requisitions; which were also used as laboratory report slips to be filed in the patients' charts. All data were stored on a random access device [26].

In 1963 the National Institutes of Health (NIH) initiated a central computing facility to provide direct data processing support to its various laboratories. By 1964 this central facility contained two Honeywell series-800 computers [54]. In 1965 NIH established its Division of Computer Research and Technology (DCRT), with Pratt as its director for intramural project development. In 1966 DCRT began to provide computer services with an IBM 360/40 machine; and then rapidly expanded to four IBM 360/370 computers that were linked to a large number of peripherally located minicomputers in NIH clinics and laboratories [74]. In 1963 Lindberg, and associates at the University of Missouri in Columbia, installed an IBM 1410 computer in their Medical Center. A major initial project was the development of a computer system for reporting all clinical laboratory test results. At that time their laboratory data already were being keypunched into cards. Other specific files of patient material being processed included tumor registry and surgical pathology [60]. In 1965 they replaced the punched card-oriented system in their clinical laboratory with IBM 1092/1093 matrix-keyboard terminals to enter test results directly into the computer. In 1965 Lindberg listed as operational the following additional applications: electrocardiogram interpretations as coded by heart station physicians, radiology interpretations as coded by the radiologists, and query-and-retrieval programs for data stored in all patient files [59]. By 1968 they had added an information system for their department of surgery which provided patient data that included laboratory, surgical pathology and autopsy reports [58]. Lindberg used the Standard Nomenclature of Diseases and Operations (SNDO) for the coding of patients' discharge diagnoses and surgical operative procedures [61] and stored these on magnetic tape for all patients admitted to the hospital between 1955 and 1965. Other categories of patient data in their system included all SNDO coded diagnoses for autopsy and surgical pathology specimens, and all coded radiology and electrocardiogram interpretations [59]. In 1969 Lindberg operated, for the Missouri Regional Medical program, a computer dedicated to the interpretation of electrocardiograms, using the 12-lead scalar system developed by Caceres within the U.S. Public Health Service (USPHS) Systems Development Laboratory. Electrocardiograms were transmitted over dial-up telephone lines to the computer center, and automated interpretations were returned to teletype printers in the doctor's office or hospital.

In the early 1960s Warner, and associates at the LDS Hospital (formerly known as the Latter Day Saints Hospital) in Salt Lake City and at the University of Utah, began to use a Control Data Corporation (CDC) 3,300 computer to support clinical applications. They used Tektronix 601 terminals capable of displaying 400 characters in a 25-column by 16-row pattern, or graphical information with a capability of 512 horizontal and 512 vertical dots. Each terminal had a decimal keyboard, and two 12-bit, octal thumbwheel switches for coding information into the computer [92]. In the 1970s they developed one of the most effective medical information systems of that decade. The HELP System at LDS Hospital had terminals located at its nursing units that allowed the nurses to select orders from displayed menus, and to review the orders entered and the results reported. In the early 1970s, MEDLAB was formed to market the clinical laboratory system they had developed that was directly interfaced to automated laboratory equipment. Special coding systems were devised to enter data from radiology. In 1971 the Systematized Nomenclature of Pathology (SNOP) code was used to enter diagnoses at a video terminal [42]. In 1975 the LDS subsystems included their clinical laboratory, multiphasic screening, and computerized electrocardiogram analysis [55]. By 1978 the LDS medical information system had outgrown its centralized computer system; during the 1980s a network of minicomputers were interfaced to the existing central computer. In the 1980s items stored in their integrated patient record database included reports from the clinical laboratory, pathology biopsies, radiology, electrocardiography, multiphasic screening, and pharmacy [75]. In the 1990s their HELP system expanded to provide comprehensive clinical support services in nine Intermountain Health Care Hospitals in Utah [41].

Since 1963 Collen and associates at Kaiser Permanente (KP) had been operating automated multiphasic health testing (AMHT) programs in both the San Francisco and Oakland medical centers [29, 30]. In 1968 a subsidiary computer center containing an IBM 360/50 computer was established in the Department of Medical Methods Research to develop a prototype MIS that included clinical laboratory and pharmacy subsystems [31]. Their multiphasic health testing system already provided patient identification data, appointment scheduling and daily patient appointment lists, specimen labels, patient and specimen registration, quality control procedures, clinical laboratory test results, physician interpretations of electrocardiograms and x-rays, clinical decision-support including alert and warning signals for findings outside of predetermined normal limits, advice rules for secondary sequential testing, consider rules for likely diagnoses. All patient data were stored in computer-based patient records and in research databases. The automated multiphasic health testing programs in San Francisco and in Oakland each entered the data for 150 patients' health checkups a day. For electrocardiogram, pathology, and radiology reports, an IBM magnetic tape/selectric typewriter (MT/ST) was used for processing written or dictated text. With slight modifications in their typing routines, secretaries used the typewriters to store on analog magnetic tape the patient identification, procedure and test data, and the physicians' reports. These data were transmitted to a receiver MT/ST located in the central computer facility. By means of a digital-data recorder and converter device, a second tape was created in a digital form acceptable for input to the patient's computer-stored medical record in the IBM 360 computer [27]. A pharmacy system was added in 1969. In the 1980s a central clinical laboratory was established and its laboratory computer system was linked to the Kaiser Permanente regional, mainframe computer center.

In 1964 the Information Systems Division of the Lockheed Missiles and Space Company in Sunnyvale, California began to apply their aerospace expertise to develop a hospital information system in the El Camino Hospital in Mountain View, California [39, 40]. In 1971 Lockheed sold its system to the Technicon Corporation, which had come to dominate automation in the clinical laboratory; and now its owner, Whitehead, saw an opportunity to extend automation from the clinical laboratory into the entire hospital information system. In March 1971 El Camino Hospital signed a contract for the installation of the Technicon MIS, a hospital information system operated with an IBM 370/155 time-shared computer located in Technicon's Mountain View offices [82]. By early 1973 the hospital had installed terminals throughout, including its clinical support services; and over the next several years continued to refine and improve the system [25]. By 1977, there were 60 terminals, each consisting of a television screen with a light-pen data selector, keyboard, and printer, located throughout the hospital, with two terminals installed at most nursing stations. The terminal's display screen was used to present lists of items, for example, orders for laboratory tests. A specific item was selected by pointing the light-pen at the desired word (or phrase), and pressing a switch on the barrel of the pen. The Technicon MIS was one of the first systems designed to allow the physician to enter his or her orders and review the results [23]. Using the light-pen, a physician could select a specific patient and then enter a full set of medical orders for laboratory work, medications, x-rays, and other procedures. The computer then stored the orders and sent appropriate laboratory requisitions, pharmacy labels, x-ray requisitions, and requests for other procedures to the appropriate hospital departments. Furthermore, physicians could generate personal order sets for particular conditions and write the complete order with a single light-pen selection [42]. Of the total number of orders, 75 % were entered into the computer by the physician [93]. Physicians, nurses, and other hospital personnel used the light-pen technique extensively and employed the keyboard only occasionally [51]. Computer-produced printouts included medication due time lists, laboratory specimen pickup time lists, cumulative test result summaries, radiology reports, and discharge summaries [17]. Physicians, on retrieving patient data from the display terminals, received clinical reminders and alerts. In 1978 they developed a library that contained information on diagnoses, recommended treatments, laboratory interpretation aids for test results, and indications for ordering diagnostic tests for certain diseases. Laboratory test results and radiology interpretations were available at the terminals as soon as they were entered into the system. A cumulative laboratory summary report printed daily showed the last 7 days of patients' test results [88]. A paper-based medical chart was maintained for all handwritten and dictated documents, since for physicians, the Technicon system was used primarily as an order entry and results reporting (OE/RR) system. Upon discharge, a complete listing of all test and procedure results, including graphic charts, were printed at the medical records department to be filed in the patient's paper charts [93].

In 1966 a system with an IBM 360/30 computer that used matrix button input terminals, similar to those at Akron Children's Hospital, was installed in the Monmouth Medical Center Hospital in Long Branch, New Jersey. These input terminals, along with keyboard typewriters, were located in the hospital's nursing stations, pharmacy, laboratory, and radiology [71]. In 1966 Barnett, and associates at the Laboratory of Computer Science, a unit of the Department of Medicine of the Massachusetts General Hospital (MGH) and the Harvard Medical School, initiated a pilot project that included a clinical laboratory reporting system and a medications ordering system [10]. Having Teletype terminals that permitted interactive order entry, Barnett was reluctant to use clerical personnel to enter physician's orders because he felt that this tended to eliminate the power and usefulness of an online computer system for checking the completeness, accuracy, and acceptability of an order; and for giving back pertinent stored current information about a specific patient. An online, interactive system could check an order against the data in the computer record for drug-drug interactions, or drug-laboratory test value interactions, or known allergic reactions to drugs. If this information was not given back immediately to the physician at the time the order was created, Barnett felt that it was less useful, since he believed that if there was a significant time delay between the writing of the order and its entry into the computer system, the responsible physician might have left the care unit and clarification of the order could then be more difficult and very time-consuming. Barnett recognized that the order entry systems generally available at that time allowed the physicians to write their orders and notes in the routine fashion, and then used clerical personnel to enter the information into the computer system. He felt that the inherent weakness in this strategy was that the computer interaction was not with the physician who was generating the order, but with a clerical staff member who had no decision making power [14].

Barnett's MGH system was soon expanded into nine patient care areas with about 300 beds and into three laboratories in the hospital; it used more than 100 standard model Teletype terminals. Computer programs were presented to the user in an interactive mode wherein the computer asked a question and the user entered a response. By 1967 Barnett reported that the computer programs in use at MGH included the entering of laboratory test results, and the printing of any selected group of laboratory tests [12]. In 1967 Barnett developed a medications ordering system at the MGH. Every hour on each patient care unit, the MGH computer generated a list of medications to be administered at that hour. It also listed laboratory test results, with weekly summaries organized in a format designed by the users to display tests in associated groups such as serum electrolytes and hematology. By 1974 there were operational at MGH the clinical laboratory and medication order processing functions; and additional modules were being developed for hematology, pathology, x-ray scheduling, x-ray film folder inventory control, and x-ray reporting. These modules were all written using the MGH Utility Multi-Programming System (MUMPS) and were implemented on several different but functionally identical computer systems. In 1971 Barnett and associates initiated the Computer-Stored Ambulatory Record (COSTAR) system for the Harvard Community Health Plan (HCHP) in Boston. COSTAR operated under the *MUMPS* language and operating system [13, 15, 45]. The health professionals in their offices manually completed structured encounter forms at the time of each patient visit. These forms were printed for the first visit and then computer-generated for subsequent visits. On these forms the physicians recorded their orders for tests, their diagnoses, and treatments. The completed forms were collected for the medical record room, and the data were entered by clerks using remote terminals connected by telephone lines to the computer located at the Laboratory of Computer Science. A status report generated after the entry of any new data to the patient's record provided an updated summary of the patient's current status, including current medications and latest laboratory test results. Barnett [11] wrote that in its design and implementation, a central objective of COSTAR was to provide information-processing support for communication of laboratory, x-ray, and electrocardiogram reports. By the late 1970s COSTAR had gone through four revisions in its system design at the HCHP [16]. By the end of the 1980s, the COSTAR system was widely disseminated in the United States, and was being used in more than 120 sites [9].

In 1967 Weed and associates at the University of Vermont College of Medicine in Burlington initiated their Problem-Oriented Medical Information System (PROMIS) [92]. In 1971 it became operational in a 20-bed gynecology ward at the University Hospital, with linkages to radiology, laboratory, and pharmacy. In 1975 Weed had a computer system that consisted of two Control Data Corporation (CDC)

1,700 series computers with CDC's operating system, and 14 Digiscribe touch-sensitive video terminals; one located in the pharmacy, and one in the x-ray department [34]. By 1977 the system had 30 touch-sensitive display terminals located in the hospital wards, in the pharmacy, clinical laboratory, and in radiology, all connected to a single minicomputer. The terminals could display 1,000 characters of information in 20 lines of 50 characters each, and had 20 touch-sensitive fields. The user selected an item by touching the screen at the position of that choice. Free-form data could be entered by typing on the keyboard attached to the terminal. In 1979 PROMIS expanded to employ a network of minicomputers [81].

In 1968 Lamson, and associates at the University of California Hospitals in Los Angeles, acquired their first computer for a clinical laboratory and surgical pathology reporting system [57]. Their initial information system was gradually expanded, and by 1975 it provided summary reports that included data received from a large number of clinical laboratory computers and also included a tumor registry [57]. In 1968 Siegel, at the New York-Downstate Medical Center in Brooklyn, described a hospital information system that used an IBM 1440–1410 computer complex connected to 40 remote typewriter-terminal printers. They entered data using punched cards, paper tape, and IBM 1092 matrix-overlay keyboards; and they used magnetic tape and disk for data storage. Terminals were placed in specialty clinics, in laboratories, radiology, and pharmacy [83]. In 1969 the nine Los Angeles County hospitals initiated a centralized information system. Beginning with an IBM 360/40 computer connected by telephone cable to remote display terminals and printers located initially in the admitting offices and pharmacies, centralized patient records were established. Pilot testing was conducted at that time by nurses for the order entry of medications, diets, and laboratory tests [77]. In 1969 Jelliffe, and associates at the University of Southern California School of Medicine, initiated at the Los Angeles County General Hospital a series of programs for clinical pharmacology to analyze dosage requirements for a variety of medications. In 1972 programs were added to analyze data from their electrocardiograms and echocardiograms [52].

In 1969 Hammond and Stead at Duke University, began to develop a minicomputer-supported, office information system [46]. Data entry methods included interactive video terminals and batch-processed mark-sense forms. They soon installed a clinical laboratory system designed to allow for the ordering and reporting of laboratory data. In 1975 their computer-stored patient record included diagnostic and treatment orders, laboratory test results, medications, and some follow-up findings [96]. They used a data dictionary to define all clinical variables, all extensively coded [49]. By 1980 their computer-based medical record system, which they called The Medical Record (TMR) system, used two PDP-11 minicomputers and was then supported by *GEMISCH* as its database management system [48]. TMR was dictionary driven, and the TMR programs were modularly constructed. The THERAPY module provided a formulary with the ability to prescribe drugs, charge for drugs dispensed in the clinic, and monitor therapies prescribed elsewhere. The STUDIES module provided for ordering tests, for entry of test results, and for viewing results, including graphics. The FLOW module provided various time-oriented presentations of the data. Their APPOINTMENT module supported a multi-specialty appointment system. When the patient arrived for the appointment, a route sheet for the collection of data, a pre-encounter medical summary, and results from tests of the previous four encounters were printed. The patient then saw the physician who recorded patient care data, orders, and prescriptions on the route sheet. The patient then reported to a clerk who entered into the computer the orders and requisitions, which were then printed in the appropriate laboratories. Laboratory data were entered, usually by the laboratory technicians, as results became available. For data entry, they displayed a full screen and then filled in blanks. The data enterer could type in the code directly or type in text; and the program would do an alphabetic search via the data dictionary and convert the text string into the proper code. Their PRINT module printed all components of the record [45]. By 1985 the Duke TMR system had increased in size to require a local area network, and linked it to the clinical laboratory system in TMR by an Ethernet connection. The laboratory could query a patient's problem list, for example, directly in TMR on the main system through the network [88]. By the late 1980s, the TMR system at Duke provided linkages to referring physicians [89].

In 1970 at the Johns Hopkins Hospital (JHH), a prototype information system was initiated to process physicians' written orders, produce work lists for ward nurses, and generate daily computer-printed, patient drug profiles for the patients' records. In 1975 a Minirecord (minimal essential record) system was initiated in the JHH Medical Clinic that used encounter forms that were filled out at each patient visit; and they contained an area for medications and procedures [63]. Work also was begun on a prototype Oncology Clinical Information System (OCIS). The OCIS contained patient care data for both hospital and clinic services, and also captured clinical laboratory test results and pharmacy data [21–23]. In 1976 a radiology reporting system was implemented at JHH using a terminal that permitted the radiologist to select phrases with which to compose descriptions and interpretations of x-ray studies. Its output was a computer-printed report which became available as soon as the radiologist completed his interpretation [95]. In 1978 a clinical laboratory information system was operational which provided the internal working documents for the laboratories, and produced the patient's cumulative laboratory report [53]. During the early 1980s, a network gradually evolved in the JHH information system. By 1986 the JHH system included IBM 3081 and 3083 computers that supported an inpatient pharmacy system with a unit dose distribution system, a clinical laboratory system which ran on three PDP 11/70 computers, and a radiology system [90].

Frey [37] and associates at Stanford Medical Center, described their ACME system that was developed with the requirements for a research database able to handle many data sets of many varieties and sizes; with some data having to be held for long periods of time; with some that require frequent updating; and able to minimize inadvertent loss of data; and be able to serve a group of medical researchers who often are inexperienced in computer techniques. ACME was a typewriter terminal-driven, time-sharing system designed to acquire, analyze, store and retrieve medical research data, and to control laboratory instruments. ACME was served by an IBM 360-50 computer, with access to 2,741 typewriter terminals, and a variety of laboratory instruments; with disc drives for storage and magnetic tape storage for backup and archival storage. Laboratory instruments were interfaced through an IBM 1800 analog-digital computer. In 1970 Grams, and associates at the University of Florida in Gainesville and the 500-bed Shands Hospital with its outpatient clinic and emergency room, began to formulate their computer-based laboratory information system that was designed to provide some clinical decision support capabilities [44]. Initially the system did not provide any reporting capabilities; the test results were manually recorded on cumulative report form. In 1975 a single computer began to service their subsystems for anatomic pathology, microscopy, chemistry, hematology, immunology, microbiology, and blood banking, in addition to their hospital admissions functions. In 1977 they installed a network to integrate their laboratory functions, hospital admissions service, and nursing stations. They used one computer for the nursing and admissions functions, linked to a second computer in the laboratory [44].

In 1972 McDonald, and associates at the Regenstrief Institute for Health Care and the Indiana University School of Medicine, began to develop the Regenstrief Medical Record System (RMRS) for the care of ambulatory patients [47]. The RMRS used a PDP 11/45 computer with a database that supported the medical record file and its associated language (CARE). Patient data was generally stored in a coded format, although some free-text entry was permitted [65]. Their database files also included their clinical laboratory system, their pharmacy system, patient appointment file, and a dictionary of terms. The RMRS was intended to complement their paper-based patient record; and for each patient served, RMRS contained a core computer-stored medical record that included laboratory, x-ray, and electrocardiography reports. A two-part patient encounter form was generated for each patient's return visit. The physician recorded numeric clinical data for later optical-machine reading into the computer. A space was provided on the form for writing orders for tests. Within the space for orders, the computer suggested certain tests that might be needed. The patient's current prescriptions were listed at the bottom of the encounter form in a medication profile. The physician refilled or discontinued these drugs by writing "R" or "D/C" next to them; and wrote new prescriptions underneath this list. The patient took a carbon copy of this section of the encounter form to the pharmacy as his prescription. Thus, the encounter form performed many of the recording and retrieving tasks for the physician. Data, recorded by physicians on the encounter forms, were entered into the computer by clerks. In McDonald's RMRS laboratory, information was acquired directly from the laboratory system. Pharmacy prescription information was captured from both the hospital and outpatient pharmacy systems. For each patient's return visit a patient summary report was generated which included historical and treatment information; and reports from laboratories, radiology, electrocardiography, and nuclear medicine in a modified flow sheet format [64]. It listed the results of the patient's laboratory tests, and the test results were presented in reverse chronological order. With this time-oriented view of the data, the physician could readily find and compare the most recent data to prior data, such as for repeated laboratory tests. An asterisk was placed beside each abnormal value for emphasis. McDonald and associates [68] reported that the

RMRS also used paper reports, rather than visual displays as its primary mechanism for transmitting information to the physician; and this mode of output was preferred since it was cheap, portable, easier to browse, and paper reports could be annotated with paper and pencil. In the early 1980s, the RMRS shared a DEC VAX 11/780 computer with the clinical laboratory and pharmacy systems; and used a microcomputer- based workstation to display forms, in which the user could enter data using a mouse to select data from menus [64]. By the mid-1980s, the RMRS's computer-based patient record contained patient's diagnoses, treatments, imaging studies, electrocardiograms; and laboratory and medication data were entered automatically from computerized laboratory and pharmacy systems [64]. In 1988 the RMRS was also linked to the laboratory, radiology, and pharmacy within the local Veterans and University hospitals [67]. By the end of the 1990s, the RMRS served a large network of hospitals and clinics [69].

In 1976 Bleich, Slack, and associates at Beth Israel Hospital in Boston initiated their clinical computing system. In 1982 they expanded their system into the Brigham and Women's Hospital. By 1984 their system ran on a network of Data General Eclipse minicomputers that supported 300 video-display terminals located throughout the hospital. The system permitted one to retrieve data from the clinical laboratories, to look up reports from the departments of radiology and pathology, look up prescriptions filled in the outpatient pharmacy, and to request delivery of patients' charts. In 1983 a survey of 545 physicians, medical students, and nurses showed that they used the computer terminals most of the time to look up laboratory test results; and 83 % said that the terminals enabled them to work faster [19]. In the 1990s their clinical computing system provided results from all laboratories and clinical departments [86]. In 1994 Brigham and Women's Hospital joined with Massachusetts General Hospital to form Partners Health Care System that included ten hospitals and more than 250 practice sites. Its clinical computing had begun with the Beth Israel system, but it was rapidly expanded to serve the entire Partners System with its clinical support subsystems. In 1979 Fetter [35] described a microcomputer-based medical information system installed at Yale University, using a Digital Equipment Corporation (DEC) 16-bit LSI-11 processor, with computer terminals installed in Yale's radiology department and its clinical laboratory.

11.3   Dietary Services

The primary function of the dietetics department of a hospital is to provide appropriate meals to inpatients. This involves menu planning, food ordering, food production, tray assembly and delivery. In the 1950s, prior to the availability of the digital computer, some hospitals used punched cards for menu selection and employed card sorters to count the numbers of meals and food items to be served [62]. In the early 1960s some hospitals used a set of punched cards with code numbers for foods prepared by the U.S. Department of Agriculture (USDA) for the machine tabulation by unit record equipment or by automated data processing with a computer. Computer-planned menus could be generated, as well as reports for food inventory, cost, and usage. In the mid-1960s Balintfy at Tulane University developed a program called Computer-Assisted Menu Planning (CAMP) for hospital dietary services. A study with 16 dieticians showed that menus planned by CAMP were significantly lower in cost (19 %) than menus planned by unassisted menu planning; they always ensured that nutritional requirements for each menu were satisfied; and would generally be acceptable to patients [7]. CAMP used a mathematical linear programming approach that attempted to optimize a balance among food cost, palatability or acceptability, and nutrition. The program required: (1) food item data such as the unit of purchase and price per unit for each food. (2) Nutrient data such as the calories, cholesterol content, percent of protein, fat, and carbohydrate; amount of sodium, magnesium, and other minerals; and vitamin content. (3) Recipe data which were the instructions for converting food into edible portions of menu items. (4) Menu item data for planning the menus for meals. Menus could be planned for a sequence of meals on a daily basis or over several weeks. They could allow some selectivity by offering a second choice of menu items; and they had to satisfy basic nutritional requirements, yet aim for lowest cost. Patients requiring special diets required special nutrients or controlled amounts of some nutrients [6]. McNabb [70] at the 8,000-bed Central State Hospital in Milledgeville, Georgia reported successfully using the program for 90-day menu planning with significant savings in costs. Reliable computer databases for food composition and nutrients, along with automated classification and coding systems for foods, were essential tools that were developed in the late 1970s. Using primarily the USDA data sources, some hospital dietary departments developed their own nutrient databases; and programs to retrieve desired food items, to calculate the latter's nutrients, and to generate menus [98]. As a part of the HIS, the dietary service program generated dietary profile records of patients, and labels or lists of diet orders for the nursing stations. By the mid-1980s computer-assisted menu planning was available from a variety of vendors. Wheeler [96] found 32 microcomputer-based programs; and reviewed and tested seven commercial programs that did one or more of the following tasks: (1) analyze diet history and compute amounts of various nutrients actually consumed daily; (2) assess adequacy of patient's diet by comparing actual with optimal nutrient intake; (3) plan a series of meals that satisfy dietary prescriptions; and (4) analyze recipes. Examples of innovative approaches included a Macintosh computer-based, interactive, self-administered dietary assessment questionnaire developed by Hernandez [50]. This program asked the patient to enter demographic data, meal habits, and dietary pattern as to types of food generally eaten, as well as specific foods eaten in the prior 24 h, with the food items pictorially prompted by displayed illustrations. Hernandez's program automatically coded food items; and was reported to be applicable to patient education and suitable for interviewing physically handicapped and aphasic patients. Ellis [32] developed an IBM PC/XT-based system using a touch-sensitive screen to select food items displayed in a hierarchical fashion for menu selection and automatic food coding. Lacson [56] described the use of mobile phones to enter into their computer in natural language the time-stamped, spoken dietary records collected from adult patients over a period of a few weeks. They classified the food items and the food quantifiers, and developed a dietary/nutrient knowledge base with added information from resources on food types, food preparation, food combinations, portion sizes, and with dietary details from the dietary/nutrient resource database of 4,200 individual foods reported in the U.S. Department of Agriculture's Continuing Survey of Food Intakes by Individuals (CSFII). They then developed an algorithm to extract the dietary information from their patients' dietary records, and to automatically map selected items to their dietary/nutrient knowledge database. They reported 90 % accuracy in the automatic processing of the spoken dietary records.

11.4   Summary and Commentary

Much work has been done to combine data from disparate departmental data systems into more "integrated ones" that support the full spectrum of data management needs of multi-hospital and ambulatory health systems. Yet efforts to support clinical users still face two key challenges, particularly with regard to CPOE and Results Reporting functions. First, the lack of data interoperability amongst the myriad of data systems, both within and across health systems, continues to be one of the most vexing problems [1, 73]. For clinicians, this lack translates into a less than complete picture of their patients who received health services in multiple settings. For health consumers (i.e., patients), this necessitates collecting and maintaining copies of records, usually paper, from each health provider. This situation will continue to worsen as health services move more from hospital and clinic settings to community and home settings. Second, the lack of a useful point of care system (POC) for clinicians makes their work harder [8] and may actually introduce errors [2]. The amount of health data was estimated at 150 Exabyte in 2011 and expected to grow. Individual patient home monitoring and testing data together with the Internet of Things sensor data [24] will increase the total health data even more dramatically. These twenty-first century data sources already exceed the capacity of most health data systems to gather and transform it into relevant information. The signal-to-noise overload will further exacerbate the ability of POC systems to provide relevant and usable information to clinicians.

Recent efforts by the Office of the National Coordinator (ONC) within the Department of Health and Human Services have focused on improving the interoperability of electronic health record systems and health information exchanges. ONC has released its 10 year vision for an interoperable health system [72]. In addition, the HL7 standards organization has released its Fast Healthcare Interoperability Resources (FHIR) specification to accelerate exchanging healthcare information electronically [36]. Taken together, funding from ONC and support for rapid standards evolution by HL7 will be a key factor in realizing data interoperability.

Realizing a POC system that provides utility and usability to clinicians, consumers and administrators (POC users) is still an unfulfilled vision. We would add several other POC user requirements to the list for both CSISs and EHRs [85]. Namely, they should:

- Know and use the POC user's context to increase the user's "cognitive window"
- Support the coordination and scheduling tasks, based on locally relevant outcomes and measures
- Be customized based on what information is entered, what the user needs to see, what the user does, and how the user thinks
- Move from device to device, installing automatically on whatever POC device is being used
- Insulate the user from the quirks of systems to which the POC sends or receives data.

In addition, ONC has funded projects that were focused on cognitive support issues. A recent report from one of these projects, SHARPC, detailed a number of features to make a better EHR [98]. The future "Smart" POC system, coupled with better EHRs and relevant, interoperable data, may realize the "much anticipated" information technology enabled transformation of the U.S. health system.

References

1. AHRQ. A robust health data infrastructure. Report prepared by JASON for the AHRQ National Resource Center; Health Information Technology: best practices transforming quality, safety, and efficiency. 2014.
2. Ash JS, Berg M, Coiera E. Some unintended consequences of information technology in health care: the nature of patient care information system-related errors. J Am Med Inform Assoc. 2004;11:104–12.
3. ASTM 1988. Standard guide for description of reservation/registration-admission, discharge, transfer (R-ADT) systems for automated patient care information systems. Philadelphia: American Society for Testing Materials; 1988. E-1239-88.
4. ASTM 1988. Standard specifications for transferring clinical laboratory data messages between independent computer systems. Philadelphia: American Society for Testing Materials; 1988. E-1238-88.
5. ASTM 1989. Standard specifications for transferring clinical observations between independent computer systems. Philadelphia: American Society for Testing Materials; 1989. E-1238-88.
6. Balintfy JL. Computer assisted menu planning and food service management. In: Spector W, editor. Handbook of biomedical information systems. Chicago: Encyclopedia Britannica; 1971. p. 85.
7. Balintfy JL, Nebel E. Experiments with computer-assisted menu planning. Hospitals. 1966;40:88–97.
8. Ball MJ, Silva JS, Bierstock S, Douglas JV, Norcio AF, Chakraborty J, et al. Failure to provide clinicians useful IT systems: opportunities to leapfrog current technologies. Methods Inf Med. 2008;47:4–7.
9. Barnett GO. The application of computer-based medical record systems in ambulatory practice. In: Orthner HF, Blum BI, editors. Implementing health care information systems. New York: Springer; 1989. p. 85–99.

10. Barnett GO. Computers in patient care. N Engl J Med. 1968;279:1321–7.
11. Barnett GO. Computer-stored ambulatory record (COSTAT). NCHSR Research Digest Series. DHEW Pub No. (HRA) 76–3145, 1976.
12. Barnett GO, Castleman PA. A time-sharing computer system for patient-care activities. Comput Biomed Res. 1967;1:41–51.
13. Barnett GO, Souder D, Beaman P, Hupp J. MUMPS: an evolutionary commentary. Comput Biomed Res. 1981;14:112–8.
14. Barnett GO. Massachusetts general hospital computer system. In: Collen MF, editor. Hospital computer systems. New York: Wiley; 1974.
15. Barnett GO, Greenes RA, Grossman JH. Computer processing of medical text information. Methods Inf Med. 1969;8:177–82.
16. Barnett GO, Justice NS, Somand ME, et al. COSTAR – a computer-based medical information system for ambulatory care. Proc SCAMC. 1978;483–7.
17. Barret JP, Hersch PL, Cashwell RJ. Evaluation of the impact of the Technicon medical information system at El Camino Hospital. Part II. Columbus: Battelle Columbus Labs; 1979.
18. Beggs S, Vallbona C, Spencer WA, Jacobs FM, Baker RL. Evaluation of a system for on-line computer scheduling of patient care activities. Comput Biomed Res. 1971;4:634–54.
19. Bleich HL, Safran C, Slack WV. Departmental and laboratory computing in two hospitals. MD Comput. 1988;6:149–55.
20. Blose WF, Vallbona C, Spencer WA. System for processing clinical research data. System design. Proc 6th IBM Symposium. 1964. pp. 463–85.
21. Blum BI, Lenhard Jr RE, McColligan EE. An integrated data model for patient care. IEEE Trans Biomed Eng. 1985;32:277–88.
22. Blum B, Lenhard Jr R. A clinical information display system. Proc SCAMC. 1977;131–8.
23. Blum BI. Design methods for clinical systems. Proc SCAMC. 1986;309.
24. Booker E. Can IoT slash healthcare costs? InformationWeek 2014 (Nov 22).
25. Buchanan NS. Evolution of a hospital information system. Proc SCAMC. 1980;1:34.
26. Campbell CM. Information system for a short-term hospital. Hosp JAHA. 1964;38:71–80.
27. Collen MF. Data processing techniques for multitest screening and hospital facilities. In: Bekey GA, Schwartz MD, editors. Hospital information systems. New York: Marcel Dekker; 1972. p. 149–87.
28. Collen MF. General requirements of a medical information system (MIS). Comput Biomed Res. 1970;3:393–406.
29. Collen MF. Computers in preventive health services research. 7th IBM Medical Symposium. 1965.
30. Collen MF. Multiphasic health testing services. New York: Wiley; 1978.
31. Collen MF. Patient data acquisition. Med Instrum. 1977;12:222–5.
32. Ellis L, Huang P, Buzzard IM. Touchscreen versus keyboard for menu-based food coding. Proc MEDINFO. 1986. pp. 999–1003.
33. Emmel GR, Greenhalgh RC. Hospital information system study (part I). Proc 4th IBM Med Symposium. 1962. pp. 443–58.
34. Esterhay Jr R, Foy JL, Lewis TL. Hospital information systems: approaches to screen definition: comparative anatomy of the PROMIS, NIH and Duke systems. Proc SCAMC. 1982;903–11.
35. Fetter RR, Mills RE. A micro computer based medical information system. Proc 2nd Annual WAMI Meeting. 1979. pp. 388–91.
36. FHIR Overview. Fast healthcare interoperability resources (FHIR) v0.0.82. Health Level Seven. 2015.
37. Frey R, Girardi S, Wiederhold G. A filing system for medical research. Int J Biomed Comput. 1971;2:1–26.
38. Gabrieli ER. Standardization of medical informatics (special issue). J Clin Comput. 1985;14:62–104.

39. Gall J. Computerized hospital information system cost-effectiveness: a case study. In: van Egmond J, de Vries Robbe PF, Levy AH, editors. Information systems for patient care. Amsterdam: North Holland; 1976. p. 281–93.

40. Gall J. Cost-benefit analysis: total hospital informatics. In: Koza RC, editor. Health information system evaluation. Boulder: Colorado Associated University Press; 1974. p. 299–327.

41. Gardner RM, Pryor TA, Warner HR. The HELP hospital information system: update 1998. Int J Med Inform. 1999;54:169–82.

42. Giebink GA, Hurst LL. Computer projects in health care. Ann Arbor: Health Administration Press; 1975.

43. Gotcher SB, Carrick J, Vallbona C, Spencer WA, Carter RE, Cornell S. Daily treatment planning with an on-line shared computer system. Methods Inf Med. 1969;8:200.

44. Grams RR. Medical information systems: the laboratory module. Clifton: Humana Press; 1979.

45. Grossman JH, Barnett GO, Koepsell TD, Nesson HR, Dorsey JL, Phillips RR. An automated medical record system. JAMA. 1973;224:1616–21.

46. Hammond WE. GEMISCH. A minicomputer information support system. Proc IEEE. 1973;61:1575–83.

47. Hammond W, Stead W, Straube M, Kelly M, Winfree R. An interface between a hospital information system and a computerized medical record. Proc SCAMC. 1980;3:1537–40.

48. Hammond WE, Stead WW, Straube MJ, Jelovsek FR. Functional characteristics of a computerized medical record. Methods Inf Med. 1980;19:157–62.

49. Hammond WE, Stead WW, Feagin SJ, Brantley BA, Straube MJ. Data base management system for ambulatory care. Proc SCAMC. 1977;173–87.

50. Hernandez T, Walker B. Innovations in microcomputer based dietary assessment. Proc MEDINFO. 1986. pp. 476–9.

51. Hodge MH. Medical information systems: a resource for hospitals. Germantown: Aspen Publishers; 1977.

52. Jelliffe RW, Schumitzky A, Rodman J, Crone J. A package of time-shared computer programs for patient care. Proc SCAMC. 1977;154.

53. Johns RJ, Blum BI. The use of clinical information systems to control cost as well as to improve care. Trans Am Clin Climatol Assoc. 1979;90:140.

54. Juenemann HJ. The design of a data processing center for biological data. Ann N Y Acad Sci. 1964;115:547–52.

55. Kuperman GJ. The pharmacy application of the HELP system. In: Kuperman GJ, Gardner RM, Pryor TA, editors. HELP: a dynamic hospital information system. New York: Springer; 1991. pp. 168–72.

56. Lacson R, Long W. Natural language processing of spoken diet records (SDRs). Proc AMIA Annu Symp. 2006. pp. 454–8.

57. Lamson BG. Mini-computers and large central processors from a medical record management point of view. International symposium on medical information systems. 1975. pp. 58–65.

58. Lindberg D. The computer and medical care. Springfield: CC Thomas; 1968.

59. Lindberg D. Electronic retrieval of clinical data. J Med Educ. 1965;40:753–9.

60. Lindberg D. A computer in medicine. Mo Med. 1964;61:282–4.

61. Lindberg D, Reese GR, Buck C. Computer generated hospital diagnosis file. Mo Med. 1964;61:581–2. passim.

62. Lowder W, Medill C. Punch cards simplify selective menus. Mod Hosp. 1958;90:90–102. passim.

63. McColligan E, Blum B, Brunn C. An automated care medical record system for ambulatory care. In: Kaplan B, Jelovsek FR, editors. Proc SCM/SAMS joint conf on ambulatory med. Washington, DC: Society for Computer Medicine; 1981. pp. 72–6.

64. McDonald CJ. The medical gopher: a microcomputer based physician work station. Proc SCAMC. 1984;453–9.

65. McDonald C, Blevins L, Glazener T, Haas J, Lemmon L, Meeks-Johnson J. Data base management, feedback control, and the Regenstrief medical record. J Med Syst. 1983;7:111–25.

66. McDonald CJ, Hammond WE. Standard formats for electronic transfer of clinical data. Ann Intern Med. 1989;110:333–5.
67. McDonald CJ, Tierney WM. Computer-stored medical records: their future role in medical practice. JAMA. 1988;259:3433–40.
68. McDonald CJ, Murray R, Jeris D, Bhargava B, Seeger J, Blevins L. A computer-based record and clinical monitoring system for ambulatory care. Am J Public Health. 1977;67:240–5.
69. McDonald CJ, Overhage JM, Tierney WM, Dexter PR, Martin DK, Suico JG, et al. The Regenstrief medical record system: a quarter century experience. Int J Med Inform. 1999;54:225–53.
70. McNabb ME. 90-day nonselective menus by computer. Hospitals. 1971;45:88–91.
71. Monmouth. Monmouth medical shapes a total system. Systems. 1966. pp. 12–48.
72. ONC/HHS. Connecting health and care for the nation. A 10 year vision to achieve an interoperable health IT infrastructure. Washington, DC: Health and Human Services, Office of the National Coordinator; 2015.
73. PCAST. Report to the president. Realizing the full potential of health information technology to improve the health of Americans: the path forward. Washington, DC: President's Council of Advisors on Science and Technology (PCAST); 2010. Available at www.thewhitehouse.gov.
74. Pratt AW. Progress towards a medical information system for the research environment. In: Fuchs G, Wagner G, editors. Sonderdruck aus Krankenhaus-Informationsysteme. New York: Schattauer-Verlag; 1972. p. 319–36.
75. Pryor TA, Gardner RM, Clayton PD, Warner HR. The HELP system. J Med Syst. 1983;7:87–102.
76. Rothrock JJ. ASTM: the standards make the pieces fit. Proc AAMSI congress. 1989. pp. 327–35.
77. Runck HM. Computer planning for hospitals-large-scale education and involvement of employees. Comput Autom. 1969;18:33.
78. Rutt TE. Work of IEEE P1157 medical data interchange committee. Int J Clin Monit Comput. 1989;6:45–57.
79. Schenthal JE. Clinical concepts in the application of large scale electronic data processing. Proc 2nd IBM medical symposium. 1960. pp. 391–9.
80. Schenthal JE, Sweeney JW, Nettleton W. Clinical application of electronic data processing apparatus: II. New methodology in clinical record storage. JAMA. 1961;178:267–70.
81. Schultz JR, Davis L. The technology of PROMIS. Proc IEEE. 1979;67:1237–44.
82. Shieman BM. Medical information system, El Camino Hospital. IMS Ind Med Surg. 1971;40:25–6.
83. Siegel SJ. Developing an information system for a hospital. Public Health Rep. 1968;83:359–62.
84. Silva J, Seybold N, Ball M. Usable health IT for physicians. Smart point-of-care and comparative effectiveness research form the true basis for meaningful use. Healthc Inform. 2010;27:40–3.
85. Simborg DW. An emerging standard for health communications: the HL7 standard. Healthc Comput Commun. 1987;4:58–60.
86. Slack WV, Bleich HL. The CCC system in two teaching hospitals: a progress report. Int J Med Inform. 1999;54:183–96.
87. Sneider RM. Using a medical information system to improve the quality of patient care. Proc SCAMC. 1978;594.
88. Stead WW, Hammond WE. Calculating storage requirements for office practice systems. Proc SCAMC. 1985;68.
89. Stead WW, Hammond WE, Winfree RG. Beyond a basic HIS: work stations for department management. Proc SCAMC. 1984;197.
90. Tolchin SG, Barta W. Local network and distributed processing issues in the Johns Hopkins Hospital. J Med Syst. 1986;10:339–53.

91. Vallbona C, Spencer WA. Texas institute for research and rehabilitation hospital computer system (Houston). In: Collen MF, editor. Hospital computer systems. New York: Wiley; 1974. p. 662–700.

92. Warner HR. A computer-based patient monitoring. In: Stacy RW, Waxman B, editors. Computers in biomedical research, vol. III. New York: Academic; 1972. p. 239–51.

93. Watson RJ. A large-scale professionally oriented medical information system – five years later. J Med Syst. 1977;1:3–21.

94. Weed LL. Problem-oriented medical information system (PROMIS) laboratory. In: Giebink GA, Hurst LL, editors. Computer projects in health care. Ann Arbor: Health Administration Press; 1975. p. 199–203.

95. Wheeler PS, Simborg DW, Gitlin JN. The Johns Hopkins radiology reporting system. Radiology. 1976;119:315–9.

96. Wheeler LA, Wheeler ML. Review of microcomputer nutrient analysis and menu planning programs. MD Comput. 1984;1:42–51.

97. Wiederhold G. Summary of the findings of the visiting study team automated medical record systems for ambulatory care. Visit to Duke University Medical Center, CDD-5 HRA Contract, June 29. 1975.

98. Witschi J, Kowaloff H, Bloom S, Slack W. Analysis of dietary data; an interactive computer method for storage and retrieval. J Am Diet Assoc. 1981;78:609–13.

99. Zhang J, Walji M. Better EHR: usability, workflow and cognitive support in electronic health records. Houston: National Center for Cognitive Informatics and Decision Making in Health Care; 2014.

Chapter 12
Clinical Laboratory (LAB) Information Systems

Morris F. Collen and Robert E. Miller

Abstract The clinical laboratory (LAB) was an early adopter of computer technology, beginning with the chemistry and hematology laboratories, which had similar information processing requirements. LAB systems in the early 1960s were primarily offline, batch-oriented systems that used punched cards for data transfer to the hospital mainframe. The advent of minicomputers in the 1970s caused a rapid surge in the development of LAB systems that supported online processing of data from automated laboratory instruments. In the 1980s, LAB systems increasingly employed minicomputers to integrate data into a common database and satisfy functional requirements, including programs for quality control, reference values, trend analyses, graphical presentation, online test interpretations, and clinical guidelines. By 1987 about 20 % of US hospitals had computer links between their LAB systems and their hospital information systems and affiliated outpatient information systems. In the 1990s, LAB systems began using client-server architecture with networked workstations, and most hospitals had a variety of specialized clinical support information systems interconnected to form a medical information system with a distributed database of clinical data that constituted the electronic patient record. By the 2000s, several hundred different clinical tests were routinely available (there had been only a few dozen in the 1950s). The need for more sophisticated and powerful LAB systems has largely been met by commercially available standalone laboratory information systems (LIS); however, there is now increasing pressure to replace these products with the lab-system functionality of the enterprise-wide integrated electronic health record system, for which there is little reported experience.

Author was deceased at the time of publication.

M.F. Collen (deceased)

R.E. Miller, M.D. (✉)
Departments of Pathology and Biomedical Engineering, Division of Health Sciences Informatics, Johns Hopkins University School of Medicine, Baltimore, MD, USA

Department of Health Policy and Management, Bloomberg School of Public Health, Johns Hopkins University, Baltimore, MD, USA
e-mail: remiller@jhmi.edu

© Springer-Verlag London 2015
M.F. Collen, M.J. Ball (eds.), *The History of Medical Informatics in the United States*, Health Informatics, DOI 10.1007/978-1-4471-6732-7_12

Keywords Clinical laboratory systems • Laboratory information systems • Chemistry laboratory systems • Hematology laboratory systems • Networked systems • Automated laboratory equipment • Minicomputer-based laboratory systems • Workstations • Clinical support information systems

This chapter on the LAB system is new to this second edition of *A History of Medical Informatics in the United States*, and reflects Dr. Morris F. Collen's meticulous scholarship in documenting the history of the application of computer technology to the clinical laboratories. The computerization of the clinical laboratories represents the earliest – and now most widely adopted – clinical application of computer technology in health care, and has evolved over the past six decades in lockstep with advances in laboratory technology and automation, and with the parallel advances in computer hardware and software.

The LAB system is the term used to describe the computer hardware and software that support the clinical laboratories, including the processing of requests for laboratory testing on patients' specimens, the internal operations of the laboratories, and the reporting of laboratory test results. The similar functions for the anatomic pathology (surgical pathology) laboratory are provided by the PATH system, which is discussed in Chap. 13.

An appreciation of the history of the LAB system provides important insights into the limitations of contemporary LAB systems and the requirements for LAB systems of the future. Additionally, an understanding of early LAB system innovations, such as rule-based processing for laboratory diagnosis or detecting hospital acquired infections, reveals many still-unfulfilled needs in clinical informatics that can be revisited and re-implemented using computer hardware and software technologies that are vastly more powerful than those available to the early LAB system pioneers.

The clinical laboratories, broadly defined, are hospital organizational units and other entities, such as commercial reference laboratories, that perform in vitro analyses on patients' specimens to aid in the diagnosis and management of the patients' health or disease. Clinical laboratory information provides unique and essential "non-sensory" input to the care process for virtually all types and categories of patients, and routine laboratory testing is now performed on millions of patients nationwide each day at a cost of only a few percent of the nation's total expenditures on health care.

Clinical laboratories historically were named for their scientific disciplines or sub-disciplines – or their technologies – making the bacteriology and pathology laboratories of more than a century ago the first true "clinical laboratories." In the ensuing decades, the hematology, chemistry and immunology laboratories, and the blood bank, all became major players. There are now laboratories named for new technologies such as flow cytometry and histochemistry; and laboratories employing molecular (nucleic acid) testing methods have become increasingly important in the rapidly evolving era of genetic and genomic medicine.

The traditional distinction between clinical pathology, which involves quantitative measurements performed by medical technologists on blood and other body fluids, and anatomic pathology, which involves the microscopic evaluation by the pathologist of tissue specimens, will diminish in the future as quantitative testing is performed more frequently on tissues, and interpretations by the pathologist are more frequently required for complex blood and body fluid analyses. For the modern LAB system, both the anatomic and clinical pathology laboratories involve the analysis of specimens removed from patients, and each may issue reports that include an interpretation by the pathologist of the findings about multiple specimens from a patient. (See Chap. 13 for more about anatomic pathology and the PATH system.)

The growth of clinical laboratories and origin of the laboratory information system (LIS or the LAB system) date back to the 1950s and the expansion of biomedical research funding by the US National Institutes of Health (NIH). The growth in NIH-funded clinical research soon resulted in discoveries about human health and disease that had clear clinical utility in managing patients' illnesses. Many of these discoveries involved measurements on blood or body fluids that were developed into practical in vitro diagnostic procedures that could be reliably performed in the hospital clinical laboratory. This, in turn, spawned the growth of clinical laboratory testing, and the subspecialty of clinical pathology, which is also known as laboratory medicine. The increasing volumes of patient testing then drove innovations in laboratory automation, and the development in the 1960s of numerous automated multichannel chemistry instruments and high-speed blood cell counters. With automated instruments, the clinical laboratories began producing large amounts of data, which created an increasing need for computerization for instrument data acquisition and to relieve the clerical burden associated with processing test requests, analyzing specimens, and reporting test results. The hospital clinical laboratories, along with the business office, became the first hospital areas to make significant use of computer technology. The "factory-like" environment of the clinical laboratories, with their stereotyped processes and numerous clerical steps, were well suited to computerized data handling using the commercially available computer technologies of the 1950s and 1960s.

Subsequent advances in information technology, with exponential increases in computer processing power and data storage capabilities, allowed more and more areas of the laboratories to be computerized over time. For example, the chemistry and hematology laboratories were the initial focus of the LAB system, as their numeric data and short alphanumeric results were well suited to early computer systems. As computers became more powerful, and computer power more affordable, the LAB system was extended to other areas of the laboratories where the data handling requirements were more complex. The microbiology laboratory, where test results often consist of text strings, and the surgical pathology laboratory, which reports large blocks of semi-structured text and free text, necessarily came later in the evolution of the LAB system.

The growth of the LAB system has followed a recurring and predictable pattern of clinically relevant biomedical discovery with subsequent innovation in laboratory methods, laboratory automation, and laboratory computer applications that can be expected to continue for at least the foreseeable future. This chapter tells the story of the LAB system, and is intended to convey Morris Collen's thoughts and perspectives as he recorded them, as it is his views and ideas on the history of the LAB system that are of the greatest value to all of us.

12.1   Introduction

The clinical laboratory traditionally is directed by a clinical pathologist, who also functions as a consultant to the clinicians. The clinical laboratory includes the divisions of chemistry, hematology, microbiology, and others; and may be associated with a blood bank. Clinical laboratory tests are one of the most frequently ordered clinical support services in the care of patients in the office and in the hospital. In each of the past six decades many new tests were added, and as the volume of laboratory testing increased, automation and computerization became essential [146]. A committee of the College of American Pathologists considered that the pathologist's role was to define the clinical laboratory (LAB) system's functions, which included: (1) maintaining proper patient identification; (2) accepting laboratory test requests; and (3) generating documents of (a) patients' test results, (b) internal laboratory reports, and (c) laboratory administrative reports [109].

Ball [8] wrote one of the first books describing the specifications for a LAB system and guidelines for selecting one. She estimated that in 1971 there were 13,500 clinical laboratories in the United States that performed 2.9 billion tests in that year. Based upon the experience at Temple University Hospital, Ball described the LAB system's main functions: (1) to relieve laboratory technical staff of clerical functions during the analysis and processing of laboratory specimens; (2) to generate collated test result data in legible and convenient formats for physicians' use; (3) to provide basic internal and external quality control programs; (4) to generate statistical summaries to aid in research and in data handling for special projects; and (5) to communicate with the main hospital computer system [10].

Lincoln [130] described the clinical laboratories as being analogous to a light industry, and estimated that in 1971 there were about 6,000 clinical laboratories in the United States, of which about 5 % had LAB systems. Experience at that time with commercial vendors confirmed that the introduction of a LAB system was a complex engineering project. Lincoln [124] and Lincoln and Korpman [130] later observed that the clinical laboratories, which were an active and full participant in the practice of medicine, functioned as a self-contained industry with a set of structured procedures directed toward the analysis of body fluids and tissues. He also noted that except for the blood bank, information was the sole medical product of a clinical laboratory.

By the early 1980s, Connelly and associates [57] at the University of Minnesota had already considered clinical laboratory computer-based information systems to be one of the first successful applications of computers in medical practice. They pointed out that microprocessor-based analyzers needed little or no understanding of computer technology; however, selection of a comprehensive LAB system demanded a high level of computer expertise.

Hicks [107] at the University of Wisconsin in Madison correctly predicted that in the 1980s computer technology would become so inexpensive that it would have a dramatic effect on the clinical laboratory.

12.2   Requirements for the LAB System

As with any clinical system or other computer application, it is essential to first define the requirements for the LAB system. This, in turn, requires careful consideration of the functions of the clinical laboratory and the demands for its analytical services, and how the laboratory meets these demands. The primary function of the laboratory is to support clinical decision making by providing specialized analyses of tissue and body-fluid specimens collected from patients for diagnosis and for monitoring therapy. To support clinical decision making, the laboratory and its information (LAB) system must be responsive to physicians and other caregivers regarding which tests are to be performed, when and how the specimens are to be collected, and in what format the test results are to be reported.

The usual reasons given for developing LAB systems were: (1) to increase the speed of the laboratory operations and reduce the turnaround time from the receipt of test requests to the delivery of the test results; (2) to improve the quality control of analytical procedures and the reliability and accuracy of the test results; (3) to reduce errors from manual transcription of data; (4) to reduce routine paper work; (5) to improve the information content of the reports of test results; (6) to improve the productivity of the laboratory staff and reduce the costs of laboratory testing; and (7) to increase the availability of data for management and for research purposes [38].

A LAB system must have functions for identifying patients; for accepting test requests; for uniquely numbering, collecting, and labeling specimens; for producing a variety of work lists and instrument load-lists; for online data acquisition from instruments; for manual entry of test results; for comprehensive quality control of analytical and other processes; for flexible reporting of test results; for data interfaces to hospital information systems and other systems; for billing and other administrative purposes; for workload, productivity, cost-accounting and management reporting; and for process improvement and research.

Morey and associates [163] at the Massachusetts Institute of Technology (MIT) published a comprehensive analysis of the chemistry laboratory at the Boston City Hospital (BCH), and defined the functional requirements for a LAB system that would be needed to handle the BCH chemistry laboratory's volume of about one million tests a year, most of which were already automated. They compared these requirements to the hardware and software characteristics for 12 LAB computer systems that were available in 1970.

Williams [241] at the Clinical Center of the National Institutes of Health advised that establishing the functional requirements for a LAB system required the collection of information regarding: (1) specimen volumes, types of tests, number of tests per specimen; (2) numbers of high-volume tests and numbers of stat or emergency tests; (3) short-term and long-term storage and retrieval requirements; (4) quality-control procedures; (5) report formats for test results, including cumulative-summary formats; (6) flagging of abnormalities on reports and comparison of patients' current test results to prior test results; (7) periodic statistical reports of workloads by categories of specimens and tests; (8) blood inventories and transfusion records for blood banks; (9) billing procedures; and (10) other specific needs of physicians, administrators, and researchers. These data could then be used to develop the functional requirements for the LAB system. Also, to ensure reliable laboratory services, backup facilities were necessary for processing laboratory data whenever there was a failure of the LAB system. Williams emphasized that although single analytical instruments could readily be connected to a computer, the laboratory operations were quite complex, and the processing of all specimens would not be identical because of variations in patients' disease states and other factors. Williams proposed some guiding principles for the LAB system: (1) laboratory tasks should be carefully divided between humans and computers to take advantage of their respective capabilities; (2) computer programs should include self-checking features; (3) computers should be used for repetitive data handling where speed and accuracy are important and computers can yield the greatest benefits; and (4) high development costs should be avoided by adapting the laboratory's processes to an existing LAB system design.

Laboratory test results must be subjected to several checking procedures, including determining if test result values are within normal limits; the flagging of abnormal values and extreme values; and checking for medical plausibility (such as unlikely combinations of test results). The LAB system has to be able to provide a variety of formatted reports of test results, including tabular and graphic printouts with cumulative-trend reports and comparisons to prior test results. Additionally, the LAB system has to be able to store all relevant patient data in a database, and to respond interactively to queries for data [241]. Blois [30] summarized the functions of LAB systems that interface with hospital information system (HIS): at the lowest level, they must receive inputs from other hospital units; at the next higher level, they must provide certain outputs of information to users; at a higher level, they must provide quality control of tests and results; and at the highest level, they must support clinical decision making.

Benson [24] proposed that the uses to which a LAB system could be applied fell into two broad categories: the improved selection of laboratory tests for diagnosis; and the improved use of laboratory test results for clinical problem solving.

Lewis [127] emphasized that a principal function of a LAB system was laboratory data management, as a modern hospital laboratory typically offered hundreds of different tests, processed thousands of patients' specimens a day with some services provided 24-h a day; and it provided many thousands of numeric or textual reports each day, often with dozens of tests per report. Lewis predicted that since clinical laboratory testing already accounted for about 8 % of the national health care expenditures in 1979, the potential cost-savings from LAB systems could be significant.

Bull and Korpman [40] wrote that a model LAB system had to be able to provide a variety of reports, including stat reports for urgently needed test results, current reports for those provided on a daily basis, and cumulative reports to be kept permanently in patients' records. The LAB system needed to help the technologists perform analyses rapidly and reliably, and make test results available to the physicians whenever, wherever, and however they could most effectively use them. Bull and Korpman estimated that 15–20 % of laboratory test data were never used in the diagnosis or treatment of a particular patient's condition, as the test results were often buried in the medical record and therefore missed by the physician; and they noted that a LAB system could provide data reporting mechanisms that would minimize such waste. They specified that the ideal LAB system should allow analyses to begin as soon as the specimens became available, and should support fast turnaround times. A variety of laboratory test report formats should be available, and test results should be accessible in a timely manner at suitably distributed electronic terminals. A LAB system should maintain a test result database and should be flexible to handle important needed or desired enhancements.

A clinical laboratory's functions involve procedures for ordering tests, collecting test specimens, preparing and analyzing the specimens, and reporting and storing the results of the analyses. Upon arrival in the laboratory, specimens are assigned unique accession numbers that are linked to the patients' identification (ID) data. Specimens may be split into aliquots, and the aliquots are then prepared for the specific analyses requested. Quantitative measurements may be made of the physical or chemical makeup of the specimens; observations and counts may be made of the numbers and types of cell constituents; or the presence of microorganisms may be assessed. These findings are then evaluated for accuracy and validity; and any errors found are corrected. Reports of the test results are provided to the clinical caregivers, administrative and accounting data are made available, and the test results are stored with other patient data in the LAB system database [135].

Bronzino [36] divided the technical requirements of a LAB system into: (1) local instrument process control, which involved of a set of computers or processors for the specimens and analytic procedures with associated specimen identification data (e.g., for a Coulter Counter or a Technicon AutoAnalyzer); and (2) central laboratory computer functions that controlled and integrated the various laboratory instruments and transferred data from analytic instruments into the computer-based patients' records. Also, a LAB system should provide clerical functions for recording, verifying, and reporting laboratory test results.

Bronzino [36] also advised that the installation of a LAB system should include consideration of: (1) the financial investment; (2) system expansion capacity to accommodate new workstations and automated instruments; (3) adequacy of system performance to provide prompt response to requests for test results; (4) operating system software reliability; (5) provisions for automatic error checking; and (6) the lack of need for computer programming experience.

Lincoln [134] advised that the acquisition of a LAB system was similar to the preparation and execution of a business plan for any new large capital investment. He suggested preparing a detailed list of specifications for software functions, hardware, installation, training, maintenance and support, in addition to assessing vendor capabilities and costs.

Weilert [235], at Wesley Medical Center in Wichita, Kansas, recommended that for a vendor-provided LAB system, it was helpful to prepare a Gantt chart to plot the timing and the estimated duration of various phases in the planning and implementation of a LAB system for a large medical center. According to Weilert, this could be expected to take about 18 months from initial planning for all of: vendor selection, contract negotiations, database preparation, site preparation, installation, training, and finally, full production operation.

Connelly and associates [56] at the University of Minnesota Health Sciences Center described a multi-attribute utility model for evaluating and selecting LAB systems offered by vendors. They assigned weights to attributes that included: (1) functionality of the applications programs; (2) maintainability and reliability; (3) performance capacity; (4) flexibility without reprogramming; (5) modifiability and programmability; (6) vendor support; and (7) vendor qualifications. They advocated such a structured approach to selecting a LAB system as they considered selection of a LAB system to be a very complex project.

For health care organizations that operate under fixed-price reimbursement arrangements or capitation payment systems, the laboratories are cost centers rather than revenue centers. With the increasing number and variety of available laboratory tests, selection of the cost effective tests for specific patient conditions and patient populations and sub-populations becomes more complicated. Accordingly, LAB systems had to be able to collect data to provide total cost and unit cost-per-test, as well as other measures of laboratory efficiency [129].

Smith and Svirbely [198] described the processing cycles of a LAB system as: an *external* cycle outside the laboratory that involved test ordering by physicians, communication of test orders and the delivery of specimens to the laboratory, and the transmission of test results back to the clinical users; and an *internal* cycle within the laboratory that included all the data-processing functions within the laboratory, such as assigning unique specimen identifiers, preparing work lists for technologists, collecting test analytic data, monitoring test data, quality control, preparing reports, and storing test results.

Since information is the principal product produced by the clinical laboratory, protecting the security and confidentiality of the information is an important requirement for a LAB system. Safeguards must be instituted to protect against loss of information, accidents, computer failures, viruses, and theft of information [226].

Before the development of computer-based clinical support information systems (CSISs), the communication of orders for laboratory testing from physicians to the laboratories, and the communication of test results from the laboratories back to physicians relied on hand-written forms and documents and typed reports. To replace these error-prone methods, a CSIS needed both computer-based physician order entry (CPOE) and results reporting (RR) functions that were capable of capable of receiving requests for laboratory procedures to be performed; and for reporting the test results after the procedures were completed. Until the 1970s, each hospital department's CSIS typically provided its own OE-RR applications, so that when a hospital implemented separate laboratory, radiology, or pharmacy subsystems, each subsystem had its own separate order entry terminal. This meant that hospital personnel had to repeatedly enter the patient's identification into separate terminals for laboratory, pharmacy, radiology, as well as for patient transfer or discharge orders, either when entering new orders, or when changing old orders for a patient. Furthermore, some types of orders required associated secondary orders to be communicated to another department, such as the dietary service; for example, an order for an upper-gastrointestinal x-ray examination to be performed on a specified day required that the procedure be scheduled in the radiology department, and also required that the nursing staff and the dietary department be notified that food and fluids should be withheld from the patient prior to the procedure, that the patient needed to be transported to the radiology department at the time of the scheduled examination, and that appropriate dietary instructions be provided for after the patient's return from the examination.

The technical design requirements for a LAB system could be developed from the functional requirements, and included computer-to-computer interoperability; that is, the LAB system had to be compatible with, and capable of communicating with other clinical support information systems (CSIS) and hospital information system (HIS) modules. The LAB system also had to include interfaces that converted analog signals generated by laboratory instruments into digital data so that high-volume data from automated and semi-automated equipment could be acquired directly by the LAB system. The LAB system also had to be capable of controlling and processing the data from all of the clinical laboratory's instruments and workstations.

In the 1980s, it became apparent that the electronic exchange of laboratory requests and results between clinical laboratories and medical care facilities required formal data exchange standards. In 1984, a task force established by the American Association for Medical Systems and Informatics (AAMSI) proposed standards for sending laboratory test requests and receiving test results, which defined multiple "levels" of information and rules for the ordering of data. As an example, dates were always to be recorded in the YYMMDD format [154].

In 1985, as a result of the increasing need for interoperability in laboratory data transfers between nations, a multi-national group proposed international standards for clinical laboratory data exchange between laboratory computer systems [75]. Additionally, laboratories began to report some test results in Système International (SI) units, so that, for example, serum glucose values would be reported in the conventional units as mg/dl, and in SI units as mmol/L [3].

In the 1990s, Logical Observation Identifier Names and Codes (LOINC) were proposed as a set of standardized names and codes for clinical laboratory tests for use in sharing laboratory test results and to assist in comparing laboratory utilization [82].

Baorto and associates [14], at Barnes Hospital at Washington University School of Medicine in St. Louis and at Columbia University Medical Center in New York, extracted raw laboratory data from LAB systems at three academic hospitals and attempted to translate the data into LOINC values. They found that coding failures were primarily due to differences in local codes or the absence of matching laboratory test names in the LOINC database. After a further 2 years of working with LOINC encoding, they found that automatic matching of the most frequent 100 laboratory tests still resulted in a number of failures, often due to ongoing changes local codes [14].

12.3 Laboratory Specimen Identification

In addition to reliable identification of patients, the clinical laboratories must ensure that a unique identification number is assigned to each specimen obtained from a patient, and that the specimens remain uniquely identified during the entirety of their time in the laboratories. Some of the challenges with the automatic reading of specimen identification numbers as specimens were being processed by automated instruments are described below.

In the 1960s, Technicon Corporation's continuous-flow chemistry analyzers used either miniature punched-cards that were attached to the specimen containers with rubber collars, or sample cups with attached barcoded labels with numbers that matched numbers on the test requisition forms. The number on the card or label was then read by a special optical reader attached to the analyzer, allowing the computer to link the specimen identification number to the test result. The National Institutes of Health (NIH) Clinical Center developed machine-readable, specimen-carrier racks that were used for both continuous-flow analyzers and for discrete-sample analyzers. Specimen numbers were read as the specimens were processed by the analyzers, and the computer then linked the test results with the specimen numbers [38].

In the 1980s, advances in barcode readers allowed streamlining of specimen workflows in ways that were not previously achievable in the clinical laboratory. Initially, barcoded labels for identifying patient specimens were generated next to the instruments used to analyze the specimens. Later, the specimens began to be labeled at the time that blood was drawn from the patient rather than at the instrument, which resulted in significant labor savings, superior services to clinicians, and reduced chances for error. Tilzer [224] at the University of Kansas reported the total integration of barcode printing for their LAB system. Brient [34], at St. Luke's Episcopal Hospital in Houston, reported moving the printing of barcode labels from the clinical laboratory to patient care locations using small, quiet, and simple-to-use barcode printers located at the nursing stations. This avoided the need to re-label specimens in the laboratory, and thereby eliminated relabeling as cause of errors. By 2010, radio frequency identification (RFID) tags, with a coiled antenna connected to an electronic chip containing patient and specimen information, were also used as an alternative to barcode labeling for the identification of clinical laboratory specimens [191].

12.4 LAB Test Results and Interpretive Reporting

Interpretive reporting, a term of art from journalism, is used to describe the use of algorithms and computer logic to enhance the value of reports of laboratory test results. Clinical laboratory (LAB system) test reports typically include four types: (1) stat reports needed for the immediate care of patients; (2) daily reports of recently completed tests; (3) cumulative summary reports that provide time-sequenced trends of laboratory results; and (4) interpretive reports that also include additional computer-generated content and that constitute an example of computer based clinical decision support.

The advent of computerized patient records made it feasible to provide computer-based clinical decision support (CDS) for a variety of purposes: reminders and alerts; evidence-based practice guidelines; guidelines for drug dosages and warnings about drug-drug interactions and adverse drug effects; and for other applications to the decision-making process in diagnosis and treatment. Information added algorithmically to interpretive reports of laboratory tests may include: reference ranges (normal values) and abnormality flags; guidelines for interpreting test results; warnings about drug-laboratory test interactions; predictive value calculations for positive and/or negative test results; recommendations for additional testing for borderline test results; and evidence-based clinical practice guidelines for the use of test results for diagnosis and treatment for specific clinical problems. Additionally, interpretive reports may be enhanced by using tables, histograms, flow charts, or graphs. (For more on decision support systems, see Chap. 17.)

Reference ranges or "normal values" accompanying test results were one of the earliest forms of clinical decision support provided by the LAB system and other systems that reported patients' test results. Reference ranges typically are defined as test values lying between the 2.5th and 97.5th percentiles in a reference population that is presumed to be representative of the patient populations that is subsequently to be tested [207], With the availability of test results from automated laboratory equipment, the frequency distributions of test results for large numbers of relatively healthy persons are often used to define "normal" reference values. With the increasing availability of computer-based patient records showing patients' data over time, the development of "normal" test values for individuals could be based on trend analyses of their own prior test values. Such were reported, among others, by Bassis [22, 23] for Kaiser Permanente Health Plan members in the San Francisco Bay Area. Cutler [62] reported on the distribution of eight serum chemistry test values for a large group of adults who had completed two multiphasic health examinations in a period of 3 years and had received a final diagnosis of "no significant abnormalities." The test results for these "healthy" persons had lower mean values and smaller standard deviations than those for a larger mixed group of examinees from the general population. Dinio and associates [66] at Perth Amboy General Hospital also developed reference test values for six age-sex categories of 2,500 hospital employees and blood donors who were free of overt illness or complaints at the time of performing 12 tests by a Technicon SMA 12. Reference test values were also developed by Reece [179] for a large private medical laboratory practice in Minneapolis, Minnesota, and by Cunnick [61] for a large life insurance population. Connelly [54] described the use of Monte Carlo simulation techniques to help improve the accuracy and value of estimating the reference range of "normal" test values.

McDonald [153] advised that for every clinical laboratory test result for a patient, the physician must consider whether a change in a current test result from the value of a prior result could be explained by a change in the patient's health status, or possibly by the effect of a patient's medication, or by some other cause. Clinical laboratory test reports usually provided interpretive statements that include a definition of the test, its normal reference levels, and alert signals for variations from normal levels or for any unexpected changes in the values from prior test results. Physicians interpreted laboratory test results that differed from standard reference normal limits as an indication that the patient may have or be developing an abnormal condition. They then initiated follow up or confirming testing and procedures to help arrive at a diagnosis, and often ordered follow up tests to monitor and manage the treatment of disease. Tables, histograms, flowcharts, time-sequenced trend analyses and other displays showing relationships between multiple test results were used to assist in interpretation of the test results.

Lindberg and associates [144] at the University of Missouri Medical Center, Columbia, studied patterns of tests that could be significant even when none of the individual test values was outside of the normal limits. They studied combinations of results of four serum chemistry tests: sodium, potassium, chloride, and bicarbonate; and found that decreased sodium and chloride concentrations associated with normal concentrations of potassium and bicarbonate constituted the most common abnormal electrolyte pattern seen in hospitalized patients. To supplement their interpretive reporting they developed a computer-based, decision support program called CONSIDER [136, 138, 217]. Lindberg and associates [143] also developed AI/COAG, a knowledge-based computer program that analyzed and interpreted blood-coagulation laboratory studies, either singly or as a group of six laboratory tests that included: the platelet count, bleeding time, prothrombin time, activated partial-thromboplastin time, thrombin time, and urea clot solubility. A printout of test results summarized abnormal findings, and the system provided possible explanations of the abnormalities and provided an interactive consultation mode for users who wished to see listing of potential diagnoses. Initial evaluation of the system revealed that more than 90 % of the coagulation studies reported by their laboratory could be successfully analyzed by the automated consultation system.

Collen and associates at Kaiser Permanente developed decision rules for alerts that automatically requested an appropriate second set of tests if abnormal laboratory test results were reported for an initial group of multiphasic screening tests. The extension of the use of the computer from the laboratory to the management of routine periodic health examinations exploited the computer's potential for supporting direct patient care. When a patient's blood and urine test results were stored in the computer along with selected physiological measurements obtained at a multiphasic health testing center, the computer could provide the physician with a summary report that contained all test results, reference values, alert flags, and likely diagnoses to be considered [48, 50].

Bleich [29] at the Beth Israel Hospital in Boston described a program written in the MUMPS language for evaluating a panel of clinical laboratory tests for acid-base disorders. On entering the test values for serum electrolytes, carbon-dioxide tension, and hydrogen-ion activity, the computer evaluated the patient's acid-base balance, provided alerts for appropriate treatment, and cited relevant references.

Wolf [244] at the University of California, San Diego wrote that the simplest procedure for computer-aided diagnosis of biochemical test results was a matching method that first compared the patient's test results to normal intervals (reference ranges), and then matched the patient data to test result patterns for 130 diseases in a computer database. The computer would report the diagnoses that matched, along with suggested further laboratory work to clarify the patient's disease status.

Klee and associates [118] at the Mayo Clinic developed a set of decision rules for a second set of tests to be requested if abnormal test results were reported for an initial group of blood tests. The patient's age, sex, Coulter-S hematology test values, and white cell differential counts were keypunched and were processed with a FORTRAN program written for a CDC 3600 computer. Patients' test results that exceeded normal reference values (standardized by age and sex) were then considered for further testing. The system was found to work best for identifying patients with anemia associated with low serum values of vitamin B12 or iron.

Groves [101] at the Medical University of South Carolina developed a computer program that automatically alerted the physician when a drug ordered for a patient could interfere with a laboratory test result. Using published information on drug-test interactions, he compiled a database of the effects of each drug listed in their formulary on a variety of laboratory tests. When drug codes were entered for medications prescribed for a patient, the computer program checked for a match between the prescribed drug and the laboratory tests ordered for the patient, so that an appropriate comment could be appended to the report of the test result.

Bull and Korpman [40] pointed out that physicians could handle large amounts of data most easily and efficiently if the data are presented in the form of a graph. Williams [238, 240] used normalized radial graphs of multiple test results to allow rapid recognition by physicians of changes in the shape and skew of the radial graphs. If all test results were within normal limits, the graph would be a regular polygon with the sides corresponding to the number of tests reported. Abnormal test results would distort the polygon and could be displayed with marks indicating the normal ranges. Williams believed that graphic displays such radial "clock" diagrams could greatly enhance the interpretation of the results of multiple tests, and may also be useful for depicting temporal trends in a series of single or multiple test results.

Connelly [52] at the University of Minnesota reported that computer-generated graphical displays for data aggregation and summarization could effectively convey the significance of laboratory results, as visual relationships portrayed by graphs and charts can be more readily grasped, and abnormal results and the degree of abnormality can be seen at a glance. He cited the Technicon SMA 12 analyzer that used this type of display. Furthermore, patients' time-trend data can be used for clinical decision-making and patient management.

Speicher and Smith [207, 208] at Ohio State University advocated interpretive reporting for clinical laboratory tests to support clinical decisions by adding specific information to reports of laboratory test results. Examples of such information included detailed descriptions of tests, normal reference levels, "alerts" for variations from normal test levels, predictive values of the laboratory test results, and "advice" regarding alternative diagnoses to be considered for reported test abnormalities. Interpretive test reporting with online processing of reported clinical laboratory test results for significant changes were recognized as important requirement for and benefit of an electronic patient record (EPR) system.

Lincoln [133, 135] emphasized that the ordering of tests and the interpretation of test results were the primary forms of interaction of the clinicians with the laboratories, and the importance of the format of the laboratory report could not be overemphasized, as the report was the principal means by which laboratories returned data to the physician. Lincoln also noted that clinical decision-making could be influenced by reporting alerts and enhancing the alerts with a display of the relevant relationships between results from multiple tests. To aid in the interpretation of the results of multiple laboratory tests, such as electrolyte or lipid panels, the results can be presented as tables, histograms, flow charts or graphic displays. Graphic displays of laboratory data with alerts are analogous to the online computer-based monitoring of heart rate, blood pressure, electrocardiogram signals, and other variables for hospitalized patients in the intensive care unit, where continuous graphic displays are also used, and where significant changes from prior values trigger immediate alerts and alarms. Other settings in which time-sequenced trend analyses of test results with alerts must be communicated to physicians (and patients) include the daily testing of blood glucose values for patients with diabetes who are taking insulin, and the monthly testing of ambulatory patients with cardiac arrhythmias who are taking Coumadin (warfarin). These conditions require regular clinical laboratory testing with standard monitoring procedures and alerts when test values are outside of specified limits. Lincoln [133] observed that with the increasing availability and importance of LAB systems, the clinical pathologist who directed the laboratory needed to be qualified as a physician, as a laboratorian, and as an informationist.

Speedie and associates [205, 206] at the University of Maryland developed a drug-prescribing review system that involved laboratory testing for monitoring therapy. The system used rules to provide feedback to physicians so that potentially inappropriate prescribing could be identified and avoided. Their Medical Evaluation of Therapeutic Orders (MENTOR) system, which was expanded in 1987, was designed to monitor inpatient drug orders for possible adverse drug events (ADEs), and also for suboptimal therapy or inappropriate. The system had rules that allowed the monitoring of whether the prescribed dosage and drug regimen were appropriate for the patient's medical condition, and whether appropriate clinical laboratory testing was obtained and the results were reviewed in a timely manner. If rules were not followed within a specified interval, an alert was triggered and a patient-specific advisory report was printed.

Salwen and Wallach [166], at the S.U.N.Y. Downstate Medical Center in Brooklyn, devised a series of algorithms for interpreting hematology data and providing clinical guidelines for the diagnostic evaluation of patients with abnormal blood counts. Their program classified the patients' blood counts as normal or abnormal, and then categorized the patients into diagnostic groups, with recommendations for further testing.

Smith and associates [199] at Ohio State University in Columbus developed a special language called Conceptual Structure Representation Language (CSRL) to facilitate interpretive reporting. They proposed that because the concept of disease hierarchy is well established in medicine in the form of disease classifications, CSRL diagnostic hierarchies could be defined that contained laboratory test values and other knowledge about specific diagnoses, against which patients' test values could be matched to determine probable diagnoses with associated levels of confidence.

Healy and associates [106] at Dartmouth Medical School used an expert system as an alternative computer-based approach to interpretive reporting. They defined an expert system as consisting of a knowledge base of rules, facts and procedures, with inferencing mechanisms for operating on the knowledge base, and facilities for providing a detailed explanation for each conclusion reached by the system. They suggested that expert systems could be more flexible and more intuitive than deterministic or statistically based interpretive systems.

Connelly [53], at the University of Minnesota, advocated embedding expert systems in the LAB system as a means of detecting important events that should be reported to clinicians and others. An expert system could automatically look for suspect results that might indicate a specimen mix-up or analytic error. Important results and their implications could be brought to the attention of clinicians through various alerting mechanisms so that critical information would not be overlooked. He described an approach in which the LAB system would notify the expert system of all changes in the status of the each laboratory specimen so that an event scanner in the expert system could look for events that were relevant to pre-stored knowledge frames and pass any appropriate information to the expert system's inference processor through instance records. If conditions specified in the knowledge frames were satisfied, an alert processor would then send a message to a file and/or an output device, such as a printer or display terminal.

Hripcsak and associates [110] at the Columbia-Presbyterian Medical Center in New York City (which had 50,000 hospital admissions and 700,000 outpatient visits a year) implemented a clinical adverse-event monitoring system. The system automatically generated alert messages for adverse events including abnormal laboratory tests and potential adverse drug-drug interactions. The system employed a set of rules and mechanisms for potential adverse clinical events; queried and checked any rules generated by the event against their rule-knowledge base; and, if indicated, triggered a pertinent alert message.

Kuperman and associates [121] at Brigham and Women's Hospital in Boston described a computer-based alerting system for abnormal clinical laboratory test results that suggested up to 12 diagnoses to be considered. Since it is important for a physician to respond in a timely manner to serious abnormal laboratory test results that occur for a patient, they reported on a controlled study that used an automatic alerting system that significantly reduced the elapsed time before appropriate treatment was ordered.

12.5 LAB Subsystems

The earliest LAB subsystems were developed for the clinical chemistry and the hematology and clinical microscopy laboratories. Because clinical chemistry lent itself readily to both instrumental automation and the processing of digital test results, more was accomplished early in the automation of operations in clinical chemistry than in other areas of the clinical laboratories [38]. As computers became more powerful and computer power became more affordable, LAB systems were developed for the microbiology, immunology (serology) and surgical pathology laboratories, which required the processing of text-based results. As LAB system software became more sophisticated, and computer processing power and data storage capabilities continued to increase, LAB subsystems were developed for other areas such flow cytometry, radioimmunoassay, gas chromatography, blood bank, genetic and molecular testing, and other LAB subspecialties.

12.5.1 Chemistry

The clinical chemistry laboratory applies the many technologies of chemistry to the analysis of human body fluids and other patient materials. In the early days, colorimetric methods involved the addition of chemical reagents to patient specimens with the intensity of the resulting color reactions compared to a set of standards. As the clinical chemistry laboratory advanced, multiple methods from inorganic, organic, and physical chemistry, as well as other quantitative techniques, were applied to the analysis of patient specimens. In addition to processing all the data from the chemical analyses, the chemistry LAB subsystem also had to provide the data processing functions described above, including processing of test requisitions, monitoring the analytic processes for quality control, providing data quality control including checks for values outside of normal reference limits, collecting and integrating the data from multiple instruments, reporting test results, maintaining a computer-stored database of its internal activities, and transferring the test results into the patients' medical records.

A key event in the history of the clinical chemistry laboratory was the invention in 1957 of an automated chemistry analyzer by Skeggs [195, 196] at the Veterans

Administration (VA) Hospital in Cleveland, Ohio. A serum sample was fed into one side of the analyzer, while precise quantities of reagents were added into the system by means of a peristaltic proportioning pump that also introduced air bubbles to separate the specimens as they flowed through long, flexible tubes. The reagents produced color changes that were measurable by a colorimeter; and the resultant signals were recorded on a moving strip chart as voltage peaks that represented the percent transmission. In 1959, using Skeggs' invention, Technicon Corporation in Tarrytown, New York, began marketing single-channel AutoAnalyzers. In 1967 the first multi-channel Technicon AutoAnalyzer was developed under contract with Kaiser Permanente's multiphasic health testing program, which performed eight blood chemistry tests on each patient's sample: albumin, calcium, cholesterol, creatinine, glucose, serum transaminase (SGOT), total protein, and uric acid [46]. Bioengineers at Kaiser Permanente connected the analog signals to an analog-to-digital voltmeter-recorder, which read the voltage peaks from the colorimeter; and punched the converted digitized test values into cards. The punched cards were then read into a computer, and the data were collated with the patient's other multiphasic test data [44]. In 1967, Technicon introduced its Sequential Multiple Analyzer (SMA) 12/60 that performed 12 different chemistry tests at the rate of 60 tests per-hour, with the time from aspiration of a sample to the finished chart-graph totaling 8 min. The SMA 12/60 came with a reader attached to the specimen sampler that read the sample-identification number from a specimen tab and printed both the number and the test results directly on to the strip-chart record [204]. Coutts and associates [60] at the VA Hospital in Los Angeles reported the use of an expanded Technicon SMA/16 that performed 16 different tests on the same sample at the rate of 30 tests per hour.

Technicon also marketed a second system that consisted of a combination of single and multiple-channel Technicon AutoAnalyzers and a minicomputer with 4K of memory, an eight-channel multiplexer, an analog-to-digital converter, a paper tape or punched card reader to input patient identification data, and a keyboard to enter the tasks to be performed and to enable retrieval of stat reports. In 1972, Technicon Corporation added a computer to its SMA system, called the SMAC (Sequential Multiple Analyzer plus Computer), that identified samples automatically, calibrated each testing channel, and calculated and reported test results. In 1973, a more advanced computer system provided process control, monitoring, analyzing, and collating that were performed on 20 or more chemistry analyses per sample at the rate of 150 samples per hour [4]. In 1974, the SMAC offered 21 different chemical analyses, and soon after added 4 more analyses [206]. In 1977, the Technicon SMA II system appeared with a computer control system for continuous curve-monitoring, automatic calibration, more flexible data output, and a built-in quality control program [126]. Bronzino [36] considered the Technicon SMAC to be an excellent example of a computerized laboratory instrument.

In the 1960s, Seligson and associates [189] at Yale University developed automated chemistry analytical instruments that performed uric acid, creatinine, or phosphate measurements on blood serum filtrates at the rate of 120 samples per hour. Automatic specimen identification was performed by a card reader at the same time that photometric readings were being on the sample. Other automated instruments measured plasma glucose and urea simultaneously at the rate of 90 samples per hour; and a flame photometer measured sodium and potassium at the rate of 120 samples per hour. Test results were punched into cards, which were read by a card reader and entered offline into a computer that then generated a variety of reports.

The LINC (Laboratory INstrument Computer) minicomputer was specifically designed for use in a laboratory environment [42]; and was used in a number of LAB systems. Evenson [80] at the University of Wisconsin in Madison used the LINC in their clinical chemistry department to process test results for their Technicon SMA 12 AutoAnalyzer. Their LINC had 16 separate channels capable of accepting instrument signals to perform online monitoring, magnetic tape storage, and a cathode-ray-tube display monitor.

In 1967, Barnett and Hoffman [15] developed a LAB system for the clinical chemistry laboratory at the Massachusetts General Hospital, which routinely processed about 1,500 test requests a day. A few months after its introduction, this LAB system had completely replaced the laboratory's previous manual processing system. A clerk would type the patient's identification number and the tests requested into a Teletype terminal, and the computer then generated the appropriate work lists for the laboratory staff. As the lab tests were completed, technicians entered the results onto work sheets and then transcribed them into the computer. The system used a DEC PDP-9 computer and was developed using the MUMPS operating system and programming language, and was later enhanced to provide direct connections to the chemistry instruments (AutoAnalyzers) to capture data and generate reports of the test results.

In the second half of the 1960s, mechanized semi-automated and fully automated chemistry instrumentation began to replace the prior manual methods for sampling, carrying out chemical reactions, and reporting the test results. Because clinical chemistry lent itself readily to both instrumental automation and the processing of digital test results, more was accomplished early in the automation of operations in clinical chemistry than in other areas of the clinical laboratories [38]. By the late 1960s, several automated analyzers were marketed in the US for chemical analyses of blood samples and were linked to a variety of computers – from minicomputers to mainframes. During the 1970s, the Technicon AutoAnalyzer was the most commonly used automated chemical analyzer in the United States. Ball [8–13] described other commercial chemistry LAB systems available in the United States in the early 1970s, all of which could interface to a variety of automated chemical analyzers. Berkeley Scientific Laboratories [38] offered four different versions of their CLINDATA Mark II series, the smallest of which employed a PDP-8/L minicomputer. Digital Equipment Corporation's Clinical Lab-12 System employed a DEC PDP-12 computer. Diversified Numeric Applications (DNA) Automated Clinical Laboratory System (ACL) used a Raytheon 703 computer.

In 1970, the AGA AutoChemist, made in Sweden for large-scale analyses, used a PDP-8 or PDP-12 minicomputer and was introduced in the United States for the Kaiser Permanente's multiphasic health testing program in Oakland, California [49]. (See Chap. 16.) It used discrete sample analyses, employing a system of pneumatically operated syringes that transferred blood serum samples and dispensed appropriate chemical solutions into separate reaction vessels. The analyzer then mixed, conveyed, pooled, read, and transmitted the electrical test readings to a computer, which calculated the final test results. It could process 100–300 specimens per hour; and could generate results for 24-test channel chemical analysis of serum specimens at a rate of 140 samples per hour [204].

In 1970, the DuPont Automatic Clinical Analyzer (ACA), made in Wilmington, Delaware, was introduced for the routine chemistry laboratory. The ACA was an easy-to-use discrete sample analyzer in which all reagents needed to perform a test on a specimen were contained in a single plastic reagent pack. The operator simply loaded the instrument with the appropriate test packs for the tests to be performed on a patient's specimen, and the instrument automatically processed the specimen, doing all the tests indicated by the test packs loaded with the specimen. The computer analyzed the results of the testing and printed a report with of the test results along with the patient's identification. The ACA was capable of performing 30 different chemistry tests, and was controlled by a special-purpose, built-in solid-state computer.

The General Medical Services-Atomic Energy Commission (GemSAEC) device, made in Fairfield, New Jersey, by Electro-Nucleonics, Inc. employed a new concept of using centrifugal force to mix samples and reagents, to sediment particulate matter, and separate liquid phases. With an interface to an external computer, it performed rapid photometric analyses of discrete micro-samples at the rate of 120 per hour [49].

In the 1970s, Kassirer and associates [116] at Tufts University School of Medicine in Boston described an automated system for processing data in their metabolic balance laboratory that included ten different AutoAnalyzer blood chemistry tests and several non-AutoAnalyzer tests. Their system converted the output of the AutoAnalyzers into digital form, carried out quality control operations, and printed out reports of the metabolic balance studies. They found that the system approximately doubled the productivity of the laboratory, and produced savings in personnel and in other costs.

Collen and associates [51] at Kaiser Permanente reported the dollar cost-per-positive laboratory test in a large health testing program; and Talamo and associates [218] at Montefiore Hospital in Pittsburgh, Pennsylvania, described a microcomputer-based system for interpretive reporting of enzyme studies in patients who had an acute myocardial infarction. Their reports included a graphic display of up to 12 blood enzyme test values, with diagnostic interpretive statements that provided useful information to cardiologists.

In the 1970s, other early automated analyzers included the Perkin-Elmer C4 Automatic Analyzer that was made in Norwalk, Connecticut, and was interfaced to an external computer. The Vickers Multichannel 300 was made in the United Kingdom, and used a PDP-8L computer as a controller for the chemical processes, with analog-to-digital conversion of test results, and output by Teletype printers. The Bausch and Lomb Zymat model 340 Enzyme Analyzer performed automatic analyses of enzymes in biological fluids, including lactic dehydrogenase (LDH), serum glutamic pyruvic transaminase (SGPT), serum glutamic oxalic transaminase (SGOT), and others. The Abbott ABA-100 used Abbott A-Gent reagents for a variety of tests including enzymes and blood lipids [38].

In the 1970s microcomputers began to be used for some chemistry LAB subsystems. Hermann and associates at the University of Pennsylvania Medical Center in Philadelphia reported using a desk-top digital microcomputer to perform off-line calculations of the test measurements from Auto-Analyzer data. In 1973 automated urinalyses using Technicon and Beckman instruments could analyze urine samples for 15 different tests performed on the same sample, including urine bilirubin, creatinine, glucose, hemoglobin, ketone, and protein.

Stauffer and associates [211] at the University of Washington School of Medicine in Seattle reported on a computer-assisted system to aid in the selection and interpretation of laboratory tests; and as an example, described its application to the diagnosis of thyroid disease. The results of multiple tests of thyroid function were entered using an interactive system written in either MUMPS or FORTRAN, after which the computer program provided a series of displays that assisted in the interpretation of the results and the selection of appropriate additional tests.

Rush [185] at the Pathologists' Service Professional Associates in Tucker, New York used three Technicon SMAC systems with a DEC PDP-11/45 computer, and evaluated their test results by comparing them to those obtained using standard reference procedures. For example, the SMAC calcium procedure was compared to a calcium procedure using an atomic absorption spectrophotometer. They were able to develop procedures that correlated acceptably between their three SMAC systems and with other standard reference methods, and they concluded that their system provided a high degree of quality control. Karcher [115] conducted a series of studies in a large clinical laboratory that compared some test results using the Technicon SMAC system with the GemSAEC and Abbott ABA-100, and found the tests results from the SMAC system to be interchangeable with the others.

In the 1980s Rodbard and associates [181] at the National Institutes of Health described a microcomputer-based system for recommending insulin dosages to patients with diabetes mellitus that were based upon daily serum glucose test values. Using an IBM PC microcomputer and a program written in BASIC that stored serum glucose test values, insulin dosages, and other relevant patient data, recommendations were provided regarding appropriate changes in insulin doses.

Klee and associates [117] at the Mayo Clinic in Rochester, Minnesota described a system for interpreting blood parathyroid hormone measurements and assisting in the diagnosis of parathyroid disorders. From a combination of blood measurements of parathyroid hormone, calcium, phosphorus, and creatinine, they developed a series of sequential tables to aid in the often complex differential diagnosis of hyperparathyroidism.

Blood gas analyses provide the physician with aids in the diagnosis and management of pulmonary and cardiac disorders, and for assessing tissue perfusion and acid-base metabolism. Blood gas analysis is typically performed using heparin-anticoagulated arterial blood samples on which measurements are made of the partial pressures of oxygen and carbon dioxide, as well as measurements of the hemoglobin concentration, pH, and temperature. A series of calculations are then made to estimate the oxygen, carbon dioxide, and bicarbonate content of the sample, as well as other calculated metabolic parameters. The hemoglobin oxygen saturation (the proportion of oxyhemoglobin to total hemoglobin) can also be estimated. It soon became evident that computer-based calculations offered the benefits of speed and precision, and in 1971 a series of publications described some of the different approaches taken.

Yoder [246] at the University of California, San Diego, reported on their BLOODGAS program, written in FORTRAN IV for an XDS Sigma 3 computer to complete these computations.

Rosner and associates [182] at the Medical Systems Development Laboratory in the US Department of Health, Education, and Welfare, reported on their pulmonary function laboratory's computer and program, which used a CDC 160A computer processed blood gas determinations that included hemoglobin, hematocrit, arterial blood pH, and oxygen and carbon dioxide tensions. Their system also included spirometry and a variety of ventilation measures, and was programmed to compute and print out a number of parameters relating to pulmonary ventilation, oxygen diffusion and gas exchange, and blood gas concentrations.

Clark and associates [43] at the University of Utah described their Computerized Automated Blood Analysis System (CABAS), that was written in assembly language and used the computers at the nearby LDS Hospital to monitor blood gases and pH, blood sodium and potassium in children in a pediatric intensive care unit.

Rowberg and Lee [184], at Cedars-Sinai Medical Center in Los Angeles, reported using a desk-top calculator to compute blood gas values.

12.5.2   *Hematology*

The hematology laboratory applies various technologies to the study of blood, including blood cells and coagulation. In a historical review of analytic methods in hematology, Wintrobe [242] noted that invention of the microscope in the 1600s and the early procedures for layering blood onto glass slides permitted visualization of blood cells. This was followed in the 1800s by procedures for staining blood smears and for counting blood cells. Wintrobe designated 1926 as the year of a revolution in hematology, as before this date hematology was essentially the science of describing the morphology of the cellular constituents of the blood, whereas after this date the methods of the physiologist and the biochemist created subdisciplines devoted to the study of hemoglobinopathies, coagulation disorders, immunohematology, and other disorders.

In the early 1960s, testing in the hematology laboratory was typically limited to the measurement of the hemoglobin concentration of the blood and the manual identification and counting the different cell types in a stained blood smear. Brittin [35] referred to hematology in the 1960s as a "cottage industry." Elbert and O'Connor [54] wrote that the hematology laboratory had more complex data acquisition and result-reporting needs than did the chemistry laboratory as the hematology laboratory had to accommodate non-numeric descriptive results. In the 1960s, hematology data-processing systems used punched cards for storing data; and used unit-record equipment for sorting and counting the punched cards and for printing out data. In the late 1960s, computers began to be used to process data from punched cards or from punched paper tape, and several automated blood-cell counters became available in the United States.

In 1965, the first Technicon AutoAnalyzer Cell Counter was used for the simultaneous determination of white and red cell counts and blood hemoglobin concentrations. Soon afterwards the Technicon Sequential Multiple Analyzer (SMA) 4A appeared and counted red and white blood cells from a 1 ml sample of whole blood, and measured the value of blood hemoglobin and the hematocrit (a measure of the packed-cell volume of the blood). The AutoAnalyzer split the blood sample into four streams. Following an automatic dilution of the white cell stream from which the red cells had been removed by a hemolysis step, the white cells entered the flow cell of the counter module, where the white cells deflected a light beam around a dark-field disc, and the deflections were registered electronically. Similarly, the red blood cell stream entered a separate flow cell, and the same electronic counting principle was employed. In a third stream, hemoglobin was converted the more stable cyanmethemoglobin, and the resulting color intensity was measured in a colorimeter. The Technicon SMA cell counter used continuous flow methods similar to those used in its chemistry AutoAnalyzer. The hematocrit was measured in the fourth stream by a "conductivity bridge" that made use of the differences in conductivity of the red cells and the free ions in the plasma, and the hematocrit could be estimated because the red cell conductivity was directly proportional to the red cell mass. Analog data from a strip-chart recorder was converted by an analog-to-digital converter that provided digital input to the computer [176]. The SMA 7A automated cell analyzer that soon followed added three red blood cell (corpuscle) indices (mean corpuscular volume, mean corpuscular hemoglobin, and mean corpuscular hemoglobin concentration), which were automatically calculated from the other four blood-cell test values. By the end of the 1960s, it was reported that 60–80 % of the workload in a large hematology laboratory could be handled efficiently and rapidly, with increased accuracy and reliability by commercially available hematology analyzers [38].

In 1971, Technicon's Hemalog system was introduced, which differed from Technicon's SMA cell analyzers as the Hemalog system had parallel analyzers with two hydraulic pumps (one blood sample pumps that delivered paired samples for each patient, and one chemical reagent pump), a multi-channel optical system with four detectors and dedicated channels for each parameter. The Hemalog system provided a hematocrit determination using an automatic packed-cell volume centrifuge. All test parameters were measured simultaneously and were processed by a digital control system, with data output on an attached printer. The system could perform ten tests simultaneously from two anti-coagulated specimens of whole blood, including red and white cell counts, hemoglobin, packed-cell volume by micro-hematocrit and conductivity, platelet count, prothrombin time, partial thromboplastin time, and the three red blood cell indices [92, 237].

During the 1970s, the most widely used automated hematology instrument was the Coulter Counter Model S, made by Coulter Electronics in Hialeah, Florida. The Coulter Model S counted and measured the sizes of individual blood cells by using the difference in electrical impedance (conductivity) between blood cells and a diluting fluid in which the cells were suspended. The instrument aspirated blood cell suspensions through a 100-μ diameter aperture across which a voltage was applied. The small voltage spikes generated as individual cells passed through the aperture were measured, and the heights of the voltage spikes could be used to determine the relative cell sizes. The Coulter Counter Model S also measured the hemoglobin concentration of each sample, and automatically calculated three red blood indices: mean corpuscular [cell] volume (MCV), mean corpuscular hemoglobin (MCH), and mean corpuscular hemoglobin concentration (MCHC). Test results were printed out on a small dedicated printer, and could be read into a remote computer in digital format [38].

Dutcher and associates [70] at the William Beaumont Hospital in Royal Oak, Michigan, reported using a computer program developed in the Clinical Pathology Department at the NIH Clinical Center to compare the Coulter Counter Model S and the Technicon SMA-7A hematology analyzers. They found that precision of each instrument was equal to, or better than, the precision of laboratory technologists, and they noted that improvements were already being made to new versions of both instruments.

The manual (visual) white blood cell differential count involves spreading a drop of blood on a glass slide and staining the blood smear with a stain that reveals the white blood cells' internal granules, and then using a microscope to visually identify and count the proportion of neutrophils, basophils, eosinophils, lymphocytes, monocytes, platelets, and any abnormal cells present, such as might be found in patients with leukemia. Training a laboratory technologist to correctly identify and count the different blood cells in a stained s blood smear usually took several months; therefore, to develop a machine that could do this automatically was a truly remarkable achievement. In the early 1970s, an electronic cell pattern-recognition instrument called Hematrak was developed by the Geometric Data Corporation in Wayne, Pennsylvania. As described by Dutcher and associates [71], the basic components of the Hematrak were a microscope, a pre-programmed electronic pattern-recognition system, a monochrome television monitor, a keyboard for data input by the operator, and a printer. The images formed by the microscope were converted to electronic signals by a slide scanner, and were then processed by a color analyzer that split the images into three color channels. The resulting color information was used to "electronically lyse" the red blood cells in the images of the blood smears, leaving only the images of the nucleated white blood cells. The images of the nucleated cells were then digitized and passed to a morphologic pattern-recognition program, where parameters such as cell nuclear shape, chromatin pattern, granularity, nuclear-to-cytoplasm ratio, and color values were used by the pattern-recognition program to identified individual white blood cell types on the basis of the morphologic characteristics. The Hematrak was able to identify normal white blood cells with an accuracy that compared favorably with the standard manual method [25], but was less reliable in identifying abnormal blood cells because of their variability – which was also a common problem for trained hematologists [72].

Ansley and Ornstein [5] described Technicon's Hemalog D, a multichannel flow analyzer for counting white blood cells subtypes based on cell size and cytochemical reactions. Identifying the white blood cell subtypes was possible because of the variety of intracellular enzymes that permitted distinctive cytochemical staining of the white cell subtypes. Dyes and cytochemical reagents stained the white cell nuclei and the specific granules in the neutrophils, basophils, eosinophils, lymphocytes, and monocytes. Suspensions of stained cells could then be they counted by photometric counters that could differentiate the white cell subtypes by their staining reactions and could count large numbers of cells – typically 10,000 per flow-analysis channel, which provided improved precision of counting. The instrument was reported to be relatively easy to operate; however, as many as 20 % of blood specimens needed further examinations by the technologist using traditional blood smears [65].

Arkin and associates [6] at the New England Deaconess Hospital in Boston, described the Corning LARC (Leukocyte Automatic Recognition Computer) Analyzer that used a "spinner" to prepare the blood slides by spreading blood on a standard glass microscope slide, which was then fixed and stained by an automatic slide stainer. The LARC Analyzer determined the characteristic morphologic features of the white blood cells (leukocytes), and classified them by processing their digital images. Slides with abnormal cells were physically sorted so that they could be reviewed by a technologist. A comparison of the results from the LARC Analyzer with those of a group of medical technologists revealed that the LARC Analyzer results were often more reproducible than those of the technologists; and that all known cases of leukemia in their study population had been detected by the LARC Analyzer.

Haug and associates [105] compared the Technicon Hemalog D automated cytochemical white blood cell differential counter, which counted 10,000 cells at the rate of 60 samples per hour, with the Corning LARC Differential Analyzer, which used a slide spinner for preparing blood smears, and counted 100, 200, or 500 white cells using a computer pattern recognition program. They concluded that the most significant difference between the two systems was analytic precision, which was a function of the differences in the numbers of cells counted.

Rosvoll and associates [183] in Atlanta, Georgia, reported a study comparing three automated differential cell counters: Technicon's Hemalog D, which used cytochemical methods; Corning's LARC, which used a pattern recognition system; and the Geometric Data Hematrak, which also used a pattern-recognition system and counted from 50 to 800 cells. They reported that all three instruments showed acceptable accuracy and flagged abnormal results for review, and that the Hemalog D exhibited the greatest analytic precision.

Schoentag and Pedersen [187] at the New York Veterans Hospital described the Perkin-Elmer Corporation's Diff3 System, which used computer pattern-recognition technology to automatically identify and count white blood cells into ten categories, and also evaluated red cell morphology and performed platelet counts. The system used a blood smear spinner and a stainer; and the stained slides were loaded into an analyzer that included microscope with a motorized stage. The images produced by the microscope were processed by a photodetector system that isolated the cell images on the slide, which were then scanned by a video camera and digitized for processing by an image-analyzing computer. Upon completion of a differential count of 100 white blood cells, a report was automatically printed. The flagging of abnormal white blood cells by the instrument was reported to be comparable in sensitivity to that of the laboratory technologists; however, the analytic specificity was less, so that a significant number of false positives were seen.

Allen and Batjer [2] at the University of Washington, Seattle, evaluated the Coulter S-Plus IV that distinguished and classified white blood cells as lymphocytes, large mononuclear cells, and granulocytes by cell volume after treatment with a special reagent. The instrument also performed a total white cell count, red cell count, and platelet count; and measured the hemoglobin concentration and calculated the hematocrit value and the red cell indices. They concluded that the usefulness of the instrument would be limited to that of a screening tool for identifying slides needing a morphologist's review.

Bollinger and associates [33] at the University of Texas, M.D. Anderson Hospital reported on a later version of Technicon's automated hematology analyzer, the Technicon H*1. It performed white blood cell, red blood cell and platelet counts; and provided hemoglobin and hematocrit values, and red blood cell indices. The system also provided a white cell differential count and was reported to have excellent performance characteristics.

Bates and Bessman [24] at the University of Texas Medical Branch at Galveston used a commercial microcomputer program, BCDE: Blood Count and Differential Evaluation, developed by Island Analytics, Galveston, and written in BASIC on an IBM-PC, to analyze automated blood cell counts and differential leukocyte counts performed on a Coulter Counter S-Plus II-VI. This analytic program was found to be useful for both triaging normal from abnormal hematologic data and for the initial analysis of abnormal data. McClure and associates [150], also at this university, used this microcomputer program to initiate a policy of not performing a manual microscopic evaluation of every blood specimen for which a blood count was done. They proposed that since normal blood counts were associated with few clinically important blood-smear abnormalities, an automated program might be useful for triaging blood counts and deciding whether a blood smear needed to be examined. They used the BCDE program to analyze the automated blood cell counts, and performed a manual white-cell differential count only if the specimen had blood cell counts from an automated cell counter that were abnormal to a stipulated degree – the so-called the "diff-if" strategy. They reported that for a population of subjects with a high percentage of hematologic disorders, the diagnostic specificity of the microcomputer program was comparable to visual examination of a blood smear in identifying hematologic abnormalities; however, it was more sensitive in predicting blood smear abnormalities and thus caused more blood smears to be examined and more manual differential cell counts to be performed. Similarly, in a population of predominantly normal subjects, the program was more sensitive in identifying elevated eosinophil counts and the presence of immature leukocytes (band cells). They concluded that the triage strategy for visual differential blood counts should be based on the laboratory's patient population.

Krause [119] at the University of Pittsburgh, reviewed the status of automated white blood cell differential counters in 1990; and concluded that the then current state-of-the-art instruments gave results equal to or better than routine manual differential counts; they could better screen for significant abnormalities; and they greatly reduced the time and expense of manual procedures. In the 1990s and 2000s advanced blood cell identifiers and counters were developed by several vendors.

Bone marrow smears were also evaluated using computer-based approaches. Wolf and associates [245] at Stanford University Medical Center developed a computer program called DIRAC (DIRectACess) to store, retrieve, and analyze bone marrow examination reports. Yountness and Drewinko [248] at the University of Texas and the MD Anderson Hospital in Houston, also reported an early computer-based system for entering and reporting results of bone marrow examinations. They developed a specialized keyboard that was labeled with descriptive terms for the various cells. The differential cell count was performed by a technologist using the keyboard, and the computer registered the accumulation of cells. When 100 nucleated cells were classified, the display monitor emitted an audio sound and displayed the differential cell count.

Red blood cell typing is a procedure routinely performed on blood donors, and is also performed by blood banks on blood transfusion recipients. Taswell and associates [219] at the Mayo Clinic in Rochester, Minnesota, reported they had used a 15-channel Technicon AutoAnalyzer for routine ABO-Rh blood typing of patients since 1968. This continuous flow AutoAnalyzer mixed red blood cells from the patient with reagent antisera, and plasma from the patient's blood sample with reagent red cells. When a patient's red cells were agglutinated by a given antiserum it was called a positive direct reaction, and the agglutination of reagent cells by the patient's plasma was called a positive indirect reaction. In each case, the agglutinated red blood cells were seen as red spots on filter paper. Weant [233], at the American National Red Cross Blood Center in Huntington, West Virginia, described their evaluation of the Technicon BG 9, a nine-channel, automated blood grouping system that required less space and performed all the tests for the ABO and Rh groups with the same accuracy. It used a sampler that held 40 blood samples and operated at a rate of 120 samples per hour. It had two proportioning pumps, a five-channel manifold, and a five-channel filter unit. Centrifuged anticoagulated blood samples were placed in the sample tray, and the cells and plasma were aspirated by two different probes. The system then suspended the blood cells in a bromelin enzyme solution that exposed additional antigen sites for reaction with reagent antibodies. Cells were subsequently mixed with antisera in four channel for anti-A, anti-B, anti-A,B, anti-D, with an additional blank control channel. The bromelin-treated cells agglutinated with the antisera, indicating a positive reactions, or remained as free cell suspensions when the reaction was negative. The reacted materials were then diluted with saline and passed through a settling tube, decanted, and deposited on moving filter paper. The plasma from the samples was split, tested against known red cell suspensions (A cells, B cells, and Group O cells); and finally decanted and deposited on to filter paper. Weant reported that a comparison of the automated results with parallel manual test results produced agreement in all instances; and the system was more reliable and less expensive than manual methods.

In 1985, Smith and associates [201] at Ohio State University reported a computer program called RED, which interpreted data related to red cell antibody identification. They described the surface of a red cell as having specific antigens that are detectable by the reactivity of the cell with antibodies corresponding to the antigen. Human red blood cells are classified as type A, B, AB, or O on the basis of the presence or absence of A and B on the surface of the red cells, and the presence of reciprocal antibodies in the patient's serum. A person of blood group A normally has anti-B antibodies in his serum; a group B person normally has anti-A; a group O person has both anti-A and anti-B; and a group AB person exhibits neither. When the immune system of a blood transfusion recipient recognizes the antigen as foreign to the recipient's system, the body's immune system sets about to destroy the antigen by developing antibodies in the serum of the recipient patient to destroy all the red cells possessing the antigen against which the antibody is directed; and the result is defined as a blood transfusion reaction. It is important to detect and identify these antibodies in the patient's serum before a blood transfusion is given by determining the patient's ABO blood group. In addition to the ABO antigens, more than 300 red cell antigens have been identified, so red cell antibody identification requires screening a patient's serum for antibodies by testing it with red cells containing selected common red cell antigens. This process is a complex one, and Smith's RED program provided a series of rules to help interpret data concerning antibodies against cell components important in transfusions [200].

Sterling [215] also developed a computer program written in BASIC for an IBM personal computer to assist in the analysis of commercial reagent red blood cell panels designed to detect "atypical" antibodies in patients' sera. The usual manual method for analyzing the data for these antibody panels involves "ruling out" or excluding a specific antibody when the corresponding antigen was present on a non-reacting cell in the panel. It was assumed that if the antibody was present in the patient's blood, agglutination or hemolysis would occur when the serum was mixed with red blood cells containing the corresponding antigen. In the system reported by Sterling, each red cell panel was represented as a matrix, with each element in the matrix representing a single red blood cell antigen. A selected red cell panel, along with the corresponding reactions from the patient's serum, was displayed on a monitor, and the possible antibody patterns were highlighted. A panel interpretation was then printed that included a list of possible non-excluded antibodies, a probability level of identification for each possible antibody, and a table of antibody characteristics to aid in the differentiation among the possible antibodies.

Blood platelets play an important role in blood coagulation; and platelet counts and platelet aggregation studies are used in the investigation of bleeding and clotting disorders. Upton [227] described the first automated blood platelet counter, which used the Technicon AutoAnalyzer technology. A whole blood sample was aspirated from a cup containing a diluent that had been automatically agitated to cause hemolysis of the red blood cells. After passing through a mixing coil and an additional dilution step, the platelets were enumerated by a cell counter. Neeley [165] used a Coulter Counter to count platelets in a sample of blood plasma. Simmons and associates [187] also used a modified Coulter Counter to count platelets; and after comparing results with those obtained using a Technicon AutoAnalyzer, they concluded that the Technicon instrument was more accurate. McHenry [158] coupled Technicon's Hemalog D automated white cell differential analyzer to a Technicon AutoCounter Instrument. A sample of whole blood was aspirated into a segment of plastic tubing, allowing the red cells to settle out. The plasma was then pipetted into a diluent, and was transferred to a particle counter that counted the platelets.

Dayhoff and associates [63] described an instrument to measure platelet aggregation, a physiologic process that occurs in vivo to stop bleeding by plugging small gaps in blood vessel walls, but may also contribute to blood clot formation in larger vessels such as occurs in coronary artery thrombosis. They used a TEXAC (TEXture Analysis Computer) whole picture image analyzer that identified and counted clumps of platelets.

Connelly et al. [55] at the University of Minnesota reported on an Expert System for Platelet Request Evaluation (ESPRE) that they had been developing since 1984 to assist physicians in determining the appropriateness of platelet transfusions. Platelet transfusions may be vital for hemostasis in critically ill patients, but they also pose risks of transfusion reactions. When ESPRE received a request for a platelet transfusion, it automatically acquired key laboratory findings from the LAB system and requested any necessary clinical information. It then provided a critique of the proposed transfusion plan with an explicit list of all platelet transfusion criteria satisfied and/or evaluated. A formal evaluation of ESPRE showed agreement with blood bank consultants' recommendations in 93 % of a group of 75 platelet transfusion requests.

In the late 1960s and early 1970s, other LAB systems that were designed to process hematology data included the LAB systems at the NIH Clinical Center, the University of Missouri at Columbia, the University of Wisconsin, the University of Alabama, Yale University, Massachusetts General Hospital, and Kaiser Permanente in San Francisco. Commercial LAB systems with hematology subsystems included the Berkeley Scientific Laboratories (BSL) CLINDATA system, which used a PDP-8 computer and was developed at the University of California, San Francisco with support from the NIH; and the Spear system [38].

By the late 1970s, almost all large clinical laboratories used automated hematology instruments linked to computerized LAB systems [69]. Lincoln [133] observed that blood counting tasks historically performed exclusively by the pathologist, and later by technologists trained to follow certain rules could now be performed using rules programmed into cell counting machines. In the 1980s and after, computer-based LAB systems continued to be improved in variety, accuracy, and efficiency; and in addition to interpretive reporting, began to add clinical decision support programs to assist with the diagnoses of anemias and other blood diseases [27, 31, 168].

12.5.3 Microbiology

Microbiology reports often require a large amount of descriptive text rather than numeric data, and because the processing of microbiology specimens may require several days or weeks before final results are available, interim reports may be needed to provide clinicians with the most current information about a specimen in process [147]. Handwritten or dictated narrative reports were often used in microbiology, and were keyed into the computer using a full-alphabetic keyboard, or by selecting codes or names for standard terms or phrases using special keyboards [241]. Computerization of descriptive test results, such as microbiology results, was typically more difficult than in chemistry or hematology, as microbiology results often require extensive English-text descriptions, and there may be several thousands of unique microorganism names. Early microbiology computer systems usually were one of two types, either having been developed primarily for computer-assisted identification of microorganisms, or for computerization of laboratory records and reports.

As early as 1958, Cordle and Boltjes [59] at the Medical College of South Carolina in Charleston began using IBM data processing equipment in their microbiology department to provide a daily laboratory control program. They used special coding schemes for specimen types and microorganisms, and 80-column punch cards for data processing. A set of cards was prepared for each specimen, and was punched with the digital code and the alphanumeric name of the specimen. The cards were then punched with the digital codes for the organisms isolated, along with the names of the microorganisms and results for other tests, which were entered as alphabetical information. At the end of the day, the cards were sorted to provide laboratory control and microbial disease survey information. Periodically the cards were sorted by date and an IBM 101 statistical machine was used to print out reports [59].

Lindberg and Reed [141] at the University of Missouri, Columbia, reported their use of a photometric device to record the rate of bacterial growth in cultures. Because it usually required a 24-h in vitro incubation of bacterial cultures before the human eye was able to see visible turbidity, the use of a photometer to periodically measure light passing through the liquid culture medium permitted an earlier detection of bacterial growth. The output voltage of the photometer was read periodically by a digital voltmeter that permitted the bacterial growth curve to be plotted. An IBM 1620 computer was used to manipulate the data to provide final bacterial growth rate curves.

In the 1970s, published reports described a variety of computerized systems for clinical microbiology. Vermeulen and associates [229] at the US Public Health Services Hospital in Baltimore described their microbiology system in which specimens types, microorganism names, test results, and other relevant data were all encoded. Using the laboratory's Teletype facilities, culture results were punched into paper tape and were transmitted to the computer center. They rented computer time on an IBM 7094 computer for reading the data on the punched paper tape, and time on an IBM 1401 for printing the final reports.

Friedman and associates [85] at the Clinical Center at the National Institutes of Health developed a computer program written in FORTRAN for a Control Data Corporation (CDC) 3300 computer to assist in the identification of dextrose-fermenting gram-negative bacteria isolated from clinical specimens. Using data from a year's experience from their laboratory in identifying organisms, they compiled a database of 38 tests most frequently used to identify 34 species of bacteria. The program then used a Bayesian probability formula that selected the most likely organism identification, and suggested additional tests that would help in further differentiating unknown bacteria. When they entered a patient's test results for an unknown specimen, the computer would retrieve the relevant probabilities from the database, and using a modified Bayes theorem (that assumed the same prior prevalence probabilities for all species), would compute the score from zero to one of the likelihood that each species in the database represented the identity of the unknown organism. The program then selected the species with the highest score as the most likely identification. In their laboratory, the program correctly identified the unknown bacteria in 99 % of cases.

In 1975 Jorgensen and associates [113] at the University of Texas Health Science Center described a computerized online microbiology record-keeping system for their annual load of approximately 100,000 culture specimens. Their goal was to promote more efficient handling of culture results within the laboratory, to provide more timely reports to the patient care areas in the hospital, and to provide an easily accessible database for use in producing laboratory statistics. They used cathode ray tube (CRT) displays for data entry and for entering culture results. CRT displays were also available in various patient care and administrative areas of the hospital for online inquiry of patients' culture reports. They used 15 screen formats designed to include the most common types of specimens, including blood, cerebrospinal fluid, other body fluids and tissues, throat cultures, urine, feces, and other specimens, as well as mycobacterial smears and cultures. The computer generated daily work lists, daily preliminary and activity reports, weekly cumulative reports, several special quality-control reports, and daily epidemiology reports for use by the Hospital Infection Control Coordinator. The computer also generated patient billing and accounting information. They used a central Burroughs 4771 computer that was shared by other hospital departments.

Lewis and Marr [128] at the Washington University School of Medicine and Barnes Hospital in St. Louis described their computer-assisted method for identifying enteric bacteria. They developed a FORTRAN program called MICROAPI that used a Bayesian statistical calculation to assist in identifying the organisms; however, it agreed with the technologists' organism identifications in only a few percent of cases.

Lupovitch and associates [147] at Holy Cross Hospital in Detroit, Michigan described their conversion of a manual reporting system to a computerized system for reports for their microbiology laboratory, which processed 9,000 specimens per year. They maintained similar report formats and updating sequences so that one system could back-up the other. They used a Hewlett-Packard programmable calculator (Model 9830) with 8K core memory, 2.5 megabytes disk memory, a line printer, and a mark-sense card reader, with programs to read the mark-sense cards written in BASIC. Observations and test results were recorded by technologists by marking the appropriate rows and columns in a series of mark-sense cards that contained both the patient's identification number and the specimen's unique number. Comments were entered from the data card using a stored dictionary of phrases that corresponded to the card column markings. Antibiotic sensitivity data and similar data could be added where appropriate. Sets of cards were collated and printed daily and when needed. They reported that the main advantage of their new system was the improved quality and ease of providing cumulative reports.

In the late 1970s, Eggert and associates [73] at the University of Wisconsin reported that they had developed a microbiology subsystem using a customized version of the LABCOM commercial LAB system from Laboratory Consulting, Inc., in Madison, Wisconsin, The system used a Digital Equipment Corporation (DEC) PDP 11/84 computer, visual-display terminals, teletypewriters and line printers that were connected with the main clinical laboratory computer, which was interfaced to the central hospital computer. This subsystem involved several programs written for microbiology. The Requisition Entry program was used to select and enter data from an array of microbiology specimen types, and test requests such as cultures, special stains, and others. The Enter Cultures program permitted the user to select and enter results for isolates from an array of options, including organism names, colony counts, comments, and antibiotic susceptibility results. One could enter numeric values, coded English, or free-text modifiers as results. Tracking the progress of the tests-in-process was supported, and finalized results of cultures were easily displayed and printed. A Microbiology Log program permitted selective reporting of the tests performed and results entered for a patient.

Hospital acquired infections, also known as nosocomial infections, represent a frequent and important type of adverse event in hospitals and involve the microbiology laboratory in multiple ways. Before the advent of hospital information systems (HISs), rates of hospital-acquired infections were generally determined from the diagnoses and notes documented in paper-based medical records. The audit procedures for programs such as those developed by the Professional Standards Review Organization (PSRO) and physician Peer Review Organization (PRO) relied on manual chart reviews by nurses with follow-up physician reviews of suspected cases. An alternative approach was to monitor laboratory microbiology reports for positive infectious organisms.

Automated infection surveillance systems began to become operational in the early 1970s, such as the one reported by Greenhalgh and Mulholland [98] at the Graduate Hospital of the University of Pennsylvania. Their system integrated the clinical microbiology laboratory's results with other patient data with the primary objectives of uncovering the etiology of infections and preventing in-hospital epidemics. A surveillance nurse used an "Infection Information Form" for computer entry of data extracted from the medical record, and from interviews with patients that were found to have positive bacterial cultures. Data were then added on organism identifications and antibiotic susceptibilities. After the data were entered into the computer, reports were generated listing patients and their demographic data, the organisms and their prevalence, and sensitivities to antibiotics; and then periodic historical and epidemiologic summaries of the data were provided.

In the early 1980s some hospitals began to use low-cost microcomputers for hospital infection surveillance systems. One example was the system developed using a RadioShack TRS-80 microcomputer for Mt. Sinai Hospital by Wise [243] at Datalab Corporation in Ohio. The system established a file for patient identification data and bed location in the hospital, and the type of infection and antibiotic treatment; and a file for organisms with records for each organism that included the body site and antibiotic sensitivity results. Data output programs provided periodic reports on patients with infections with their hospital services, body sites of infections, sensitivities of organisms, and counts and frequencies.

Lyman and associates [148] at the New York University Medical Center's Bellevue Hospital described the use of a natural-language text processing system that stored narrative hospital discharge summaries. The system allowed retrieval of cases with, for example, acute bacterial meningitis listed in pediatric discharges, and provided details such as counts and frequencies, signs, symptoms, types of treatment, and some outcome results.

Dove and Hierholzer [68] at Yale New Haven Hospital designed and deployed software for an infection control system that ran on IBM-XT/AT or DEC microcomputers. Their system was designed to integrate data from several hospital departments to support utilization review, risk management, and quality assurance. The system was found to be quite flexible and was adapted for use at St. Joseph's Hospital in Syracuse, New York.

With the development of hospital information systems (HISs) with software for automated extraction of data from computer-based patient records, Streed and Hierholzer [216] at the University of Iowa Hospitals reported on 5 years' experience with a HIS using an IBM mainframe computer that had light-pens with visual display terminals. In 1980, this HIS had an online infection management system that replaced a punch card system purchased in 1976, and that conformed more closely to the requirements of the Joint Commission on Accreditation of Healthcare Organizations' (JCAHO) mandated infection monitoring and infection control programs. A series of phased enhancements to the system allowed comparisons of recent and past infection rates. Cost-evaluation software provided useful financial data related to nosocomial infections, and data from the microbiology and the pharmacy systems were merged to provide follow-up correlations of antibiotic use with the appearance of antibiotic resistance.

Using the HELP system they had developed at LDS Hospital, and linking their computer-based microbiology laboratory to the HELP system, Warner's group was able to develop a Computerized Infectious Disease Monitoring System to identify hospital-acquired infections [89]. In 1986, they described the system's main features: microbiology test results combined with other information such as pharmacy and radiology data; a knowledge base created by infectious disease physicians; automatic medical decision-making capabilities activated by patients' test results; and timely reporting of computer-based medical findings to infectious disease personnel [79]. As each microbiology test result was stored in the computer-based patient record, it was processed by a program that screened the result for selected information, and, for example, if a blood culture was positive, the program automatically activated algorithms that determined whether the bacterium isolated was a likely pathogen, whether the patient's current antibiotic therapy was appropriate based on the organism's antibiotic susceptibility results, and listed the most effective and lowest cost treatment considering any patient allergies or medical contraindications. A report containing this information was printed automatically each day, or could be printed manually. The researchers concluded from a 12-month study in 1986–1987 that computer-assisted monitoring of antibiotic therapy provided an efficient method for identifying and remedying inappropriate use of antibiotics, and lowering rates of hospital-acquired infections [78].

12.5.4   Other LAB Subsystems

There are other LAB subsystems and laboratory computer applications that are not discussed in detail in this chapter. The anatomic pathology or surgical pathology subsystem (PATH system) is described in Chap. 13. The blood bank or transfusion medicine subsystem, which assists the blood bank in providing safe blood products for transfusion, differs from other LAB subsystems because of US Food and Drug Administration (FDA) regulations. The examples below illustrate additional ways in which computer technology has been applied to laboratory automation.

Electrophoresis measures the migration rates of protein particles in an electric field. In the late 1960s Gelman Corporation in Ann Arbor, Michigan developed an electrophoresis instrument that measured the migration rates of protein particles that had been placed on a cellulose polyacetate membrane. The instrument scanned an eight-sample separation strip and printed out a graph for each of the eight samples. The computer module of this instrument, the Digiscreen C, integrated the area under the curve of each graph and printed out the value. It also could be connected online to a LAB system [38].

Gas chromatography is used to separate and identify the components of complex gas mixtures based on the different distribution coefficients between a moving gas phase and a stationary liquid phase, which is either coated on small particles which fill a tube or is coated as a thin film on the wall of a capillary tube. Because the transit time of a particular compound at a given gas flow rate and liquid stationary phase is a reproducible parameter for a compound, Bieman [25] at the Massachusetts Institute of Technology combined a gas chromatograph with a mass spectrometer, and used an IBM 1800 computer to continuously record the mass spectra of the effluent of the gas chromatograph to generate three-dimensional chromatogram reports. Bronzino [36] described the Finnagin 4021 system, which also connected a gas chromatograph and a mass spectrometer to a computer. The gas chromatograph separated the chemical constituents in patient specimens; for example, mixtures of drugs, and the separated components were then introduced into the mass spectrometer, which generated characteristic spectra for the individual components. The minicomputer controlled the process and stored the data from the spectrometer, and matched the spectrum of the sample to those already stored in the computer.

12.6   Examples of Early LAB Systems

The LAB system was one of the earliest applications of computers in direct patient care in the late 1950s and early 1960s, as some laboratory tests were already automated and merely needed to be interfaced to a digital computer. The initial growth of the LAB system involved predominantly the clinical laboratories, but pathologists also began working on the pathology information (PATH) system, which is discussed separately in Chap. 13.

In the early years of LAB systems, the clinical laboratory usually could not justify a dedicated computer system, so the laboratory typically shared the facilities of a central hospital mainframe computer that was otherwise used for accounting applications. As these mainframe systems provided only batch processing functions using punched-card inputs, the usual work flow at the time was for a hospital ward secretary to take the paper laboratory requisition – on which the physician had ordered chemistry, hematology, or other tests – and punch the request information along with the patient's identification number into one or more cards. The punched cards would be passed through a card reader that was connected to the central computer, which then generated specimen-collection schedules and work lists for the laboratory technologists, along with specimen labels and punched cards for each test ordered. The punched cards and the patient's specimens were then carried to the appropriate laboratory where the tests were to be performed. When the tests were completed, the technologists wrote the test results on the appropriate card; and a clerk keypunched the test result into the card. The cards were then batched and transmitted to the central computer, where periodic reports were printed that listed completed test results that were available up to that time for each patient. Periodically, a final cumulative-summary report of all test results was printed [58].

In the late 1950s, Rappaport and associates at the Youngstown Hospital Association in Youngstown, Ohio, began developing software for a LAB system that used IBM computers, was punch-card oriented, and operated primarily in a batch-processing mode [38]. Physicians marked laboratory test orders on preprinted forms from which a clerk or nurse transcribed the orders onto two-part punch cards with patients' identification numbers imprinted on the cards, and with preprinted and pre-punched specimen accession numbers. These cards then served as the laboratory test requisitions for chemistry, hematology, and urinalyses. The cards were sent to the laboratory where one part of the card was punched with the information that had been written or stamped on the card, thus providing machine-readable data for the automated laboratory instruments. The second part of the card served as the specimen collection list for the hospital wards, where pre-punched and encoded card stubs could be attached to the specimens. Initially, the laboratory used single-channel AutoAnalyzers for serum glucose determinations, with dual channel analyzers added later for glucose and urea nitrogen tests done on the same sample. In 1960, they created a central automated chemistry unit, and in 1963 they added a four-channel AutoAnalyzer unit for electrolyte testing. In 1964, they installed an IBM 1440 computer; and in the 1970s they added more instruments to provide 17 automated chemical procedures. In this LAB system, data from the Technicon AutoAnalyzers were collected by an IBM 1080 Data Acquisition System that read the analog and digital signals for the 15 chemistry tests performed by the AutoAnalyzers. The system had a punch card reader that read the specimen accession numbers on the attached card stubs. Hematology test results from the Coulter Coulters were transmitted through an interface to the IBM Data Acquisition System, as were data from other semi-automated laboratory instruments. Any test results that had been manually recorded were later keypunched into punch cards. Urgently required (stat) tests were reported automatically to the hospital nursing units. All laboratory data were transmitted to a central IBM 370 computer that provided a variety of summary reports. All patient data were then stored in the patient medical record on magnetic disk storage [175].

In 1959, Vallbona and Spencer [228] at the Texas Institute for Research and Rehabilitation (TIRR) Hospital in Houston used punch cards for their clinical laboratory test data. In 1961 they began to use IBM 1401 and 1620 computers. In 1965 they initiated online operations using an IBM 1410 computer; and in 1967 they installed an IBM 360/50 computer. By 1972 their LAB system was providing computer-generated online reports for blood gas calculations; and cumulative reports for blood and urine chemistry, microbiology, urinalyses, spinal fluid tests, and others.

In the early 1960s, Warner and associates at the Latter Day Saints (LDS) Hospital in Salt Lake City used a Control Data Corporation (CDC) 3200 computer for their cardiovascular research laboratory. They soon added a CDC 3300 computer, and extended their system into several other areas, including the clinical laboratory, beginning with clinical chemistry [173]. They used Tektronix 601 terminals that were capable of displaying either 400 characters in a 25-column by 16-row pattern, or graphical information with 512 horizontal and 512 vertical dots. Each terminal had a decimal keyboard and two 12-bit octal thumbwheel switches for coding information into the computer) [230]. Cards were keypunched with patients' names and identification numbers and were then read into the computer. Manually performed tests from chemistry, hematology, and urinalyses were entered into the computer by clerks using remote terminals. A Technicon SMA 12/30 chemistry analyzer was directly interfaced to the computer. All patient data were stored in the patient's computer-based record. A daily printout showed all of the patient's test results, and was placed in the patient's chart. Upon discharge from the hospital, the patient's file was transferred from the disk storage to magnetic-tape storage [38]. In the early 1970s, a company called MEDLAB, which was formed to market the LDS LAB system, was acquired by the Control Data Corporation. In 1971 at LDS, Systematized Nomenclature of Pathology (SNOP) codes were used to enter diagnoses at a video terminal [91]. By 1975, LDS subsystems included clinical laboratory, multiphasic screening, and computerized electrocardiogram analysis [115]. In 1982, as their patient load increased, they converted from a dual CDC computer system to a TANDEM computer system. By the 1980s, all clinical laboratory results were stored in coded form, and were available in their HELP system [88].

In 1962, Barnett and associates at the Laboratory of Computer Science, a unit of the Department of Medicine of the Massachusetts General Hospital (MGH) and the Harvard Medical School, initiated a major project with the MGH clinical laboratories to begin developing a LAB system. By 1967, this LAB system software included functions for entering test results, and for selective printing of results by test or test group [15, 16, 19, 97]. Two Digital Equipment Corporation (DEC) PDP-9 minicomputers were used; one for the production LAB system, and the other was used for software development and served as a backup for the production LAB system. All data were stored on magnetic disks, with daily incremental data transfers to magnetic tape storage. Additionally, a copy of all data was made weekly to magnetic tape storage. Teletype terminals were used for inputting test requests from paper requisitions, and medium-speed printers provided reports of the laboratory tests results. When the requisitions and patients' specimens arrived in the laboratory, clerks entered the patient data and test requests into the computer through the Teletype terminals. The system provided the specimen accession numbers and generated the laboratory work lists. When all the test results were obtained for a given work list, the technologists used Teletype terminals to enter the results and any comments into the patients' computer files, which were stored on (random-access) disk storage. By 1967, the MGH LAB system supported 9 patient care areas with about 300 beds and 3 clinical laboratories that were processing a daily volume of about 1,500 routine test requests. More than 100 standard model Teletype terminals were connected to the system for interactive data entry and data retrieval, including entering laboratory test results and the printing laboratory reports [15].

In 1968, Barnett described the entry of structured narrative text, such as pathology reports, into patients' records using an interactive conversational technique with a predetermined branching structure and a fixed vocabulary for data entry. The user entered patient information by selecting the desired items from a list on a display screen [18, 20].

In the 1970s, automated instruments such as Technicon AutoAnalyzers were interfaced to the MGH system. Daily and weekly cumulative reports of test results were printed. Listings of the charges for tests done were prepared and punched into paper tape for accounting purposes. Utilization reports were produced daily and summarized monthly for administrative purposes that time. In 1971, Grossman [99] and associates wrote that the MGH's most successful project was the reporting system for clinical chemistry laboratory tests that included the summarization of results by test category and the flagging of abnormal test results. Their online interactive system also could check an order against a computer database for drug-drug interactions or drug-laboratory test interactions, and could appropriately flag normal and abnormal test results [16, 97].

In 1962, Lamson at the University of California, Los Angeles, began entering uncoded full English text pathology diagnoses into a magnetic file system.

Information was keypunched in the exact text form supplied by the pathologists, and was then coded using a dictionary look-up process, with the coded reports stored on disk. Lamson's data dictionary was generated by accumulating new diagnostic terms encountered in the reports [124]. To avoid manual coding and to facilitate data retrieval, Lamson used 3 years of patient data to develop a thesaurus of all words that had identifiable relationships. A computer query program then matched the terms in users' queries and retrieved the patients' records containing the appropriate words. In 1965, his patients' files contained about 16,000 words and the thesaurus contained 5,700 English words. Lamson [125] recognized that more programming would be necessary to address problems of syntactic and semantic nature. Working with Jacobs at IBM, Lamson went on to develop a natural language retrieval system that used a data dictionary for looking up pathology records, including surgical pathology and bone-marrow examinations, autopsy reports, nuclear medicine reports, and reports of neuroradiology findings – all of which used unique numeric codes for each English word [111, 169]. Patients' records were maintained in text master files, with data for new patients merged into the text master files in medical record-number order.

In the 1960s, Robinson [180] entered narrative surgical pathology reports using an IBM Magnetic Tape/Selectric Typewriter (MT/ST) system that was interfaced to a magnetic tape drive connected to a computer. As reports were transcribed, the system stored information on the magnetic tape that was later transferred to the computer for processing, so that neither the pathologist nor the transcriptionist was dependent on direct access to a time-sharing computer. The program that processed the pathology reports matched each word against a standard vocabulary, and identified new or misspelled words for later human editing.

In 1963, Lindberg and associates [142] at the University of Missouri in Columbia installed an IBM 1410 computer in their Medical Center for a project to develop a system for reporting clinical laboratory test results. As each patient was admitted to the hospital, a deck of 30 punched cards with printed and pre-punched patient identifiers was created and accompanied the patient to their hospital ward. Requests for laboratory tests for a patient were written onto the pre-punched cards for the patient that then accompanied the patient's specimens to the laboratories. In the laboratories, other pre-punched-cards were used to designate 44 different types of specimens and tests. Test results were written onto the cards and then keypunched, and decks of punched cards containing chemistry, bacteriology, and serology data were read into the computer using an IBM 1912 card reader located in the laboratory. Prior to using this new computer system, official reports of laboratory tests were generated using (punch card) unit-record equipment, and were transmitted to the hospital wards where they were printed on Teletype terminals. The punched cards in the laboratories were then read into an IBM 1620 computer that generated summary records for the laboratories, and billing documents for the accounting office. Laboratory data were then stored on magnetic tapes for future retrieval, primarily for research purposes, with queries performed using either punched cards read in at the computer center, or through remote IBM 1014 input-output typewriters connected to the computer by telephone lines [144].

In 1965, Lindberg and associates replaced the punch card-oriented system in their clinical laboratory with IBM 1092/1093 matrix-keyboard terminals that were used to enter test results directly into the computer. By depressing one or more of 260 buttons, test results in the chemistry, bacteriology, and hematology laboratories were entered using the matrix keyboards. The meaning of each button was indicated by an English-language description that appeared next to the button. The descriptions were printed on sheets of opaque plastic that overlaid each keyboard, so that the meaning of each button could be defined according to which plastic overlay was placed on the keyboard, and the keyboards had micro-switches that sensed notches in the plastic overlays that uniquely coded each type of overlay. The IBM 1092/1093 matrix-keyboard terminals were linked to an IBM 1410 computer equipped with direct-access disk memory. Test results entered into the computer were processed by a LIMITS program that categorized them as reasonable, abnormal, or as unreasonable. This program then evaluated factors including age, sex, race of the patient; previous diagnoses; changes in test results from earlier results; expected normal ranges of test values; and the pattern of results across tests. Test results within normal limits were transmitted via a teleprocessing system and immediately printed out at the nursing stations. Abnormal or questionable results were transmitted to the clinical laboratory office for review by a pathologist before being released to the wards. All test results were stored for 1 day on direct-access disk storage, and were sorted and merged with previous laboratory results. The next day, the laboratory data were transferred to magnetic tape storage [139, 144]. In 1965 Lindberg also listed the following additional applications as being operational: electrocardiogram interpretations coded by heart station physicians, and radiology interpretations coded by the radiologists. Query and retrieval programs were available for all data stored in the patient files; other patient data processed included tumor registry and surgical pathology [140].

By 1968, Lindberg and associates had added an information system for their department of surgery that provided patient data including laboratory, surgical pathology and autopsy reports [137]. Lindberg used the Standard Nomenclature of Diseases and Operations (SNDO) for coding patients' discharge diagnoses and surgical operative procedures [146], which were stored on magnetic tape for all patients admitted to the hospital between 1955 and 1965. Other categories of patient data in their system included all SNDO coded diagnoses for autopsy and surgical pathology specimens, and all coded radiology and electrocardiogram interpretations [138]. Their LAB system was programmed to recognize patterns of laboratory test results and other findings recorded in the patient's record; and to provide some clinical decision support to physicians.

In 1963, Collen and associates at Kaiser Permanente (KP) introduced an automated multiphasic health testing system (AMHTS) for ambulatory patients at their Oakland and San Francisco medical centers [44, 45, 47]. The systems at each center processed the results from a battery of clinical laboratory tests, initially performed on Technicon AutoAnalyzers and later on a Jungner AutoChemist, both of which were interfaced to card punch machines. The punched cards with the test results were read into an IBM 1440 computer located in Oakland that then printed out summary reports of test results for the clinicians. In 1968, KP's Department of Medical Methods Research installed an IBM 360/50 computer in Oakland to develop a prototype medical information system (MIS) that included LAB subsystems [45]. KP's earlier automated multiphasic health-testing system (AMHTS) was already processing 3,000 tests a day, and provided patient-identification data, laboratory specimen labels, patient and specimen registration, quality control data, and clinical laboratory test results. Additionally, clinical decision-support was provided that included alerts and warning signals for findings outside of predetermined normal limits, as well as rules and advice for secondary sequential testing, and rules for likely diagnoses. All patient data were stored in computer-based patient records, and also in research databases [49, 223]. In 1969, a manual punched-card system was installed at the San Francisco KP Hospital. In 1972, a computer-based LAB system was installed and was integrated into the hospital information system. The LAB system included a LOGIN subsystem for test requisitions and for assigning accession numbers to specimens, and for compiling a set of appropriately identified prepunched test cards. The deck of cards was then read into a card-reader terminal, permitting the computer to generate listings of patients' names and identifiers. Chemistry test results from a Technicon AutoAnalyzer, and hematology test results from a Coulter Counter automatically generated punched cards that were read into card readers and stored in the patients' computer-based patient records. Other test results were inscribed on the test cards for subsequent data entry into the central computer (Terdiman and Collen [222]). In the 1980s, a central regional clinical laboratory was established by KP; in the 1990s the standalone multiphasic testing systems were absorbed into the national KP Health Connect system.

In 1964, Williams [241], at the Clinical Pathology Department of the National Institutes of Health, developed a patient and specimen identification system for their LAB system. The patient's name and identification number were preprinted and punched onto 25 mark-sense test-request cards at the time of admission to hospital. The cards were kept with the patient's medical record at the nursing station so that physicians could mark the cards when laboratory testing was desired. The cards then accompanied the patient's specimens to the laboratory, where they were keypunched and then sent to the computer room to be read into the computer. The laboratory also developed a novel accessioning station at which specimen tubes were inserted into a rack, causing accession numbers to be generated that corresponded to the rack positions. At the same time, the patient identification and test request information on the accompanying cards were read by an attached mark-sense card reader. This combination of a specialized accessioning station, sample racks, and carriers represented the first attempt to provide computer-readable specimen identification [38].

In 1964, the Information Systems Division of the Lockheed Missiles and Space Company in Sunnyvale, California began to develop a hospital information system (HIS) at the El Camino Hospital in Mountain View, California [86, 87]. In 1971, Lockheed sold the system to Technicon Corporation, and the El Camino Hospital signed a contract for the installation of the Technicon HIS [183]. By 1973, El Camino had installed terminals throughout the hospital, including terminals for a

LAB system [39]. The terminals' display screens were used to present lists; for example, of orders for clinical laboratory tests. A specific item was selected by pointing the light-pen at the desired word (or phrase), and pressing a switch on the barrel of the pen. The Technicon HIS was one of the first systems designed to allow the physician to directly enter orders for laboratory tests, and review the test results online [32]. Using the light-pen, a physician could select a patient and then enter orders for laboratory work and other procedures. Physicians, nurses, and other hospital personnel made extensive user of the terminals' light-pens, and only occasionally had to use the keyboards. The computer stored the orders and sent laboratory test requests and other orders to the appropriate hospital departments [91]. Computer printouts included laboratory specimen pickup lists, cumulative test summaries, and other reports. Test results were available at the terminals as soon as they were entered into the system by the laboratories. Physicians also received clinical reminders and alerts when retrieving patient data from the display terminals. A cumulative laboratory summary report was printed each day which showed the last 7 days of patients' test results. Upon discharge, a complete listing of all test results was printed at the medical records department to be filed in the patient's paper chart. In 1978, they developed a library containing information about interpretation of test results, as well as diagnoses and recommended treatments [21, 108, 203, 231].

In 1964, Tatch, in the Surgeon General's Office of the US Army, reported the automatically encoding of clinical diagnoses by punching paper tape as a by-product of the typing of a clinical record summary sheet. The computer program operated upon words within selected blocks of text, one at a time, and then operated on each letter to produce a unique number that replaced the word. The number was matched to an identification table, and an identity code was appended to the number. Using a special syntax, the numbers were used to generate a diagnostic code. This diagnosis code was then added to the clinical record summary [220].

In 1965, Lamson, at the University of California, Los Angeles, reported that they had developed a prototype LAB system for their clinical chemistry laboratory, which had automated chemistry analyzers; and that computer-based data processing was already operational in their hospital. Initially, data from hand-written test requisitions were transferred to punched cards by a manual keypunch, but this was soon replaced by terminals on the hospital nursing units that transmitted laboratory requests to automatic card-punch machines in the laboratory. Initially, test results were recorded on mark-sense cards until laboratory instruments provided direct digital readouts, or computers with analog-to-digital conversion capabilities could provide test results in digital form. At the end of each day, the computer printed out individual summaries of each patient's tests results [125]. In 1968, Lamson acquired a computer system for both the clinical laboratories and for a surgical pathology reporting system [123]. Their initial information system was gradually expanded, and by 1975 it provided summary reports that included data received from a large number of clinical laboratories [122].

In 1967, Weed and associates at the University of Vermont's College of Medicine in Burlington introduced their Problem-Oriented Medical Information System (PROMIS). By 1971, the system was used on a 20-bed gynecology ward at the

University Hospital, with linkages to the clinical laboratory. By 1977, the system had 30 touch-sensitive display terminals located on hospital wards and in the clinical laboratory that were connected to a single minicomputer. The terminals could display 1,000 characters of information in 20 lines of 50 characters each, and had 20 touch-sensitive fields. The user could select an item by touching the screen, and free-form data could be entered by typing on the keyboard attached to the terminal [77, 188].

In 1968, Siegel at the New York-Downstate Medical Center in Brooklyn described their hospital information system, which used an IBM 1440–1410 computer connected to 40 remote typewriter-terminal printers. They entered data using punched cards, paper tape, and IBM 1092 matrix-overlay keyboards; and used magnetic tape and disk for data storage. Terminals were placed in specialty clinics and the clinical laboratories [192].

In 1969, Pratt at the National Institutes of Health (NIH) reported on the use of automatic coding of autopsy diagnoses using the Systematized Nomenclature of Pathology (SNOP). He wrote that in the creation of a computer-based natural language processing (NLP) system, it was necessary to provide for the morphological, syntactic, and semantic recognition of input data. He used SNOP in his semantically organized dictionary, and subdivided the SNOP codes into four major semantic categories: Topography [T], Morphology [M], Etiology [E], and Function [F]. He also developed semantic subcategories and morphemes (smallest meaningful parts of words) to permit the coding of words not found in the SNOP dictionary, and for the recognition of medical-English synonyms [171]. Pratt developed parsing algorithms for morphological, syntactic, and semantic analysis of autopsy diagnoses; and developed a series of computer programs that processed medical text to produce a linguistic description and a semantic interpretation of the text [172]. This medical text analysis included translation of the text into the four field types (T, M, E, F) defined in the SNOP dictionary.

In 1969, Hammond and Stead [102–104] at Duke University began to develop a minicomputer-supported medical information system (MIS) known as The Medical Record (TMR) system. In the 1970s, with the availability of mass storage devices for minicomputers, they developed a distributed network of minicomputers, implemented a clinical laboratory (LAB) system designed to support the ordering and reporting of laboratory data, and used a data dictionary to define the codes for their LAB system. Data entry methods included both interactive video terminals and batch-processed mark-sense forms. By 1974, they used a Digital Equipment Corporation (DEC) PDP-11 minicomputer to interface their system to their University Health Services Clinic (UHSC) and to the Duke hospital information system.

By the late 1970s, Hammond [104] stated that their system contained all the features of a computer-based patient record so that when a patient saw a physician who recorded data and test orders on the paper encounter sheet, a clerk could enter the orders into the system so they could be printed out in the appropriate clinical laboratories. By 1984, the Duke HIS was linked to 18 clinical service departments and 64 laboratories [213]. Clinical laboratory data were entered by the laboratory technologists as the test results became available. For data entry, they displayed a full screen and then filled in blanks. The data enterer could type in the appropriate laboratory test code or type in text and the program would do an alphabetic search via the data dictionary and convert the text string into the proper code. By 1985, Duke's TMR system had increased in size to require a local area network that linked to their LAB system by an Ethernet connection, which allowed the laboratory to query a patient's problem list directly in the patient's electronic record. By the late 1980s their LAB system provided linkages to referring physicians for clinical services [104, 212].

Frey and associates [83] at Stanford Medical Center described their Advanced Computer for Medical Research Project. Known as the ACME system, it was developed as a flexible research database able to handle multiple data sets of varying types and sizes – with some data having to be held for long periods of time, and other data requiring frequent updating. The system included features designed to minimize inadvertent data loss, and to provide a simple user interface for medical researchers who were inexperienced in the use of computers. ACME was a typewriter-terminal driven, time-sharing system designed to acquire, analyze, store, and retrieve medical research data, and to control clinical laboratory instruments. The system was hosted on an IBM 360/50 computer, with IBM 2741 typewriter terminals, and interfaces to a variety of laboratory instruments that were interfaced through an IBM 1800 computer that had analog-to-digital data conversion capabilities. Disc drives were used for working storage and magnetic tapes were used for backup and archival storage.

In 1970 Myers and associates [164] at the University of Pennsylvania reported a system in which a pathology report was translated into a series of data elements that were encoded using arbitrarily assigned numbers. While the typist entered routine pathology reports using a program that also controlled by a paper tape punch as an output device, the data in the report was automatically coded and a punched paper tape was produced as a by-product of typing. The data on the punched paper tapes were then transferred to either magnetic tapes or to a disk storage system.

In 1970 Grams and associates at the University of Florida in Gainesville and at the 500-bed Shands Hospital began developing a computer-based laboratory information (LAB) system, which was designed to provide some clinical decision support capabilities [93]. Initially the computer system did not have any capabilities for reporting test results, and the test results were manually recorded on cumulative report forms. Also, a portable punch card (Port-A-Punch) system was used initially for ordering laboratory procedures. The cards were batch processed to create blood-drawing lists, labels for specimens, and work sheets; following which they were sent to an IBM 370 computer system for billing the laboratory charges. In 1975 a more comprehensive system was used to support their chemistry, hematology, immunology, and microbiology laboratories, and their blood bank. In 1977, they installed a network to integrate their laboratory functions with their hospital admitting office and nursing stations. They used one computer for the nursing units and the admitting office that was linked to a second computer in the laboratory [95].

   In the early 1970s, several commercial LAB systems were being marketed that used minicomputers [8, 11]. Berkeley Scientific Laboratories described in some detail four commercially developed, operational LAB systems marketed by Spear Computers, Inc, Digital Equipment Corporation (DEC), Diversified Numerical Applications (DNA), and BSL's own CLINDATA Mark II system [38].

   The Spear Computers Class 300 LAB system controlled the gathering and testing of patients' specimens; and collected and analyzed the data from both automated and manually performed test procedures in the chemistry, hematology, and microbiology laboratories.

   Clerks entered the patient's identification (ID) data and hospital-assigned ID number into the system by keyboard. The computer generated lists for specimen pickup and laboratory work lists. The computer automatically assigned a five-digit accession number to each specimen, and printed pressure-sensitive labels with the patient's name, hospital number and specimen number. Digitized data from test results were entered into the system's LINC computer and were stored in its data files, and test results were printed out on report forms. Spear Computers developed the basic software used by its system, with some programming for the version of its LAB system installed at the Perth Amboy General Hospital in New Jersey developed by the Medical Development Corporation [38].

   Digital Equipment Corporation (DEC) derived its CLINI-LAB 12 system from the LABCOM data acquisition system developed at the University of Wisconsin in Madison. The patient's hospital number, the laboratory test type, and the accession numbers of the specimens were entered into the computer either manually using Teletype terminals, or by punched cards passed through a punched-card reader. Automated laboratory instruments such as Technicon Auto-Analyzers were connected to analog-to-digital converters that allowed the PDP-12 computer to capture digitized data. The system had both random-access disk and magnetic tape storage. A cathode ray tube (CRT) display was available, and a line printer provided a variety of laboratory reports. The LAB system software included a central patient file from which patients' stored laboratory data were accessible by users through the Teletype terminals [38].

   The Berkeley Scientific Laboratories (BSL) CLINDATA system used a PDP-8 computer with random-access disk storage for patient data files, and magnetic-tape storage for long-term retention of patient data. BSL developed software that acquired data from both AutoAnalyzers in the chemistry laboratory and Coulter Counters in the hematology laboratory, and also allowed data to be input for manually performed laboratory procedures. The system also accepted free-text comments entered through keyboards. Test requests could be manually entered directly into the system using a keyboard, or they could be punched into cards which were then read into the system by a card reader. The system generated specimen collection lists (such as blood drawing lists), and adhesive-backed labels that displayed the patient's name, hospital number, and names of the tests to be performed. The system also produced worksheets that specified the tests to be performed on each specimen. Analog signals from AutoAnalyzers were monitored to detect voltage peaks which were converted to digital values for computer input. Output data from a Coulter counter were entered into the computer, and computations were performed to provide the various red blood-cell indices. A variety of test reports were printed, including daily and cumulative-summary reports, and also for stat or an on-demand query basis [38].

In the early 1970s, the State University of New York at its Upstate Medical Center in Syracuse, New York, developed a LAB system as a subsystem of its hospital information system. Upon a patient's entry into hospital, the admitting office typed up an admission form using a keyboard with a cathode-ray tube (CRT) display connected to a Systems Engineering Laboratories (SEL) 810A computer. A deck of punched cards, physician-order forms, and specimen-identification labels were then generated. A physician-order form that requested a desired test was attached to a punched card, and with appropriate specimen labels was sent to the clinical laboratory. The punched card was then read into the computer, and the patient data were displayed on a cathode-ray terminal. After visual verification of the displayed data by a clerk, the computer printed out a specimen-collection list and laboratory worksheets. AutoAnalyzer test results were entered online through an interface to the computer. Non-automated test results were entered into the LAB system using keyboard-display terminals. At the end of each day all completed test data were transferred to a second central SEL computer that printed daily and 7-day cumulative reports [38].

In the early 1970s at The Johns Hopkins Hospital (JHH), a prototype clinical information management system was developed that processed physicians' written orders, generated work lists for nurses, and produced computer-printed patient drug profiles that were filed in patients' charts [193]. In 1975, a Minirecord (minimal essential record) system was developed for the JHH Medical Clinic with encounter forms for each patient visit with lists of medications and procedures [151]. By 1978, an internally developed LAB system written in MUMPS provided specimen collection lists, work lists and instrument load-lists for the laboratory staff, and acquired online data from automated laboratory instruments. The LAB system also produced cumulative summaries of patient's test results and billing and administrative reports [112, 162]. By the mid-1980s, the JHH system included IBM 3081 and 3083 computers linked to the MUMPS LAB system which ran on three PDP-11/70 minicomputers and served both the clinical and surgical pathology laboratories [161, 214, 225].

In 1971, Barnett's Computer-Stored Ambulatory Record (COSTAR) system was developed for the Harvard Community Health Plan (HCHP) in Boston. The COSTAR system used remote terminals connected by telephone lines to computers located in the Laboratory of Computer Science at MGH. HCHP physicians ordered clinical laboratory tests on a special order form which the patient took to the laboratory for specimen collection, and where test results were entered into the computer as soon as the results were available. Physicians then received daily reports of their patients' tests results that had been completed during the prior 24 h, and they also could review test results on the system's display terminals. Additionally, status reports generated after the entry of any new data into patients' records provided updated summaries, including current medications and latest clinical laboratory test results [17, 96, 100].

Morey and associates [163] at the Massachusetts Institute of Technology, published a comprehensive analysis of the chemistry laboratory at the Boston City Hospital and described the functional requirements for a LAB system to handle its load of about one-million tests a year, most of which were already automated. They evaluated the hardware and software characteristics of 12 computer systems that were available in 1970, and recommended as a suitable turnkey LAB system either a system from Digital Equipment Corporation or one from Spear.

In 1971, Elbert and associates [74] at the University of Ohio Hospitals installed a Technicon Hemalog-8 hematology analyzer that employed continuous-flow stream hydraulics to aspirate whole blood samples and directly measure the hemoglobin, hematocrit, red blood cell count and platelet count; and calculate the red blood cell indices. In 1974, they added a Hemalog D automated white blood cell differential counter that also was based on continuous-flow technology; and in 1976 they installed a LABCOM laboratory information system that used a Digital Equipment Corporation (DEC) PDP-11/45 minicomputer for online data acquisition from both the Hemalog-8 and the Hemalog D systems. Test request and test result codes of up to four characters were set up to match the requirements of the analyzers, and clerks entered test request codes into the computer system from paper requisition forms so that specimen collection labels and processing labels could be generated. Tubes of blood with specimen labels were placed on the Hemalog-8 system, and as the specimens were processed by the instrument, the results were printed by a built-in printer and were captured by the LABCOM computer. A Teletype printer also could be used to print reports of test results. Similarly, the Hemalog D system provided a total white blood cell count and the percentages of each white blood cell subtype using its built-in printer, with the instrument data also captured by the LABCOM computer. The computer then compared the total white blood cell counts from the two systems before printing out the cell count from the Hemalog-8, which was normally the default print value. When there were significant differences between the total white blood cell counts from the two instruments, or when abnormal cells were reported, a manual (visual) white blood cell differential cell count was performed.

In 1972, McDonald and associates at the Regenstrief Institute in Indianapolis deployed the Regenstrief Medical Record System (RMRS), which included a LAB system running on a Digital Equipment Computer (DEC) PDP-11/45 located in the Regenstrief Health Center [157]. This LAB system had connections to a variety of terminals located in the clinical laboratories that allowed data entry and subsequent retrieval of test results directly from the system [156, 157]. For each patient's visit to a physician, a patient summary report was generated that included data from the clinical laboratories, with data from other clinical subsystems also displayed in a modified flow sheet format [156]. This report listed the patient's laboratory results in reverse chronological order, which allowed the physician to readily find and compare the most recent laboratory data to any prior data for repeated laboratory tests. Additionally, an asterisk was placed beside each abnormal test value for emphasis.

McDonald [156] reported that the RMRS used paper reports – rather than visual displays – as its primary mechanism for transmitting information to physicians, as paper reports were economical, portable, easy to browse, and could be annotated with a pen or pencil. In the early 1980s, the RMRS shared a DEC VAX 11/780 computer with the clinical laboratories and used microcomputer-based workstations to display forms into which the user could enter data using a mouse to select choices from menus [152]. By the mid-1980s, the RMRS's computer-based patient record contained patients' clinical laboratory data entered automatically from their LAB system [152]. In 1988, the RMRS was also linked to the clinical laboratories in the local Veterans and University hospitals [154].

In the 1970s, the most common topology for a LAB system was a minicomputer with 10–50 terminals that were directly connected to the computer in a "star" configuration. The typical data processing requirements for such a LAB system were to accept data entered through an input terminal, and to have that data processed by the computer as it arrived and then written to a magnetic disk for subsequent retrieval from the disk for printing at an output terminal. Each time the minicomputer exchanged data with a terminal or disk, a different program might be handle the transaction; for example, the order entry program would collect data from the laboratory requisition, and the specimen-collection-list program would print it. Since there would usually be more programs than could fit into the computer's main memory, programs were swapped to-and-from the disk, and the large size of the programs often resulted in a substantial overhead that affected system performance. The replacement of batch processing of test result reports with online processing by minicomputers greatly shortened test-reporting turnaround times, and facilitated the timely reporting of urgent and stat reports.

In the 1970s, distributed LAB system architectures began to be developed; and by the 1980s distributed LAB systems were available that consisted of a collection of workstations, each with its own microcomputer and local data storage that communicated with each other using a local area network or LAN [97]. This design allowed data traffic to be spread out over more disks than was possible with a centralized, single-computer system [160].

Genre [90] described several alternative architectures for implementing a LAB system: (1) completely freestanding; (2) linked to a hospital information system but issuing its own reports; or (3) functioning as a subsystem of a large hospital information system. It soon became evident that implementing a LAB system, with its multiple subsystems and connections, could be a difficult and complex project.

Enlander [76], at Stanford University, noted that although LAB systems had been available for more than a decade that used central computers for most laboratory data processing functions including instrument data acquisition, an alternative LAB system architecture would be to use microprocessors to preprocess data at each laboratory analyzer. The advantages of a front-end microprocessor-based architecture included increased flexibility in analyzer usage, increased efficiency in the use of the central computer, economy in software development, more flexibility in coping with changes in laboratory instrumentation and methods, better technologist control, and hardware redundancy for backup in case of system failure. In

1968, Stanford Medical Center's ACME research database system, which was hosted on an IBM 360/50 computer, used an IBM 1800 data acquisition computer to process data from their Technicon SMA-12/60 chemistry analyzer. By 1975, they were using microprocessors for converting the signals from the SMA analyzer to digital data.

Wertlake [236] at Children's Hospital of San Francisco proposed that laboratories wishing to use computers but not desiring the expense of a turn-key vendor's LAB system could begin with an advanced programmable calculator and gradually develop programs for laboratory calculations, and could use dedicated microprocessors for instrument data acquisition. Wertlake used a Hewlett-Packard 9830 programmable calculator that had 8K of core memory and a BASIC language interpreter that allowed laboratory personnel to write programs for calibration of automated analyzers and for performing selected clerical functions and reporting of laboratory test results. The advantages of using these calculators for both batch processing and for online instrument data acquisition were the ease of programming and the low-cost input/output devices. They also used a Hewlett-Packard 9821 calculator connected to a four-channel electrolyte analyzer to provide automated interpretation and output of the analyzer data. Wertlake and colleagues subsequently added a central minicomputer that used the programmable calculators as preprocessors.

In 1975, Blois [30] reported that that some LAB systems were beginning to satisfy perceived functional and technical requirements, even though the majority were "homemade;" and many required that the test requests and results be keypunched, and many provided only batch-processed summary reports for physicians and for billing. Some LAB systems employed a dedicated small computer that interfaced directly with automated instruments. Blois estimated that about 15 commercial companies had installed about 150 turnkey LAB systems over the prior 6–7 years. In a few large hospital information systems, the LAB system functioned as a subsystem and as a laboratory data management system rather than an instrument control system. Blois stated that these LAB systems were often the most successful.

The Diversified Numerical Applications (DNA) Automated Clinical Laboratory System used special-purpose keyboards to enter test request information from handwritten requisition forms. AutoAnalyzers were connected through an analog-to-digital converter to a Raytheon 703 computer, which also accepted digitized data directly from other automated instruments. The DNA software supported a computer-based patient file on disk storage, and provided a variety of printed laboratory reports [174].

In 1976, Bleich, Slack, and associates at Beth Israel Hospital in Boston introduced their clinical computing system. In 1982, they expanded the system to the Brigham and Women's Hospital. By 1984, the system ran on a network of Data General Eclipse minicomputers that supported 300 video-display terminals located throughout the hospitals, including the clinical laboratories. The system permitted one to retrieve data from the clinical laboratories, to look up reports from the departments of radiology and pathology, to look up prescriptions filled in the outpatient pharmacy, and to request delivery of patients' charts. A 1983 survey of 545 physicians, medical students, and nurses revealed that they used the computer terminals mostly to look up laboratory test results, and 83 % said that the terminals enabled them to work faster [28]. In the 1990s, their clinical computing system provided results from all their laboratories and clinical departments [197]. In 1994, Brigham and Women's Hospital joined with Massachusetts General Hospital to form Partner's Health Care System that included 10 hospitals and more than 250 practice sites with their clinical laboratories and clinical support subsystems [221].

In 1979, Fetter [81] described a microcomputer-based medical information system installed at Yale University that used a Digital Equipment Corporation (DEC) 16-bit LSI-11 processors with computer terminals installed in Yale's clinical laboratory.

In 1979, the PathNet LAB system was marketed by Cerner Corporation, and used a DEC VAX minicomputer to provide order-entry and results-reporting functions, a patient-data file, and laboratory functions including the printing of specimen labels, specimen-collection lists, work lists, and a variety of reports. Microbiology and blood bank subsystems supported the processing for these laboratories, and included textual reports [201].

Also in the 1970s, early LAB systems were installed at the University of Pennsylvania Hospital, at the University of Washington in Seattle, the Hopkins Medical Laboratories in Providence, Rhode Island, and at the University of Vermont Medical Center in Burlington [36].

In 1980, Williams and associates at the Mercy Hospital in Urbana, Illinois, developed a distributed LAB system in which clusters of terminals used for similar functions (such as a cluster used for order entry) were connected to Motorola 68000 microcomputers, each with its own memory and disk storage. A file-server program managed data storage and retrieval on the disk, and handled communications with other terminal clusters in the local-area network. Only the user-programs directly required by a terminal cluster were stored in that cluster. One data-storage cluster handled each major LAB subsystem, such as hematology or chemistry [160].

Norbut and associates [167] at the University of Pittsburgh Health Center used a North Star Horizon II microcomputer, with programs they wrote in North Star BASIC, that was interfaced to a cathode ray display terminal for structured data input and for rapid inquiry. Their variable-length patient files contained strings of numeric codes with associated free-text comments. A printer generated a daily work list for each laboratory area, and printed interim and cumulative reports, workload statistics, quality control summaries, and other reports. They planned to expand their system using a distributed network of low-cost minicomputers, with mark-sense cards for data entry from the individual workstations.

During the 1970s and 1980s, many articles were published on how to select a vendor-supported LAB system, including how to develop a statement of required specifications, how to evaluate available vendor-supported LAB systems, how to choose a LAB system vendor, and how to negotiate a contract [13, 131].

By the mid-1980s, some large laboratories used a distributed network of micro-computers and minicomputers to provide LAB system functions and to maintain computer-based patient records. One or more micro- or minicomputers processed the data from the various laboratory divisions and transmitted the data to the minicomputer maintaining the patient records [201]. This distributed LAB system architecture provided a more predictable response times, better performance per dollar, easier expansion, and greater reliability [160].

Lincoln [129] described distributed computer architectures that served serve both the hospital and the clinic using networked workstations with connections to the clinical laboratory. Enterprise-wide systems that served several hospitals had local area networks and distributed database management software that linked the various LAB systems' databases and integrated the patient data to provide patient medical records that were usable by the clinicians.

In the 1980s, systems with knowledge bases were described that had special tools for guiding users. Demuth [65] described a knowledge-based system that included "experts'" knowledge, such as pathology, where the system attempted to mimic the reasoning and logic of the pathologist by using simple queries and responses to navigate hierarchies (decision trees).

After the 1980s, advanced text-processing systems used both syntactic and semantic approaches, and added knowledge bases that controlled how parsers interpreted the meaning of words in particular contexts, such as in the processing of pathology reports [1].

By the end of the 1980s, most clinical laboratories used a commercial vendor-supported LAB information system that provided direct data acquisition from automated instruments, and generated reports for chemistry, hematology, and urinalysis tests. These systems also printed specimen-collection lists and technologists' work lists, monitored quality control, and provided a variety of reports for physicians and laboratory managers, and for accounting functions [198].

In the 1990s, Citation Computer Systems was reported to be one of the largest vendors of LAB systems, controlling nearly 20 % of the market, with a family of local-area network-based, menu-driven systems designed to support the clinical laboratories [201].

12.7 Evaluations of Early LAB Systems

The evaluation of a LAB system usually involved comparing the operational efficiency of the laboratory before and after the installation of a LAB system; and comprehensive evaluations often considered comparisons with a previously installed LAB system or with alternative LAB systems. Longitudinal studies of the efficiency of LAB systems were conducted when significant changes occurred in the laboratory, such as changes in the laboratory work load, the installation of new laboratory technologies such as automated instruments, or changes in the requirements for communicating laboratory test requests and reports; or to assess the effects of a LAB system on personnel and their functional relationships within the laboratory.

In 1965, the clinical chemistry laboratory at the Mount Sinai Hospital in New York City performed about 260,000 tests annually, and employed a total of 22 people who took hours-to-days to complete all of their work. After installing a

Technicon SMAC multi-channel computer-based chemistry analyzer, they were able to process approximately 10,000 tests a day with most of them completed by mid-afternoon [36].

In 1971, Berkeley Scientific Laboratories (BSL) reported a study of the laboratory operations in five large Chicago-area hospitals that compared their annual costs for five consecutive years. They reported that batch data processing was the key to an efficient, high-volume, day-shift operation; and that LAB systems that used a hospital information system generally reported lower costs for their laboratory data-processing functions, as the LAB system usually did not include the full costs of computer programming and communication networks. They found that the LAB system improved laboratory scheduling, reduced lost billings, and greatly improved information reporting system for management decision-making. They noted that the justification for a standalone LAB system rested primarily on anticipated further growth in the demand for laboratory services; the extent to which organizational weaknesses would not allow that demand to be met; the ability of the existing LAB system to provide acceptable turn-around times and adequate laboratory quality control; and the capability of the LAB system to integrate its data with other hospital patient information. They stated that many of the anticipated benefits from a LAB system were dependent upon integration with a hospital information system, and recommended coordinating the development of a laboratory data system with a total hospital information system [38].

Ball [13] surveyed a group of pathologists using a LAB system and found that speed, accuracy, and storage capabilities were three major advantages common to most LAB systems. Also, computer generated reports were of great value, as the laboratory personnel spent less time at clerical work, and the LAB system provided faster service and communication of test results, as well as improved management of the laboratory. The major deterrents to using a LAB system were system cost, time-consuming installation, personnel training time, and the need for high reliability and suitable back-up procedures for system down-times. Connectivity with a central hospital computer system also was an advantage, as the efficiency of a LAB system was greatly influenced by its association with a hospital information system, whether it was a subsystem of a hospital information system, or if it was a stand-alone LAB system with telecommunication linkages to the hospitals and the physicians' offices that it served.

McLaughlin [159] provided an early detailed economic analysis of a LAB system. He described the costs of laboratory services per patient as dependent upon the patient mix in the population served, the technology used, the organization of the laboratory, the definition of the costs, and how they varied over time with variations in the workload. A basic measure of the internal operational efficiency of a clinical laboratory is its cost per test. This is determined by collecting all of the direct and the indirect costs that were incurred in a specified period of time (such as for a month) for laboratory space, equipment, supplies, and personnel needed to do the testing. This total cost is then divided by the numbers of the tests performed in that time, and the result is a measure of the average per-test cost for that period. In determining laboratory costs, it is important to distinguish between the actual costs to the laboratory and the charges to the patient, since charges usually include added profit, or may be fixed by external agencies such as Medicare. The definition of the number of tests performed is not a simple one when the test is included in a panel of several tests that are done automatically by automated chemical analyzers and where some of the tests were not requested and therefore may not be reported. Additional efficiency measures may include the laboratory's operating costs per-patient or hospital-day, and the average number of tests completed per technician-hour. Another important measure – and a major determinant of the physician satisfaction with the laboratory services, is the response time or turnaround time from the receipt of the test request by the laboratory to the reporting of the test result to the physician, which is dependent on both the internal operations of the LAB system and its tele-communication facilities. Finally, without a benefits-realization program involving the physician customers of the laboratory, just getting data to physicians faster may not produce any improvements in quality of care or reductions in costs without an appropriate changes in physicians' behavior.

Rappaport [175] published a detailed economic analysis of his LAB system, and reported that in 1971 the average direct-cost per-test for all of his automated equipment was 15.5 cents. Barnett [19] at the Massachusetts General Hospital reported that the cost of their computer system for processing and reporting the chemistry procedures was approximately nine cents per test. Waxman [210, 232] summarized their costs per laboratory test as follows: the average cost of a clinical laboratory test in a manual mode was about 52 cents, based on a daily volume of 250 tests. For this same test volume, the introduction of automated procedures, with manual documentation, reduced the cost per test to 24 cents; and above 2,500 tests per day, the cost per-test was less than 7 cents.

Raymond [177, 178] at the University of Pennsylvania in Philadelphia reported that the LAB system installed in the William Pepper Laboratory at the Hospital of the University of Pennsylvania decreased stat test requests from about 100 per day to less than 30 per day, even though no special effort was made to discourage stat requests. Raymond [177, 178] proposed that an important measure for evaluating a LAB system was a reduction in service time; such as times taken to service routine and stat test requests. Another evaluation criterion is the accuracy of the results reported, which involves using test-assay quality control procedures to assure the accuracy of test measurements, and data quality control procedures to reduce clerical errors in the recording and reporting of test results. Additional factors that influence the satisfaction of users with clinical laboratory services are the formatting of the test reports, and the provision of clinical decision-support functions such as test normal limits, alerts for abnormal test results, and comments by the clinical pathologist to assist in the interpretation of some test results. The effectiveness of a LAB system is also influenced by connections to other medical information systems, such as hospital information systems, or office information systems serving physicians' offices.

Grams [94] published a detailed cost analysis of the LAB system installed at the University of Florida and reported the cost-per-test was between 13 and 17 cents. Wertlake [236] at Cedars-Sinai Medical Center in Los Angeles wrote that computerizing the laboratory was an indispensable means of solving many problems in the laboratory, including: 19 problems with patient registration and identification, 14 with patient location and chart location, 10 with physician ordering, 13 associated with transposition or other editing errors of physician orders by hospital personnel, 12 with specimen collection, 5 associated with transporting specimens to the laboratory, 4 associated with specimen accessioning, 3 performance characteristics that could be helped by a LAB system; and 22 other problems associated with major laboratory activities.

Lewis [127] estimated that approximately 8 % of national health care expenditures were for clinical laboratory testing, and because laboratory costs in the 1960s and 1970s reflected a large amount of clerical labor, the potential increased productivity and cost-savings from a LAB system could be enormous.

Lincoln and Korpman [135] reviewed selected publications reporting the effects of a LAB system on the performance of the clinical laboratory. They concluded that a LAB system could improve the throughput of laboratory testing; for example, the completion rate of white blood-cell differential counts before the installation of the LAB system averaged 10 differential counts per-hour, and with a LAB system averaged 34 per-hour. The turnaround time for a routine complete blood count averaged 4.5 h before the LAB system, and 1.6 h after the LAB system was installed. The turnaround time for routine chemistry analysis of blood electrolytes averaged 4.0 h before the LAB system, and 2.1 h with the LAB system. The clerical staff required to respond to telephone queries for test results decreased from nine clerks per ten million work units to two clerks, due to more rapid completion of laboratory tests and more effective dissemination of laboratory test results by the LAB system. They concluded that the greatest expense avoidance provided by the LAB system resulted from automation of clerical procedures.

12.8 Summary

The LAB system has evolved rapidly over the past half-century as a result of the growth of clinical laboratory testing and laboratory automation. The urinalysis as the first laboratory test dates back thousands of years, and physicians have routinely used clinical laboratory testing to supplement the physical examination of patients for more than a century; however, advances in biomedical science and the invention of automated chemical analyzers and cell counters starting in the 1950s revolutionized the clinical laboratories and initiated the cycle of automation and computerization that has given rise to the modern LAB system.

The clinical laboratory was an early and very successful example of the application of computer technology in clinical medicine. Williams [240] wrote that the use of the computer in the clinical laboratory was the first use of the computer in any clinical area; and the initial use of computers in the laboratory served to distinguish clinical computing from hospital computing, which was then concerned largely with financial and administrative data processing. The earliest computer applications in the laboratory were limited by the computer technology then available, and were based upon the computing experiences and applications that had been developed for business and industry – under the assumption that laboratory operations were standardized, stable, and definable [239].

The chemistry laboratory was the first clinical laboratory discipline to employ computers in day-to-day operations as the chemistry laboratory typically produced data consisting of small numeric values that were frequently available in digital form from analytical instruments. The hematology laboratory and clinical microscopy followed soon afterwards, where the data also included short alphabetic strings used to report the results of the examination of blood smears and urine specimens. The microbiology laboratory, on the other hand, posed greater challenges for early LAB computer systems because of the high proportion of textual data in the microbiology reports. Lincoln [132] wrote that the early LAB systems were first deployed in the chemistry and hematology laboratories because the chemistry and hematology laboratories had very similar information processing requirements, and these laboratories were profitable revenue centers that could support the development costs of early LAB systems.

In the early 1960s, the typical clinical laboratory could not justify a dedicated computer system, so the laboratory often shared the facilities of a central hospital mainframe computer that was otherwise used for accounting applications. As these mainframe systems usually provided only batch processing functions using punched card inputs, early LAB systems were primarily offline, batch-oriented systems that used punched cards for data transfer to the mainframe, with periodic printing of final cumulative summary reports of test results [58]. It was noted that although that LAB systems using shared mainframe computers were suitable for some routine test reporting functions, they often did not satisfy physicians' needs for immediate test reports for the emergency care of patients.

In the second half of the 1960s, the availability of affordable minicomputers caused a rapid surge in the development of LAB systems, with DEC PDP-8, PDP-11 and PDP-12 minicomputers used for standalone LAB systems, as well as IBM 1130 and 1800 computers, and CDC 3200 and 3300 computers. The increasingly widespread use of LAB systems was made possible by minicomputers, which were less costly than mainframe computers, but still powerful enough to meet the laboratory's computing needs.

By the end of the 1960s, advances in science and technology, socioeconomic pressures, and changes in the organization of medical care all helped to generate an increased demand for laboratory services [146]. By then, most hospitals of 100 beds or more had automated equipment in their chemistry and hematology laboratories, with online processing by a computer system that permitted the real-time entry of data as it was generated, and that provided visual feedback for verifying that the data entered were correct, and computer-based quality control (QC) for detecting analytical errors and for ensuring conformance with established QC limits.

In the 1970s, the clinical laboratory underwent great changes in information processing. The increasing use of computers was facilitated by the fact that much of the data processed in the laboratory was numeric, with relatively little English-language text. Some large laboratories still used time-sharing, mainframe computers to address the growing workloads and the demands for accuracy and rapid-reporting of test results needed to support clinical decision making; however, increasing numbers of clinical laboratories were making use of special purpose minicomputers, which extended the capabilities of the LAB system to include a greater variety of test data, more flexible online interfaces for automated instruments, additional calculations for test assays and quality control functions, and more convenient long-term storage and retrieval of test result data.

In the 1970s, the majority of new LAB systems used dedicated minicomputers, mostly the DEC PDP series, although some used Hewlett-Packard, Wang, or Data General Nova computers; or IBM 1130/1800 or CDC 3200 and 3300 systems. Some large LAB systems still used IBM 360 and IBM 370 mainframe computers, with huge visual-display terminals, extensive magnetic-disc storage, and high-speed line printers. These large mainframe computers also were linked to automated laboratory instruments in the laboratories, though often through smaller computers that captured the digital output from instruments. LAB system software typically was programmed in the FORTRAN, BASIC or MUMPS programming language.

In 1971, Berkeley Scientific Laboratories (BSL) concluded that in addition to large and comprehensive laboratory computer systems for large centralized laboratories, there would be a growing need for smaller, modular computer systems and semi-automated instruments to support urgent "stat" or emergency testing [38].

In the mid-1970s, a survey of computer applications in approximately 100 US hospitals revealed that only about one third had clinical laboratory (LAB) systems [209]. At the end of the 1970s, a survey conducted by Maturi and DuBois [149] for the National Center for Health Services Research and Development (NCHSRD) to assess the state of commercially available LAB systems reported that the major vendors of LAB systems at that time were Becton Dickenson (BD), Technicon, Medlab, and Community Health Computing (CHC). They also noted that the pharmacy system market was dominated by BD, International Business Machines (IBM), and Shared Medical Systems (SMS); and the major vendors of radiology systems were Siemens and General Electric (GE). At the end of the 1970s, Young and associates [247] at the University of Southern California conducted a survey of minicomputer-based laboratory systems in hospitals of 100–300 beds. They found that less than a quarter of these hospitals had laboratory applications that included the preparation of laboratory worksheets and schedules, and very few supported the two-way data transmission of laboratory orders and test results. They concluded that smaller hospitals' systems with minicomputers fell short of the more sophisticated systems in larger hospitals with mainframe computers.

It became increasingly evident that although large centralized LAB systems could provide acceptable services for routine testing procedures, they could not readily provide the immediate stat test reporting required for the care of acutely ill and emergency room patients because of inefficient workflows and/or manual data entry. But at the same time, the evolving hospital information systems (HISs) could readily integrate the laboratory data generated by their local LAB systems into their electronic patient records (EPRs). Since most of the information collected and processed by the clinical laboratory was essential in the diagnosis and treatment of patients, it became evident that the EPR was essential for good patient care, and the clinical laboratory became a major contributor of clinical data to the EPR. Also evident during the past five decades was that physicians had become increasingly dependent upon on laboratory data, the clinical laboratory, and its LAB system. In the 1950s only a few dozen clinical laboratory tests were routinely available, but by the 2000s, several hundred different tests were available. As the demand for laboratory testing increased and new analytical methodologies and laboratory instruments were developed, it became necessary to employ more sophisticated and powerful LAB systems to meet these demands, as the nature of most laboratory tests made them ideal for automation and computerization [37].

In 1980, a survey by Ball and Jacobs [7] of hospital information system (HIS) vendors found that 18 vendors provided computer support for some or all of the laboratory, pharmacy, and radiology functions. By 1987 about 20 % of US hospitals had computer links between their hospital information systems (HISs) and affiliated physicians' offices and outpatient information systems (OISs). Some had workstation terminals that enabled data to be exchanged, copied, and modified; and some permitted direct access to laboratory and radiology reports from an office information system [166]. Linkages of hospital and laboratory information systems to physicians' offices were motivated by the desire to make test results available to physicians [154]. In 1987, a Medical Software Buyer's Guide listed more than 900 products that included software for the laboratory, pharmacy, and radiology [170]. Dorenfest [67] reported that the number of hospitals using computer systems for other than financial applications had risen dramatically as computer applications moved into patient registration, pharmacy and nursing applications, and into the clinical laboratory.

In the 1980s, LAB systems increasingly employed minicomputers that could integrate data from all of the laboratory areas into a common database, and could satisfy most of a LAB system's functional requirements. LAB systems included programs to provide improved quality control, reference values, trend analyses, graphical presentation of data, online laboratory test interpretations, and clinical guidelines.

In the 1990s, LAB systems began using a client-server architecture with networked personal computer (PC) workstations distributed throughout the laboratories. By this time, the functions of the LAB systems were well understood and had evolved to the point that they provided comprehensive computer support for the laboratories' internal specimen analysis and test reporting functions, and also had the capability providing a variety of ad hoc reports for quality and management purposes, and provided efficient data retrieval for research and other needs [84].

Also by the 1990s, most hospitals had installed a variety of specialized clinical support information systems (CSISs) for the clinical laboratories, pathology, pharmacy, radiology/imaging, electrocardiography (ECG), and other ancillary services. Although these CSISs had separate patient databases, and some operated as independent systems, most were interconnected to form a medical information system (MIS) with a distributed database of clinical data that constituted the "electronic patient record" (EPR).

Genre [90] predicted that LAB systems would soon be able to automatically accept orders generated by physicians at the patients' bedsides using an order-entry module of the hospital information system. The LAB system would receive test requests from the hospital information system, and the laboratory would receive positively-identified patient specimens that could be placed in random order on analytical instruments, which would then download individual test requests from the LAB system; and the LAB system would make laboratory data available seamlessly across all venues of care, including remote locations such as physicians' offices and elsewhere.

12.9   Closing Comments

In this chapter, Morris Collen chronicles the rich history of the use of computer technology in the clinical laboratories with details that have not previously been systematically documented. This half-century history the LAB system helps us understand the strengths and limitations of contemporary LAB systems, it helps define new strategies and architectures for LAB systems of the future, and it informs us about other novel applications of information technology to biomedical science and to patient care.

In recent decades, the LAB systems installed in most US hospitals and large health care organizations have been commercial products marketed by a handful of laboratory information system (LIS) vendors whose systems typically use dedicated mid-level computer servers with desktop personal computer (PC) workstations. These commercial systems provide extensive functionality for the internal operations of the clinical laboratories, and typically are interfaced to electronic health record (EHR) systems and other systems for communicating test orders, for reporting test results, and for billing.

However, these standalone LIS products are now being disrupted by increasing pressures to replace departmental LAB systems with the lab-system functionality of so-called enterprise-wide integrated electronic health record systems (EWS). Enterprise-wide EHR systems are single-vendor products that provide comprehensive EHR support across the continuum of care: inpatient, outpatient, emergency department, home care, long-term care and elsewhere. These enterprise-wide systems have a single patient database and integrated "departmental" sub-systems for the laboratories, pathology, pharmacy, radiology, oncology and others.

The pressures to replace the standalone LAB system arise from the new emphasis on integrated EHR systems as US health care moves from volume-based, fee-for-service reimbursement to a patient-outcome centric reimbursement system with bundled and/or capitated payments, where provider organizations must assume financial risk for patient outcomes and population health. Risk-based payment systems place new demands on the EHR for coordination of all aspects of patient care, for maintaining patient registries for disease management and preventive care programs, and for supporting comprehensive clinical and financial analytics.

Historically, in volume-based fee-for-service environments, the usual EHR architecture was a "best-of-breed" configuration, with multiple departmental computer systems and other EHR building blocks, typically supplied by multiple vendors and each with a separate patient database. Communications between these best-of-breed systems used Health Level 7 (HL7) asynchronous messaging, with messaging between subsystems limited to selected data only, and with patient database queries and other data queries normally not feasible across the multiple best-of-breed platforms.

The anticipated advantages of replacing standalone departmental LAB systems with the LAB system functions of enterprise-wide or integrated EHR systems include: simplified test ordering, specimen tracking, and result reporting; improved embedded clinical decision support (CDS) for test selection and test interpretation; fewer patient identification problems; reduced software licensing costs; reduced IT staffing and support costs; and comprehensive and powerful clinical and financial analytics – including novel applications such as real-time detection of healthcare-associated infections (HAIs), and others. However, there is little accumulated experience with "integrated" LAB systems and no published data on either the benefits of this strategy or the potential disadvantages, such as loss of internal laboratory functionality that may adversely affect laboratory productivity, service levels, or costs.

Other disruptive forces affecting both the clinical laboratories and the LAB system include the rapidly evolving technologies of genetic and genomic medicine, as well as bedside and other point-of-care (POC) testing devices, wearable and implantable monitoring equipment, and other personal testing technologies. The data and knowledge management requirements of genetic and genomic medicine exceed the capabilities of both current LAB systems and EHRs, and will require new information processing strategies, and new LAB system and EHR system architectures and applications. Additionally, advances in point-of-care and other personal testing technologies may change the venue of some patient testing and reduce the number of specimens that must be transported to the clinical laboratories; although for at least the foreseeable future, the clinical laboratory will continue to perform a broad range of specialized in vitro testing. And irrespective of whether the LAB system of the future becomes part of the comprehensive EHR or remains a standalone platform, the key functions of the LAB system will continue to evolve through a recurring cycle of biomedical discovery followed by the development of practical in vitro analytic methods, advances in laboratory automation and instrumentation, and the ongoing development of novel LAB system applications.

References

1. Adams LB. Three surveillance and query languages. MD Comput. 1986;3:11–9.
2. Allen JK, Batjer JD. Evaluation of an automated method for leukocyte differential counts based on electronic volume analysis. Arch Pathol Lab Med. 1985;109:534–9.
3. Aller RD. Impact of Systeme International conversion on laboratory information systems. Arch Pathol Lab Med. 1987;111:1130–3.

4. Amar H, Barton S, Dubac D, Grady G. SMAC: the computer controller analyzer. In. Advances in automated analysis. Technicon International Congress 1972. Tarrytown: Mediad; 1973. p. 41–6.
5. Ansley H, Ornstein L. Enzyme histochemistry and differential white cell counts on the Technicon Hemalog D. In; Advances in automated analysis. Technicon International Congress 1970. Tarrytown: Mediad; 1971. p. 437–46.
6. Arkin CF, Sherry MA, Gough AG, Copeland BE. An automatic leukocyte analyzer. Validity of its results. Am J Clin Pathol. 1977;67:159–69.
7. Ball MJ, Jacobs SE. Hospital information systems as we enter the decade of the 80s. Proc SCAMC. 1980;1:646–50.
8. Ball MJ. An overview of total medical information systems. Methods Inf Med. 1971;10:73.
9. Ball MJ. Introduction. Chapter 1. In: Ball MJ, editor. Selecting a computer system for the clinical laboratory. Springfield: Thomas; 1971. p. 3–4.
10. Ball MJ. Specifications for a laboratory data processing system. Appendix E. In: Ball MJ, editor. Selecting a computer system for the clinical laboratory. Springfield: Thomas; 1971. p. 96–106.
11. Ball MJ. Available computer systems. In: Ball MJ, editor. Selecting a computer system for the clinical laboratory. Springfield: Thomas; 1971. p. 54–73.
12. Ball MJ. Survey of pathologists' experiences in computerization. In: Ball MJ, editor. Selecting a computer system for the clinical laboratory. Springfield: Thomas; 1971. p. 14–20.
13. Ball MJ. Selecting a computer system for the clinical laboratory. Springfield: Thomas; 1971.
14. Baorto DM, Cimino JJ, Parvin CA, Kahn MG. Using Logical Observation Identifier Names and Codes (LOINC) to exchange laboratory data among three academic hospitals. Proc AMIA. 1997;96–100.
15. Barnett GO, Hofmann PB. Computer technology and patient care: experiences of a hospital research effort. Inquiry. 1968;5:51–7.
16. Barnett GO, Castleman PA. A time-sharing computer system for patient-care activities. Comput Biomed Res. 1967;1:41–51.
17. Barnett GO, Souder D, Beaman P, Hupp J. MUMPS – an evolutionary commentary. Comput Biomed Res. 1981;14:112–8.
18. Barnett G, Greenes RA. Interface aspects of a hospital information system. Ann N Y Acad Sci. 1969;161:756–68.
19. Barnett GO. Massachusetts general hospital computer system. In: Collen MF, editor. Hospital computer systems. New York: Wiley; 1974.
20. Barnett GO, Greenes RA, Grossman JH. Computer processing of medical text information. Methods Inf Med. 1969;8:177–82.
21. Barrett JP, Hersch PL, Caswell RJ. Evaluation of the impact of the implementation of the Technicon Medical Information System at El Camino Hospital. Part II: economic trend analysis. Final report 1972; p. 27.
22. Bassis ML, Collen M. Normal chemistry values in an automated multiphasic screening program. In; Proc Technicon Symposium 1986. Automation in Analytical Chemistry. White Plains: Mediad; 1987. p. 309–12.
23. Bates JE, Bessman JD. Evaluation of BCDE, a microcomputer program to analyze automated blood counts and differentials. Am J Clin Pathol. 1987;88:314–23.
24. Benson ES. Research and educational initiatives in improving the use of the clinical laboratory [proceedings]. Ann Biol Clin (Paris). 1978;36:159–61.
25. Benzel JE, Egan JJ, Hart OJ, et al. Evaluation of an automated leukocyte counting system. II. Normal cell identification. Am J Clin Path. 1974;62:530–6.
26. Biemann K. The role of computers in conjunction with analytical instrumentation. Proc IEEE. 1979;67:1287–99.
27. Birndorf NI, Pentecost JO, Coakley JR, Spackman KA. An expert system to diagnose anemia and report results directly on hematology forms. Comput Biomed Res. 1996;29:16–26.

28. Bleich HL, Beckley RF, Horowitz GL, Jackson JD, Moody ES, Franklin C, et al. Clinical computing in a teaching hospital. N Engl J Med. 1985;312:756–64.
29. Bleich H. Computer evaluation of acid-based disorders. J Clin Invest. 1969;48:1689–96.
30. Blois MS. In: Enlander D, editor. Incorporation of clinical laboratory information systems into the hospital information system. New York: Academic; 1975.
31. Blomberg DJ, Ladley JL, Fattu JM, Patrick EA. The use of an expert system in the clinical laboratory as an aid in the diagnosis of anemia. Am J Clin Pathol. 1987;87:608–13.
32. Blum BI. A history of computers. In: Blum B, editor. Clinical information systems. New York: Springer; 1986. p. 1–32.
33. Bollinger PB, Drewinko B, Brailas CD, Smeeton NA, Trujillo JM. The technicon H* 1 – an automated hematology analyzer for today and tomorrow. Complete blood count parameters. Am J Clin Pathol. 1987;87:71–8.
34. Brient K. Barcoding facilitates patient-focused care. Healthc Inform. 1995;12:38. 40, 42.
35. Brittin GM. The impact of automation in hematology on patient care. New York: Technicon International Congress; 1972.
36. Bronzino JD. Computerization concepts in the clinical laboratory. In: Bronzino JD, editor. Computer applications for patient care. Menlo Park: Addison-Wesley; 1982. p. 117–37.
37. Bronzino JD. Computers and patient care. In: Bronzino JD, editor. Technology for patient care. Saint Louis: C.V. Mosby; 1977. p. 57–102.
38. BSL. Berkeley Scientific Laboratories. A study of automated clinical laboratory systems: US health services and mental health administration. Available from National Technical Information Service, Springfield; 1971.
39. Buchanan NS. Evolution of a hospital information system. Proc SCAMC. 1980;1:34–6.
40. Bull BS, Korpman RA. The clinical laboratory computer-system-who is it for? Arch Pathol Lab Med. 1980;104:449–51.
41. Bush IE. Trouble with medical computers. Perspect Biol Med. 1979;600–20.
42. Clark WA, Molnar CE. A description of the LINC. In: Stacy RW, Waxman BD, editors. Computers in biomedical research, vol. II. New York: Academic; 1965. p. 35–65.
43. Clark JS, Veasley LG, Jung AL, Jenkins JL. Automated PO2, PCO2, and pH monitoring of infants. Comp Biomed Res. 1971;4:262–74.
44. Collen MF, Rubin L, Davis L. Computers in multiphasic screening. In: Stacy RW, Waxman BD, editors. Computers in biomedical research, vol. I. New York: Academic; 1965.
45. Collen MF. The Permanente Medical Group and the Kaiser Foundation Research Institute. In: McLean ER, Soden JV, editors. Strategic planning for MIS. New York: Wiley; 1977. p. 257–71.
46. Collen MF. Machine diagnosis from a multiphasic screening program. Proc of 5th IBM Medical Symposium; 1963. p. 1–23.
47. Collen MF. Multiphasic health testing services. New York: Wiley; 1978.
48. Collen MF. Periodic health examinations using an automated multitest laboratory. JAMA. 1966;195:830–3.
49. Collen MF, Terdiman JF. Technology of multiphasic patient screening. Annu Rev Biophys Bioeng. 1973;2:103–14.
50. Collen MF, Rubin L, Neyman J, Dantzig GB, Baer RM, Siegelaub AB. Automated multiphasic screening and diagnosis. Am J Public Health Nation Health. 1964;54:741–50.
51. Collen MF, Feldman R, Sieglaub AB, Crawford D. Dollar cost per positive text for automated multiphasic screening. New Engl J Med. 1970;283(9):459–63.
52. Connelly D. Communicating laboratory results effectively; the role of graphical displays. Proc AAMSI Cong. 1983;113–5.
53. Connelly DP. Embedding expert systems in laboratory information systems. Am J Clin Pathol. 1990;94:S7–14.
54. Connelly DP, Willard KE. Monte Carlo simulation and the clinical laboratory. Arch Pathol Lab Med. 1989;113:750–7.
55. Connelly DP, Sielaff BH, Scott EP. ESPRE – expert system for platelet request evaluation. Am J Clin Pathol. 1990;94:S19–24.

56. Connelly DP, Glaser JP, Chou D. A structured approach to evaluating and selecting clinical laboratory information systems. Pathologists. 1984;38:714–20.
57. Connelly DP, Gatewood LC, Chou DC. Computers in laboratory medicine and pathology. An educational program. Arch Pathol Lab Med. 1981;105:59.
58. Constandse WJ. The use of a computer installation for a general purpose laboratory information system. Proc of the 6th IBM Medical Symposium. 1964. p. 495–544.
59. Cordle F, Boltjes BH. Electronic data logging and statistical evaluation in medical microbiology. Proc of the San Diego Biomedical Symposium. 1962;2:100.
60. Coutts A, Hjelm VJ, Kingsley GR, Betz GP. Multiple laboratory testing in a large federal hospital. Autom Anal Chem. 1968;1:151.
61. Cunnick WR, Cromie JB, Cortell R. Value of biochemical profiling in a periodic health examination program: analysis of 1000 cases. In: Davies DF, Tchobanoff JB, editors. Health evaluation: an entry to the health care system. New York: Intercontinental Medical Book Corp; 1973. p. 172–88.
62. Cutler JL, Collen MF, Siegelaub AB, Feldman R. Normal values for multiphasic screening blood chemistry tests. Adv Autom Anal. 1969;3:71.
63. Dayhoff RE, Ledley RS, Zeller JA, Park CM, Shiu MR. Platelet aggregation studies using TEXAC whole picture analysis. Proc SCAMC. 1978;31–6.
64. Debauche R, De Laey P. Evaluation of the Hemalog D system in a hospital clinical laboratory. In: Barton EC, editor. Advances in automated analysis. Tarrytown: Mediad; 1976. p. 294–311.
65. Demuth AI. Automated ICD-9-CM coding: an inevitable trend to expert systems. Health Care Commun. 1985;2:62–5.
66. Dinio RC, Ramirez G, Pribor HC. Pattern recognition of SMA 12 values as a diagnostic tool. In: Barton ED, et al., editors. Advances in automated analysis. Miami: Thurman Associates; 1970. p. 201–9.
67. Dorenfest SI. The decade of the 1980s: large expenditures produce limited progress in hospital automation. US Healthc. 1989;6:20–2.
68. Dove HG, Hierholzer Jr W. An integrated, microcomputer based infection control system. Proc MEDINFO. 1986;486–7.
69. Drewinko B, Wallace B, Flores C, Crawford RW, Trujillo JM. Computerized hematology: operation of a high-volume hematology laboratory. Am J Clin Pathol. 1977;67:64–76.
70. Dutcher TF, Desmond SA, Greenfield L. A computer program for use in the evaluation of multichannel laboratory instruments. Am J Clin Pathol. 1971;55:302.
71. Dutcher TF, Benzel JE, Egan JJ, Hart DJ, Christopher EA. Evaluation of an automated differential leukocyte counting system. I. Instrument description and reproducibility studies. Am J Clin Pathol. 1974;62:525.
72. Egan JJ, Benzel JE, Hart DJ, Christopher EA. Evaluation of an automated differential leukocyte counting system. 3. Detection of abnormal cells. Am J Clin Pathol. 1974;62:537–44.
73. Eggert AA, Emmerich KA, Spiegel CA, Smulka GJ, Horstmeier PA, Weisensel MJ. The development of a third generation system for entering microbiology data into a clinical laboratory information system. J Med Syst. 1988;12:365–82.
74. Elbert EE, O'Connor M. Combined use of the Hamalog 8 and hemalog D online to a laboratory computer system. In: Barton EC, editor. Advances in automated analysis. Tarrytown: Mediad; 1976. p. 365–75.
75. Elevitch FR, Boroviczeny KG. A proposed international standard for interlaboratory information exchange. Arch Pathol Lab Med. 1985;109:496–8.
76. Enlander D. Computer data processing of medical diagnoses in pathology. Am J Clin Pathol. 1975;63:538–44.
77. Esterhay Jr R, Foy JL, Lewis TL. Hospital information systems: approaches to screen definition: comparative anatomy of the PROMIS, NIH and Duke systems. Proc SCAMC. 1982;903–11.
78. Evans RS, Gardner RM, Burke JP, Pestotnik SL, Larsen RA, Classen DC, et al. A computerized approach to monitor prophylactic antibiotics. Proc SCAMC. 1987;241–5.

79. Evans RS, Larsen RA, Burke JP, Gardner RM, Meier FA, Jacobson JA, et al. Computer surveillance of hospital-acquired infections and antibiotic use. JAMA. 1986;256:1007–11.
80. Evenson MA, Hicks GP, Keenan JA, Larson FC. Application of an online data acquisition system using the LINC computer in the clinical chemistry laboratory. In; Automation in analytical chemistry. White Plains: Mediad; 1968. p. 137–40.
81. Fetter RR, Mills RE. A micro computer based medical information system. Proc 2nd Annual WAMI Meeting. 1979. p. 388–91.
82. Forrey AW, McDonald CJ, DeMoor G, Huff SM, Leavelle D, Leland D, et al. Logical observation identifier names and codes (LOINC) database: a public use set of codes and names for electronic reporting of clinical laboratory test results. Clin Chem. 1996;42:81–90.
83. Frey R, Girardi S, Wiederhold G. A filing system for medical research. Int J Biomed Comput. 1971;2:1–26.
84. Friedman BA. Informating, not automating, the medical record. J Med Syst. 1989;13:221–5.
85. Friedman RB, Bruce D, MacLowry J, Brenner V. Computer-assisted identification of bacteria. Am J Clin Pathol. 1973;395–403.
86. Gall J. In: van Egmond J, de Vries Robbe PF, Levy AH, editors. Computerized hospital information system cost-effectiveness: a case study. Amsterdam: North Holland; 1976. p. 281–93.
87. Gall J. Cost-benefit analysis: total hospital informatics. In: Koza RC, editor. Health information systems evaluation. Boulder: Colorado Associated University Press; 1974. p. 299–327.
88. Gardner RM, Pryor TA, Warner HR. The HELP hospital information system: update 1998. Int J Med Inform. 1999;54:169–82.
89. Gardner RM, Pryor TA, Clayton PD, Evans RS. Integrated computer network for acute patient care. Proc SCAMC. 1984;185–8.
90. Genre CF. Using the computer to manage change in the clinical pathology lab. In: Ball MJ et al., editors. Healthcare information management systems. New York: Springer; 1995. p. 267–82.
91. Giebink GA, Hurst LL. Computer projects in health care. Ann Arbor: Health Administration Press; 1975.
92. Gralnick HR, Abrams E, Griveber H, Koziol J. Evaluation of the hemalog system. In: Advances in automated analyses. Proc Technicon International Congress 1972. Tarrytown: Mediad; 1972. p. 9–14.
93. Grams RR, Johnson EA, Benson ES. Laboratory data analysis system. VI. System summary. Am J Clin Pathol. 1972;58:216–9.
94. Grams RR, Thomas RG. Cost analysis of a laboratory information system (LIS). J Med Syst. 1977;1:27–36.
95. Grams RR. Medical information systems: the laboratory module. Clifton: Humana Press; 1979.
96. Greenes RA, Pappalardo AN, Marble CW, Barnett GO. Design and implementation of a clinical data management system. Comput Biomed Res. 1969;2:469–85.
97. Greenes RA, Barnett GO, Klein SW, Robbins A, Prior RE. Recording, retrieval and review of medical data by physician-computer interaction. N Engl J Med. 1970;282:307–15.
98. Greenhalgh PJ, Mulholland SG. An automated infection surveillance system. Hospitals. 1972;46:66. passim.
99. Grossman JH, Barnet GO, McGuire MT, Swedlow DB. Evaluation of computer-acquired patient histories. JAMA. 1971;215:1286–91.
100. Grossman JH, Barnett GO, Koepsell TD, Nesson HR, Dorsey JL, Phillips RR. An automated medical record system. JAMA. 1973;224:1616–21.
101. Groves WE, Gajewski WH. Use of a clinical laboratory computer to warn of possible drug interference with test results. Proc of the 16th annual Southeast regional conference. 1978. p. 192–200.
102. Hammond WE. GEMISCH. A minicomputer information support system. Proc IEEE. 1973;61:1575–83.

103. Hammond WE, Stead WW, Straube MJ. Planned networking for medical information systems. Proc SCAMC. 1985;727–31.

104. Hammond WE, Stead WW, Straube MJ. An interface between a hospital information system and a computerized medical record. Proc SCAMC. 1980;3:1537–40.

105. Haug HH, Muller H, Schneider W. Comparative study of differential white cell counting with histochemical (Hemalog D) and morphologic methods. In: Barton EC, editor. Advances in automated analysis. Proc Technicon International Congress. Tarrytown: Mediad; 1977. p. 325–9.

106. Healy JC, Spackman KA, Beck JR. Small expert systems in clinical pathology: are they useful? Arch Pathol Lab Med. 1989;113:981–3.

107. Hicks GP. Chip technology. Its influence on the distribution of laboratory data and procedures in the 1980s. Arch Pathol Lab Med. 1981;105:341.

108. Hodge MH. Medical information systems: a resource for hospitals. Germantown: Aspen Publishers; 1977.

109. Hosty TA, Lundberg GD, Krieg AF, Marquardt VC, Sinton EB, Wertman B. So a laboratory computer system sounds like a good idea? Pathologists. 1979;33:293–6.

110. Hripcsak G, Allen B, Cimino JJ, Lee R. Access to data: comparing AccessMed with query by review. J Am Med Inform Assoc. 1996;3:288–99.

111. Jacobs H. A natural language information retrieval system. Methods Inf Med. 1968;7:8.

112. Johns CJ, Simborg DW, Blum BI, Starfield BH. A minirecord: an aid to continuity of care. Johns Hopkins Med J. 1977;140:277–84.

113. Jorgensen JH, Holmes P, Williams WL, Harris JL. Computerization of a hospital clinical microbiology laboratory. Am J Clin Pathol. 1978;69:605–14.

114. Jungner I, Jungner G. The autochemist as a laboratory screening instrument. In: Benson ES, Strandjord PE, editors. Multiple laboratory screening. New York: Academic; 1969. p. 71–9.

115. Karcher RE, Foreback CC. A comparison of selected SMAC channels to other commonly utilized laboratory instruments. In: Barton EC et al., editors. Advances in automated analysis. Proc Technicon International Congress. Tarrytown: Mediad; 1977. p. 191–6.

116. Kassirer JP, Brand DH, Schwartz WB. An automated system for data processing in the metabolic balance laboratory. Comput Biomed Res. 1971;4:181–96.

117. Klee GG, Cox C, Purnell D, Kao P. Use of reference data in the interpretation of parathyroid hormone measurements. Proc SCAMC. 1984;398–1.

118. Klee GG, Ackerman E, Elveback LR, Gatewood LC, Pierre RV, O'Sullivan M. Investigation of statistical decision rules for sequential hematologic laboratory tests. Am J Clin Pathol. 1978;69:375–82.

119. Krause JR. Automated differentials in the hematology laboratory. Am J Clin Pathol. 1990;93:S11–6.

120. Kuperman GJ, Gardner RM, Pryor TA. The pharmacy application of the HELP system. In: Kuperman GJ, Gardner RM, Pryor TA, editors. HELP: a dynamic hospital information system. New York: Springer; 1991. p. 168–72.

121. Kuperman GJ, Jonathan M, Tanasijevic MJ, Ma'Luf N, Rittenberg E, Jha A, et al. Improving response to critical laboratory results with automation results of a randomized controlled trial. J Am Med Inform Assoc. 1999;6:512–22.

122. Lamson BG. Mini-computers and large central processors from a medical record management point of view. International Symposium on Medical Information Systems. 1975. p. 58–65.

123. Lamson BG, Russell WS, Fullmore J, Nix WE. The first decade of effort: progress toward a hospital information system at the UCLA Hospital, Los Angeles, California. Methods Inf Med. 1970;9:73–80.

124. Lamson BG. Storage and retrieval of medical diagnostic statements in full English text. Proceedings of the First Conference on the Use of Computers in Radiology. 1966. p. D34–43.

125. Lamson BG. Computer assisted data processing in laboratory medicine. In: Stacy RW, Waxman BD, editors. Computers in biomedical research. New York: Academic; 1965. p. 353–76.
126. Levine JB. SMA II: the quiet revolution. Advances in automated analysis. Proc Technicon International Congress. Tarrytown: Mediad; 1977. p. 112–20.
127. Lewis JW. Commentary: clinical laboratory information systems. Proc IEEE. 1979;67:1299–300.
128. Lewis JW, Marr JJ. Use of a small laboratory computer for identification of the Enterobacteriaceae. J Med Syst. 1977;1:23–6.
129. Lincoln TL. Health care and the sociotechnical workplace. Arch Pathol Lab Med. 1986;110:306–7.
130. Lincoln TL. Computers in the clinical laboratory: what we have learned. Med Instrum. 1978;12:233–6.
131. Lincoln TL, Aller RD. Acquiring a laboratory computer system. Vendor selection and contracting. Clin Lab Med. 1991;11:21–40.
132. Lincoln T. An historical perspective on clinical laboratory systems. In: Blum BI, Duncan KA, editors. A history of medical informatics. New York: Addison-Wesley; 1990. p. 267–77.
133. Lincoln TL. Hospital information systems what lies behind friendliness and flexibility? Inform Health Soc Care. 1984;9:255–63.
134. Lincoln TL. Medical information science: a joint endeavor. JAMA. 1983;249:610–2.
135. Lincoln TL, Korpman RA. Computers, health care, and medical information science. Science. 1980;210:257–63.
136. Lindberg D. Impact of public policy on the development, adoption, and diffusion of medical information systems technology. Washington, DC: U.S. Govt. Print. Office; 1978.
137. Lindberg D. The computer and medical care. Springfield: CC Thomas; 1968.
138. Lindberg D. Electronic retrieval of clinical data. J Med Educ. 1965;40:753–9.
139. Lindberg D. Operation of a hospital computer system. J Am Vet Med Assoc. 1965;147:1541–4.
140. Lindberg D. A computer in medicine. Mo Med. 1964;61:282–4.
141. Lindberg D, Reese GR. Automatic measurement and computer processing of bacterial growth data. Biomedical sciences instrumentation. Proc of the 1st National Biomedical Sciences Instrumentation Symposium. 1963. p. 11–20.
142. Lindberg DA, Van Pelnan HJ, Couch HD. Patterns in clinical chemistry. Am J Clin Pathol. 1965;44:315–21.
143. Lindberg D, Gaston LW, Kingsland LC. A knowledge-based system for consultation about blood coagulation studies. In: The human side of computers in medicine. Proc Soc for Computer Med 10th Annual Conf. 1980. p. 5.
144. Lindberg D, Vanpeenen HJ, Couch RD. Patters in clinical chemistry. Low serum sodium and chloride in hospitalized patients. Am J Clin Pathol. 1965;44:315–21.
145. Lindberg D, Reese GR, Buck C. Computer generated hospital diagnosis file. Mo Med. 1964;61:581. 2 PASSIM.
146. Lucas FV, Lincoln TL, Kinney TD. Clinical laboratory science. A look to the future. Lab Investig. 1969;20:400–4.
147. Lupovitch A, Memminger J, Corr RM. Manual and computerized cumulative reporting systems for the clinical microbiology laboratory. Am J Clin Pathol. 1979;72:841–7.
148. Lyman M, Chi E, Sager N. Automated case review of acute bacterial meningitis of childhood. Proc MEDINFO. 1983;790–3.
149. Maturi VF, DuBois RM. Recent trends in computerized medical information systems for hospital departments. Proc SCAMC.1980;3:1541–49.
150. McClure S, Bates JE, Harrison R, Gilmer PR, Bessman JD. The "diff-if". Use of microcomputer analysis to triage blood specimens for microscopic examination. Am J Clin Pathol. 1988;90:163–8.

151. McColligan E, Blum B, Brunn C. An automated care medical record system for ambulatory care. Proc SCM/SAMS Joint Conf on Ambulatory Care. 1981. p. 72–6.
152. McDonald CJ. The medical gopher: a microcomputer based physician work station. Proc SCAMC. 1984;453–9.
153. McDonald CJ. Action-oriented decisions in ambulatory medicine. Chicago: Year Book Medical Publishers; 1981.
154. McDonald CJ, Tierney WM. Computer-stored medical records: their future role in medical practice. JAMA. 1988;259:3433–40.
155. McDonald CJ, Murray R, Jeris D, et al. A computer-based record and clinical monitoring system for ambulatory care. Am J Public Health. 1977;67:240–5.
156. McDonald CJ, Wilson G, Blevins L, Seeger J, et al. The Regenstrief medical record system. Proc SCAMC. 1977;168-9.
157. McDonald CJ, Overhage JM, Tierney WM, et al. The Regenstrief medical record system: a quarter century experience. Int J Med Inform. 1999;54:225–53.
158. McHenry LE, Parker PK, Branch B. Simultaneous platelet counts, in conjunction with Hemalog D analyses, utilizing the Technicon AutoCounter system. Advances in Automated Analysis. Proc Technicon International Congress. Tarrytown: Mediad; 1977. p. 376–80.
159. McLaughlin. Alphanumeric display terminal survey. Datamation. 1973;20:71–92.
160. Michalski RS, Baskin AB, Spackman KA. A logic-based approach to conceptual data base analysis. Inform Health Soc Care. 1983;8:187–95.
161. Miller R, Causey J, Moore G, Wilk G. Development and operation of a MUMPS laboratory information system: a decade's experience. Proc SCAMC. 1988;654–8.
162. Miller RE, Steinbach GL, Dayhoff RE. A hierarchical computer network: an alternative approach to clinical laboratory computerization in a large hospital. Proc SCAMC. 1980;32–8.
163. Morey R, Adams MC, Laga E. Factors to be considered in computerizing a clinical chemistry department of a large city hospital. Proc AFIPS. 1971;477–90.
164. Myers J, Gelblat M, Enterline HT. Automatic encoding of pathology data. Computer-readable surgical pathology data as a by-product of typed pathology reports. Arch Pathol. 1970;89:73.
165. Neeley WE. Computer calculation of electronic platelet counts. Am J Clin Pathol. 1972;58:33–6.
166. Newald J. Hospitals look to computerization of physician office linkage. Hospitals. 1987;61:92–4.
167. Norbut AM, Foulis PR, Krieg AF. Microcomputer reporting and information system for microbiology. Am J Clin Pathol. 1981;76:50–6.
168. O'Connor M, McKinney T. The diagnosis of microcytic anemia by a rule-based expert system using VP-Expert. Arch Pathol Lab Med. 1989;113:985–8.
169. Okubo RS, Russell WS, Dimsdale B, Lamson BG. Natural language storage and retrieval of medical diagnostic information: experience at the UCLA hospital and clinics over a 10-year period. Comput Prog Biomed. 1975;5:105–30.
170. Polacsek RA. The fourth annual medical software buyer's guide. MD Comput. 1987;4:23–136.
171. Pratt AW, Pacak M. Automatic processing of medical english. Reprinted by US Dept HEW, NIH 1969; 1969a.
172. Pratt AW, Pacak M. Identification and transformation of terminal morphemes in medical English. Methods Inf Med. 1969;8:84–90.
173. Pryor TA. A note on filtering electrocardiograms. Comput Biomed Res. 1971;4(5):542–7.
174. Quam K. The DNA, automated clinical laboratory system. Am J Med Technol. 1975;41:228–31.
175. Rappaport AE, Gennaro WD. The economics of computer-coupled automation in the clinical chemistry department of the Youngstown Hospital Association. In: Stacy RW, Waxman BD, editors. Computers in biomedical research. New York: Academic Press; 1974. p. 215–24.

176. Ratliff CR, Casey AE, Kelly J. Use of the SMA 4 AutoAnalyzer in a central hematology service. Automation in analytical chemistry. Proc Technicon Symposium. Whites Plains: Mediad; 1968. p. 193–9.
177. Raymond S. Criteria in the choice of a computer system. I. The computer in theory. JAMA. 1974;228:591–4.
178. Raymond S. Criteria in the choice of a computer system. II. The computer in practice. JAMA. 1974;228:1015–7.
179. Reece RL, Hobbie RK. Computer evaluation of chemistry values: a reporting and diagnostic aid. Am J Clin Pathol. 1972;57:664–75.
180. Robinson III RE. Acquisition and analysis of narrative medical record data. Comput Biomed Res. 1970;3:495–509.
181. Rodbard D, Jaffe M, Beveridge M, Pernick N. A data management program to assist with home monitoring of blood glucose and self adjustment of insulin dosage for patients with diabetes mellitus and their physicians. Proc SCAMC. 1984;321–4.
182. Rosner SW, Palmer A, Caceres CA. A computer program for computation and interpretation of pulmonary function data. Comput Biomed Res. 1971;4:141–56.
183. Rosvoll RV, Mengason AP, Smith L, Patel HJ, Maynard J, Connor F. Visual and automated differential leukocyte counts. A comparison study of three instruments. Am J Clin Pathol. 1979;71:695–703.
184. Rowberg A, Lee S. Use of a desk-top calculator to interpret acid-base data. Am J Clin Pathol. 1973;59:180.
185. Rush RL, Nabb DP. Bringing it all together on three SMAC systems. In: Barton EC, editor. Advances in automated analysis. Proc Technicon Congress. Tarrytown: Mediad; 1977. p. 376–80.
186. Salwen M, Wallach J. Interpretative analysis of hematologic data using a combination of decision making technologies. MEDCOMP. 1982;3:428.
187. Schoentag RA, Pedersen JT. Evaluation of an automated blood smear analyzer. Am J Clin Pathol. 1979;71:685–94.
188. Schultz JR, Davis L. The technology of PROMIS. Proc IEEE. 1979;67:1237–44.
189. Seligson D. Observations regarding laboratory instrumentation and screening analysis. In: Benson ES, Strandjord PE, editors. Multiple laboratory screening. New York: Academic; 1969. p. 87–119.
190. Shieman BM. Medical information system, El Camino Hospital. IMS Ind Med Surg. 1971;40:25–6.
191. Shim H, Uh Y, Lee SH, Yoon YR. A new specimen management system using RFID technology. J Med Syst. 2011;35:1403–12.
192. Siegel SJ. Developing an information system for a hospital. Public Health Rep. 1968;83:359–62.
193. Simborg DW, Macdonald LK, Liebman JS, Musco P. Ward information-management system: an evaluation. Comput Biomed Res. 1972;5:484–97.
194. Simmons A, Schwabbauer M, Earhart C. A fully automated platelet counting apparatus. In: Advances in automated analysis. Proc Technicon International Congress. Miami: Thurman Associates. 1971. p. 413–5.
195. Skeggs LT. An automatic method for colorimetric analysis. Am J Clin Pathol. 1957;28:311–22.
196. Skeggs LT, Hochstrasser H. Multiple automatic sequential analysis. Clin Chem. 1964;10:918–36.
197. Slack WV, Bleich HL. The CCC system in two teaching hospitals: a progress report. Int J Med Inform. 1999;54:183–96.
198. Smith Jr JW, Svirbely JR. Laboratory information systems. MD Comput. 1988;5:38–47.
199. Smith Jr JW, Speicher CE, Chandrasekaran B. Expert systems as aids for interpretive reporting. J Med Syst. 1984;8:373–88.

590   M.F. Collen and R.E. Miller

200. Smith Jr JW, Svirbely JR, Evans CA, Strohm P, Josephson JR, Tanner M. RED: a red-cell antibody identification expert module. J Med Syst. 1985;9:121–38.
201. Smith JW, Svirbely JR. Laboratory information systems. In: Shortliffe EH, Perreault LE, editors. Medical informatics: computer applications in health care. Reading: Addison-Wesley; 1990. p. 273–97.
202. Smythe WJ, Shamos MH, Morgenstern S, Skeggs LT. SMA 12/60: a new sequential multiple analysis instrument. Automation in analytical chemistry. Proc Technicon Symposium. White Plains: Mediad; 1968. p. 105–13.
203. Sneider RM. Using a medical information system to improve the quality of patient care. Proc SCAMC. 1978;594–7.
204. Snyder LR, Leon LP. New chemical methods for SMAC. In: Barton EC, editor. Advances in automated analysis. Tarrytown: Mediad; 1977. p. 186–90.
205. Speedie SM, Palumbo FB, Knapp DA, Beardsley R. Evaluating physician decision making: a rule-based system for drug prescribing review. Proc MEDCOMP. 1982;404–8
206. Speedie SM, Skarupa S, Blaschke TF, Kondo J, Leatherman E, Perreault L. MENTOR: integration of an expert system with a hospital information system. Proc SCAMC. 1987;220–4.
207. Speicher CE, Smith JW. Communication between laboratory and clinician: test requests and interpretive reports. In: Speicher CE, Smith JW, editors. Choosing effective laboratory tests. Philadelphia: Saunders; 1983. p. 93–108.
208. Speicher CE, Smith JW. Interpretive reporting in clinical pathology. JAMA. 1980;243:1556–60.
209. Spencer WA. An opinion survey of computer applications in 149 hospitals in the USA, Europe and Japan. Inform Health Soc Care. 1976;1:215–34.
210. Stacy RW, Waxman BD. Computers in biomedical research. New York: Academic; 1974.
211. Stauffer M, Clayson KJ, Roby RJ, Strandjord PE. A computer-assisted system: thyroid disease. Am J Clin Pathol. 1974;62:766–74.
212. Stead WW, Hammond WE. Computer-based medical records: the centerpiece of TMR. MD Comput. 1988;5:48–62.
213. Stead WW, Hammond WE, Winfree RG. Beyond a basic HIS: work stations for department management. Proc SCAMC. 1984; 197–9.
214. Steinbach G, Miller R. A dual processor standard MUMPS system with load-sharing and provision for rapid hardware backup. MUMPS Users Group Q. 1981;11:32–8.
215. Sterling RT, O'Connor M, Hopkins 3rd M, Dunlevy BE. Red blood cell antibody identification and confirmation using commercial panels. A computer program for the IBM personal computer. Arch Pathol Lab Med. 1986;110:219–23.
216. Streed SA, Hierholzer WJ. Analysis of five years' experience using an on-line infection data management system. Proc MEDINFO. 1986;86:26–30.
217. Takasugi S, Lindberg D. Information content of clinical blood chemistry data. Proc MedINFO. 1980;432–5.
218. Talamo TS, Losos 3rd F, Kessler GF. Microcomputer assisted interpretative reporting of protein electrophoresis data. Am J Clin Pathol. 1982;77:726–30.
219. Taswell HF, Nicholson LL, Cochran ML. Use of a 15-channel blood grouping AutoAnalyzer for patient typing. Technicon International Congress. 1973. p. 57–8.
220. Tatch D. Automatic encoding of medical diagnoses. 6th IBM Medical Symposium. 1964. p. 1–7.
221. Teich JM, Glaser JP, Beckley RF, Aranow M, Bates DW, Kuperman GJ, et al. The Brigham integrated computing system (BICS): advanced clinical systems in an academic hospital environment. Int J Med Inform. 1999;54:197–208.
222. Terdiman JF, Collen MF. Kaiser-Permanente patient computer medical record-past experience and future goals. Proc Assoc Inf Sci. 1976;13:27.
223. Terdiman JF. Mass random storage devices and their application to a Medical Information System (MIS). Comput Biomed Res. 1970;3:528–38.

224. Tilzer LL, Jones RW. Use of bar code labels on collection tubes for specimen management in the clinical laboratory. Arch Pathol Lab Med. 1988;112:1200–2.
225. Tolchin SG, Barta W. Local network and distributed processing issues in the Johns Hopkins Hospital. J Med Syst. 1986;10:339–53.
226. Ulirsch RC, Ashwood ER, Noce P. Security in the clinical laboratory. Guidelines for managing the information resource. Arch Pathol Lab Med. 1990;114:89–93.
227. Upton RC, Spaet TH, La Mantia J. Automatic platelet counting with the AutoAnalyer. In; Automation in analytical chemistry. Proc Technicon Symp 1967, Vol 1. White Plains: Mediad; 1967. p. 197–9.
228. Vallbona C, Spencer WA. Texas institute for research and rehabilitation hospital computer system (Houston). In: Collen MF, editor. Hospital computer systems. New York: Wiley; 1974. p. 662–700.
229. Vermeulen GD, Schwab SV, Young VM, Hsieh RK. A computerized system for clinical microbiology. Am J Clin Pathol. 1972;57:413–8.
230. Warner HF. A computer-based information system for patient care. In: Bekey GA, Schartz MD, editors. Hospital information systems. New York: Marcel Dekker; 1972. pp 293–332.
231. Watson RJ. A large-scale professionally oriented medical information system – five years later. J Med Syst. 1977;1:3–21.
232. Waxman BD. Biomedical computing: 1965. Ann NY Acad Sci. 1966;128:723–30.
233. Weant BD. Evaluation of the Technicon B G automated blood grouping systems. Proc 1976 Technicon Internatl Congress. Tarrytown: Mediad; 1977. p. 438–45.
234. Weed LL. The patient's record as an extension of the basic science training of the physician; rules for recording data in the clinical record; presentation of case examples and flow sheets. Cleveland: Cleveland Metropolitan General Hospital, School of Medicine, Western Reserve University; 1967.
235. Weilert M. Implementing an information system. Clin Lab Med. 1983;3:233–50.
236. Wertlake PT. Integrated hospital and laboratory computer system vital to hospital laboratory. 7th Technicon Internatl Congress 1976. Tarrytown: Mediad; 1977. p. 438–45.
237. Weschler W, Allens S, Negersmith K. Hemalog: an automated hematology laboratory system. In: Advances in automated analysis. Proc 1970 Technicon Internatl Congress. Miami: Thurman Associates; 1971. p. 431–6.
238. Williams BT, Foote CF, Galassie C, Schaeffer RC. Augmented physician interactive medical record. Proc MEDINFO. 1989;779–83.
239. Williams BT, Chen TT, Schultz DF, Moll JD, Flood JR, Elston J. PLATO-based medical information system – variable keyboards. Proc 2nd Conference on Medical Info Systems. 1975. p. 56–61.
240. Williams BT. Computer aids to clinical decisions. Boca Raton: CRC Press; 1982.
241. Williams GZ, Williams RL. Clinical laboratory subsystem. In: Collen M, editor. Hospital computer systems. New York: Wiley; 1974. p. 148–93.
242. Wintrobe MM. The clinicians' expectation of the laboratory in the remote and recent past and in the future. In: Advances in automated analysis. Proc 1976 Technicon International Congress. Tarrytown: Mediad; 1977. p. 288–93.
243. Wise WS. Microcomputer infection surveillance system. Proc SCAMC. 1984;215–9.
244. Wolf PL. Utilization of computers in biochemical profiling. In: Enlander D, editor. Computers in laboratory medicine. New York: Academic; 1975. p. 81–101.
245. Wolf PL, Ludwig HR, Vallee JF. Progress toward a direct-access hematology data-base. Arch Pathol. 1971;91:542–9.
246. Yoder RD. Computational augmentation of blood gas measurements. Proceedings of the 1971 26th annual conference. 1971. p. 701–5.
247. Young EM, Brian EW, Hardy DR, Kaplan A, Childerston JK. Evaluation of automated hospital data management systems (AHDMS). Proc SCAMC. 1980;1:651.
248. Yountness E, Derwinko B. A computer-based reporting system for bone marrow evaluation. Am J Clin Pathol. 1978;69:333–41.

Chapter 13
Anatomic Pathology Information Laboratory Information Systems and Natural Language Processing: Early History

Alexis B. Carter, Michael J. Becich, and Morris F. Collen

Abstract Anatomic Pathology laboratories began to encode and retrieve diagnoses from paper reports using punched cards in the 1960s. When Anatomic Pathology Laboratory Information systems (APLIS) began to be used in the 1970s, pathology departments found that searching free text for diagnoses was hindered by the variability of terms for the same concept and by the amount of computer resources required. Consequently, system developers began to engineer natural language processing (NLP) algorithms to translate computationally ambiguous written language into coded concepts. At the same time, pathologists began to develop the Systemized Nomenclature of Pathologists (SNOP), which eventually developed into the internationally utilized ontology called the Systematized Nomenclature of Medicine Clinical Terms (SNOMED-CT). Systems in the 1970s used keywords based on concepts to encode reports and the development of query languages to retrieve them. By the 1980s, the user was guided through decision trees to the best matching concept code from data dictionaries that linked pathology systems with medical record systems, and linguistic analysis that converted natural language into a structured database. At that time, some advanced NLP systems had knowledge bases that indicated how experts would interpret the meaning of words in particular contexts, but most query languages were still based on the search and retrieval of encoded terms. Much has occurred since then, including the recognition of Pathology Informatics as a discipline and the use of many NLP algorithms as well as algorithms to scrub identifiers from free text reports for research purposes.

Author was deceased at the time of publication.

M.F. Collen (deceased)

A.B. Carter, M.D., F.C.A.P., F.A.S.C.P. (✉)
Department of Pathology and Laboratory Medicine, Emory University,
1364 Clifton Road NE, Room F149A, Atlanta, GA 30322, USA
e-mail: abcart2@emory.edu

M.J. Becich, M.D., Ph.D.
Department of Biomedical Informatics, University of Pittsburgh School of Medicine,
Pittsburgh, PA, USA
e-mail: becich@pitt.edu

© Springer-Verlag London 2015
M.F. Collen, M.J. Ball (eds.), *The History of Medical Informatics in the United States*, Health Informatics, DOI 10.1007/978-1-4471-6732-7_13

Keywords Anatomic pathology • Anatomic Pathology Laboratory Information Systems (APLIS) • Natural language processing (NLP) • Systemized Nomenclature of Pathologists (SNOP) • Systematized Nomenclature of Medicine Clinical Terms (SNOMED-CT) • Linguistic analysis • Knowledge bases • Algorithms • Pathology informatics

Anatomic Pathology is the branch of medicine that studies the structural (histologic) and functional (disease-related) disturbances caused by pathophysiologic changes in tissues and organs of the body. The pathologist in a medical center traditionally directs both the anatomic pathology (AP) department and the clinical pathology (CP) or laboratory medicine. In an anatomic pathology department, several types of reports are produced including surgical pathology, molecular pathology, hematopathology, cytology and autopsy reports which are managed by an Anatomic Pathology Laboratory Information System (APLIS). This chapter focuses on AP systems and not CP systems. Details on the CPLIS or clinical pathology systems are provided in Chap. 12.

Surgical pathology is a pathology subdiscipline of Anatomic Pathology that receives either tissue specimens with an accompanying requisition for gross examination or specimen slides (usually as part of secondary consultation) for microscopic examination [59]. After completing the examination, the pathologist transmits back a surgical pathology report that is a description of the macroscopic and microscopic characteristics of a tissue specimen, with an interpretation of the pathologist's findings, and provides a diagnosis as well as guiding comments to the treating physician. Traditionally, the recording, processing, and storage of surgical pathology reports had been carried out by manual as well as automated methods. In the 1960s, punched cards were used for data entry and for requests for data retrieval [40]. By the 1970s, interactive cathode ray tube (CRT) terminals with keyboards were the usual mode for entering and retrieving data for APLIS systems. By the 1980s, computer-based natural language processing (NLP) systems were beginning to appearing in APLIS systems [8]. After the 2000s, surgical pathology reports were mostly dictated, transcribed and stored in APLIS systems. ·

A cytology report by a pathologist describes the microscopic findings of stained smears of fluids, secretions, fine needle aspirates of solid tissue as well as tissue brushings from the body; except that blood and bone marrow smears are usually examined and reported from the hematopathology (or hematology) division of the laboratory. An autopsy report is a detailed description of the postmortem examination of the various organs and tissues of the body [60, 66, 67].

13.1 Requirements of an APLIS System

Functional requirements of an APLIS system are to: (1) provide a means for communicating a requisition for services to the pathology department; (2) enter the pathologist's report; (3) store the data in a way to enable its use for clinical, administrative, and research purposes; (4) generate pathology reports that provide information of value to the care of the patient; and (5) permit retrieval of pathology data that are also useful for medical research and education. As for any system within or interfacing with an electronic health record (EHR), an APLIS system requires a method for placing orders for AP services in the pathology department, and traditionally these orders have been manually transcribed from paper requisitions that accompany the specimen or slide(s) into the APLIS. This is still in common practice today, although more and more systems are enabled to accept electronic orders from an EHR. Whether on paper or electronic, orders for AP services must contain appropriate patient identification and clinical information as well as a description of where each of the specimens obtained from an individual patient was derived.

Technologic requirements of an APLIS system include the ability to process the pathologist's reports that are largely in free form, natural language, narrative text, just as are many other physicians' notes found in patients' medical records. Traditionally, pathologists dictated their reports which were transcribed by a medical transcriptionist or secretary, who then filed the signed paper reports in the patient's paper chart. From the viewpoint of quality control and editing, the most desirable approach to narrative text acquisition is the entry of the dictated report directly into the computer system by use of an interactive terminal, but reliable speech recognition would not become available until the 1990s [60]. It soon became evident that the large amount of free text used in pathologists' reports created a major problem for computer-based information systems since narrative text required more storage space than did numbers, was sometimes difficult to interpret due to variability in meaning behind the same words, and was usually difficult to search and retrieve for information. To overcome the first problem, systems were developed which converted medical concepts into shorter computer language codes. The second problem required the development of standardized terminology for diagnoses and other concepts. The third problem required the development of special query and retrieval languages.

13.2   Encoding and Retrieval of Anatomic Pathology Text

Natural language processing (NLP) of pathologists' dictated and transcribed reports was developed to overcome difficulties in searching free text reports for concepts. Reports containing certain concepts had shorter computer language codes assigned to each relevant concept, and each concept was defined in data dictionaries with uniform agreement of vocabulary and meaning. Special query and retrieval languages were developed. In the 1980s, Bishop [5] defined the requirements for an ideal coding system which, in the 1980s, did not exist; namely, that there should be a unique concept code for each term (word or phrase), each concept code should be defined, each concept should be independent, synonyms of terms should be equitable to their assigned concept, each concept code should be linked to codes of related terms, the system should encompass all of medicine and be in the public domain, and the format of the knowledge base should be described completely in functional terms to make it independent of the software and hardware used. A concept is a single one-to-one representation of the thing, idea, or condition that exists, while a term is a word or phrase that represents that concept. A concept may have one to multiple synonymous terms (e.g., myocardial infarction and heart attack are different terms for the same concept). Although it is possible to search and retrieve computer-stored text by matching desired words or sets of words, it is much simpler to search and retrieve by numbers and letters and symbols. Thus, to facilitate storage and retrieval of diagnostic terms but also to facilitate retrieval of reports which may have synonymous terms for the same concept, the terms in a data dictionary are usually represented by the numerical code for its corresponding concept. The coding of terms has the advantage of presenting data to the computer in a compact and consistent format. The disadvantages of coding are that users have to be familiar with the coding system, codes have a tendency to reduce and stereotype information, and they require frequent revisions to avoid becoming obsolete [60]. To develop and use standard concepts requires the development of a data dictionary, which is a lexicon of standard, accepted, defined, and correctly spelled concepts and terms. Such a data dictionary has to list all data items stored in the computer database, with their definitions and their codes, and any associated relevant information required for their storage and retrieval, and for their linkage to other data items and files. A data dictionary for pathology was usually initiated by selecting commonly used terms from a standard medical dictionary and from related medical literature. It then continually added new terms as they were entered from the APLIS database itself. The design of the data dictionary had to provide expandability for incorporating new data items introduced by new procedures. As these lexicons became the basis for automated natural language processing (NLP), they included *syntactical* information (information defining attributes about the term such as to whether the word was a noun, verb, or other) as well as *semantical* information (the meaning of the word in the language of medicine) [46].

Medical terminology is the compilation of standard medical terms by their meaning, and medical nomenclature provides a systemized way of generating new terms for the terminology. Medical ontology is a compilation of concepts, each of which may have more than one term, which are formally named and which additionally have definitions regarding attributes of the concept such as type, properties and relationships with other concepts such as by disease type.

A common method used for early medical information systems to simplify the coding problem was to standardize medical textual data, and to simplify its entry, storage, and retrieval by using special-purpose, structured, and pre-coded data entry forms. However, this approach decreased the flexibility and richness of textual entry. It was relatively simple to type words and sentences into the computer by using the keyboard, and then to retrieve such text by matching letter-by-letter, word-by-word, or sentence-by-sentence. One way of accomplishing this in the 1960s was by using IBM's Magnetic Tape/Selectric Typewriter (MT/ST) that interfaced an office typewriter to a magnetic tape drive. By the late 1960s, this could be connected directly to a digital computer. Robinson [58] used such a system to enter narrative surgical pathology reports, and at the time of the transcription, the system permitted the information to be acquired for computer processing, so the user was not dependent on access to a time-sharing computer. His program matched each word against a standard vocabulary, and thus identified new or misspelled words for human editing.

The earliest work on classifying and codifying diseases by systematic assignment of related diagnostic terms to classes or groups was done by the World Health Organization (WHO). WHO took over from the French the classification system that had been adopted in 1893 and was primarily based upon body site and etiology of diseases [14]. The first International Classification of Diseases (ICD) published under WHO sponsorship was in its sixth revision in 1948. In the 1950s, medical librarians manually encoded ICD-6 codes for diagnoses. In the 1960s, ICD-7 codes were generally key punched into cards for electronic data processing. The International Classification of Diseases, Adapted (ICDA) used in the United States for indexing hospital records, was based on ICD-8 that was published in 1967. Beginning in 1968, ICDA began to serve as the basis for coding diagnostic data for official morbidity and mortality statistics in the United States. In addition, the payors of insurance claims began to require ICDA codes for payment, which encouraged hospitals to enter into their computers the hospital discharge diagnoses and the appropriate ICDA codes. The ninth revision of ICD appeared in 1977. Since ICD was originally designed as an international system for reporting causes of death, ICD-9 was revised to better classify diseases. In 1978, its Clinical Modification (ICD-9-CM) included more than 10,000 terms and permitted six-digit codes plus modifiers. ICD-9-CM also included in its Volume III a listing of procedures. From the 1980s through the 2010s (30 years), the ICD-9-CM was the nationwide classification system used by medical record librarians and pathologists for the coding of diagnoses in the United States. As of late 2014, ICD-10 was expected to be required for use in the United States in October 2015.

The Standard Nomenclature of Diseases and Operations (SNDO) was developed by the New York Academy of Medicine. It was published by the American Medical Association in 1932 and was used in most hospitals in the United States for three decades. SNDO listed medical conditions in two dimensions: the first was by anatomic site or topographic category (as examples, body as a whole, skin, musculoskeletal, respiratory, cardiovascular); the second was by etiology or cause (for example, due to prenatal influence, due to plant or parasite, due to intoxication, due to trauma by physical agent). The two-dimensional SNDO was not sufficiently flexible to satisfy clinical needs, so its fifth (and last) edition appeared in 1961.

A four dimensional nomenclature, intended primarily for pathologists, was developed by a group led by Arthur H. Wells, within the College of American Pathologists. It was called the Systemized Nomenclature of Pathologists (SNOP). First published in 1965, SNOP coded medical terms into four major semantic categories: Topography (T) for the body site affected; Morphology (M) for the structural changes observed; Etiology (E) for the cause of the disease; and Function (F) for the abnormal changes in physiology [71]. Thus a patient with lung cancer who smoked cigarettes and had episodes of shortness of breath at night would be assigned the following string of SNOP terms: T2600 M8103 (bronchus, carcinoma); E6927 (tobacco-cigarettes); F7103 (paroxysmal nocturnal dyspnea) [55]. The use of SNOP was readily adopted by pathologists in the 1960s, as it was well suited for coding for computer entry when using punched cards. In 1969 Pratt, at the National Institutes of Health (NIH), began to report on the automatic SNOP coding of autopsy diagnoses. He wrote that in the creation of a computer based natural language processing system, it was necessary to provide for the morphological, syntactic and semantic recognition of input messages. He used SNOP as his semantically organized dictionary. As part of this work, the above categories were split into semantic subcategories and morphemes (the smallest meaningful parts of words) to permit the successful identification of word forms that were not found in the SNOP dictionary, and for the recognition of medical English synonyms [56]. He developed parsing algorithms for morphological, syntactic, and semantic analysis of autopsy diagnoses; and a series of computer programs which when given as input a body of medical text, produced as output a linguistic description and semantic interpretation of the given text [57]. The result of the analysis was the translation of medical text into the four fields (T, M, E, and F) as they were listed in the SNOP dictionary. In the 1970s, it was the basis for the development of computer programs to permit automatic SNOP encoding of pathology terms [53, 55]. At the National Institutes of Health, Pratt's contribution to this field was lauded by Wells [71]. Pratt [54] soon concluded that SNOP was not the ideal semantic lexicon for medical linguistics, though it presented many desirable features that could be incorporated in any new medical lexicon. Complete as well as multiple TMEF statements were considered to be necessary for pathologist's purposes [26]. The successful use of SNOP by pathologists encouraged Cote, Gantner, and others to expand it to attempt to encompass all medical specialties.

As a result of the expansion of SNOP, the Systemized Nomenclature of Medicine (SNOMED) was first published in 1977 [68]. In addition to SNOP's four attributes of Topography (T), Morphology (M), Etiology (E), and Function (F), it contained three more attributes: Disease (D), Procedure (P), and Occupation (O). Disease (D) was used to encode classes of diseases, complex disease entities, and syndromes, which made SNOMED as suitable for statistical reporting as the ICD. Procedure (P) was used to describe diagnostic, therapeutic, preventive, or administrative procedures, and Occupation (O) was used to encode the patient's occupational and industrial hazards [9, 10, 20]. Some reports comparing SNOMED and ICD advocated SNOMED as superior for the purposes of medical care and research, since ICD was designed primarily for statistical reporting and was often too general to identify specific patient problems. In addition, SNOMED defined the logical connections between the categories of data contained in the final coded statement. Furthermore, SNOMED codes could be used to generate ICD codes, but not vice versa [27].

An important contribution to the standardization of medical terminology was made by Burgess Gordon who headed a committee of the American Medical Association to develop Current Medical Terminology (CMT) for the alphabetical listing of terms with their definitions and simplified references [25]. The first edition of CMT was published in 1962 with revisions in 1964 and 1965 [24]. In 1971, the fourth edition was expanded into the Current Medical Information and Terminology [22] to attempt to provide a "distillate" of the medical record by using four-digit codes for such descriptors as symptoms, signs, laboratory test results, x-ray, and pathology reports [21, 23]. Referred to as CMIT, it was available in machine-readable form and was an excellent source of structured information for over 3,000 diseases. It was used by Lindberg et al. [44] as a computer aid to diagnosis in his CONSIDER program for searching CMIT by combinations of attributes and then listing the diseases in which these attributes occurred.

The importance of identifying medical procedures and services, in addition to diagnoses, for the payment of medical claims led to the development of special systems for terminology and coding of medical services and procedures. In 1967 the first edition of Current Procedural Terminology (CPT) was published with a four-digit coding system, but it was soon revised and expanded to five-digit codes to facilitate the frequent addition of new procedures [13]. Subsequently, the American Medical Association provided frequent revisions of CPT, such that in the 1970s and 1980s CPT-4 was the most widely accepted system of standardized descriptive terms and codes for reporting physician-provided procedures and services under government and private health-insurance programs. In 1989, the new Health Care Financing Organization began to require every physician's request for payment for services to patients in the office to include ICD-9-CM codes and also required reporting procedures and services using CPT-4 codes [61].

Although CMIT had defined its diagnostic terms, a common deficiency of systems such as SNOP, SNOMED, and ICD was that they lacked a common dictionary that defined their terms and concepts precisely. As a result, the same condition could be defined differently and assigned different codes by different coders [32]. An important benefit from using data dictionaries was their ability to encourage the standardization of medical terms through their definitions, and thereby facilitate the interchange of medical information among different health professionals, and also among different medical databases. Since the data stored in patients' records came from multiple databases, such as from the pathology system, the laboratory system, the pharmacy system, and others, standards for exchanging such data had to be established before they could be readily transferred into a computer-based, integrated patient record.

The National Library of Medicine (NLM) met the problem of variances in medical terminology by instituting its own standard controlled vocabulary called Medical Subject Headings (MeSH) which was used by librarians for indexing NLM's stored literature citations. However, MeSH was not designed to serve as a vocabulary for patient records. In the 1980s, the NLM began to develop a Unified Medical Language System (UMLS) to compensate for differences in terminology among different systems, such as for MeSH, CMIT, SNOP, SNOMED, and ICD [33]. UMLS was not planned to form a single vocabulary, but rather to unify terms from a variety of standardized vocabularies and codes for the purpose of improving bibliographic retrieval, and to provide standardized data terms for computer-based records. It was still evident at the end of the 1980s, that an ideal coding system was not yet available which would satisfy all the requirements of an ideal system as defined by [5].

Automated text processing soon offered the formalized structuring and encoding of standardized medical terms in an automated fashion that would provide a great savings of storage space and would improve the effectiveness of the search and retrieval process for text. Since the manual coding of text was tedious, time-consuming, and led to inconsistent coding, efforts were soon directed to develop software for the automated encoding by computer. As early as 1962, Lamson at the University of California, Los Angeles, began to enter uncoded surgical pathology diagnoses in full English text into a magnetic file system. The information was key-punched in English in the exact form supplied by the pathologists. The patient record was recalled by patient name or identification number, and a full prose print-out of the diagnosis was provided. To avoid manual coding, Lamson [41, 42] col-lected 3 years of patient data into a thesaurus that related all English words that had identifiable relationships. His computer program then matched significant words present in a query and retrieved patients' records containing these words. In 1965, his patients' files contained about 16,000 words, and his thesaurus contained 5,700 English words. However, he recognized that more programming would be neces-sary to provide syntactic tests that could clear up problems of a semantic and syn-tactic nature. Working with Jacobs and Dimsdale from IBM, Lamson went on to develop a natural language retrieval system that contained a data dictionary for pathology records which contained unique numeric codes for each English word, including surgical pathology and bone-marrow examinations, autopsy reports, nuclear medicine, and neuroradiology findings [50]. The extensive thesaurus con-tained hierarchical and synonymous relationships of terms; as for example, to iden-tify that dyspnea and shortness-of-breath were acceptable synonyms [34, 35, 37]. Patient records were maintained in master text files, and new data were merged, in order of patient medical record numbers, into the master text files. A set of search programs produced a document that was a computer printout of the full English text of the initial record in an unaltered, unedited form [41].

In 1963 Korein [38, 39] at New York University Medical Center designed a method for storing a physician's dictated narrative text in a variable-length and variable-field format. The narrative data were then subjected to a program that gen-erated first an identifier and then the location for each paragraph in the record. The next step reformatted the data on tape such that the content of the document was made into a list of words with a set of desired synonyms. On interrogation, the pro-gram would search for the desired words or synonyms and would retrieve the selected text. This technique, which identified key words, also later served as one approach to automatic retrieval of literature documents. In 1964 Tatch [70], in the Surgeon General's Office of the U. S. Army, reported automatically encoding diag-noses by punching paper tape as a by-product of the normal typing process for the clinical record summary sheet (not the pathology report; a study on this came later). The computer program operated upon actual words within selected blocks, one at a time, and then produced a unique numeral for each letter resulting in a composite set of unique numerals that represented each word. The combined numeral was matched to an identification table, and an identity code was appended to the numeral. Based on a syntax code, the numerals were added one-at-a-time, until a diagnostic classification was determined. The diagnostic code related to the final sum was retrieved from memory and added to the clinical record summary.

In 1966, Buck [7], with Lindberg's group at the University of Missouri at Columbia, developed a program for retrieving patients' records from computer files that included the patients' coded discharge medical diagnoses, surgical operations, surgical pathology and cytology interpretations, autopsy diagnoses, and the interpretations of electrocardiograms and roentgenograms. The diagnosis files were stored on magnetic tape in a fixed-field format and processed by an IBM 1410 computer system. Queries were entered from punched cards with the code numbers of the diagnoses to be retrieved. The computer searched the magnetic tape records for the diagnoses, which in 1966 contained more than 500,000 records, and then identified the medical record numbers of the patients who had the diagnoses of interest.

Similar approaches to automated encoding of diagnoses were applied using CPT and ICD-9-CM. The diagnosis, or the procedure, was entered into the system as an English word or phrase. The search for and retrieval of coded items was simple, but the retrieval of uncoded textual items was more difficult. The approaches to automatic encoding of entered text led to the retrieval of stored text by the matching of words and phrases, such as used for a key-word-in-context (KWIC) search [36] or by pattern matching of word strings [73]. Early systems attempted to match the term with one in their data dictionary or lexicon, and if no direct match was found, the system then searched for a synonym that could be accepted by the user.

In 1970 Myers and associates [48] at the University of Pennsylvania, reported a system in which a pathology report was translated into a series of keyword or data elements encoded using arbitrarily assigned numbers. Similar to the technique reported by Tatch in 1964, the typist entered the routine pathology report using a typewriter controlled by a paper tape program, the data elements were automatically coded, and a punched paper tape could be produced as a by-product of typing. The report was stored on either magnetic tape or a disk storage system.

Enlander [12] developed a computer program that searched for certain pre-established key words in each diagnostic sentence according to a hierarchical structure that was based on the four-digit SNOP code. When this mode was applied to 500 diagnostic sentences, the automated keyword search encoded 75 % of the sentences. In a pilot clinical information system at Kaiser Permanente in Oakland, California, Enlander used a visual display terminal equipped with a light pen to select and enter a diagnosis, and the SNOP-coded diagnosis was then automatically displayed.

By the 1980s, more advanced systems added knowledge to guide the user by displaying queries and responses through decision trees that led to the best matching concept code. The search for words in a dictionary made their retrieval easy. However, it was more difficult to search for and retrieve exact meaningful expressions from such text. That is, although it was easy to enter and store words, it was not always easy for the retriever to figure out what they had meant to the person who had entered the words. Blois described the problem by saying that computers were built to process the symbols fed to them, in a manner prescribed by their programs, where the meaning of the symbols was known only to the programmers but rarely to the program and never to the computer. Consequently one could transfer everything except the meaning. Blois further pointed out that the available symbols (codes) rarely matched the clinical data precisely, so that the user frequently had to "force" the data into categories that might not be appropriate [6]. Ideally, what was needed was a natural language processing system that could interact with the computer in ordinary language, and through these decades this was an important objective. Certainly the fluidity of spoken and written language was markedly different from formal, structured computer languages. Computers readily surpassed humans at processing strings of numbers or letters; however, people found it more effective to communicate using strings of words. The approach of matching words and phrases was useful for processing a highly structured text. However, this method ignored the syntax of sentences and missed the importance of the positions of words in a sentence and the relations between words including negation. Obermeier [49] at Battelle Laboratories, Columbus, Ohio, defined natural language processing as the ability of a computer to process the same language that humans use in normal discourse. He believed that the central problem for natural language processing was how to transform a potentially ambiguous phrase into an unambiguous form that could be used internally by the computer system. This transformation, called parsing, was the process of combining words or symbols into groups that could be replaced by a more general symbol. Different types of parsers evolved which were based on pattern-matching, syntax or grammar, semantics or meaning, knowledge bases, and combinations of these approaches.

Hendrix [31], at SRI International, described the complex nature of natural language research as requiring the study of sources of lexical knowledge (concerned with individual words, the parts of speech to which they belong, and their meanings), syntactic knowledge (concerned with the grouping of words into meaningful phrases), semantic knowledge (concerned with composing the literal meaning of large syntactic units from the semantics of their subparts), discourse knowledge (concerned with the way clues from the context being processed are used to interpret a sentence), and domain knowledge (concerned with how medical information constrains possible interpretations). Clearly natural-language processing had to consider semantics since medical language was relatively unstandardized, it had many ambiguities, ill-defined terms, and multiple meanings of the same word or term (synonyms). Wells [71] offered an example of "…semantically equivalent phrases …muscle atrophy, atrophy of muscle, atrophic muscle, muscular atrophy." In addition, natural language processing had to consider syntax, or the relation of words to each other in a sentence. When searching for strings of words such as mitral stenosis and aortic insufficiency, the importance of the ordering of the words was evident since mitral insufficiency and aortic stenosis had a very different meaning. The phrase "time flies for house flies" made sense only when one knows that the word flies is first a verb and then a noun. Another common problem with computer word searches by exact letter-by-letter matches was the handling of inconsistent spelling and typographic errors.

In addition to automatic encoding of diagnoses, the retrieval of text required the development of automated processing programs to facilitate the retrieval of stored text. In 1968 Barnett, and associates at the Massachusetts General Hospital, began to structure the narrative text, such as progress notes, by using an interactive, conversational technique with a predetermined branching structure of the data and a fixed vocabulary. The user entered the information by selecting the desired items from a list on a display screen [2, 3]. Later Barnett's group reported the development of a Medical Query Language (MQL) for the retrieval and analysis of data from their COSTAR ambulatory patient records. An MQL query was made up of a series of statements; each statement began with a keyword. MQL queries could be indefinitely long, or could be broken down into a series of subqueries, each designed to accomplish some portion of the total problem. A statement was scanned and passed on to a parser that matched the scanned symbols to rules in the MQL grammar; and then the program went on to execute the query [47].

Hammond and Stead at Duke University used a data dictionary to define the codes for their CP system that was linked to their The Medical Record (TMR) system [29]. Their dictionary permitted modification and updating of specific functions and allowed for differences between various medical specialties and clinics. Major sections of the dictionary were devoted to system specifications, problems, procedures, providers, supplies, and therapies. In addition, there were demographic and examination data and also professional fees, accounting, messages, and report controls. An alphabetically arranged thesaurus permitted synonym definitions. Where appropriate for free text input, all codes and their text equivalents were defined in the dictionary. The user could enter the code directly or could type text and let the program do an alphabetic search in the dictionary and convert the text string to the appropriate code [30].

In the late 1970s, Sager and associates at New York University, initiated their Linguistic String Project that converted the natural language of medical records into a structured database [62, 64, 65, 69]. Whereas earlier attempts at automated encoding systems dealt with phrases that were matched with terms in a dictionary, Sager first performed a syntactic analysis of the input, then mapped the analyzed sentences into a tabular arrangement of the syntactic segments, in which the segments were labeled according to their medical content. In the resultant table (called an information format) the rows corresponded to the successive statements in the documents and the columns to the different types of information in the statements [64]. Thus Sager's automatic-language processor parsed each sentence and broke the sentence into components such as subject-verb-object; and the narrative statements into six statement types, such as general medical management, treatment, medication, test and result, patient state, and patient behavior. The processor then transformed the statements into a structured tabular format. This transformation of the record was more suitable for their database-management system; it also simplified retrieval of the records that were then transformed back for the users into a narrative form. Sager et al. [63] reported that they had applied the methods of linguistic analysis to a considerable body of clinical narrative that included pathology reports. They successfully tested their approach for automatic encoding of narrative text in the Head and Neck Cancer Database maintained at that time at the Roswell Park Memorial Institute. In 1985 they reported that their medical-English lexicon, which gave for each word the English and medical classification, numbered about 8,000 words [45]. By 1986 they reported that they had applied the methods of linguistic analysis to a considerable body of clinical narrative: hospital discharge summaries, initial histories, clinic visit reports, and radiology and clinical-pathology reports [63].

In the 1980s, Gabrieli, and associates at Buffalo, New York, developed an office information system called Physicians' Records and Knowledge Yielding Total Information for Consulting Electronically (PRAKTICE) for processing natural language and other elements in medical records [17, 19]. He developed his own computer-compatible medical nomenclature by a numeric representation, where the location of a term in a hierarchical tree served as the code. For example, the diagnosis of polycythemia was represented by 4-5-9-1-2, where 4 = clinical medicine, 4-5 = a diagnostic term, 4-5-9 = hematologic diagnostic term, 4-5-9-1 = red cell disorder, and 4-5-9-1-2 = polycythemia [18]. Gabrieli developed his own lexicon that contained more than 100,000 terms and used his nomenclature for processing medical text. He described his method for processing free text as beginning with a parser that recognized punctuation marks and spaces, breaking down each sentence into individual words while retaining the whole sentence intact for reference. Each word was numbered for its place in the sentence, and then matched against a Master Word Lexicon. Each word was given a grammatical classification (noun, verb, etc.) and a semantic characterization (grouped among "clue [medical] words", "modifiers", or "others"). Next, the system looked for any words near to the medical term that might be modifiers altering its meaning (usually adjectives). Thus, the term "abdominal pain" might be preceded by a modifier, such as "crampy abdominal pain". In the third step, the remaining words were analyzed for their relationship to other words in the sentence [16].

Thus, the early natural language, text-processing systems were primarily syntax based, and identified words and phrases as subjects or predicates, nouns or verbs. After completing the syntax analysis, semantic-based systems attempted to recognize the meanings of words, and used dictionaries and rewrite rules to generate the stored text. By the 1980s, some advanced text-processing systems used both syntactical and semantical approaches, with knowledge bases that indicated how expert parsers would interpret the meaning of words in particular contexts, such as in the processing of the discharge summaries in the patients' records. Yet even in the 1980s, most query languages for retrieving data from computer-based patient records were still based on the search and retrieval of encoded terms. Demuth [11] described the two approaches that had been used to develop automated coding systems: (1) A language-based system that matched English words against a dictionary, and if a match or an accepted synonym was found, assigned a code, and (2) A knowledge-based or expert system that included the universe of knowledge of the "experts" for whom the particular system was intended. The expert system attempts to mimic the reasoning and logic of the pathologist by using hierarchical (decision tree-based systems) that attempted to automate human reasoning and logic using simple queries and responses. The decision tree design mandated the nature and order of the questions to be asked, and how they were to be answered. Demuth concluded that an automated coding system must possess characteristics of both a language-based and

Table 13.1   Chronological timeline of efforts at coding system development

Year	Encoding/NLP event
1893	French classification system adopted for classification of diseases based upon body site and etiology (predecessor of ICD)
1932	Standard Nomenclature of Diseases and Operations (SNDO) is published by the American Medical Association (closes in 1961)
1948	WHO publishes 6th revision of ICD (ICD-6)
1962	Current Medical Terminology (CMT) is published
1965	Systemized Nomenclature of Pathology (SNOP) is published (predecessor of SNOMED)
1967	International Classification of Diseases Adapted (ICDA) is published
1967	Current Procedural Terminology (CPT) is first published
1971	CMT is expanded to Current Medical Information and Terminology (CMIT)
1977	ICD-9 is published
1977	Systemized Nomenclature of Medicine (SNOMED) is published (derived from SNOP)
1978	ICD-9 Clinical modification (ICD-9-CM) is published (still being used as of 2014)
1980s	National Library of Medicine builds the Unified Medical Language System (UMLS)

a knowledge-based system in order to provide the feedback necessary to help the medical record professional arrive at the correct codes. After the 1980s, some advanced text-processing systems used both syntactical and semantical approaches, and added knowledge bases that indicated how expert parsers would interpret the meaning of words in particular contexts, such as in the processing of pathology reports [1]. A chronological sequence of coding system development, coding system implementation and retrieval efforts are in Tables 13.1, 13.2, and 13.3.

13.3   Summary and Commentary

This early history of the APLIS with particular relevance to biomedical informatics is truly a comprehensive look at Pathology Informatics in the AP laboratory. Much has happened since the 1980s, where Dr. Collen's excellent synopsis leaves off. In the mid-1980s, Bruce Friedman at the University of Michigan, began a national meeting Automating Information Management in the Clinical Laboratory (AIMCL) which was the foundation for Pathology Informatics, a term first introduce in the 1990s, [15]. As a result of the pioneering work of Dr. Friedman, a team at the University of Pittsburgh launched a companion meeting, Advancing Pathology Informatics, Imaging and the Internet in 1996 (see http://www.pathologyinformat-ics.com). Drs. Becich and Friedman then co-founded the Association for Pathology Informatics (API) in 1999 (see http://www.pathologyinformatics.org). These two meetings have subsequently merged to form the Pathology Informatics Summit. These key events were the catalyst for the foundations of the discipline of Pathology Informatics. Many improvements in the modern CPLIS as well as the APLIS have

Table 13.2 Chronological timeline of efforts at coding system implementation

Year	Encoding/NLP event
1960s	IBM MT/ST typewriter to magnetic tape system
1960s	ICD-7 used to encode electronic data
1962	Lamson entered UNcoded full English text into magnetic tape file system
1963	Korein and Tick develop method to store dictated narrative text in variable length and variable field format
1964	Tatch in US Surgeon General's Office reports automatic coding of diagnoses by punching paper tape as a byproduct of the normal typing process for clinical record summary sheets
1966	Buck and Lindberg develop program to store coded data for pathology, notes, surgical operations, etc.
1968	ICDA is the coding basis for diagnostic, morbidity and mortality data
1968	Barnett develops manual coding system with predetermined branching structure and fixed vocabulary
1969	Pratt uses SNOP encoding of autopsy diagnoses
1970	Robinson uses IBM MT/ST to encode pathology reports
1970	Myers reports encoding of pathology reports using arbitrarily assigned numbers as a by-product of typing pathology reports
1980s	Demuth uses decision tree-based system to automate pathologists' reasoning and logic using simple queries and responses
1980s	Gabrieli et al. develop information system "Physician's Recrods and Knowledge Yielding Total Information for Consulting Electronically (PRAKTICE)" for NLP
1981	Hendrix described NLP and its various knowledge categories required
1985	Hammond and Stead report coding CP system terms in TMR system
1987	Obermeier defines NLP and parsing
1989	C. Bishop defines requirements for the ideal text coding system
1989	US HCFO begins to require that every physician's request for payment include an ICD-9-CM code

Table 13.3 Chronological timeline of efforts at retrieval of encoded text

Year	Encoding/NLP event
1966	Kent uses key-word-in-context to retrieve data
1970s (late)	Sager linguistic string project (automated language parsers) initiated
1975	Enlander reports computer program that searches for certain pre-established keywords based on SNOP code
1978	Yianilos uses pattern matching of word strings for retrieval
1981	Barnett develops Medical Query Language (MQL) to retrieve and analyze COSTAR ambulatory patient records

as their roots these early initiatives in biomedical informatics in the domain of Pathology which continue to have broad implications for the practice, research, and training of future generations of Pathology Informaticians. In 2010, API in coordination with Drs. Liron Pantanowitz and Anil Parwani (co-editors-in-chièf) launched the *Journal for Pathology Informatics* (JPI, see http://www.jpathinformatics.org). Over 200 manuscripts focused on Pathology Informatics, the CPLIS and the APLIS have been peer reviewed and published today. One of the most downloaded papers from JPI is by Park et al. [52] which describes the History of Pathology Informatics in the modern era and describes global as well as the US modern history. This manuscript is a nice adjunct to this early history, and its reading is encouraged.

In addition, there has been significant innovation in the United States in Pathology Informatics in the last three decades including the pathology informatics role in bioinformatics [4], imaging informatics including whole slide imaging [51, 72], molecular pathology informatics [28], telepathology [72], tissue banking informatics [4] as well as many of the more modern innovations to the LIS that have occurred since the pioneering work described by Dr. Collen For an in depth look at the current innovations going on in Pathology Informatics see the *Journal of Pathology Informatics* (http://www.jpathinformatics.org). An important example of this is Pathology Informatics' instrumental role and also the American Board of Pathology's joint sponsorship with the American Board of Preventative Medicine for the new Clinical Informatics board certification under the American Board of Medical Specialties [43]. The future of Pathology Informatics is extremely bright and we are grateful to Dr. Collen for so accurately reflecting its early history and foundations in biomedical informatics.

References

1. Adams LB. Three surveillance and query languages. MD Comput. 1986;3:11–9.
2. Barnett G, Greenes RA. Interface aspects of a hospital information system. Ann N Y Acad Sci. 1969;161:756–68.
3. Barnett GO, Greenes RA, Grossman JH. Computer processing of medical text information. Methods Inf Med. 1969;8:177–82.
4. Becich MJ. The role of the pathologist as tissue refiner and data miner: the impact of functional genomics on the modern pathology laboratory and the critical roles of pathology informatics and bioinformatics. Mol Diagn. 2000;5:287–99.
5. Bishop CW. A name is not enough. MD Comput. 1988;6:200–6.
6. Blois MS. Information and medicine: the nature of medical descriptions. Berkeley: University of California Press; 1984.
7. Buck CR J, Reese GR, Lindberg DA. A general technique for computer processing of coded patient diagnoses. Mo Med. 1966;63:276–9. passim.
8. Connelly DP, Gatewood LC, Chou DC. Computers in laboratory medicine and pathology. An educational program. Arch Pathol Lab Med. 1981;105:59.
9. Cote RA. Architecture of SNOMED: its contribution to medical language processing. Proc SCAMC. 1986; 74–84.
10. Cote RA. The SNOP-SNOMED concept: evolution towards a common medical nomenclature and classification. Pathologist. 1977;31:383.
11. Demuth AI. Automated ICD-9-CM coding: an inevitable trend to expert systems. Healthc Comput Commun. 1985;2:62.
12. Enlander D. Computer data processing of medical diagnoses in pathology. Am J Clin Pathol. 1975;63:538–44.
13. Farrington JF. CPT-4: a computerized system of terminology and coding. In: Emlet H, editor. Challenges and prospects for advanced medical systeams. Miami: Symposia Specialists; 1978. p. 147–50.

14. Feinstein AR. ICD, POR, and DRG: unsolved scientific problems in the nosology of clinical medicine. Arch Intern Med. 1988;148:2269–74.
15. Friedman BA. Informatics as a separate section within a department of pathology. Am J Clin Pathol. 1990;94(4 Suppl 1):S2–6.
16. Gabrieli ER. Computerizing text from office records. MD Comput. 1986;4:44–9.
17. Gabrieli ER. Automated processing of narrative medical text: a new tool for clinical drug studies. J Med Syst. 1989;13:95–102.
18. Gabrieli ER. A new electronic medical nomenclature. J Med Syst. 1989;13:355–73.
19. Gabrieli ER. The medicine-compatible computer: a challenge for medical informatics. Methods Inf Med. 1984;9:233–50.
20. Gantner GE. SNOMED: the systematized nomenclature of medicine as an ideal standardized language for computer applications in medical care. Proc SCAMC. 1980; 1224–6.
21. Gordon BL. Linguistics for medical records. In: Driggs MF, editor. Problem-directed and medical information systems. New York: Intercontinental Medical Book Corp; 1973. p. 5–13.
22. Gordon BL, Barclay WR, Rogers HC. Current medical information and terminology. Chicago: American Medical Association; 1971.
23. Gordon BL. Terminology and content of the medical record. Comput Biomed Res. 1970;3:436–44.
24. Gordon BL. Biomedical language and format for manual and computer applications. Methods Inf Med. 1968;7(1):5–7.
25. Gordon BL. Standard medical terminology. JAMA. 1965;191:311–3.
26. Graepel PH, Henson DE, Pratt AW. Comments on the use of the systematized nomenclature of pathology. Methods Inf Med. 1975;14:72–5.
27. Graepel PH. Manual and automatic indexing of the medical record: categorized nomenclature (SNOP) versus classification (ICD). Inform Health Soc Care. 1976;1:77–86.
28. Gullapalli RR, Desai KV, Santana-Santos L, Kant JA, Becich MJ. Next generation sequencing in clinical medicine: challenges and lessons for pathology and biomedical informatics. J Pathol Inform. 2012;3:40. doi:10.4103/2153-3539.
29. Hammond WE, Stead WW, Straube MJ. Planned networking for medical information systems. Proc SCAMC. 1985; 727–31.
30. Hammond WE, Stead WW, Straube MJ, Jelovsek FR. Functional characteristics of a computerized medical record. Methods Inf Med. 1980;19:157–62.
31. Hendrix GG, Sacerdoti ED. Natural language processing: the field in perspective. Byte. 1981;6:304–52.
32. Henkind SJ, Benis AM, Teichholz LE. Quantification as a means to increase the utility of nomenclature-classification systems. Proc MEDINFO. 1986; 858–61.
33. Humphreys BL, Lindberg D, D. Building the unified medical language system. Proc SCAMC 1989: 475-80.
34. Jacobs H. A natural language information retrieval system. Proc 8th IBM Medical Symp, Poughkeepsie. 1967; 47–56.
35. Jacobs H. A natural language information retrieval system. Methods Inf Med. 1968;7:8.
36. Kent A. Computers and biomedical information storage and retrieval. JAMA. 1966;196:927–32.
37. Korein J. The computerized medical record: the variable-field-length format system and its applications. Proc IFIPS TCH Conf. 1970: 259–91.
38. Korein J, Goodgold AL, Randt CT. Computer processing of medical data by variable-field-length format. JAMA. 1966;196:950–6.
39. Korein J, Tick LJ, Woodbury MA, Cady LD, Goodgold AL, Randt CT. Computer processing of medical data by variable-field-length format. JAMA. 1963;186:132–8.
40. Krieg AF, Henry JB, Stratakos SM. Analysis of clinical pathology data by means of a user-oriented on-line data system. In: Enslein K, editor. Data acquisition and processing in biology and medicine, Proc Rochester Conf, vol. 5. Oxford: Pergamon Press; 1968. p. 163–72.
41. Lamson BG. Methods for computer storage and retrieval of medical free text from the medical record. South Med Bull. 1969;57:33–8.

42. Lamson BG, Glinsky BC, Hawthorne GS, et al. Storage and retrieval of uncoded tissue pathology diagnoses in the original English free-text. Proc 7th IBM Med Symp. Poughkeepsie, NY; 1965: 411–26.
43. Lehmann CU, Shorte V, Gundlapalli AV. Clinical informatics sub-specialty board certification. Pediatr Rev. 2013;34:525–30.
44. Lindberg DA, Rowland LR, Buch WF. CONSIDER: a computer program for medical instruction. Proc 9th IBM Med Symp. Yorktown Heights; 1968: 59–61.
45. Lyman M, Sager N, Freidman C, Chi E. Computer-structured narrative in ambulatory care: its use in longitudinal review of clinical data. Proc SCAMC. 1985; 82–6.
46. McCray AT, Sponsler JL, Brylawski B, Browne AC. The role of lexical knowledge in biomedical text understanding. Proc SCAMC. 1987; 103–7.
47. Morgan MM, Beaman PD, Shusman DJ, Hupp JA, Zielstorff RD, Barnett GO. Medical Query Language. Proc SCAMC. 1981; 322–5.
48. Myers J, Gelblat M, Enterline HT. Automatic encoding of pathology data. Computer-readable surgical pathology data as a by-product of typed pathology reports. Arch Pathol. 1970;89:73.
49. Obermeier KK. Natural-language processing. Byte. 1987;12:225–32.
50. Okubo RS, Russell WS, Dimsdale B, Lamson BG. Natural language storage and retrieval of medical diagnostic information: experience at the UCLA Hospital and Clinics over a 10-year period. Comput Programs Biomed. 1975;5:105–30.
51. Pantanowitz L, Valenstein PN, Evans AJ, Kaplan KJ, Pfeifer JD, Wilbur DC, et al. Review of the current state of whole slide imaging in pathology. J Pathol Inform. 2011;2:36. doi:10.4103/2153-3539.
52. Park S, Parwani AV, Aller RD, Banach L, Becich MJ, Borkenfeld S, et al. The history of pathology informatics: a global perspective. J Pathol Inform. 2013;4:7. doi:10.4103/2153-3539.112689.
53. Pratt AW. Automatic processing of pathology data. Leaflet published by National Institutes of Health, Bethesda, Maryland 1971.
54. Pratt AW. Representation of medical language data utilizing the systemized nomenclature of pathology. In: Enlander D, editor. Computers in laboratory medicine. New York: Academic; 1975. p. 42–53.
55. Pratt AW. Medicine, computers, and linguistics. In: Brown J, Dickson JFB, editors. Biomedical engineering. New York: Academic; 1973. p. 97–140.
56. Pratt AW, Pacak M. Automatic processing of medical English. Preprint No. all, Classification:IR 3.4. Reprinted by USHEW, NIH; 1969a.
57. Pratt AW, Pacak M. Identification and transformation of terminal morphemes in medical English. Methods Inf Med. 1969;8:84–90.
58. Robinson RE. Acquisition and analysis of narrative medical record data. Comput Biomed Res. 1970;3:495–509.
59. Robinson RE. Surgical pathology information processing system. In: Coulson W, editor. Surgical pathology. Philadelphia: JB Lippincott; 1978. p. 1–20.
60. Robinson RE. Pathology subsystem. In: Collen M, editor. Hospital computer systems. New York: Wiley; 1974. p. 194–205.
61. Roper WL. From the health care financing administration. JAMA. 1989;261:1550.
62. Sager N, Tick L, Story G, Hirschman L. A codasyl-type schema for natural language medical records. Proc SCAMC. 1980; 1027–33.
63. Sager N, Friedman C, Chi E, Macleod C, Chen S, Johnson S. The analysis and processing of clinical narrative. Proc MEDINFO. 1986; 1101–5.
64. Sager N, Bross I, Story G, Bastedo P, Marsh E, Shedd D. Automatic encoding of clinical narrative. Comput Biol Med. 1982;12:43–56.
65. Sager N, Hirschman L, Lyman M. Computerized language processing for multiple use of narrative discharge summaries. Proc SCAMC. 1978; 330–43.
66. Smith J, Melton J. Automated retrieval of autopsy diagnoses by computer technique. Methods Inf Med. 1963;2:85–90.

67. Smith JC, Melton J. Manipulation of autopsy diagnoses by computer technique. JAMA. 1964;188:958–62.
68. SNOMED. Systematized nomenclature of medicine. Skokie: College of American Pathologists; 1977.
69. Storey G, Hirschman L. Data base design for natural language medical data. J Med Syst. 1982;6:77–88.
70. Tatch D. Automatic encoding of medical diagnoses. 6th IBM Medical Symposium, Poughkeepsie; 1964; 1–7.
71. Wells AH. The conversion of SNOP to the computer languages of medicine. Pathologists. 1971;25:371–8.
72. Williams S, Henricks WH, Becich MJ, Toscano M, Carter AB. Telepathology for patient care: what am I getting myself into? Adv Anat Pathol. 2010;17:130–49.
73. Yianilos PN, Harbort RA, Buss SR, Tuttle Jr EP. The application of a pattern matching algorithm to searching medical record text. Proc SCAMC. 1978; 308–13.

Chapter 14
Pharmacy Information (PHARM) Systems

Morris F. Collen and Stuart J. Nelson

Abstract Computer-based pharmacy (PHARM) systems have notably improved the quality and safety of medical care. By the 1980s automated ward-based medication cabinets were available to support drug administration and pharmacy management, overcoming problems encountered when drugs were stocked in nursing stations, administered to patients at different hospital locations, and recorded in different paper-based records. When the growing use of prescribed drugs in patient care resulted in an increasing number of adverse drug events (ADEs), PHARM systems were used together with computer-based physician order entry/results reporting systems (CPOE/RRs) systems to prevent and detect such events. With greater computer storage capabilities and much larger databases, PHARM systems were better able to discover and monitor ADEs in inpatient and outpatient care for prescription drugs and over-the-counter medications. With links to comprehensive patient data within a defined population database, they could calculate rates of diseases and rates of ADEs. Medication reconciliation and interoperability standards such as RxNorm and Health Level 7 messaging supported sharing information across institutions. User-centered design focused on making systems more effective and reducing alert fatigue. Pharmacogenomics is expected to influence medication therapy and improve the safety and effectiveness of prescribed drugs; the interactions which occur in polypharmacy will lead to fewer medication complications in the elderly; and better understanding of pharmacokinetics will lead to improved dosing and timing of medications.

Keywords Computer-based pharmacy systems • Drug administration • Pharmacy management • Adverse drug events • Medication reconciliation • Pharmacogenomics • Polypharmacy • RxNorm • Interoperability • Physician order entry

---

Sections of this chapter are reproduced from author Collen's earlier work *Computer Medical Databases*, Springer (2012).

Author was deceased at the time of publication.

M.F. Collen (deceased)

S.J. Nelson, M.D., FACP, FACMI (✉)
Health Sciences Library and Informatics Center, University of New Mexico,
Albuquerque, AZ, USA
e-mail: stuart.james.nelson@gmail.com

© Springer-Verlag London 2015
M.F. Collen, M.J. Ball (eds.), *The History of Medical Informatics in the United States*, Health Informatics, DOI 10.1007/978-1-4471-6732-7_14

611

Almost every visit to a physician by a patient results in an order, a re-order (refill), or a change in one or more prescribed drugs for the patient. Prior to computer-based patient records, at the end of an office visit, the physician usually gave the patient one or more paper-based prescriptions to take to a pharmacy. In a hospital visit, the physician entered orders for prescribed drugs on an order sheet in the patient's paper-based record. In both settings, it was time consuming for the physician if a review of the patient's record was needed.

With the advent of electronic patient records in hospital information systems (HISs) that had computerized provider order entry/results reporting (CPOE/RR) and a computer-based pharmacy information (PHARM) system, the order entry function in the HIS transmitted the prescriptions the physician ordered for a patient to the PHARM system; the PHARM system then generated and sent the list of prescriptions for the patient with orders for any alerts to the appropriate nursing station. When each prescribed medicine had been given to a hospital patient, nurses entered into the information system the date, time, dose, and the method of its administration. These systems greatly facilitated the process of providing and monitoring drug therapy; they also supported a high quality of patient care by advising guidelines for optimal drug therapy for each patient, and by alerting the health care providers of any potential adverse drug events (ADEs).

14.1 Requirements of a PHARM System

The primary functional requirements of a PHARM system were to improve the quality, safety, and efficiency of the drug-therapy process by providing accurate information for each drug, reducing errors in prescribing and administering drugs, providing alerts of any potential ADEs, and monitoring overall drug usage. According to Heller [81], a Director of the U.S. Pharmacopeia, a PHARM system was required to furnish alerts to medication orders that were outside the dosage ranges accepted for the prescribed drug; reject orders for a drug to be administered by an inappropriate route; provide alerts for possible drug-drug interactions, drug allergies, and known adverse drug effects on ordered laboratory tests; and give timely reminders when best to observe a patient's response to a prescribed drug.

Gouveia [68, 69] an associate in pharmacy at the Massachusetts General Hospital (MGH), defined the medication portion of a PHARM system as including the ordering, supplying, distributing, charting, controlling, and satisfying the legal and accounting requirements for dispensing medications; its objectives were to reduce medication errors, decrease nurses' record-keeping duties, and provide a comprehensive audit of drug therapy.

The medication process was expected to include planning the drug therapy, providing data on usual and optimal dosage of drugs by patient's age and gender, and calculating mixtures of intravenous solutions or of ingredients when ordered for parenteral feedings. It was also expected to include the indications for and contraindications against the use of a drug; any appropriate advice if better alternative therapy was available; alerts for potential ADEs such as from prescribing errors, drug-drug interactions, drug-laboratory-test interactions, drug allergies and toxic – effects. It was essential to document the drug therapy, evaluate the results of the therapy, and modify or terminate the drug therapy as indicated. Seed [179], at the Montefiore Medical Center in Bronx, New York, enumerated a detailed listing of objectives for computer-assisted writing of prescriptions that could grow into a full PHARM system.

A survey of hospital pharmacists listed the important functions of a PHARM system as including its ability to interface with the HIS and to provide 24-h a day service, drug-allergy alerts and intravenous solutions support, inventory control, and access to future enhancements [75]. Williams [223], at the University of Chicago Medical Center, identified basic management functions of a PHARM system that were readily computerized; these included prescription label production, drug billing and accounting, statistics and reporting, drug utilization and inventory control, and legal requirements. A PHARM system also needed to maintain a continuing database that could provide a patient's prior history for any drugs administered and any past ADE, and monitor the patient population for ADEs to help assure the quality and safety of drug therapy [3, 210].

Bootman [19] classified the main functions of a PHARM system as (1) dispensing functions that included preparing and printing of prescription labels, maintaining patient medication profiles, providing medication warning statements, monitoring and preparing refill prescriptions, maintaining formulary files; (2) clinical services functions that included contraindications to drugs, drug-drug interaction screening, drug-disease interaction monitoring, drug-allergy screening, patient compliance monitoring for over- and under-use, and printing of dispensed medication package inserts for patient education; (3) management and accounting activities that included sales analysis by product and manufacturer, inventory control for controlled and non-controlled substances, accounts receivable and payable, personnel records, and automatic production of periodic management reports; and (4) support for the pharmacist in providing an efficient, reliable, and professional practice for improved patient care.

Fritz [60] reported that some of the most comprehensive pharmacy systems at that time were developed around a unit-dose drug distribution concept that reduced drug errors and provided relatively strict drug control. In such a system each medication dose was individually packaged and labeled to retain its identity up to the time it was administered to the patient. Computer systems kept track of doses, drug inventory, accurate medication listings, and charges; the pharmacy system security was password-protected to restrict the type of activity permitted to a specific person and to allow individual transactions to be traced to that person.

Technical requirements of a PHARM system included its ability to operate as a standalone system or as a subsystem within a clinic, hospital, or a comprehensive MIS. Within an integrated comprehensive information system, its requirements were generally similar to those of other subsystems. Turner [213] described some specific programming requirements for a hospital PHARM system that included an accounting process not only for financial transactions, but also for every dispensed dose of a narcotic or controlled drug. A PHARM inventory program had to track thousands of different drugs, with their expiration dates and lot numbers, and drugs distributed from multiple vendors. In a PHARM system, automated printing of labels was a great time saver, especially in a hospital, where the time of administration might require the medication to be given as often as every few hours, and a patient might receive each day several different medications administered in different manners. Turner noted that an important requirement for a hospital PHARM system was the preparation of labels for the intravenous administrations of solutions that were frequently reconstituted. In an outpatient or hospital information system, a PHARM system needed to communicate closely with a CPOE/RR program.

Drug standards for medications, their names, terms, and codes are essential. Since 1820 the United States Pharmacopeia (USP) has set standards for drugs designed to meet the needs of both health professionals and the public. These standards related to preparation and purity of products. In 1961 the USP and the American Medical Association established the United States Adopted Name (USAN) program for giving unique nonproprietary names (commonly referred to as generic names) for pharmaceuticals. In 1980, the first edition of the USP Drug Index (USP-DI) became available in electronic form [225].

Provision of approved prescribing information was established by the Food and Drug Administration (FDA). Some of these drug labels were made available in the *Physicians' Desk Reference* (*PDR*), published annually by Thompson Health Care, Inc. in Montvale, New Jersey. Commonly used by medical practitioners, the PDR has been available on CD-ROM and via the Internet since the year 2000. The FDA established a structured product labeling (SPL) guideline for submission of proposed and publication of approved labels. In 2003, the FDA and the National Library of Medicine (NLM) developed a system for publishing the labels as they were approved and updated. The labels became freely available on the internet at a NLM website called DailyMed, with a mechanism for downloading electronic versions of SPLs.

Cimino [35] pointed out that the FDA's National Drug Codes (NDC) were assigned by individual drug suppliers, rather than by a central authority. The Health Level Seven (HL7) Vocabulary Technical Committee proposed using a group of terms as standards. Using the terms obtained from knowledge bases maintained by three leading vendors of pharmacy systems, the Committee found that their terms matched fairly well with samples of drug terms from several commercial products. The NLM and the Veterans Administration (VA) held an experiment with developing standard names for clinical drug products [156]. From this effort the NLM began a project known as *RxNorm*, which provided standard, normalized names for clinical drug products, defined as ingredient(s), strength(s), and dose form. Including in the information in their naming database were such things as the names used by commercial PHARM system vendors, the VA, and information, including National Drug Codes (NDCs), from the FDA [155].

Standardized technology of a PHARM subsystem was required so that it could be integrated with the clinical laboratory, radiology, pathology, and other information subsystems into a comprehensive MIS, with a common database that contained the patients' electronic health records. A PHARM system had to have the ability to be enhanced and expanded to accept new technology, as it did in the 1970s when medication orders began to be entered by light-pen selection from menu-driven computer display terminals, and again in the 1990s when CPOE became available in HISs and provided online alerts for possible drug-drug interactions [11].

14.2 Examples of Early PHARM Systems

Since 1966 the Mayo Clinic in Minnesota has administered its Rochester Epidemiology Program Project, containing the medical records of the population of most of the 90,000 residents of Olmstead County, for more than 40 years. Kurland and associates [109] at the Mayo Clinic, conducted a series of population-based, case-control, and cohort follow-up studies of the long-term effects of drug exposures. Their many published reports included studies of relationships between long-range drug therapy and subsequent development of cancers, and between drug therapy during pregnancy and subsequent congenital abnormalities of children.

Barnett and associates at the Massachusetts General Hospital (MGH) reported in 1966 that their computer-based programs at the hospital included recording of medication orders, automatic printing of up-to-date lists of prescribed drugs to be administered to patients, charting of medications given, and preparation of summaries of prior drug orders and drug administrations [5]. Additional PHARM system functions allowed the user to examine the medication formulary, and permitted the pharmacist to add new drug entities to the formulary file. When a drug was ordered for a patient, the system's drug ordering program automatically checked the patient's identification data and the spelling and dosage limits for the drug ordered; it listed all active medication orders for the patient, and provided important drug information that had been entered by the pharmacist into the hospital formulary. The online interactive system could check an order against the data in the patient's computer record for any likely drug-drug interactions, or for drug-laboratory test-value interactions, or for known allergic reactions to drugs. Barnett advocated that this information be given immediately to the physician at the time of the initial creation of the order, since after the responsible physician left the patient care unit a needed change in the medication order would be more time consuming [6]. At each patient care unit the MGH computer generated a list of medications to be administered every hour. It also listed laboratory test results, with weekly summaries organized in a format designed by the users to display tests in associated groups, such as serum electrolytes, hematology tests, and others.

The earliest computer used in their medication cycle was a Digital Equipment Corporation (DEC) PDP-1-d, with a UNIVAC drum memory, serving 64 input-output teletypewriter terminals [68, 69]. In 1974, Barnett's MUMPS-based PHARM system was implemented on a patient care unit of the MGH, using cathode-ray display entry terminals. Souder [203] reported the results of a 13-month evaluation comparing two patient care units, with similar patients as to their ages, length of hospital stay, and number of medications ordered. One used the new PHARM system; the other did not. The completeness, legibility, and clarity of the computer-based orders were judged significantly better, and provided better records than the manual orders of the control care unit. However, due to the slow response time, inadequate number of entry terminals, and other causes for the dissatisfaction of physician users, this medication system was terminated after 1 year of operation.

Since 1969 the Harvard Community Health Plan had used the Computer Stored Ambulatory Record (COSTAR) developed by Barnett [5]. Approximately 90 % of its patients received prescription drugs from their pharmacy. Since 1988 the pharmacy records were linked to the patients' COSTAR records. The Health Plan's PHARM system maintained the patients' medication records; from 1988 to 1992 their automated pharmacies dispensed 6.0 million prescriptions to 391,000 people. Members over 65 years of age were prescribed a median of seven different drugs per person. Physicians used two-part prescription forms; the top copy was given to the patient or sent directly to the pharmacy; the other copy was attached to the patient's visit encounter form, coded by the medical record department, and entered in the patient's computer-based record [162].

In 1994 Harvard Community Health Plan merged with Pilgrim Health Care and in 1998 joined with the Harvard Vanguard Medical Group. The largest inpatient facility for their hospitalized patients was Brigham and Women's Hospital in Boston, with 720 beds, where an internally developed HIS, the Brigham Integrated Computing System, that was built using Datatree MUMPS [199]. It had a patient database that already contained medical records for more than one million people, and a PHARM system that contained some pharmacy data since 1981 and some laboratory data since 1986 [99]. By 1998, as a result of these mergers, ambulatory patients with Harvard Community Health Plan could have their outpatient pharmacy data linked with their inpatient pharmacy data from their records with the Brigham and Women's Hospital [33].

In 1967 Maronde and associates [132, 134] at the University of Southern California School of Medicine and the Los Angeles County Hospital initiated a computer-based, drug dispensing system to process more than 600,000 outpatient prescriptions per year. The objectives for the system were to limit excess drug quantities specified in individual prescriptions, undesirably frequent prescriptions for the same drug, and inappropriate concurrent prescriptions for different drugs. Each prescription was entered into the system by a pharmacist who typed in the prescription using a computer terminal. The prescription labels were then printed by remote printers in the local pharmacies, with information as to medication refills, a summary of the patient's current medication history, and if there was any conflict or potential drug-drug interactions in medications prescribed by the various clinics.

They reported that of 52,733 consecutive prescriptions for the 78 drug products most frequently prescribed to outpatients by 870 different physicians representing more than 80 % of all outpatient prescriptions, 13 % were for excessive quantities of drugs, with some outpatients receiving as many as 54 prescriptions during a 112-day period; and there were numerous examples of concurrent prescriptions of two different drugs that could result in serious drug-drug interactions. They concluded that an adequate PHARM system with a CPOE/RR program could alert physicians to risks of possible ADEs and needless drug expenditures.

In 1969 an information system with centralized computer-based patient records for the nine Los Angeles County hospitals was initiated, using an IBM 360/40 computer connected by telephone cable to visual display terminals and to printers located initially in the admitting offices and pharmacies; the pilot testing was conducted by nurses for the order entry of medications, diets, and laboratory tests [26, 91, 132, 134, 175, 180]. In 1969 Jelliffe and associates at the University of Southern California School of Medicine also initiated at the Los Angeles County General Hospital a series of pharmacology programs to analyze dosage requirements for a variety of medications [92].

In 1967 Weed and associates at the University of Vermont College of Medicine in Burlington, initiated their Problem Oriented Medical Information System (PROMIS). It became operational in 1971 for a 20-bed gynecology ward at the University Hospital, with linkages to the pharmacy. By 1975 Weed's PROMIS included a Digiscribe touch-sensitive video terminal located in the pharmacy [48].

In 1968 Collen and associates at the Kaiser Permanente Northern California (KPNC) Region, began operating in their San Francisco medical center a prototype medical information system that included a PHARM subsystem. By 1973 the data from 1,200 prescriptions daily in the outpatient pharmacy were entered by pharmacists directly into the appropriate patients' computer-stored medical records by using online electric typewriters connected by telephone lines to the central computer, where the records resided in a direct-access mode. The prescription data included patient and physician identification, and the name, dose, and method of administration of each prescribed drug. For prescription refills, upon entering the prescription number, a new prescription label was printed and the cumulative number of prior dispensed prescriptions was automatically recorded [41]. Between 1969 and 1973 computer-stored records included 1.3 million prescriptions for more than 3,400 drug products dispensed to almost 150,000 patients; and an adverse drug reaction monitoring system was begun under a contract with the FDA. A region-wide pharmacy database was established in 1986; and in 1991 the KPNC program initiated a region-wide, Pharmacy Information Management System (PIMS) that by 1994 was operational in 108 pharmacies. By the year 2000 several pharmacoepidemiology research projects were being conducted.

In 1971 all KPNC patients' hospital and outpatient diagnoses began to be stored on computer tapes. By 1992 laboratory, pathology, and radiology diagnostic data, and by 1994 clinical data for outpatient visits were all being stored in computer databases. By the year 2000, computer-stored patient data were available for 2.8 million KP members [54, 55].

In 1969 Hammond and Stead, and their associates at Duke University, began to develop a minicomputer-supported outpatient information system (OIS). Data entry methods included interactive video terminals and batch-processed mark-sense forms. By 1975 their computer-stored patient records included medications [77, 222]. Prescriptions dispensed at a peripheral Duke clinic's pharmacy were entered into a Digital Equipment Corporation PDP 11/45 minicomputer using The Medical Record (TMR) system developed at Duke University. In a study reported by Gehlbach [65], the medication system provided feedback encouraging physicians to prescribe lower-cost generic drugs rather than brand-name drugs, thereby significantly increasing the use of generic drugs.

In 1970 Spencer and associates at the Texas Institute for Rehabilitation and Research (TIRRIS) in the Texas Medical Center initiated a medication scheduling program and a pharmacy inventory program that generated the charges for each drug and for all pharmacy charges within their HIS, which contained about 2,000 patient records.

In 1970 the Johns Hopkins University Hospital initiated a prototype PHARM system in a single, 31-bed, acute medical ward. It used an IBM 1620 computer that had been installed earlier to process physicians' written orders, to produce work lists for ward nurses, and to generate daily computer-printed, patient drug profiles [185]. Physicians wrote medication orders for hospital patients on order sheets coupled with carbon paper for copies that were then collected by pharmacy personnel and brought to a pharmacy, where the orders were entered into the system using a computer terminal, along with the identifying data for new patients as well as their known allergies. The system was used to evaluate their unit-dose medication system, and to monitor drug therapy for potential ADEs. They found that the system increased the nursing time available for direct patient care activities, and decreased errors in carrying out physicians' orders.

A detailed analysis of the operation resulted in a new set of requirements for an enhanced unit-dose system; and in May 1974 a new version of their PHARM system went into operation, using IBM 360–370 computers, and 3,278 cathode ray tube terminals with light-pen selectors for data input by a medical professional or a clerk located at the nursing stations or in the pharmacy. The system edited orders, rejected inappropriate drug doses or drug administration routes; and a pharmacist then reviewed the orders. The system printed unit-dose envelopes that contained the name and location of the patient, the time of the scheduled drug administration, the drug description, and any special instructions; after the envelopes were filled and checked, they were placed in a tray for delivery to the nursing station [197, 198].

In 1975 Simborg reported on version II of the hospital medication system, which had been upgraded with display terminals using keyboard and light-pen selection input [197]. Orders were entered by clerks and verified by pharmacists. This computer-based, unit-dose system was compared to the noncomputer-based, traditional multidose system on a similar size (30-bed) adult medical nursing unit at Johns Hopkins Hospital. In the traditional nursing unit, the error rate was 4.6 times greater (105 errors out of 1,428 doses compared to 20 errors out of 1,234 doses), and medication-related activities consumed more than twice as much registered nurses' time (39.9 % compared to 17.7 %). For 250 beds the total costs were 7 % higher using the computer unit-dose system; for 450 beds the total costs were 14 % lower using the computer system. The authors concluded that the computer-based, unit-dose system was more efficient than was the traditional multidose system; however, they made no statement about the added benefits to the unit-dose system alone, without adding the computer system.

Johns [98] repeated a cost evaluation of the unit-dose, drug-distribution system that was operational in 1978 at the Johns Hopkins Hospital, and found a similar decrease in the medication error rate with the unit-dose system. He also reported that the time spent by registered nurses on medication-related activities was reduced from 40 to 18 %. Although this 22 % reduction in nursing effort provided a potential cost savings, the reduction in nursing effort was not actually accompanied by a reduction in nurse staffing. As a consequence of the lack of a benefits-realization effort, the automated system cost $1.83 more per bed per day than the conventional system. Johns' conclusion was similar to that of many hospital administrators at that time: the failure to realize the potential savings these systems could provide had led to considerable skepticism about such claims in hospital management circles.

In 1979 the PHARM system at the Oncology Center, originally one of three satellites of the central unit-dose PHARM system for the Johns Hopkins Hospital, became a standalone PHARM system; data from inpatient medication profiles and from outpatient clinical notes were manually extracted and entered by clinical data coordinators in the Oncology Center. However, because of the manual work involved only a limited set of drugs were recorded and data accuracy was difficult to achieve.

In 1984 an independent, standalone, outpatient prescription system was purchased, and the PHARM system was fully integrated with the Oncology Center's clinical information system. It provided computerization of medication records, prescription label generation, formulary updates, billing, and statistical data. In addition, clinical interfacing with the PHARM system permitted review of the appropriateness of the drug therapy based on clinical diagnoses that the pharmacist could independently access from any computer terminal in the clinic or pharmacy areas [79].

In 1971 the Yale-New Haven Hospital in Connecticut implemented a computer-based formulary service that contained a listing of all dosage forms of each drug used in the hospital, with cross-index listings of common synonyms and proprietary names. Since only formulary drugs were maintained in the hospital, the result was that approximately one-half of the drugs and dosage forms that previously were used at the hospital were eliminated. A Formulary Catalog was published periodically listing newly added drugs. In 1972 a Connecticut Regional Drug Information Service was established to assist participating hospitals in the development of viable formulary systems, and two-thirds of the hospitals in the state participated in a shared formulary service that contained all drugs and dosage forms on the formulary of any participating hospital. One of the hospitals used a computer with punched card input to prepare and print the distributed formulary [124].

In 1971 the El Camino Hospital in Mountain View, California, initiated installation of the Technicon Medical Information System (MIS) [61, 62, 186]. The hospital information system employed an IBM 370/155 time-shared computer located in Technicon's Mountain View offices. By 1973 the Technicon MIS had installed terminals throughout the hospital's clinical services [27]. The terminal's display screen was used to present lists of items, including the various orders for prescribed medications. A specific medication item was selected by pointing the terminal's light-pen selector at the desired word or phrase on the display, and then pressing a switch on the barrel of the pen. The Technicon MIS was one of the first systems designed to allow the physicians themselves to enter orders and review the results [16]. The computer stored the orders and sent appropriate drug requisitions to the pharmacy. Computer-produced printouts also included medication time-due lists [7]. The pharmacy received all drug orders as they were entered into the system, printed dispensing labels that included known drug allergies, and provided daily drug profiles of all medications being taken by each patient.

In 1972 Platiau and associates at the Rhode Island Hospital in Providence [161] described their PHARM system that used punch cards for servicing more than 30 cost centers in the hospital pharmacy. Each cost center had a data file of all pharmacy items it received, including its fiscal history, unit cost, unit of issue, dosage form, and package size; an item file containing a full English description of each drug; and a master work sheet that contained a list of all items distributed to the patient care area. The list was generated by selecting the appropriate pre-punched card that indicated the drug description and drug code, the patient's identification, the date, the cost center, and the sequence number of the request [161]. Periodic reports were produced that included the activity of each item distributed to each patient care area, compiled by drug-category for each item (unit cost, unit of issue, dosage form), and the totals for all care areas combined. The final report generated was the inventory-release form showing the total dollar value charged to each cost center; a punched card with this information was produced for input to the hospital's general ledger system. This system resulted in a 50 % reduction in the accounting department's workload for processing pharmacy transactions [161].

In 1972 the VA began developing in its Southern California facilities a PHARM system for processing information on patients, prescriptions, and management information, called APPLES (Automated Prescription Processing, Labeling and Editing System). In 1974 the VA expanded the APPLES PHARM system to process more prescriptions per day by using visual-display terminals and printers installed in eight pharmacies and connected by a network to a computer center located 125 miles away [88]. By the early 1990s, the VA had implemented its Decentralized Hospital Computer Program (DHCP) in each of its 170 medical centers, which included a PHARM system in addition to LAB and RAD systems [99]. Graber and associates [70] at the VA Hospital and Vanderbilt University in Nashville, Tennessee, extracted prescription and clinical laboratory data from the VA-DHCP patient database, and established a separate drug use database to monitor patient laboratory data during drug therapy in addition to drug utilization.

In 1972 the National Institutes of Health (NIH) implemented the PROPHET System, a time-shared system using a DEC PDP-10 computer, accessible remotely by graphics-display terminals communicating over dedicated voice-grade telephone lines, connected to 13 academic centers in the United States. The system supported research promoting the emergence of a predictive science regarding drugs and drug-related phenomena. NIH offered biomedical scientists throughout the nation an opportunity to evaluate computer-based information-handling methods in searching for chemical-biological relationships [168]. Rubin [174], at Bolt, Beranek and Newman, described the PROPHET system as a specialized computer resource developed by NIH to aid scientists who studied the mechanisms of drug actions and other chemical/biological interrelationships. The system could be used to analyze data using its graphing and statistics commands, and by manipulating models of molecular structures. A users group of pharmacology-related scientists selected statistical tools and developed algorithms that best fitted their needs.

In 1972 McDonald and associates at the Regenstrief Institute for Health Care and the Indiana University School of Medicine began to develop the Regenstrief Medical Record System (RMRS) for the care of ambulatory patients. In 1976 they initiated a PHARM system when a group of their patient care clinics was moved from the Wishard Memorial Hospital into a new building; prescription information was captured from both the hospital and the outpatient pharmacy systems. Their new pharmacy was staffed by seven pharmacists and processed up to 1,200 prescriptions a day. A drug distribution system was implemented that used automated aids for the prescription filling and dispensing processes [139].

The Regenstrief PHARM system was initially serviced by a minicomputer located in the Regenstrief Health Center Building. It employed a set of table-driven computer programs written in the BASIC-PLUS language; the database managed the tables that contained the formulary and prescription information, and the patients' medication profiles. The RMRS database files also included their pharmacy system. The patients' current prescriptions were listed at the bottom of an encounter form in a medication profile. The physician refilled or discontinued these drugs by writing "R" or "D/C" next to them, and wrote new prescriptions underneath this list. The patients took a carbon copy of this section of the encounter form to the pharmacy as their prescriptions. Data, recorded by physicians on the encounter forms, were entered into the computer by clerks. An ambulatory patient's prescription was entered using a computer terminal; and the patient's identification, the medication's strength and dosage were checked, the patient's medication record was reviewed for possible drug-drug interactions, and the prescription labels were printed. If the patient had a computer-based medical record, then the prescriptions were also printed on the paper encounter forms. Their PHARM system also provided all of the required pharmacy inventory, management, and accounting functions [31]. After implementing the PHARM system in the outpatient pharmacy of the Regenstrief Health Center, that processed up to 1,500 prescriptions each day and where physicians entered their prescriptions directly into microcomputer work stations, it was found that pharmacists spent 12.9 % more time correcting prescription problems, spent 34 % less time filling prescriptions, 46 % more time in problem-solving activities involving prescriptions, and 3.4 % less time providing advice [135]. It concluded that computer-based prescribing resulted in major changes in the type of work done by hospital-based outpatient pharmacists.

McDonald [141] reported that the RMRS still used paper reports rather than visual displays as its primary mechanism for transmitting information to the physician; this mode of output was preferred since it was cheap, portable, easier to browse, and paper reports could be annotated with paper and pencil. However, Murray [150] described the prior writing of paper prescriptions as a somewhat painful prescribing medium for pharmacists, patients, and especially for physicians who needed to recall which medication and dosage for more than 20,000 products, and then write each legible prescription. McDonald [136] also instituted computer-generated suggestions for the treatment of some common medical conditions in an attempt to reduce medication errors. Pharmacy prescription information was captured from both the hospital and outpatient pharmacy systems. For each patient's return visit a patient summary report was generated which included medication and treatment information in a modified flow sheet format [141]. In the early 1980s the RMRS shared a DEC VAX 11/780 computer with the pharmacy and other sub-systems; and used microcomputer-based workstations to display forms, in which the user could enter data using a mouse to select data from menus [140]. By the mid-1980s the RMRS's computer-based patient records contained medication data that were entered automatically from the pharmacy systems [140].

In 1988 the RMRS was also linked to the pharmacies within the local VA and University hospitals. By the end of the 1990s the RMRS served a large network of hospitals and clinics [137, 138]. In 1994 the Regenstrief Medical Record System (RMRS) contained in its database more than 750,000 patients from the Wishard Memorial Hospital, Indiana University Hospital, the Roudebush VA Hospital, and other sites linked to Indiana University in Indianapolis; it accounted for more than 700,000 outpatient visits per year [99].

In 1973 Blois and associates at the University of California San Francisco Medical Center initiated the pharmacy module of their HIS that was operational with eight cathode ray tube (CRT) terminals and assorted printers connected to their central Four-Phase Systems of minicomputers, using their own-developed operating system and applications software. It generated a drug list for each hospital patient, automatically captured drug billing items, printed the medication schedules for the nursing services, provided a database to support a warning system for drug allergies and drug-drug interactions, and maintained the pharmacy inventory [15].

In 1974 the Tri-Service Medical Information System (TRIMIS) of the Department of Defense (DoD) was initiated for all of the inpatients and outpatients of the medical facilities of the United States armed services. In 1977 TRIMIS selected the Naval Regional Medical Center in Charleston, South Carolina, as the test and evaluation site for its PHARM system, beginning with the outpatient pharmacies and then adding the inpatient pharmacies in September 1978 [212]. This pilot test used a time-sharing Data General minicomputer located in Atlanta, Georgia; the system was tested and became operational in 5 days.

Subsequently, the TRIMIS Initial Operating Capability PHARM systems were installed at the US Air Force Regional Hospital in Carswell AFB, Texas; at the Watson Army Community Hospital at Fort Dix, New Jersey; and at the Naval Regional Medical Center Portsmouth, Virginia [4, 152, 153]. The fully operational TRIMIS PHARM system provided order entry specifications for identifying authorized health care providers and eligible patients. It provided patients' prescription drug profiles, reviews for drug sensitivities and for potential drug-drug interactions, retrieval of clinical drug information, displays for requesting new and refill prescriptions, the ability to modify, cancel, or reorder existing pharmacy prescriptions, and to chart and report medications administration. The system also supported pharmacists' work functions by preparing lists for filing, labeling and dispensing medications. It maintained records of all prescriptions ordered for each patient; and displayed, when requested, an inpatient's laboratory test results, medication data, and dietary orders. In addition, the system provided management functions that included stock inventories, any required reports for controlled substances (narcotic drugs); it maintained a drug formulary, and supported an appropriate level of system security and patient data confidentiality [14, 154, 211]. A cost-benefit analysis of implementing and operating a TRIMIS PHARM system as compared to the traditional manual system operating in a generic Military Treatment Facility, including personnel, supplies, inventory, automated PHARM system services and maintenance, concluded that the automated PHARM system was the more effective method [130].

In 1974 the Appalachian Regional Hospitals health care system, that included ten community hospitals and several primary care centers, established at its central site in Lexington, Kentucky, its Computerized Pharmaceutical Services Support System (CPSSS) that was written in house in COBOL language. It used a Univac 9480 central processing unit with associated disc and tape drives; and with privately leased phone lines, it provided online services to its various pharmacies. Specially trained, non-pharmacist, computer terminal operators entered all required prescriptions and patient related data; prescription labels were automatically printed, with dosage instructions; and a pharmacist reviewed the patient's profile for potential ADEs. The system maintained its various needed files in its computer database. By the end of 1975, they dispensed about 1,300 prescriptions per day, and the database maintained records on approximately 40,000 ambulatory patients [220].

In 1976 Lassek and associates [110] at the Johns Hopkins University reported the establishment of the Public Health Service Ambulatory Care Data System designed for the use in their national system of 8 hospitals and 26 outpatient clinics. In addition to coded clinical data, dispensed drugs were coded by pharmacists using a three-digit number derived from the coding system used in the American Pharmaceutical Association Directory. The early use of the system reported studies of medication use by diagnoses and by physicians.

Since 1977 Group Health Cooperative of Puget Sound, a health maintenance organization, maintained a computer-based record for every prescription drug and over-the-counter medicine dispensed by its outpatient pharmacies, and since 1989 for its dispensed inpatient prescription drugs. In 1986 it added its patients' laboratory and radiology data to its database. A computer-based record was created for every medication at the time the prescription was filled; and the record contained selected information about the patient, the prescriber, and the prescription. The pharmacy database was frequently used for postmarketing drug surveillance and for pharmacoepidemiology studies [178].

Since 1977 the Beth Israel Hospital in Boston, with 452 beds, had maintained a patients' computer-stored database using a network of Data General computers, and had a PHARM system since 1979 with six cathode ray tube terminals and two printers in the pharmacy. Pharmacists entered information in response to a series of displayed prompts indicating the medication, dosage, disposing form, time and method of administration, and other needed data. It provided 24-h inpatient services that included unit-dose medications, and mechanisms for dispensing intravenous mixtures of solutions and parenteral solutions for nutrition. In addition it processed approximately 40,000 outpatient prescriptions and refills per year [164]. By 1988, they had increased to 504 beds, and had more than 800,000 electronic records that included inpatient and outpatient pharmacy and laboratory data. They used ClinQuery to access their patient data [99].

A review of computer applications in hospital pharmacies prior to 1975 was made by Knight [103] and Conrad. Most of the earliest computer applications in pharmacies used punch cards for establishing medication files and drug formularies. In a comprehensive literature review of computer applications in institutional pharmacies from 1975 to 1981, Burleson [28] described the introduction of automated medication distribution systems that provided pharmacists access to online computer systems programmed to help calculate the amounts of drugs to add to complex intravenous solutions; and of the various ingredients for parenteral nutrition solutions; and how to facilitate the online use of computer databases, including the NLM's MEDLINE. Braunstein [21]), of National Data Corporation in Charleston, South Carolina, estimated that in 1982 computer technology was used in about 75 % of pharmacies providing services to nursing homes, in 20 % of pharmacies providing outpatient services, and in 10 % providing services in hospitals. A 1982 national survey reported by Stolar [208] found that 17.6 % of hospital-based pharmacies had PHARM systems (almost double the number reported in 1978); with about 70 % that functioned as a part of a HIS, and 30 % operated as standalone PHARM systems.

In 1982 the University of Minnesota Hospitals, Department of Pharmaceutical Services, mailed a questionnaire survey to vendors of commercial PHARM systems; 30 companies responded that they marketed a hospital pharmacy system, 20 reported they had done so for 2 years or longer; and 16 claimed to have contracts with more than 20 health care institutions. The majority of companies reported they provided a database, and screened for duplicate ordering of a same drug, some type of automated drug-interaction screening, accounting of controlled substances, some inpatient dispensing functions, and management and inventory functions [209].

Brown [24] reported using, in a dermatologist's office, a 16-bit microcomputer with video terminals and keyboard to write drug prescriptions and patient instructions. Drug dosages, directions, and labeling phrases were retrieved from a diagnosis-oriented formulary of 300 drug products. Therapy summaries were automatically composed and printed for the paper-based medical records.

Ricks [170] described a commercial medication computer system developed by Datacare, Inc., as a part of its evolving hospital information system, that employed IBM computers installed for a group of three hospitals operated by the Fairfax Hospital Association in Falls Church, Virginia. The Fairfax Hospital included 656 acute care beds; and its pharmacy department was staffed by 16 full-time pharmacists that filled more than one million medication orders per year. A computer-based, unit-dose medication system became the core of its evolving PHARM system to improve the quality and efficiency of its drug distribution and record keeping.

Siegel reported a study of the Drug Exception Reporting System (DERS), a commercial drug prescription monitoring system used in conjunction with their computerized drug ordering PHARM system, in 40 New York State mental health facilities. Every time an order involving a drug was given or discontinued, a prescription was completed and served as the data entry instrument to their PHARM system. DERS reviewed every drug order against a set of guidelines for prescribing; and it flagged and produced a listing of all drug orders for which there was an exception to an established guideline. In a study period of the prescribing habits of clinicians in six psychiatric centers, for periods from 6 to 18 months, they reported that their system significantly reduced the number of drug orders written in exception to the guidelines; and that physicians' acceptance of the system was high. Siegel [195, 196] also reported a later study conducted in 11 psychiatric facilities of the drug ordering practices of 73 clinicians with similar demographics; and they compared 31 clinicians who used only the drug ordering system with 42 clinicians who used both the drug ordering system and the DERS monitoring system. They concluded that the added monitoring system improved prescribing practices of physicians and increased their knowledge of pharmacotherapy. Although 75 % of physicians felt the guidelines should be monitored, only 12 % felt the challenge to physicians' autonomy to be beneficial; and over half reported that when they received exception reports that their most common response was to justify an exception. It was concluded that attention to some human factors' components might help to alleviate some negativism among physicians.

Anderson and associates [3] at the University of Nebraska College of Pharmacy in Omaha, described using an Apple II+ microcomputer to manage their records of controlled substances and also to manage financial and personnel information for their University Hospital pharmacy department.

In a series of articles published in 1984 that reported on the use of microcomputers for specialized pharmacy applications, Turner [213] described how a microcomputer in the Department of Defense TRIMIS PHARM subsystem was used for information processing of intravenous solutions that required multiple programming modules for the various involved functions; such as making appropriate calculations during the formulation and preparation of intravenous solutions, and for performing pharmacokinetic calculations for tailoring doses of the medications that varied with the patient's age, gender, weight and height; combined with the characteristics of the drug such as its half-life, elimination rate, its initial dose, and its maintenance doses to be given at specified time intervals.

Honigman and associates [84] at the Denver General Hospital used the commercially available MICROMEDEX Clinical Information System, which included the DRUGDEX system that was developed at the University of Colorado Medical Center. It provided information concerning drug therapy, dosage, usage, contraindications, drug interactions, and adverse effects.

Fireworker and associates [53] at the hospital pharmacy in the 350-bed hospital of St. John's University in Jamaica, New York, reported a modular installation of their PHARM system using a microcomputer with a floppy disk drive for each of four modules (controlled substances, investigational drugs, intravenous medications, and inventory control), all connected to a common, hard disk storage device. The multi-computer system was developed to provide a higher level of reliability, and to separate the PHARM subsystem from the rest of the hospital information system.

In 1985 a published review of commercially available pharmacy computer systems listed 29 vendors, the great majority of which provided either standalone or integrated systems with drug-drug interaction programs; six of these were listed as having more than 100 installations [125]. A published review by Raymond [169] listed a total of 52 commercial computer-based PHARM systems; a few reported having more than 1,000 systems installed in 1986, and the majority provided drug interaction functions.

Mackintosh [128] described the microcomputer-based PHARM system they obtained for correctional facilities in Falls Church, Virginia; and that they had obtained by mail order directly from the vendor, a commercial EX/2 RX System from Signature Software Systems for less than $500. The system satisfied their functional requirements. Outpatient medical care was provided 24-h a day to 8,000 residents. Since most of the residents were young and not taking many medications, ADEs were not as prevalent as in the average community pharmacy; although clinical factors, such as diabetes and allergies, would be noted in a patient's profile. Medications were dispensed repeatedly in small doses to the same patients. The system did not need any billing and accounting functions at the correctional facilities.

A review of the diffusion of the major vendors of PHARM systems during the past few decades reveals interesting details. In the 1970s the major vendors were Becton Dickenson, IBM, and Shared Medical Systems. By the 1990s the importance of computerized drug information systems began to be widely recognized, yet pharmacists still felt more strongly than physicians and nurses that such systems would readily fit into their daily work routines [194]. Humphrey [87] reported that the St. Jude Children's Hospital in Memphis, Tennessee, replaced their system developed in-house with Cerner's PharmNet system interfaced to Cerner's clinical systems, linking to the laboratory system to monitor for drug-lab interferences in addition to the usual other PHARM system functions. In a 1995 published review, 23 vendors were listed as having more than 100 installations of their pharmacy systems; 5 of these were listed as having more than 1,000 installations [44]. A later study of community pharmacists, university pharmacists, and pharmacy students found them to be generally positive about the computer systems, the accuracy of online information services, and their usefulness for pharmacists [193]. In the 1990s several vendors provided decentralized, full-dose medication dispensing systems that allowed barcode scanning of medications and of patients' wrist bands, all integrated with the patient's drug profile via interfaces to a hospital's centralized PHARM system [129, 157].

In a study of the accuracy of medication records stored in electronic patient records of an outpatient geriatric center of the University of Pittsburgh School of

Medicine, Wagner and Hogan [217] found that 83 % represented correctly the drug, dose, and schedule of the current medication. The most frequent cause of errors was the patient misrepresenting a change in medication. The failure to capture drugs ordered by outside physicians accounted for 26 % of errors; transcription errors were relatively uncommon.

By the year 2000 the prescribing functions of a PHARM system could be fulfilled by using a small, pocket-size, portable handheld device, containing stored-programs that could display on its screen the relevant drug formulary information and potential drug-drug interactions; and that communicated wirelessly with a central PHARM system that could automate the process of ordering prescribed drugs, screen for drug-drug interactions, display the patient's insurance coverage, display drug charges, and print the prescription at a local pharmacy of the patient's choice [219].

14.3   Identification, Surveillance, and Prevention of Adverse Drug Events

Identification and surveillance of ADEs are primarily the responsibility of the U.S. Food and Drug Administration (FDA), whereas real-time monitoring for ADEs during active patient care is primarily the responsibility of the health care provider. The frequent occurrence of undesirable effects of drugs on patients has always been an important threat to their health and is a substantial burden to medical practice. With the general increase in the age of patients and with the introduction in each decade of new drugs, the risks of ADEs have increased. Ruskin [176], a former director of the Adverse Reactions Task Force of the FDA, defined an ADE as a substantiated noxious pathologic and unintended change in the structure (signs), function (symptoms), and chemistry (laboratory data) of a patient that was not a part of the disease; and was linked with any drug used in the prophylaxis, diagnosis, or therapy of disease, or for the modification of the physiologic state of a patient. Karch [100] defined an adverse drug reaction (ADR) as any response to a drug that was noxious and unintended, such as a toxic or side effect of a drug, a drug allergy, or an undesired drug-drug interaction; and that occurred at customary doses used in patients for prophylaxis, diagnosis, or therapy. The more general term, adverse drug events (ADEs), includes adverse drug reactions, errors of drug dosage and administration, uses of a drug for therapy despite its contra-indications, adverse drug effects on laboratory tests, and any other undesired effects of a drug on a patient; and the term generally excluded therapeutic failures, poisonings, and intentional overdoses. The FDA considers an ADE to be a serious one if it resulted in hospitalization, in a prolongation of hospitalization, in a persistent or significant disability, or in death.

In the 1950s the FDA and the American Medical Association (AMA) began to collect voluntary reports on ADEs, and the FDA established *ADE registries* for the voluntary reports from physicians and hospitals of suspected ADEs. In the 1960s the FDA began a continuous surveillance of ADEs; in 1965 it initiated its computerized

Spontaneous Reporting System (SRS) [131]. Kerr [102] estimated that, in the 1 year of 1988, about 55,000 ADEs were filed with the FDA. DuMouchel [47] at AT&T Labs used the FDA's Spontaneous Reporting System (SRS) database, and described it to be a computerized database of adverse drug reactions that were primarily reported by health professionals to search for ADEs that were unusually frequent. By the 1990s the SRS contained more than one million reports, with the earliest dating back to 1969, all collected after the marketing of the drugs. DuMouchel emphasized that the full value of this warning system was not realized because of the difficulty in interpreting its reported frequencies, since the FDA's SRS did not allow calculations of incidence rates or dose-response curves for the combination of a given drug and its ADEs, as such a rate would require an appropriate denominator with which to report the frequency of the reported drug-ADE combination. He used a modified Bayesian approach with an internally derived-baseline frequency as the denominator for calculating rates for drug-event combinations; and then compared the reported frequency of a drug-event combination to the internally derived baseline frequency to compute a relative-risk measure for the ADE. He pointed out that this method of screening for ADEs in the SRS did nothing to minimize reporting bias; he advocated appropriate epidemiological studies before making any final decisions on any ADE rate.

In the 1960s Visconti [216] noted that about 5 % of hospital admissions were reported to be due to ADEs. The 1962 Kefauver-Harris amendments to the Food, Drug and Cosmetic Act began to require pharmaceutical firms to report to the FDA all ADEs encountered in premarketing clinical trials of their drugs under investigations. In 1962 the World Health Organization (WHO) initiated an international program for the promotion of the safety and efficacy of drugs that led to the implementation of the WHO Pilot Research Project for International Drug Monitoring. In 1968 the WHO International Drug Monitoring Project moved to Alexandria, Virginia, where its International Drug Surveillance Center evaluated voluntary reporting systems for ADEs, and developed a drug dictionary and a cross-reference system between drug names. In 1971 this Center moved to WHO Headquarters in Geneva [82]. In 1972 the WHO reported that the frequency of adverse reactions in seven hospitals in the United States and Canada ranged from 10 to 18 % [173]. In 1992 the Prescription Drug User Fee Act (PDUFA) was passed providing FDA with fees from manufacturers submitting a new drug application (NDA), and financing additional reviewers to expedite the processing of new drugs.

Cuddihy [42] at Sandoz Pharmaceutical reported using a commercially available program, General Retrieval System from Information Science, Inc. of New York that provided the monitoring, search, and retrieval capabilities needed for the management and reporting of ADEs. Due to the increasing complexity of satisfying FDA requirements, by 1977 Sandoz had installed an IBM 360/65 system, and was using a more sophisticated data management system [221]. Windsor [224] of Norwich Pharmaceutical Company, reported that in the 1 year of 1972, at least 1,968 articles in the medical literature reported ADEs.

Caranasos and associates [30] at the University of Florida reported that in a series of 7,423 medical inpatients, 12.5 % had at least one ADE; and 16 patients

(0.22 %) died of drug-associated causes, of which 11 had been seriously or terminally ill before the fatal drug reaction occurred. Porter [163] reported that for 26,462 medical inpatients in collaborating hospitals from seven countries 24 (0.09 %) were considered to have died as a result of ADEs from one or more drugs; this drug induced death rate was slightly less than 1-per-1,000, and was a rate considered to be consistent in the collaborating hospitals. Most who died were very ill prior to the event, and over half had cancer or alcoholic liver disease.

In 1991 a survey conducted of 1,100 clinical pharmacists in 500 hospitals in the United States and Canada that were enrolled in the Drug Surveillance Network to perform post-marketing surveillance of drugs found that more than 85 % had PHARM systems and had implemented spontaneous reporting systems for the identification of ADEs. Since the drug information was volunteered, it generally failed to identify many ADEs; and it did not provide adequate data to quantify the relationships between drug therapy and drug toxicity, or of the incidence rates of ADEs [73].

In 1993 an international multidisciplinary conference was held to develop standardized terms to facilitate international drug surveillance. The conference recommended that a dictionary of clinical data be collected for drug surveillance and for pharmacoepidemiology research; and a minimum drug-therapy data-set be collected for patients before and during their hospitalization [108]. In 1993 the FDA established MEDWATCH, a voluntary Medical Products Reporting Program for health professionals to notify FDA of any adverse events from the use of medical products. In November 1997 the FDA initiated its Adverse Event Reporting System (AERS) designed as a pharmacosurveillance tool. AERS used *MeDDRA* (Medical Dictionary for Drug Regularity Affairs) as its primary tool to classify and search for medically significant adverse events. AERS had the capability to receive electronic submissions of ADEs, and to provide automatic signal-generation capabilities, and improved tools for the analysis of potential adverse event signals. By the year 2000 AERS contained almost two million reports since 1969 [101].

Premarketing drug testing is conducted before a new drug is marketed in the United States for its efficacy and safety. Carson [32] reviewed the process of testing drugs by the FDA prior to their approval for marketing; and advised that the background risk of an ADE was considered to be high if it occurred in greater than one per 200 cases per year; and it was considered to be low if it occurred in less than 1 per 10,000 cases per year; and intermediate if the rate of an ADE was in between these values.

In the premarketing phases of a drug evaluation, clinical trials are often limited by the relatively small numbers of selected patients studied and the short time period over which the patients are observed; so that even when clinical trials are conducted with large enough numbers to detect events that occur relatively frequently, they do not always identify rare ADEs. Randomized controlled clinical trials have been generally accepted as the best methods for evaluating the efficacy and safety of a drug, and most pre-market drug testing uses this method. Patients included in pre-approval clinical trials were typically well monitored for concomitant drug use, and were closely followed for early signs of adverse events; in contrast to post-marketing studies where patients could have multiple diseases, and could take multiple prescription drugs in addition to over the counter medications. The strength of randomized clinical trials is that randomization is more likely to distribute the levels of unanticipated confounding variables more evenly in the control and intervention groups, making it less likely that confounding rather than intervention is responsible for the effects found in the analysis of the data. An alternative to randomization is to perform a time-series trial in which the drug intervention is turned on and off multiple times, and this has the advantage of controlling for underlying secular trends [171].

Canfield and associates [29] at the University of Maryland described the complex FDA drug application process that drug developers and manufacturers had to follow to request approval of a drug product, and how the process required much inter-organizational data flow. They developed new software for the FDA's generic drug application process that produced a more scalable and flexible architecture that could be generalized to other contexts in inter-organizational, health care information systems. They reported that 3 years of experience with the new system showed an improvement over the prior system. Guess [76] at Merck Research Laboratories wrote of the difficulties of studying drug safety prior to marketing when relevant studies were often unpublished; and described some of the criteria used to relate adverse experiences in premarketing clinical trials, that studied the relative risk of users of the drug compared to non-users. The consistency of the reports from multiple clinical trials of the drug, and the time interval between the drug administration and the occurrence of the ADE were found to be helpful.

The identification and quantification of potentially important risks have generally been conducted in postmarketing evaluation of intended beneficial effects of drugs, and also of unintended and undesired effects of the drugs. Post-marketing strategies for the detection, surveillance, and the online monitoring of known ADEs, and for the discovery of previously unknown ADEs, are conducted indefinitely at some level after the marketing of a new drug; and a variety of post-marketing strategies have been reported. The identification and quantification of potentially important risks of ADEs are conducted in the post-marketing evaluation of the intended beneficial effects of drugs, and of the unintended and undesired effects of the drugs. In addition, the effects of concomitantly administered drugs and of patients' associated diseases are generally not fully explored prior to marketing, and are usually conducted as a part of post-marketing drug surveillance. As a result ADEs are usually identified by post-marketing clinical observations of a series of treated patients [207]. Lesko [115] also emphasized the differences between premarketing drug studies that involve a few thousand individuals; and post-marketing surveillance cohort studies that involve tens of thousands of exposed individuals in order to be able to reliably detect rare ADEs. He asserted that randomized controlled clinical trials were generally accepted as the best methods to study the safety and efficacy of drugs.

Strom [206, 207] described the requirements of large electronic bases for ADE surveillance. The requirements were to contain records of a large enough population to discover rare events for the drugs in question, to include inpatient and outpatient care with each patient's data linked with a unique identifier, to include all laboratory tests, radiology and other procedures, and to have all prescribed and over-the-counter medications. Strom periodically published comprehensive monographs on pharmacoepidemiology and ADEs monitoring systems; and described a pharmaco-epidemiologic approach as one that generally required studying the association between drug experience and disease incidence; and determining the sensitivity (the proportion correctly classified as having the ADE) and the specificity (the proportion correctly classified as not having the ADE) of the approach. A simple measure used was the proportional reporting ratio that was the ratio of the proportion of an event reported for the drug being studied to the proportion of the same event for all other drugs in the same database. Descriptive epidemiology studies included the relative risk-ratio that compared the incidence and prevalence of an event following the administration of a drug to its incidence and prevalence before the use of the drug. Bayesian statistical methods compared the probability of an ADE occurring after the administration of a drug, to its prior probability of occurring.

Drug surveillance was defined by Finney [52] as a process for the systematic collection of information associated with the use of drugs, and the analysis of the information with the objective of obtaining evidence for and about adverse events, and had the capacity to detect both known and previously unsuspected drug-event associations. Finney defined an *event* as an undesirable happening experienced by the patient in the context of the patient's disease, irrespective of whether the event was thought to be wholly or partially caused by the drug, and that occurred in the time-interval between the drug administration and the appearance of the event. Finney proposed that the aim of monitoring was to study serious ADEs; although he stated that opinions would differ about the lower limits of the class of events to be regarded as serious. He advocated the use of computers for maintaining the records of the monitored population, and that the population had to be large enough to provide statistically significant rates of detected ADEs. Finney described, as the simplest statistical procedure to use, comparing totals of events in two successive periods of equal length, and if there was a significant increase in the rate of the event in the later period, than a closer study would be desirable. He advocated monitoring the incidence rates of paired drug-event trends over adequate periods of time, and as soon as any difference between the two rates exceeded a pre-defined critical value, the computer would be programmed to provide an alert warning that further scrutiny was warranted. Finney cautioned that the method was not ideal; that it was not likely to detect anything other than gross effects under the usual conditions of patient care; and that detecting a difference in rates that exceeded the pre-defined critical value was not necessarily proof of a harmful effect of a drug; but could be a false-positive alert. He cautioned that some events reported would be due to overdose or errors of drug administration, rather than an adverse reaction to the drug. He pointed out that the ascertainment of patients' records of events would be more readily obtained in a hospital environment, and event-types would be more clearly recognizable there.

In 1966 the Boston Collaborative Drug Surveillance Program (BCDSP) was initiated in the Lemuel Shattuck Hospital in Boston. Nurses were trained to collect the information from medical records, and from patients and their physicians. For each drug ordered by a physician, the nurse filled out a form with the name of the drug, the dose, the frequency, route of administration, and the specific therapeutic indication. When the drug was stopped the date was recorded, and the reason for discontinuing the drug, including any ADE. When the patient was discharged, then the discharge diagnoses were recorded; and all the information was then transferred to punch cards [200]. In 1966 Jick and associates at Tufts University School of Medicine joined the BCDSP and implemented an ADE monitoring program for hospitalized patients [95]. They reported that during their first 9 months, about 300 ADEs were reported for the 900 patients studied, of which 67 % were believed to be due to the implicated drug, and 25 % of these were believed to be life threatening. By 1970 the BCDSP involved eight hospitals and reported that in six of them 6,312 patients had 53,071 drug exposures; 4.8 % had ADEs, and in 3.6 % of patients the drug was discontinued due to the ADE [96].

Jick [93, 97] summarized their experience with monitoring ADEs, and reported that the BCDSP had collaborated for 10 years in a program of monitoring ADEs in 40 hospitals in seven countries on about 38,000 inpatients and more than 50,000 outpatients. Jick further summarized their experience by defining the relationship between the risk of the baseline illness and the risk of a drug induced illness. With the drug risk high and the baseline risk of illness low, the ADE would be detected readily. If the drug added slightly to a high baseline risk then the effect would not be detectable. When both risks were low, intermediate, or high, then systematic evaluations such as by case-control studies would be needed. By 1982 their database had collected data on over 40,000 admissions in general medical patients in 22 participating hospitals [218].

Shapiro [181] reported that in a series of 6,199 patients in the medical services of six hospitals who were monitored for ADEs, deaths due to administered drugs in the hospitals were recorded in 27 patients (0.44 %). Miller [147] described the monitoring of ADEs from commonly used drugs in eight collaborating hospitals, and reported that ADEs occurred in 6 % of all patients exposed to drugs; about 10 % of these ADEs were classified as being of major severity, and 4 % of these ADEs had either caused or strongly influenced hospital admission.

Leape and associates [113] in Boston reviewed more than 30,000 hospital records and they identified 3.7 % with problems caused by medical treatment and reported that drug complications were the most common type of adverse events, occurring in 19 % of patients. In another 6-month study of medication errors that were the cause of 247 ADEs occurring in a second group of hospital patients, they found that most medication errors occurred in physician orders (39 %) and in nurse administration (38 %), with the remainder nearly equally divided between transcription and pharmacy errors. They reported that, overall, nurses intercepted 86 % of medication errors, and pharmacists 12 %. They concluded that system changes to improve dissemination and display of drug and patient information should make less likely any errors in the use of drugs [112].

Samore [170] reported that by specifying an adverse event and collecting appropriate periodic data, one could determine the prevalence of the adverse event in a defined population. In studies where the occurrence of reported ADEs could be related to a defined denominator population, a percentage, or a rate of ADEs could be computed. By establishing an upper limit (for example, two standard deviations greater than the mean prevalence rate), a cluster of the events could indicate an increased incidence rate, and serve as an alert for a possible adverse event. Since registries generally lacked population information that could be used as a denominator, they could not provide a measure of relative risk of an ADE.

Bates and associates [8, 9] at the Brigham and Women's Hospital in Boston, reported their studies to evaluate the incidence of ADEs; the incidence of potentially injurious ADEs (those with a potential for injury related to a drug); the number of ADEs that were actually prevented, such as when a potentially harmful drug order was written but was intercepted and cancelled before the order was carried out; and the yields of several strategies for identifying ADEs and potential ADEs. They concluded that ADEs occurred frequently, were usually caused by physicians' decision errors, and were often preventable by appropriate alerts. They then evaluated the potential for identifying or preventing each adverse event using a computerized event-monitor that was a program used to search databases to identify specific events. They defined three levels of patient data in accordance with their information content: level (1) included demographics, drugs, and laboratory tests; level (2) included all orders; and level (3) included problem lists and diagnoses. In a group of 3,138 patients admitted to their medical service with 133 ADEs, 84 (63 %) were judged to be severe, 52 (37 %) were judged to be preventable, and 39 (29 %) were judged to be both severe and preventable. In addition each ADE was rated as to its identifiability and preventability, on a 6-point scale; where "1" meant little evidence, and "6" meant certain evidence They did not find any event monitor that was highly sensitive or highly specific; but the use of combinations could decrease false-positive rates [9]. The Brigham and Women's Integrated Computer System also added a program to automatically screen patients' medication profiles for pairs of interacting drugs, and to provide alerts of possible interactions between two prescribed drugs, or between pairs of drug families or classes; and they continued their studies in detecting and preventing ADEs with increasingly larger patient groups. They concluded that ADEs were a major cause of provider (iatrogenic) injury; and they advocated improving the systems by which drugs are ordered, administered, and monitored [12, 107].

Bates [11] also evaluated an intervention program, where computer providers included physicians, nurses, and pharmacists who used a computer provider order entry/results reporting (CPOE/RR) system with an ADEs monitoring program; and reported a significant decrease in failures to intercept serious medication errors (from 10.7 to 4.9 events per 1,000 patient days). Bates [10] further reported that during a 4-year period of studying the effects of computer provider order entry (CPOE) on ADEs; and after excluding medication errors in which doses of drugs were not given at the time they were due and these comprised about 1 % of all ADEs, the remaining numbers of ADEs decreased 81 %, from 142 per 1,000 patient days in the baseline period to 26.6 per 1,000 patient days in the final period.

By 1998 the Brigham and Women's Hospital Integrated Computer System included a computer-based, event detection application that used a set of screening rules to detect and monitor ADEs. They studied ADEs over an 8-month period for all patients admitted to nine medical and surgical units; and compared ADEs identified by their computer-based monitor, with intensive chart review, and with stimulated voluntary reporting by nurses and pharmacists. They reported that computer monitoring identified 2,620 alerts, of which 275 were determined to be ADEs (45 % of all the ADE); and the ADEs identified by the computer monitor were more likely to be classified as being severe; chart review found 398 (65 % of the ADEs); and 76 ADEs were detected by both computer monitor and chart review; and (d) voluntary reports detected only 23 (4 %) of the ADEs. The positive- predictive value of computer-generated alerts was 23 % in the final 8 weeks of the study. The computer strategy required 11 person-hours per week to execute, whereas the chart review required 55 person-hours per week, and voluntary report strategy required five person-hours per week [94]. With the addition of a CPOE/RR subsystem enhanced with a decision-support program to help detect drug-drug interactions, they found a further substantial decrease in the rate of serious medication errors [10].

Del Fiol [43] described the BCDSP collaboration with a large hospital in Brazil, using real-time, alert-notification system, and a knowledge base of drug-drug interactions that included 326 rules focused on detecting moderate and severe drug-drug interactions of the common drug categories of cardiovascular drugs, oral anticoagulants, antiviral drugs and antibiotics. In this study they reported the system had detected that 11.5 % of the orders had at least one drug-drug interaction, of which 9 % were considered to be severe. They suggested that since only 16 % of their rules were actually used in this trial study, a small but carefully selected group of rules should be able to detect a large amount of drug-drug interactions.

In 1970 Cohen and associates at Stanford University began to develop a computer-based PHARM system called Monitoring and Evaluation of Drug Interactions by a Pharmacy-Oriented Reporting (MEDIPHOR) system, with the objective of providing appropriate information regarding ADEs to physicians for their hospital patients. The goals of their system included: (1) establish procedures for collecting drug interaction information from the medical literature, and assessing the scientific validity and clinical relevance of the information; (2) create and implement computer technology capable of prospective detection and prevention of clinically significant drug interactions; (3) develop procedures that utilize the capabilities of the MEDIPHOR system to identify patients receiving specific drug combinations in order to study the incidence and clinical consequences of drug-drug interactions; and (4) evaluate the effects of the MEDIPHOR system on medication use, on physician prescribing practices. Their system initially used a time-sharing computer at Stanford University; by 1973 they had acquired two Digital Equipment PDP-11 computers, and had programmed the MEDIPHOR system in the MUMPS language. Prior to the introduction of the MEDIPHOR system, prescriptions had been entered using typewriters for all prescriptions dispensed from the central hospital pharmacy. With the advent of the computer-based system, each typewriter was replaced by a video terminal and a label printer. As each new prescription was entered, the computer updated the patient's drug profile, printed a prescription label, checked for potentially interacting drug combinations, and maintained a record of all patients' medications. Information on drugs dispensed directly at nursing stations was sent to the pharmacy for entry there by pharmacy personnel. Every new prescription was checked for possible interactions with the components of each medication. They reported that some hospital patients had received concurrently more than 40 drugs.

They developed a large computer-stored database of drug-interaction information that had been collected from the literature by clinical pharmacologists, and entered the data interactively into their computer using a computer display terminal located in a central hospital pharmacy. They maintained a Drug Index that described the components of each drug and the drug class to which it belonged, and an Interaction Table that contained for each possible pair of interaction classes whether there was evidence that drugs in these two classes could interact with each other. Their Drug Index and Interaction Table constituted the drug-interaction database of the MEDIPHOR system. By 1973 their database contained more than 4,000 pharmaceutical preparations; and programs were initiated for the MEDIPHOR system to provide automatic online monitoring alerts to pharmacists, physicians, and nurses when potentially interacting drug combinations were prescribed. Query programs could be used to provide information on drug interactions that were currently on record for a given drug or a class of drugs, or to produce a data profile for any drug-drug interaction. The system generated drug-interaction reports for physicians and nurses that assigned an alert class that ranked the urgency of the report as to its immediacy and severity: from number (1), the most serious and life threatening, and immediate action is recommended; to number (5), when the administration of both drugs could produce organ toxicity [38–40].

In 1974 a version of the MEDIPHOR system was developed for outpatient services, where patients could obtain their drugs from different outpatient pharmacies [38]. Physicians at Stanford University Medical Center were surveyed to evaluate their responses to the computerized, drug-interaction warning system; of 862 respondents, 25 % had received at least one warning report, and 44 % of physicians who had received reports indicated that they had changed their behavior in response to the information [149].

In 1987 the Division of Clinical Pharmacology at Stanford University had expanded MEDIPHOR into a system called MINERVA (Monitoring and INtERVention of therapeutic Actions) to apply computer-monitoring techniques to other than drug interactions. In addition to prescription data and drug profiles from the pharmacy, an intermediary system called MONITOR was initiated when laboratory test results began to be collected by a direct link to the clinical laboratory computer system that was established in 1976. With the addition of current patient census data obtained from the hospital's computerized accounting system, the MINERVA subsystem became operational and it also provided MINERVA TM (therapy monitoring) rules as guidelines in order to prospectively monitor and detect potential therapy problems, and to evaluate the impact of MINERVA on physician processes and patient outcomes [39].

In 1975 Warner and associates at the University of Utah initiated their PHARM system at the LDS Hospital in Salt Lake City, as a subsystem of their HELP (Health Evaluation through Logical Processing) information system. The PHARM system was designed to monitor all drug orders as they were entered into the computer, and to present a message to the user if potential problems were detected involving drug-drug, drug-allergy, drug-lab, drug-disease, drug-diet, drug-dose, or drug-interval interactions. The drug monitoring system was embedded in the medication ordering software and was used by nurses and pharmacists as they entered drug orders into the system [80]. They used a unit-dose dispensing system; drug orders were sent from the nursing stations to the pharmacy, where a pharmacist used a computer terminal to enter the orders into the patients' computer records. Upon entering the patient's identification number, the patient's name was displayed; the pharmacist then entered the drug (or drug code) number and the dose, route and schedule of administration. A computer-based medication profile was kept for each patient that allowed the pharmacist to review, from a computer terminal, all drugs currently given to the patient, all discontinued drug orders, and any drug allergies of the patient. Medication profiles could also be provided for the entire nursing division.

In 1976 they had 149 drug-monitoring HELP sectors. They advised that there was an important need to integrate laboratory data with drug data in order to monitor drug therapy, since they found that 44.8 % of all warning messages were for drug-laboratory alerts. Using their HELP decision-support program that contained rules established by physicians and pharmacists, they monitored drug orders online for ADEs, including adverse drug effects on laboratory tests. When a drug, or history of a drug allergy, was entered into the computer, it was checked automatically for any "alert" conditions. ADEs alerts were reported for 5.0 % of patients; 77 % of the warning messages resulted in changes of therapy. They reported using an algorithm with ten weighted questions to produce a score that estimated the probability of an ADE; characterized the severity of an ADE as mild, moderate, or severe; and classified ADEs as type A (dose-dependent, predictable and preventable) that typically produced 70–80 % of all ADEs; or type B (idiosyncratic or allergic in nature, or related to the drug's pharmacological characteristics) and that usually were the most serious and potentially life threatening of all ADEs. In the first 16 months a total of 88,505 drug orders for 13,727 patients were monitored; 690 (0.8 %) drug orders resulted in a warning on 5 % of all patients; and 532 (77.1 %) of the warning messages resulted in a change in therapy [86].

Evans [49] reported following almost 80,000 LDS patients for a 44 month period and concluded that alerts to physicians of ADEs detected early was associated with a significant reduction of ADEs. Classen [36] described a larger group of 91,574 LDS hospital patients that were followed for a 3-year period, during which 2.43 per 100 admissions developed ADEs. The average time from admission to development of an ADE was 3.7 days; and the average number of different drugs given to patients before they experienced the ADE was 12.5. They concluded that ADEs were associated with a prolonged length of hospital stay, and about a twofold increased risk of death.

In the 1980s, they redefined the HELP programs for their PHARM system using "frames" as the basic unit of information application in order to enhance the order entry process, and to apply predictive knowledge frames. Their menu-based, order entry program then used the complete clinical patient profile for the dynamic creation of patient-adjusted, order entry screens. Such information relied on their centralized patient database and a medical knowledge base; and used an inference machine that combined these two information sources to create data entry screens that fitted the needs of the patient. When a medication order was entered, the display suggested drug dosage and administration schedule based on such relevant data as the patient's age, weight, and laboratory test results, that were obtained from the computer-stored patient's record; it also advised alternative medications that should be considered [166].

In the 1990s medication orders were still written by physicians, transcribed by unit clerks, and entered into the HELP system by clinical pharmacists and nurses. Their PHARM system used logic criteria to review automatically every drug order and, with other data from the HELP system determined if the new drug order might result in a drug-drug, drug-laboratory, or other ADEs [80, 106]. They further enhanced their HELP system with a computerized ADEs monitoring system [49]. Intermountain Health Care, Inc., the parent company of the LDS Hospital, then installed their PHARM and HELP systems in ten of its larger hospitals in Utah [99].

Lindberg and associates [121, 122] at the University of Missouri School of Medicine reported developing in the 1960s a computer database system that provided a quick reference source for drugs, their interactions, and for basic pharmacological principles that they had abstracted from AMA Drug Evaluations, manufacturer's drug inserts such as listed in the Physician's Desk Reference (PDR), and also from the medical literature. Their drug database was organized to be readily accessed in accordance with alternate drug names, indications, contraindications, adverse reactions, drug-drug interactions, laboratory tests, route of administration, drug dosage, pharmacologic and physiologic actions, and by other items. Their IBM 360/50 database management system supported up to 20 simultaneous users, with terminals located conveniently for physicians to use. They could access their database using CONSIDER, a general-purpose storage and retrieval program for formatted text they had developed. At that date they estimated that 15 % of all patients entering a hospital at that time could expect to have an ADE that would prolong their hospital stay; that one-seventh of all hospital days were devoted to treating drug toxicity; and that during a typical hospital stay a patient might be given as many as 20 drugs simultaneously, in which case the patient had a 40 % chance of having an ADE. By 1977 their system was online, and was also accessible by computer terminals located in a variety of sites in the state of Missouri [63, 64].

In the 1960s Collen and associates at the Kaiser Permanente Northern California region initiated a computer-based surveillance system for detecting early warning signals of known and of unknown potential ADEs in outpatients from a defined membership of several hundred thousand persons [57, 58]. Prescriptions filled in the outpatient pharmacies, and diagnoses recorded by physicians in the hospitals and clinics, were stored in a central computer. The epidemiologic approach to monitoring ADEs described by Finney [52] was applied. Supported by a contract from the FDA between 1966 and 1973, they monitored ADEs; in 1973 these computer-stored records contained more 1.3 million prescriptions for 3,446 drug products dispensed to 149,000 patients. With data collected between 1969 and 1973, their initial efforts at data analysis consisted primarily of a search for associations between drugs and subsequent ADEs, by comparing incidence rates of a known or of a suspected ADE in users of a drug, or of a group of drugs, to the rates of the ADE in the drug non-users. Friedman [56, 59] also used case-control methods for identifying possible associations of specific diseases and the prior use of specific drugs. By identifying a group of patients with specific cancers and a control group without these cancers, he compared prior exposure rates to specific drugs in both groups. Friedman advocated monitoring both outpatients and inpatients for ADEs since patients moved in and out of both settings as needed for their care.

In 1977 Friedman [56, 59] added a study of drug carcinogenesis using the computer-based hospital and outpatient records to relate outpatient drug use in 1969–1973 to the subsequent incidence rates of cancer. Kodlin [104] and Ury [214], also at Kaiser Permanente, described a mathematical, response-time model as a possible method of detecting ADEs. They compared the observed number of event-occurrences before and after a drug was administered, and used base frequency rates of events that were derived from medical records of patients who did not report having these events.

Melmon [144] at the University of California in San Francisco wrote that although prescribed drugs usually contributed to the physician's ability to influence favorably the course of many diseases, their use created a formidable health problem since, at that time, 3–5 % of all hospital admissions were primarily for ADEs; 18–30 % of all hospitalized patients had an ADE while in the hospital, and the duration of hospitalization for those patients was almost doubled as a result; about one-seventh of all hospital days were devoted to the care of drug toxicity at an estimated annual cost of $3 trillion.

Maronde [133] advised that an assessment of chemical mutagenesis should also be included when available such as objective data of chromosomal breaks, deletions, or additions, since they felt that the possible role of drugs in producing mutations had not been given sufficient attention. They advised that monitoring for chemical mutagenesis would entail chromosomal staining and study of chromosome morphology, and assessment of the incidence of discernible autosomal dominant and sex-linked recessive mutations.

In 1972 a Pharmacy Automated Drug interaction Screening (PADIS) System was initiated at the Holy Cross Hospital in Fort Lauderdale, Florida, with a database to operate its unit-dose drug system, and integrate its existing computer system to detect and prevent potential drug-drug interactions. It was designed to function as a batch-process system that was run once daily to screen and print all patient-medication profiles for drug interactions for that day. In a study conducted in 1974, a manual review of 13,892 daily patient-medication profiles found a 6.5 % incidence rate of possible drug interactions per patient-day, lower than the 9 % incidence rate per patient-day detected by their computer-based system [74].

Reporting on the assessment of ADEs from commonly used drugs in eight collaborating hospitals, Miller [147] found that ADEs occurred in 6 % of all drug exposures and in 28 % of all patients. About 10 % of the ADEs were classified as being of major severity; and in about 4 % an ADE had either caused or strongly influenced hospital admission. Although some ADEs might be unavoidable, Morrell [149] estimated that 70–80 % were potentially preventable. In 1973 pharmacists at Mercy Hospital in Pittsburgh, Pennsylvania, developed a database incorporating a list of 10,000 drug-drug interactions and 7,000 individual drug-laboratory test interferences from ADEs reported in the literature.

Pharmacists dictated patients' drugs and laboratory tests into a recording device; at the end of a day the recording was re-played and pre-punched cards for each drug and for each lab test were assembled with the patients' identification cards. A pharmacist reviewed the printout in conjunction with the patients' charts, and reported any significant potential interactions to the physicians. Daily reviews of patients' charts resulted in entry of all drugs used and laboratory test data reported; and a list was printed of potential drug-drug interactions and drug-lab interferences. COBOL programs were written to update, search, list, and revise data [20].

Naranjo and associates [151] from the University of Toronto considered a major problem in drug evaluation studies was the lack of a reliable method of assessing the causal relation between drugs and ADEs. They developed an ADEs probability scale and studied the degree of agreement between raters of ADEs using definitions of definite, probable, possible, and doubtful ADEs. The between-raters agreement for two physicians and four pharmacists who independently assessed 63 randomly selected alleged ADEs was 38–63 %; these scores were maintained on re-testing. The between-raters agreement of three attending physicians who independently assessed 28 other cases of alleged ADEs was 80 %, and this was considered to be very high. Michel and Knodel [145] at the University of South Carolina, Columbia, used Naranjo's method of probability-scale algorithms to evaluate and score 28 ADEs in 5 months in 1984 to check on the consistency in evaluating ADEs and concluded that it compared favorably with other scoring methods.

Speedie and associates [204, 205] at the University of Maryland developed a CPOE/RR drug-prescribing review program that used a set of rules to provide feedback to physicians when prescribing drugs, in an attempt to identify drug orders that were potentially inappropriate. Their system was expanded in 1987; and their MENTOR (Medical Evaluation of Therapeutic Orders) system was designed to monitor inpatient drug orders for possible ADEs and for suboptimal therapy. They developed a set of rules that judged if the drug, dosage, and regimen were appropriate given the patient's condition and laboratory results; if the drug was appropriate and timely laboratory results were obtained; and if appropriate periodic monitoring of laboratory results were being performed. The failure to follow any of these rules within a specified time triggered an alert signal and printed a patient-specific advisory.

Blum [17] studied methods for the computer modeling of clinical causal relationships, such as occurred with ADEs. He considered medical systems to be inherently probabilistic in nature and emphasized that the task of demonstrating a casual relationship was non-spurious (that is, not a false positive or false negative) was the most difficult task in deriving causal relationships from large clinical databases, due to confounding variables, lack of size and intensity of the finding, and its validity. Blum further advised that a true causal relationship was best established by controlled clinical trials.

With the developing interest in using lower-cost microcomputers for medical computing applications, Harrison and Ludwig [78], at the University of California, San Francisco, developed a drug-drug interaction system designed to run on an Apple II microcomputer with 48K RAM and one Apple floppy disc. Using published lists of drug interactions for individual drugs or drug classes, the physician could enter the list of drugs prescribed for the patient; their program then searched the indexed lists for all classes of drugs that each drug referenced and reported all drug interactions it found.

Ludwig and Heilbronn [126] described an algorithm that combined Bayesian and heuristic approaches to non-independent observations of multiple conditions. With a database containing many attributes (that could be drugs) and diagnoses (that could be ADEs), they evaluated a variety of statistical approaches; they reported that a causal network model was inferior to a logistic regression model but was comparable to that of a linear discriminant function, and could provide inferences not possible with other simpler statistical methods.

Roach and associates [172] at Virginia Polytechnic Institute developed an expert system for evaluating ADEs from taking drug combinations. To facilitate clinician users, they allowed natural language communication with the system. They provided a database of eight commonly used drugs, containing information on potential interactions, with explanations on the mechanisms on why these interactions occurred, as to whether these were chemicophysical, pharmacodynamic, pharmacokinetic, or physiologic; and what corrective action could be taken to minimize interactions. They used PROLOG, a logic programming language that provided a means for representing facts about the drugs, and rules that could manipulate those facts. They developed an expert system for pharmacological information to assist in decisions involving combination drug therapy. They organized and encoded pharmacological information in rules and frames for systemic retrieval of mechanisms responsible for drug interactions, including interactions between drug classes.

In 1986 the Joint Commission on Accreditation of Healthcare Organizations (JCAHO) mandated a program of criteria-based, *drug use evaluation* (DUE) for patients receiving medications in hospitals, with the goal of monitoring the appropriateness and effectiveness of drug use; and it included the pharmacists intervention in medication dosage recommendations, medication order clarification, identification of drug-drug interactions, and of other ADEs [127]. In 1987 the Drug Surveillance Network, a nation-wide network of hospital-based clinical pharmacists was established to serve as a rapid response mechanism for identifying and clarifying early warning signals of possible problems reported to the pharmaceutical industry or to the FDA, and to determine the incidence of specific adverse events associated with certain drugs in hospitalized patients. In 1994 approximately 400 hospitals participated in this Network, and had collected data on more than 10,000 patients [72].

Lesar [114] found in a study conducted at the Albany Medical Center Hospital, a large tertiary teaching hospital in Albany, New York, that from a total of more than 289,000 medication orders written in a 1-year study at that time, the overall detected error rate was 1.81 significant errors per 1,000 written orders. Brennan [23] reported that the Harvard Practice Group found that an examination of the medical records of a representative sample of more than 2.6 million patients in hospitals in New York State revealed that the statewide incidence of adverse events was 3.7 %; of these 19 % were drug-related. In 1991 a survey conducted of 1,100 clinical pharmacists in 500 hospitals in the United States and Canada that were enrolled in the Drug Surveillance Network to perform post-marketing surveillance of drugs found that more than 85 % had PHARM systems and had implemented spontaneous reporting systems for the identification of ADEs. Since the drug information was volunteered, it generally failed to identify many ADEs; and it did not provide adequate data to quantify the relationships between drug therapy and drug toxicity, or of the incidence rates of ADEs [73].

Dolin [46], at Kaiser Permanente's Southern California region, began developing in 1989 an automated medical record on an IBM-PC in the Internal Medicine Clinic at the Harbor-UCLA Medical Center. In 1990 the clinic added a Pascal interface to a commercially available drug-interaction program that listed 808 drug interactions, including some for over-the-counter medications. It was programmed so that, without the user's having to exit the patient automated record, pressing on the F3 key would flag any prescribed drug in the patient's record that had been found to interact with another prescribed drug, and next pressing on the F4 key would provide comments and recommendations.

Carson [32] reviewed the use of cohort studies that followed a group of patients exposed to a new drug and compared their experience with that of an unexposed group or exposed to another drug of the same class.

In 1994 Miller and associates at the Washington University Medical School and the Barnes-Jewish Hospital in St. Louis, Missouri, began operating their computer-based pharmacy system for seven pharmacies that annually filled 1.6 million medication orders and dispensed six million doses of drugs. They used two commercial pharmacy expert systems that provided alerts for possible ADEs in real time to pharmacists. The first system, DoseChecker, examined medication orders for potential under-dosing or over-dosing of drugs that were eliminated in the body primarily by the kidneys; and gave a recommended new dose for the drug that had caused the alert. The second, PharmADE, provided alerts for orders of contraindicated drug combinations, and listed the drugs involved and described the contraindications. When a potentially dangerous combination was identified, an alert report was sent via facsimile to the pharmacy responsible for providing the patient's drugs; and a daily list of alert reports for patients was prepared and batch processed [146].

Grams [71], at the University of Florida, reviewed the medical-legal experience with ADEs in the United States and recommended that it should be standard practice to implement a sophisticated, computer-based pharmacy system for every outpatient service and deliver the most acceptable drug in a safe and efficacious manner. The value of automated surveillance of ADEs soon became widely recognized, as large computerized databases facilitated the capabilities to monitor and investigate trends of known ADEs, and to provide alerts and early warning signals of possible or potential ADEs [13].

Hripcsak and associates [85], at the Columbia-Presbyterian Medical Center in New York, developed a generalized clinical event monitor that would trigger a warning about a possible ADE in clinical care, including possible medication errors, drug allergies, or side effects; and then generate a message to the responsible health care provider. Their objective was to generate alerts in real time in order to improve the likelihood of preventing ADEs.

McMullin [142, 143] reported that, between May and October 1995, the PHARM system at a large university hospital electronically screened 28,528 drug orders and detected dosage problems in 10 % of patients; it then recommended lower doses for 70 % of the patients and higher doses for 30 %. After pharmacists alerted the physicians, the doses were appropriately adjusted.

Anderson and associates [2] at Purdue University and the Indiana University School of Medicine, found that drug orders entered into the medical information system (MIS) at a large private teaching hospital had an error rate of 32 per 1,000 orders; and could be significantly reduced by involving pharmacists in reviewing drug orders; and that a PHARM system and a hospital CPOE/RR program could detect a significant percent of medication errors and could save a substantial number of excess hospital days by preventing ADEs. They also developed a simulation model for evaluating alternative systems for detecting and preventing ADEs. They projected that a computer-based PHARM system that could detect 26 % of medication errors during the stages of prescribing, dispensing, and administering drugs could save a large number of excess hospital days and patient care costs.

By 1997 the United Health Group (founded in 1974) consisted of 12 affiliated health plans in the United States; and it began to study adverse drug events that were already identified by FDA's Spontaneous Reporting System (SRS). They had approximately 3.5 million members representing commercial, Medicaid, and Medicare patient groups. Their pharmacy database consisted of pharmacy claims typically submitted electronically by a pharmacy at the time a prescription was filled; and it included full medication and provider information. They identified denominator data in order to calculate the rates of adverse events, and to conduct postmarketing studies of utilization and adverse events in their health plans' populations. As an example, from their claims data they were able to study the comparative rates of diarrhea following administration of seven different antibiotics [182].

Raschke and associates [167] at the Good Samaritan Regional Medical Center in Phoenix, Arizona, using its Cerner hospital information system, developed a targeted program for 37 drug-specific ADEs that provided an alert when a physician wrote an order that carried an increased risk of an ADE, such as a prescription with inappropriate dosing. During a 6-month study period, their alerting system provided 53 % true-positive alerts, of which 44 % had not been recognized by the physicians prior to the alert notification.

Choi [34] reviewed six drug information databases designed primarily for educating consumers and available at that time on CD-ROMs, evaluating the information given by each for 20 frequently prescribed drugs. The databases were then ranked for accuracy and completeness of their prescription information when compared to the 1998 edition of USP Advice for Patients. The Mayo Clinic Family Pharmacist had the highest score, followed in descending order by Medical Drug Reference, Pharm-Assist, Home Medical Advisor, The Corner Drug Store, and Mosby's Medical Encyclopedia.

Hennessy [83] wrote that drug utilization review programs were an important approach to improving quality and decreasing costs of patient care, and could be used also for identifying adverse drug events (ADEs). Strom [207] noted that drug utilization data was an important source of insight into disease and treatment patterns of clinicians; and that the *National Disease and Therapeutic Index* was generally the most useful in its reporting four times a year on more than 400,000 office-based physicians for all contacts with patients during a 48-h period.

Payne [159] described two medical care centers in the VA Puget Sound Health Care System that used a clinical event monitor developed by the Veterans Affairs Northwest Network (VISN20) to prevent and detect medication errors. They reported that during a typical day their event monitor received 4,802 messages, 4,719 (98 %) of which pertained to medication orders, and concluded the monitor served an important role in enhancing the safety of medication use.

In the year 2000 the Institute of Medicine estimated that annually about 80,000 people in the United States were hospitalized and died from ADEs; and the report, *To Err is Human: Building a Safer Health System* (Institute of Medicine 2000), increased the attention of the nation to the important need for improving the safety of drug therapy and for better drug monitoring [105].

As systems for identifying potential ADEs and drug interactions grew, a new phenomenon, known as *alert fatigue*, began to be recognized. Brown and associates [25] described RADARx, a Veterans Administration (VA) VistA-compatible software that integrated computerized ADE screening and probability assessment; and they reported that overall, only 11 % of RADARx alerts were true positives. A literature review by van der Sijs [215] found rates of override of drug alerts varied from 49 % to 96 %. Isaac [89] suggested that the current alert systems may be inadequate to protect patient safety. Phansalkar [160] described an expert panel consensus development on improving alert procedures and reducing alert fatigue.

14.4 Polypharmacy

In 1991 the Joint Commission on Accreditation of Healthcare Organizations (JCAHO) developed a set of indicators to assess various drug use activities; as, for example, the number of patients over 65 years of age who were discharged with seven or more prescription drugs [99].

Reports of ADEs usually described studies of adverse reactions in patients from using one or two drugs. The advent of computer-based surveillance of patient data permitted the use of strategies designed for the data mining of large patient databases, not only to identify known ADEs, but also to provide an early warning alert for unknown possible ADEs. However, many hospital patients and most elderly patients take multiple prescription drugs (*polypharmacy*), and are thereby more often exposed to potential ADEs. Ouslander [158] pointed out that the elderly are more susceptible to ADEs, they take multiple combinations of drugs, and recommended more research to help make drug therapy in the elderly safer and more effective. An effective ADE surveillance system for a group of patients, such as the elderly, who take multiple drugs requires both a very large, longitudinal database of the total care, inpatient and outpatient, of a very large defined population, in order to be able to include rare ADEs, and to provide denominators for ADE rates, and a very powerful computer capable of data mining very large numbers of data items.

Cluff and associates [37] at the Johns Hopkins Hospital developed an early surveillance system for ADEs. From a medication order form, patient and prescription data for hospital patients were recorded on punched cards; and the data were then stored on magnetic tape for computer entry. During the initial 1-year of 1965, from the surveillance of 900 patients they reported that 3.9 % were admitted with ADEs, and 10.8 % acquired ADEs after admission to the hospital. Those who received multiple drugs had more ADEs, occurring in 4.2 % of patients who received five or less drugs, and in 24.2 % of patients who received 11–15 drugs [201, 202].

Fassett [51] noted that in any recent year, drugs have been prescribed for nearly 60 % of the United States population, with the highest exposure rate being in the very young and in the very old. After age 60 years the average American receives nearly 11 prescriptions per year. With the access to very large patient databases and very effective data mining and computer analytics, the likelihood increases of discovering previously unknown ADEs between multiple prescribed drugs.

Monane and associates [148] at Merck-Medco Managed Care program provided prescription drug benefits through retail and mail pharmacy services for approximately 51 million Americans. They estimated that individuals aged 65 years and older constituted 12 % of the United States population, and consumed approximately 30 % of prescribed medications. They reported a study from April 1, 1996, through March 31, 1997, when 2.3 million patients aged 65 years and older filled at least one prescription through their mail-service pharmacy. They developed a drug database and surveillance system with an ADE alerting program programmed to identify the most dangerous drugs for the elderly. Of more than 23,000 patients aged 65 years and older who received prescription drugs during this 12 month period, a total of 43,000 prescriptions generated alerts to pharmacists and triggered phone calls to physicians, resulting in a significant change in the medication orders. A meta-analysis of deaths resulting from ADEs indicated that it was between the fourth and sixth leading cause of death in the United States [111].

14.5 Pharmacotherapy Systems

The ability to use computer programs to assist in the decision making process that involved complex drug therapies began to be recognized in the 1960s. Pratt and associates [165] at the National Cancer Institute reported studying the interrelationships of drug dose schedule, drug toxicity, tumor growth, and mortality rates of mice with an experimental strain of leukemia that were given different doses of an experimental drug. They developed a mathematical model, and used their computer to predict survival time and determine optimum dose schedule.

Bonato [18] at the George Washington University Biometric Laboratory reviewed some of their collaborative studies, conducted with the VA's Cooperative Studies of Chemotherapy in Psychiatry and with the Psychopharmacology Service Center of the National Institute of Mental Health (NIMH). These studies were of psychoactive drugs and their effects on behavior. Bonato described how the computer made possible complex studies that were not previously feasible by allowing statistical analyses of large collections of data stored on magnetic tape, collected from 37 collaborating VA hospitals over multiple months for several drugs; including data from instruments such as those converting analog to digital electroencephalograms; and also included 2-year follow-up studies conducted by the NIMH of drugs given to a group of schizophrenic patients.

Lindberg [120, 123] at the University of Missouri in Columbia described a computer program to assist in the selection of antibacterial drugs therapy. In assays of the sensitivity of bacteria to drugs, it was necessary to identify the bacteria, and then consider the effects of an antibacterial drug, including its bactericidal power, its rate of action, the susceptibility of the organism, and its pharmacological efficiency. Lindberg advocated computer-based approaches to analyze rapidly the multiple factors involved; and he reported studies of the effects of different doses of a variety of antibiotics on different periods of bacterial growth in cultures, as related to measurements of blood and tissue concentrations of the drugs, to help to determine optimal intervals between doses of the drugs for patients.

Sheiner and Rosenberg [184] at the University of California at San Francisco developed a pharmacokinetic model to try to better determine the optimal dosage of a toxic drug for an individual patient in order to improve its desired beneficial effect and decrease its rate of adverse drug events. For drugs where blood levels were regularly related to the desired drug effects, such as digitalis preparations, antiarrhythmic drugs, and antimicrobial drugs, they developed a computer-based system that allowed the physician to better produce desired targeted blood levels for these drugs They used prediction rules derived from studies of the general population for estimating the volume of distribution of the drug from calculations of the body surface area of the patient being treated based on the patient's height and weight; and by estimating pharmacokinetic parameters such as rate of drug elimination from the body and the resultant drug blood level. Using programs written in Fortran IV and run on a CDC 6400 computer, tests of the system were conducted on patients treated with digoxin; and subsequent improved models of the system produced a significant decrease in the toxicity rate of this drug [183].

Lincoln and associates [116] at the Rand Corporation in Santa Monica, California began to develop computer-based mathematical models of the treatment of leukemia. With associates at the University of Southern California, Baylor College of Medicine, University of Oklahoma, and University of Washington, they developed CLINFO, a prototype computer system to help analyze laboratory and clinical data on patients treated for leukemia by using graphical displays of data and statistical analyses. CLINFO employed a Data General Eclipse minicomputer connected to cathode-ray-tube display terminals. They described their initial use of the CLINFO system in monitoring the treatment of leukemia patients in the Children's Hospital in Los Angeles [117]. They subsequently reported the great usefulness of CLINFO in the development of a protocol for the methotrexate treatment of cancers that required monitoring the clearance of the drug from the blood and careful adjusting of the intravenous drug dose to prevent toxicity [118]. They concluded that some of their most successful applications resulted from studies concerning the dynamic distribution of drugs in body fluids, particularly of drugs used in the treatment of cancer chemotherapy where frequent critical decisions with respect to drug dosage, therapeutic effectiveness, and toxic side effects must be made [119].

In 1972 computer-assisted pharmacotherapy was advanced by Shortliffe and associates [187–190] at the Stanford University School of Medicine when they developed the MYCIN system to serve as a clinical consultation aid in selecting antibiotic therapy for patients with infections. In 1979 the success of Shortliffe's group with MYCIN led them to develop ONCOCIN, an oncology protocol management consultant designed to assist physicians in the treatment of cancer patients [191, 192].

Jelliffe and associates [90–92] at the University of Southern California School of Medicine developed computer programs for clinical pharmacology to analyze a patient's optimal dosage requirements for a variety of drugs, including cardiac, antibiotic, anesthetic, and others. A diverse multi-purpose library of programs provided rapid and easy computations on demand; and by using a network of time-shared computers, other community and teaching hospitals were permitted to use their programs whenever desired. A quantitative mathematical approach to individualized regimens for drug therapy programs considered the patient's kidney function, the blood serum drug levels from past doses; it allowed the selection of desired therapeutic goals or serum levels; and then printed out dosage regimens to achieve and maintain the desired clinical goals, with the option to rerun the program with selection of different therapeutic goals if desired [66]. More advanced computer programs were then developed for the adaptive control of pharmacokinetic models in drug therapy since the patient does not always respond to the drug as desired. The initial dose regimen was chosen based on best estimates of the model parameters; and the real patient's response was then compared to the simulated model's response; and the difference was used to advise a new dosage regimen; and the cycle was then repeated until the desired therapeutic result was obtained [92].

In 1978 a computer program to aid in the use of digitalis drug preparations was developed by a group in New England led by Gorry and associates [67]. The program constructed a patient-specific model upon which to base the determination of drug dosage, and then used feedback information about a variety of clinical aspects of the patient's response. It assessed the therapeutic and the toxic effects of the drug on the patient, and then made any needed modifications in its recommendations.

Inherited differences in drug effects had begun to be described in the 1950s, and it was recognized that adverse drug reactions could be caused by specific drug metabolizer phenotypes. This gave rise to the field of *pharmacogenetics*, which focused on genetic polymorphisms in drug metabolizing enzymes and how they translated into inherited differences in drug effects. With the establishment of the Human Genome Project in 1990, the term *pharmacogenomics* began to be used to relate adverse drug reactions to specific drug metabolizer phenotypes; and also referred to the entire spectrum of genes that determine drug behavior and sensitivity. This new field of study of the impact of genomic variability on drug response, efficacy, and metabolism, facilitated the discovery of new therapeutic targets and interventions, and helped to elucidate groups of genes that determined the efficacy and toxicity of specific medications [50]. The development of DNA microarrays, microscopic physically ordered arrays of thousands of DNAs of known sequences, attached to solid surfaces, began to be used to study gene expression patterns and to provide clues of the functions of specific genes. Microarray-based gene expression analyses were expected to facilitate the more rapid identification of disease-specific genes and reveal the cellular pathways involved in their pathophysiology; and the discovery of disease-specific genes and their pathways had implications for facilitating the development of more effective and less toxic drugs [45].

A study of two commercially available online computer services of drug information, BRS Colleague and Dialog Medical Connection, used as drug information sources by physicians, nurses, and pharmacists, reported that less than one-third of 1,118 search sessions completely answered the questions, and errors occurred in 81 % of the searches that retrieved incomplete information [1].

14.6   Summary and Commentary

The increasing use of prescribed drugs in patient care has resulted in an increasing number of adverse drug events (ADEs). One of the most important contributions computers have made to the quality and safety of medical care was in pharmacotherapy and in adverse drug event monitoring. Whereas prior to the 1960s, hospitals stocked full lines of medications at patient care units in cabinets managed by nurses, with the advent in the 1970s of automated medication dispensing from unit-dose machines, this led in the 1980s to automated, ward-based medication cabinets. Prior to the introduction of hospital unit-dose systems, drugs were sometimes obtained out of general sources in nursing stations; their administration to patients could be given at different hospital locations, and were often recorded in different paper-based records.

Whereas the earliest PHARM systems were primarily used to support drug administration and pharmacy management functions, it soon became apparent that the prevention and detection of ADEs needed to be a very important function of a PHARM system and of a computer provider order entry/results reporting (CPOE/RR) system. The advent of larger computer-stored databases allowed PHARM systems to better meet the information needs for discovering and monitoring ADEs in inpatient and outpatient care for prescription drugs and over-the-counter medications; and also to provide linkage to all of a patient's data by a unique patient identifier; preferably within a defined population database in order to provide a denominator necessary to calculate rates of diseases and rates of ADEs.

The earliest PHARM systems were used for improving drug administration, but it was soon realized that the most important application of the increasing computing power, associated with the greatly expanding data storage capacities, needed to be applied to the development of automated PHARM systems for monitoring and detecting and preventing ADEs in order to improve the quality and safety of patient care; and could be especially useful for hospitalized patients who usually have accessible a full record of information on all events occurring for each patient; and especially important for patients over the age of 60 years who take multiple prescription drugs (polypharmacy) and for whom ADEs are more common.

Beginning in the 1960s, it was realized that developing computer-based drug monitoring systems for studying, detecting and preventing ADEs could be especially useful for hospitalized patients who usually have accessible a full record of information on all events occurring for each patient; and especially important for patients over the age of 60 years who take multiple prescription drugs and for whom ADEs are more common.

The advent of computer-based surveillance of patient data permitted the use of strategies designed for the data mining of large patient databases, not only to identify known ADE, but also to provide an early warning alert for unknown possible ADEs.

Issues arising from the widespread adoption of CPOE systems, clinical decision support in prescribing, and the sharing of information have led to new concerns with continuing improvement in medication management and prevention of drug errors. In some cases it appeared that CPOE systems were having little effect on reducing drug errors, thus increasing the interest in usability, and, in particular, user-centered design principles. *Alert fatigue* was also recognized as a major concern, as clinicians were unable to deal with the flood of alerts arising from the systems. Sharing information among institutions, enabled by such standards as RxNorm and HL7 messaging, known as semantic and syntactic *interoperability*, and *medication reconciliation*, assuring that lists of current medications for patients are complete and accurate at the time of transfer of care, are also issues that have arisen.

Hopefully in the next years advances in pharmacogenomics will influence medication therapy and further improve the safety and effectiveness of prescribed drugs; improvements in understanding human factors and interface design will reduce the amount of alert fatigue; the interactions which occur in polypharmacy will lead to fewer medication complications in the elderly; and better understanding of pharmacokinetics will lead to improved dosing and timing of medications.

References

1. Abate MA, Shumway JM, Jacknowitz AI. Use of two online services as drug information sources for health professionals. Methods Inf Med. 1992;31:153–8.

2. Anderson JG, Jay SJ, Anderson M, Hunt TJ. Evaluating the potential effectiveness of using computerized information systems to prevent adverse drug events. Proc AMIA. 1997; 228–32.

3. Anderson RJ, Young WW. Microcomputers as a management tool for hospital pharmacy directors. Proc SCAMC. 1984; 231–3.

4. Barnett GO, Justice NS, Somand ME. A computer-based medical information system for ambulatory care. Proc SCAMC. 1978; 486–7.

5. Barnett GO, Castleman PA. A time-sharing computer system for patient-care activities. Comput Biomed Res. 1967;1:41–51.

6. Barnett GO. Massachusetts General Hospital computer system. In: Collen MF, editor. Hospital computer systems. New York: Wiley; 1974.

7. Barret JP, Hersch PL, Cashwell RJ. Evaluation of the impact of the Technicon medical information system at El Camino Hospital. Part II. Columbus: Battelle Columbus Labs; 1979.

8. Bates DW, Leape LL, Petrycki S. Incidence and preventability of adverse drug events in hospitalized adults. J Gen Intern Med. 1993;8:289–94.

9. Bates DW, O'Neil A, Boyle D, Teich J, Chertow GM, Komaroff AL, et al. Potential identifiability and preventability of adverse events using information systems. JAMIA. 1994;1:404–11.

10. Bates DW, Teich JM, Lee J, Seger D, Kuperman GJ, Ma'Luf N, et al. The impact of computerized physician order entry on medication error prevention. JAMIA. 1999;6:313–21.

11. Bates DW, Leape LL, Cullen DJ, Laird N, Petersen LA, Teich JM, et al. Effect of computerized physician order entry and a team intervention on prevention of serious medication errors. JAMA. 1998;280:1311–6.

12. Bates DW, Cullen DJ, Laird N, Petersen LA, Small SD, Servi D, et al. Incidence of adverse drug events and potential adverse drug events: implications for prevention. JAMA. 1995;274:29–34.

13. Berndt DJ, Hevner AR, Studnicki J. CATCH/IT: a data warehouse to support comprehensive assessment for tracking community health. Proc AMIA. 1998; 250–4.

14. Bickel RG. The TRIMIS planning process: decisions, decisions, decisions. In: Emlet HE, editor. Challenges and prospects for advanced medical systems. Miami: Symposia Specialists; 1978. p. 175–81.

15. Blois MS, Wasserman AI. The integration of hospital information subsystems. San Francisco: Office of Medical Information Systems, University of California, San Francisco Medical Center; 1974.

16. Blum BI. A history of computers. In: Blum B, editor. Clinical information systems. New York: Springer; 1986. p. 1–32.

17. Blum RL. Machine representation of clinical causal relationships. Proc MEDINFO. 1983; 652–6.

18. Bonato RR. In: Stacy RW, Waxman BD, editors. Computer analysis of psychopharmacological data. New York: Academic; 1965. p. 315–30.

19. Bootman JL. Community pharmacy. In: Levinson D, editor. Computer applications in clinical practice. New York: Macmillan; 1985. p. 167–72.

20. Bouchard RE, Tufo HM, Van Buren H, et al. Everything you always wanted to know about the POMR. In: Walker HK, Hurst JW, Woody MF, editors. Applying the problem-oriented system. New York: Medcom Press; 1973. p. 47–61.

21. Braunstein ML. Applications of computers in pharmacy: an overview. Proc AMIA. 1982;7–9.

22. Braunstein ML. Applications of computers in pharmacy. Mobius: J Contin Educ Prof Health Sci. 1983;3:37–9.

23. Brennan TA, Leape LL, Laird NM, Hebert L, Localio AR, Lawthers AG, et al. Incidence of adverse events and negligence in hospitalized patients: results of the Harvard Medical Practice Study I. N Engl J Med. 1991;324:370–6.

24. Brown GA. Patient care information system: a description of its utilization in Alaska. Proc SCAMC. 1980;2:873–81.
25. Brown S, Black K, Mrochek S, Wood A, Bess T, Cobb J, et al. RADARx: recognizing, assessing, and documenting adverse Rx events. Proc AMIA. 2000; 101–5.
26. Brunjes S. Pharmacy information systems. So Med Bull. 1969;57:29–32.
27. Buchanan NS. Evolution of a hospital information system. Proc SCAMC. 1980;1:34–6.
28. Burleson KW. Review of computer applications in institutional pharmacy: 1975–1981. Am J Health Syst Pharm. 1982;39:53–70.
29. Canfield K, Ritondo M, Sponaugle R. A case study of the evolving software architecture for the FDA generic drug application process. JAMIA. 1998;5:432–40.
30. Caranasos GJ, May FE, Stewart RB, Cluff LE. Drug-associated deaths of medical inpatients. Arch Intern Med. 1976;136:872–5.
31. Carlstedt B, Jeris DW, Kramer W, Griefenhage R, McDonald CJ. A computer-based pharmacy system for ambulatory patient care. Indiana Pharm. 1977;58:92–8.
32. Carson JL, Strom BL, Maislin G. Screening for unknown effects of newly marketed drugs. In: Strom BL, editor. Pharmacoepidemiology. 2nd ed. New York: Wiley; 1994. p. 431–47.
33. Chan KA, Platt R. Harvard Pilgrim Health Care/Harvard Vanguard Medical Associates. In: Strom BL, editor. Pharmacoepidemiology. 3rd ed. New York: Wiley; 2000. p. 285–93.
34. Choi J, Sullivan J, Pankaskie M, Brufsky J. Evaluation of consumer drug information databases. JAPHA-Wash. 1999;39:683–7.
35. Cimino JJ, McNamara TJ, Meredith T, Broverman CA, Eckert KC, Moore M et al. Evaluation of a proposed method for representing drug terminology. Proc AMIA. 1999; 47–51.
36. Classen DC, Pestotnik SL, Evans RS, Lloyd JF, Burke JP. Adverse drug events in hospitalized patients. Excess length of stay, extra costs, and attributable mortality. JAMA. 1997;277:301–6.
37. Cluff LE, Thornton GF, Seidl LG. Studies on the epidemiology of adverse drug reactions. I. Methods of Surveillance. JAMA. 1964;188:976–83.
38. Cohen SN, Armstrong MF, Briggs RL, Chavez-Pardo R, Feinberg LS, Hannigan JF, et al. Computer-based monitoring and reporting of drug interactions. Proc MEDINFO. 1974;74:889–94.
39. Cohen S, Kondo L, Mangini RJ et al. MINERVA: a computer-based system for monitoring drug therapy. NCHSR research series. DHHS Pub No (PHS) 87-3376. National Center for Health Services Research and Health Care Technology Assessment; 1987.
40. Cohen SN, Armstrong MF, Crouse L, Hunn GS. A computer-based system for prospective detection and prevention of drug interactions. Drug Inf J. 1972;6:81–6.
41. Collen MF. The Permanente Medical Group and the Kaiser Foundation Research Institute. In: McLean ER, Soden JV, editors. Strategic planning for MIS. New York: Wiley; 1977. p. 257–71.
42. Cuddihy RV, Ring WS, Augustine NF. Modification of a management information system software package to process drug reaction data. Methods Inf Med. 1971;10:9.
43. Del Fiol G, Rocha BH, Kuperman GJ, Bates DW, Nohama P. Comparison of two knowledge bases on the detection of drug-drug interactions. Proc AMIA. 2000; 171–5.
44. DePietro S, Tocco M, Tramontozzi A. 1995 pharmacy review. Pharmacy systems: keeping pace. Healthc Inform. 1995;12:29–30. 2, 34 passim.
45. Diehn M, Alizadeh AA, Brown PO. Examining the living genome in health and disease with DNA microarrays. JAMA. 2000;283:2298–9.
46. Dolin RH. Interfacing a commercial drug-interaction program with an automated medical record. MD Comput. 1992;9:115–8.
47. DuMouchel W. Bayesian data mining in large frequency tables, with an application to the FDA spontaneous reporting system. Am Stat. 1999;53:177–90.
48. Estherhay RJ, Walton PL. Clinical research and PROMIS. Proc SCAMC. 1979; 241–54.
49. Evans RS, Pestotnik SL, Classen DC, Horn SD, Bass SB, Burke JP. Preventing adverse drug events in hospitalized patients. Ann Pharmacother. 1994;28:523–7.

50. Evans WE, Relling MV. Pharmacogenomics: translating functional genomics into rational therapeutics. Science. 1999;286:487–91.

51. Fassett WE, MBA RP. Drug related informatics standards. Proc AAMSI. 1989; 358–62.

52. Finney DJ. The design and logic of a monitor of drug use. J Chronic Dis. 1965;18:77–98.

53. Fireworker RB, Esposito V. Computerization of a hospital pharmacy. Proc SCAMC. 1984; 246–50.

54. Friedman GD. Kaiser Permanente Medical Care Program: northern California and other regions. In: Strom BL, editor. Pharmacoepidemiology. New York: Wiley; 1994. p. 187–97.

55. Friedman GD, Habel LA, Boles M, McFarland BH. Kaiser Permanente Medical Care Program. In: Strom BL, editor. Pharmacoepidemiology. New York: Wiley; 2000. p. 263–83.

56. Friedman GD. Computer data bases in epidemiological research. Proc AAMSI Symp. 1984; 389–92.

57. Friedman GD. Screening criteria for drug monitoring: the Kaiser-Permanente drug reaction monitoring system. J Chronic Dis. 1972;25:11–20.

58. Friedman GD, Collen MF, Harris LE, Van Brunt EE, Davis LS. Experience in monitoring drug reactions in outpatients: the Kaiser-Permanente drug monitoring system. JAMA. 1971;217:567–72.

59. Friedman RB, Huhta J, Cheung S. An automated verbal medical history system. Arch Intern Med. 1978;138:1359–61.

60. Fritz WL. Hospital pharmacy. In: Levinson D, editor. Computer applications in clinical practice. New York: Macmillan; 1985. p. 173–9.

61. Gall J. Computerized hospital information system cost-effectiveness: a case study. In: van Egmond J, de Vries Robbe PF, Levy AH, editors. Information systems for patient care. Amsterdam: North Holland; 1976. p. 281–93.

62. Gall J. Cost-benefit analysis: total hospital informatics. In: Koza RC, editor. Health information system evaluation. Boulder: Colorado Associated University Press; 1974. p. 299–327.

63. Garten S, Falkner RV, Mengel CE, Lindberg D. A computer based drug information system. Med Electron Dig. 1977;2:4–5.

64. Garten S, Mengel CE, Stewart WE, Lindberg DA. A computer-based drug information system. Mo Med. 1974;71:183–6.

65. Gehlbach SH, Wilkinson WE, Hammond WE, Clapp NE, Finn AL, Taylor WJ, et al. Improving drug prescribing in a primary care practice. Med Care. 1984;22:193–201.

66. Goicoechea FJ, Jelliffe RW. Computerized dosage regimens for highly toxic drugs. Am J Health Syst Pharm. 1974;31:67–71.

67. Gorry GA, Silverman H, Pauker SG. Capturing clinical expertise: a computer program that considers clinical responses to digitalis. Am J Med. 1978;64:452–60.

68. Gouveia WA. Computer applications in the hospital pharmacy. Hosp JAHA. 1971;45:80–3.

69. Gouveia WA, Diamantis C, Barnett GO. Computer applications in the hospital medication system. Am J Hosp Pharm. 1969;26:141–50.

70. Graber SE, Seneker JA, Stahl AA, Franklin KO, Neel TE, Miller RA. Development of a replicated database of DHCP data for evaluation of drug use. JAMIA. 1996;3:149–56.

71. Grams RR, Zhang D, Yue B. A primary care application of an integrated computer-based pharmacy system. J Med Syst. 1996;20:413–22.

72. Grasela TH. Clinical pharmacy drug surveillance network. In: Strom BL, editor. Pharmacoepidemiology. New York: Wiley; 1994. p. 289–300.

73. Grasela TH, Walawander CA, Kennedy DL, Jolson HM. Capability of hospital computer systems in performing drug-use evaluations and adverse drug event monitoring. Am J Health Syst Pharm. 1993;50:1889–95.

74. Greenlaw CW, Zellers DD. Computerized drug-drug interaction screening system. Am J Health Syst Pharm. 1978;35:567–70.

75. Grohman G. Evaluating a hospital pharmacy computer system. Comput Healthc. 1983;4:42–3.

76. Guess HA. Premarketing applications of pharmacoepidemiology. In: Strom BL, editor. Pharmacoepidemiology. New York: Wiley; 2000. p. 450–62.
77. Hammond WE. GEMISCH. A minicomputer information support system. Proc IEEE. 1973;61:1575–83.
78. Harrison PB, Ludwig D. Drug interactions on a microcomputer. Proc AAMSI Symp. 1983; 479–83.
79. Harwood PM, Causey JP, Goldberger S. Pharmacy system. In: Enterline JP, Lenhard RE, Blum BI, editors. A clinical information system for oncology. New York: Springer; 1989. p. 139–60.
80. Haug PJ, Gardner RM, Tate KE, Evans RS, East TD, Kuperman G, et al. Decision support in medicine: examples from the HELP system. Comput Biomed Res. 1994;27:396–418.
81. Heller WM. Drug distribution in hospitals. Data processing in drug distribution systems. Hospitals. 1968;42:73.
82. Helling M, Venulet J. Drug recording and classification by the WHO research centre for international monitoring of adverse reactions to drugs. Methods Inf Med. 1974;13:169–78.
83. Hennessy S, Strom BL, Soumerai SB. Drug utilization review. In: Strom BL, editor. Pharmacoepidemiology. New York: Wiley; 2000. p. 505–23.
84. Honigman B, Rumack BH, Pons PT, Conner CS, Prince J, Rann L et al. A computerized clinical information system for physicians, pharmacists and nurses. Proc SCAMC. 1984; 308–13.
85. Hripcsak G, Allen B, Cimino JJ, Lee R. Access to data: comparing AccessMed with query by review. JAMIA. 1996;3:288–99.
86. Hulse RK, Clark SJ, Jackson JC, Warner HR, Gardner RM. Computerized medication monitoring system. Am J Health Syst Pharm. 1976;33:1061–4.
87. Humphrey W. Pharmacy computing reaches maturity. Healthc Inform. 1992;9:38–41.
88. Huntington ED. A multi-user, single data base pharmacy system. Proc SCAMC. 1979; 892–6.
89. Isaac T, Weissman JS, Davis RB, Massagli M, Cyrulik A, Sands DZ, et al. Overrides of medication alerts in ambulatory care. Arch Intern Med. 2009;169:305–11.
90. Jelliffe RW, Bayard D, Schumitzky A, Milman M, Van Guilder M. Pharmaco-informatics: more precise drug therapy from 'multiple model' (MM) adaptive control regimens: evaluation with simulated vancomycin therapy. Proc MEDINFO. 1994;8:1106–10.
91. Jelliffe RW. Computers in cardiotherapeutics. In: Cady LD, editor. Computer techniques in cardiology. New York: Marcel Dekker; 1979. p. 261–322.
92. Jelliffe RW, Schumitzky A, Rodman J, Crone J. A package of time-shared computer programs for patient care. Proc SCAMC. 1977; 154–61.
93. Jick H. In-hospital monitoring of drug effects: past accomplishments and future needs. In: Ducrot H, editor. Computer aid to drug therapy and to drug monitoring. New York: North-Holland; 1978. p. 3–7.
94. Jha AK, Kuperman GJ, Teich JM, et al. Identifying adverse drug events. JAMIA. 1998;5:305–14.
95. Jick H. Drug surveillance program. Med Sci. 1968;18:41–6.
96. Jick H, Miettinen OS, Sharpiro S, et al. Comprehensive drug surveillance. JAMA. 1970;213:1455–60.
97. Jick H. The discovery of drug-induced illness. N Engl J Med. 1977;296:481–5.
98. Johns RJ, Blum BI. The use of clinical information systems to control cost as well as to improve care. Trans Am Clin Climatol Assoc. 1979;90:140–52.
99. Jones JK. Inpatient databases. In: Strom BL, editor. Pharmacoepidemiology. New York: Wiley; 1994. p. 257–76.
100. Karch FE, Lasagna L. Adverse drug reactions: a critical review. JAMA. 1975;234:1236–41.
101. Kennedy DL, Goldman SA, Little RB. Spontaneous reporting in the United States. In: Strom BL, editor. Pharmacoepidemiology. New York: Wiley; 2000. p. 151–74.
102. Kerr S. IS-the best medicine for drug-monitoring. Datamation. 1988;34:41.

103. Knight JR, Conrad WF. Review of computer applications in hospital pharmacy practice. Am J Hosp Pharm. 1975;32:165–73.
104. Kodlin D, Standish J. A response time model for drug surveillance. Comput Biomed Res. 1970;3:620–36.
105. Kohn LT, Corrigan JM, Donaldson MS. To Err is human: building a safer health system. Washington, DC: National Academies Press; 2000.
106. Kuperman GJ, Gardner RM, Pryor TA. The pharmacy application of the HELP system. In: Kuperman GJ, Gardner RM, Pryor TA, editors. HELP: a dynamic hospital information system. New York: Springer; 1991. p. 168–72.
107. Kuperman GJ, Bates DW, Teich JM, Schneider JR, Cheiman D. A new knowledge structure for drug-drug interactions. Proc AMIA. 1994; 836–40.
108. Kurata JH, Overhage M, Gabrieli E, Jones JK. International data standards for hospital-based drug surveillance. MD Comput. 1994;12:50–7.
109. Kurland L, Annegers JF, O'Fallon W. Utilization of Mayo Clinic records for population-based long-term evaluations of drug exposure. In: Ducrot H, editor. Computer aid to drug therapy and to drug monitoring. New York: North-Holland; 1978. p. 69–76.
110. Lassek W, Rendell M, Ross D, Smith C, Kernek S, Williams J et al. Epidemiologic and clinical use of pharmaceutical profiles in an ambulatory care data system. Proc SCAMC. 1982; 346–50.
111. Lazarou J, Pomeranz BH, Corey PN. Incidence of adverse drug reactions in hospitalized patients: a meta-analysis of prospective studies. JAMA. 1998;279:1200–5.
112. Leape LL, Bates DW, Cullen DJ, Cooper J, Demonaco HJ, Gallivan T, et al. Systems analysis of adverse drug events. JAMA. 1995;274:35–43.
113. Leape LL, Brennan TA, Laird N, Lawthers AG, Localio AR, Barnes BA, et al. The nature of adverse events in hospitalized patients: results of the Harvard Medical Practice Study II. N Engl J Med. 1991;324:377–84.
114. Lesar TS, Briceland LL, Delcoure K, Parmalee JC, Masta-Gornic V, Pohl H. Medication prescribing errors in a teaching hospital. JAMA. 1990;263:2329–34.
115. Lesko SM, Mitchell AA. The use of randomized controlled trials for pharmaco-epidemiology studies. In: Strom BL, editor. Pharmacoepidemiology. New York: Wiley; 2000. p. 539–52.
116. Lincoln T, Aroesty J, Sharpiro NZ. Cancer chemotherapy – an example of physician decisionmaking. Proc San Diego Biomed Symp. 1972;11:177–81.
117. Lincoln TL, Groner GF, Quinn JJ, Lukes RJ. The analysis of functional studies in acute lymphocytic leukaemia using CLINFO: a small computer information and analysis system for clinical investigators. Inform Health Soc Care. 1976;1:95–103.
118. Lincoln TL, Aroesty J, Groner GF, Willis KL, Morrison PF, Isacoff WH. Decision-making in high-dose methotrexate cancer chemotherapy. Inform Health Soc Care. 1977;2:163–72.
119. Lincoln TL, Korpman RA. Computers, health care, and medical information science. Science. 1980;210:257–63.
120. Lindberg D. Medical informatics/computers in medicine. JAMA. 1986;256:2120–2.
121. Lindberg D. The computer and medical care. Springfield: CC Thomas; 1968.
122. Lindberg DAB, Rowland LR, Buch WF et al. CONSIDER: a computer program for medical instruction. In: 9th IBM med symposium 1968:59–61.
123. Lindberg D, Reese GR. Automatic measurement and computer processing of bacterial growth data. Biomedical Sciences Instrumentation, vol 1. Proc 1st National Biomedical Sciences Instrumentation Symp. 1963; 11–20.
124. Lipman AG, Madeux B. Computer-based formulary service reduces costs, eliminates confusion. Hospitals. 1977;51:109.
125. Lloyd SS, Rissing JP. Physician and coding errors in patient records. JAMA. 1985;254:1330–6.
126. Ludwig D, Heilbronn D. The design and testing of a new approach to computer-aided differential diagnosis. Methods Inf Med. 1983;22:156–66.
127. MacKinnon G, Wuller W. Using databases in pharmacies. Healthc Inform. 1993;10:34–6. 38, 40.

128. Mackintosh DR. A microcomputer pharmacy system for correctional facilities. Proc AAMSI Cong. 1989; 200–3.
129. Marietti C. Robots hooked on drugs: robotic automation expands pharmacy services. Healthc Inform. 1997;14:37–8. 40, 42.
130. Marino CA. Cost-benefit analysis of an automated pharmacy system. Proc SCAMC. 1979; 873–7.
131. Marlin RL. Reliability factors in adverse drug reaction reporting. Methods Inf Med. 1981;20:157.
132. Maronde RF, Siebert S. Electronic data processing of prescriptions. In: Bekey GA, Schwartz MD, editors. Hospital information systems. New York: Marcel Dekker; 1972. p. 73–110.
133. Maronde RF, Rho J, Rucker TD. Monitoring for drug reactions including mutations, in outpatients. In: Ducrot H, editor. Computer aid to drug therapy and to drug monitoring. New York: North-Holland; 1978. p. 63–8.
134. Maronde RF, Lee PV, McCarron MM, Seibert S. A study of prescribing patterns. Med Care. 1971;9: 383–95.
135. McDonald CJ. The medical gopher: a microcomputer based physician work station. Proc SCAMC. 1984; 453–9.
136. McDonald CJ. Protocol-based computer reminders, the quality of care and the non-perfectability of man. N Engl J Med. 1976;295:1351–5.
137. McDonald CJ, Hammond WE. Standard formats for electronic transfer of clinical data. Ann Intern Med. 1989;110:333–5.
138. McDonald CJ, Blevins L, Tierney WM, Martin DK. The Regenstrief medical records. MD Comput. 1987;5:34–47.
139. McDonald CJ, Murray R, Jeris D, Bhargava B, Seeger J, Blevins L. A computer-based record and clinical monitoring system for ambulatory care. Am J Public Health. 1977;67:240–5.
140. McDonald CJ, Hui SL, Smith DM, Tierney WM, Cohen SJ, Weinberger M, et al. Reminders to physicians from an introspective computer medical record: a two-year randomized trial. Ann Intern Med. 1984;100:130–8.
141. McDonald CJ, Wilson G, Blevins L, Seeger J, Chamness D, Smith D et al. The Regenstrief medical record system. Proc SCAMC. 1977b; 168–9.
142. McMullin ST, Reichley RM, Kahn MG, Dunagan WC, Bailey TC. Automated system for identifying potential dosage problems at a large university hospital. Am J Health Syst Pharm. 1997;54:545–9.
143. McMullin ST, Reichley RM, Watson LA, Steib SA, Frisse ME, Bailey TC. Impact of a Web-based clinical information system on cisapride drug interactions and patient safety. Arch Intern Med. 1999;159:2077–82.
144. Melmon KL. Preventable drug reactions – causes and cures. N Engl J Med. 1971;284:1361.
145. Michel DJ, Knodel LC. Comparison of three algorithms used to evaluate adverse drug reactions. Am J Health Syst Pharm. 1986;43:1709–14.
146. Miller JE, Reichley RM, McNamee LA, Steib SA, Bailey TC. Notification of real-time clinical alerts generated by pharmacy expert systems. Proc AMIA. 1999; 325–9.
147. Miller RR. Drug surveillance utilizing epidemiologic methods. A report from the Boston Collaborative Drug Surveillance Program. Am J Health Syst Pharm. 1973;30:584–92.
148. Monane M, Matthias DM, Nagle BA, Kelly MA. Improving prescribing patterns for the elderly through an online drug utilization review intervention: a system linking the physician, pharmacist, and computer. JAMA. 1998;280:1249–52.
149. Morrell J, Podlone M, Cohen SN. Receptivity of physicians in a teaching hospital to a computerized drug interaction monitoring and reporting system. Med Care. 1977;15:68–78.
150. Murray MD, Loos B, Tu W, Eckert GJ, Zhou X, Tierney WM. Effects of computer-based prescribing on pharmacist work patterns. JAMIA. 1998;5:546–53.
151. Naranjo CA, Busto U, Sellers EM, Sandor P, Ruiz I, Roberts EA, et al. A method for estimating the probability of adverse drug reactions. Clin Pharmacol Ther. 1981;30:239–45.
152. Nazarro JT. Looking at a computerized pharmacy in the military sector. Comput Hosp. 1980;1:29–32.

153. Nazarro JT, Barnett WA. Pharmacy Information System, the Charleston Experience. Proc SCAMC. 1979; 878–9.
154. NDC. National Drug Code. Functional description for pharmacy (Rev. 1.0). Rockville, MD: NDC Federal Systems, Inc;1983; 1.0–4.4.
155. Nelson SJ, Zeng K, Kilbourne J, Powell T, Moore R. Normalized names for clinical drugs: RxNorm at 6 years. Rockville, MD: JAMIA. 2011;18:441–8.
156. Nelson SJ, Brown SH, Erlbaum MS, Olson N, Powell T, Carlsen B et al. A semantic normal form for clinical drugs in the UMLS: early experiences with the VANDF. Proc AMIA. 2002; 557–61.
157. Neuenschwander M. New technology. Healthc Inform. 1994;11:48–54.
158. Ouslander JG. Drug therapy in the elderly. Ann Intern Med. 1981;95:711–22.
159. Payne TH, Savarino J, Marshall R, Hoey CT. Use of a clinical event monitor to prevent and detect medication errors. Proc AMIA. 2000; 640–4
160. Phansalkar S, van der Sijs H, Tucker AD, Desai AA, Bell DS, Teich JM, et al. Drug-drug interactions that should be non-interruptive in order to reduce alert fatigue in electronic health records. JAMIA. 2013;20:489–93.
161. Platiau PE, Gallina JN, Jeffrey LP. Computer improves record keeping. 1. Hospitals. 1972;46:90–5.
162. Platt R. Harvard community health plan. In: Strom BL, editor. Pharmacoepidemiology. New York: Wiley; 1994. p. 277–87.
163. Porter J, Jick H. Drug-related deaths among medical inpatients. JAMA. 1977;237:879–81.
164. Pope RA, Slack WV, Janousek, Mattson CJ. A computer-based IV admixture. Methods Inform Med. 1982;21:65–9.
165. Pratt AW, White WC, Wall DD. A study in experiment cancer chemotherapy. Proc 4th IBM Med Symp. 1962; 319–25.
166. Prokosch HU, Pryor TA. Intelligent data acquisition in order entry programs. Proc SCAMC. 1988; 454–8.
167. Raschke RA, Gollihare B, Wunderlich TA, Guidry JR, Leibowitz AI, Peirce JC, et al. A computer alert system to prevent injury from adverse drug events: development and evaluation in a community teaching hospital. JAMA. 1998;280:1317–20.
168. Raub WF. The PROPHET system and resource sharing. In: Computers in life science Research. FASEB Monographs vol 2. New York: Springer; 1974. p. 189–94.
169. Raymond T. Pharmacy systems review. Healthc Comput Commun. 1987;4:28–38. 54.
170. Ricks TD. A community hospital unit dose medication system for pharmacy and nursing stations. Proc SCAMC. 1981; 624–9.
171. Rind DM, Davis R, Safran C. Designing studies of computer-based alerts and reminders. MD Comput. 1995;12:122–6.
172. Roach J, Lee S, Wilcke J, Ehrich M. An expert system for information on pharmacology and drug interactions. Comput Biol Med. 1985;15:11–23.
173. Royal BW, Venulet J. Methodology for international drug monitoring. Methods Inf Med. 1972;11:75–86.
174. Rubin AD, Risley JF. The PROPHET system: an experiment in providing a computer resource to scientists. Proc MEDINFO. 1977; 77–81.
175. Runck HM. Computer planning for hospitals-large-scale education and involvement of employees. Comput Autom. 1969;18:33.
176. Ruskin A. Storage and retrieval of adverse reaction data (and the international monitoring program). Proc 8th IBM Medical Symp. 1967; 67–8.
177. Samore M, Lichtenberg D, Saubermann L et al. A clinical data repository enhances hospital infection control. Proc AMIA. 1997; 56–60.
178. Saunders KW, Stergachis A, Von Korff M. Group health cooperative of Puget Sound. In: Strom BL, editor. Pharmacoepidemiology. New York: Wiley; 1994. p. 171–85.
179. Seed JC. Restricted data formats. Ann NY Acad Sci. 1969;161:484–526.

180. Seibert S, Brunges S, Soutter JC, Maronde RF. Utilization of computer equipment and techniques in prescription processing. Drug Intell. 1967;1:342–50.
181. Shaprio PA, Stermole DF. ACORN: (automatic coden report narrative). An automated natural language question answering system for surgical reports. Comput Autom. 1971;20:13–8.
182. Shatin D, Drinkard C, Stergachis A. United Health Group. In: Strom BL, editor. Pharmacoepidemiology. New York: Wiley; 2000. p. 295–305.
183. Sheiner LB, Rosenberg B. Individualizing drug therapy with a feedback-responsive computer system. Proc MEDINFO. 1974; 901–7.
184. Sheiner LB, Rosenberg B. Pharmacokinetic modeling for individual patients: a practical basis for computer-aided therapies. Proc San Diego Biomed Symp. 1972; 183–7.
185. Shephard RH. Plans for developing a computational facility at the Johns Hopkins Medical Institutions. Proc 3rd IBM Med Symp. 1961; 191–6.
186. Shieman BM. Medical information system, El Camino Hospital. IMS Ind Med Surg. 1971;40:25–6.
187. Shortliffe EH, Axline SG, Buchanan BG, et al. An artificial intelligence program to advise physicians regarding antimicrobial therapy. Comp Biomed Res. 1973;6:544–60.
188. Shortliffe EH, Axline SG, Buchanan BG, Cohen SN. Design considerations for a program to provide consultations in clinical therapeutics. Proc San Diego Biomed Symp. 1974;3:313–9.
189. Shortliffe EH, Davis R, Stanton G, et al. Computer-based consultations in clinical therapeutics: explanation and rule acquisition capabilities of the MYCIN system. Comput Biomed Res. 1975;8:303–20.
190. Shortliffe EH. A rule-based approach to the generation of advice and explanations in clinical medicine. In: Schneider/Sagvall Hein, editors. Computational linguistics in medicine. New York: North-Holland; 1977. pp 101–8.
191. Shortliffe EH, Scott AC, Bischoff MB, Campbell AB, Van Melle W, Jacobs CD. An expert system for oncology protocol management. In: Buchanan BG, Shortliffe, editors. Rule based expert systems: the Mycin experiments of the Stanford Heuristic programming project. Reading: Addison-Wesley; 1984. p. 653–65.
192. Shortliffe EH, Scott AC, Bischoff MB. ONCOCIN: an expert system for oncology protocol management. 1991; 876–81.
193. Shumway JM, Jacknowitz AI, Abate MA. Attitudes of community pharmacists, university-based pharmacists, and students toward on-line information resources. Methods Inf Med. 1996;35:142–7.
194. Shumway JM, Jacknowitz AI, Abate MA. Analysis of physicians', pharmacists', and nurses' attitudes toward the use of computers to access drug information. Methods Inf Med. 1990;29:99–103.
195. Siegel C, Alexander MJ, Dlugacz D, Fischer S. Evaluation of a computerized drug review system: impact, attitudes, and interactions. Comput Biomed Res. 1984;17:149–35.
196. Siegel C, Alexander MJ, Dlugacz YD, Fischer S. Evaluation of a computerized drug review system: impact, attitudes, and interactions. In: Anderson JG, Jay SJ, editors. Use and impact of computers in clinical medicine. New York: Springer; 1987. p. 238–56.
197. Simborg DW. Medication prescribing on a university medical service-the incidence of drug combinations with potential adverse interactions. Johns Hopkins Med J. 1976;139:23–6.
198. Simborg DW, Derewicz HJ. A highly automated hospital medication system: five years' experience and evaluation. Ann Intern Med. 1975;83:342–6.
199. Sittig DF, Franklin M, Turetsky M, Sussman AJ, Bates DW, Komaroff AL, et al. Design and development of a computer-based clinical referral system for use within a physician hospital organization. Stud Health Technol Inform. 1998;52(Pt 1):98–102.
200. Slone D, Jick H, Borda I, Chalmers T, Feinleib M, Muench H, et al. Drug surveillance utilising nurse monitors: an epidemiological approach. Lancet. 1966;288:901–3.
201. Smith JW. A hospital adverse drug reaction reporting program. Hospitals. 1966;40:90.
202. Smith RM. How to automate a hospital. Mana Serv 1966; 48–53.

203. Souder DE, Zielstorff RD, Barnett GO. Experience with an automated medication system. In: Ducrot H et al., editors. Computer aid to drug therapy and to drug monitoring. New York: North-Holland; 1978. p. 291–301.

204. Speedie SM, Palumbo FB, Knapp DA, Beardsley R. Evaluating physician decision making: a rule-based system for drug prescribing review. Proc MEDCOMP. 1982; 404–8.

205. Speedie SM, Skarupa S, Blaschke TF, Kondo J, Leatherman E, Perreault L. MENTOR: Integration of an expert system with a hospital information system. Proc SCAMC. 1987; 220.

206. Strom BL. Pharmacoepidemiology. 2nd ed. New York: Wiley; 1984.

207. Strom BL. Other approaches to pharmacoepidemiology studies. In: Strom BL, editor. Pharmacoepidemiology, 3rd edition. New York: Wiley; 2000. p. 387–99.

208. Stolar MH. National survey of hospital pharmaceutical services – 1982. Am J Hosp Pharm. 1983;40:963–9.

209. Swanson DS, Broekemeier RL, Anderson MW. Hospital pharmacy computer systems: 1982. Am J Health Syst Pharm. 1982;39:2109–17.

210. Tayloe DR. The pharmacy computer and the physician. Proc AMIA Congress 1982; 25–6.

211. Trusty RD. TRIMIS approach to automation (pharmacy information). Proc SCAMC. 1979; 869–72.

212. Trusty RD, Nazzaro JT. A Tri-Service regionalized pharmacy information system test and experience. Proc MEDINFO. 1980; 921–3.

213. Turner GH. Microcomputers in pharmacy: current applications. Proc SCAMC. 1984; 205–7.

214. Ury HK. A new test statistic for the Kodlin-Standish drug surveillance model. Comput Biomed Res. 1972;5:561–75.

215. van der Sijs H, Aarts J, Vulto A, Berg M. Overriding of drug safety alerts in computerized physician order entry. JAMIA. 2006;13:138–47.

216. Visconti JA, Smith MC. The role of hospital personnel in reporting adverse drug reactions. Am J Hosp Pharm. 1967;24:273–5.

217. Wagner MM, Hogan WR. The accuracy of medication data in an outpatient electronic medical record. JAMIA. 1996;3:234–44.

218. Walker AM, Cody RJ, Greenblatt DJ, Jick H. Drug toxicity in patients receiving digoxin and quinidine. Am Heart J. 1983;105:1025–8.

219. Walsh PJ. E-pharmacy systems. Prescription and medication fulfillment come of age. MD Comput. 1999;17:45–8.

220. Weissman AM, Solomon DK, Baumgartner RP, Brady JA, Peterson JH, Knight JL. Computer support of pharmaceutical services for ambulatory patients. Am J Health Syst Pharm. 1976;33:1171–5.

221. Westin AF. A policy analysis of citizen rights: issues in health data systems. US Dept. of Commerce, National Bureau of Standards: for sale by the Supt. of Docs., United States Government Printing Office; 1977.

222. Wiederhold G. Summary of the findings of the visiting study team automated medical record systems for ambulatory care. Visit to Duke University Medical Center, CDD-5 HRA Contract, June 29. 1975.

223. Williams FL, Nold EG. Selecting a pharmacy information system. Proc SCAMC. 1983; 200–2.

224. Windsor DA. Adverse-reactions literature: a bibliometric analysis. Methods Inf Med. 1977;16:52–4.

225. Zuckerman AE, Johnson KW. Converting a reference textbook into a computer searchable database: the experience with the USP DI. Proc SCAMC. 1984; 341.

Chapter 15
Imaging Information Systems

Bradley James Erickson, Ronald L. Arenson, and Robert A. Greenes

Abstract The earliest radiology information systems (RISs) were developed in the late 1960s to support administrative tasks such as scheduling and workflow; in 1978, leading developers joined together to form what became the dominant RIS. Widely deployed today, the RIS is being integrated into the electronic health record; reporting functions are supported by speech recognition or by structured reporting. The 1980s saw the development of picture archival and communication systems (PACS) to store the multiplicity of images generated by new technologies, notably computerized tomography (CT) and magnetic resonance imaging (MRI), and make them available for interactive viewing on special display terminals. In the early 1990s, PACSs were installed in Department of Defense and Veterans Administration facilities. Today, PACS are blending with teleradiology to support subspecialists in interpreting examinations 24 h a day. Workflow systems that manage RIS and PACS information across multiple hospitals require routing much like the PACS of the early days. Vendor neutral archives can offer centralized storage and respond to queries from any PACS/RIS. In radiology, the image component is governed by the standard known as Digital Communications in Medicine (DICOM); activities such as orders, reports, and billing are communicated by Health Level 7. As imaging information systems continue to evolve, preferred implementations for specific tasks are being defined under the Integrating the Healthcare Enterprise (IHE); computer algorithms are being developed to aid in the adoption of Computer Aided Diagnosis (CAD); and visualization and measurements based on 3D imaging hold promise for some diagnostic and therapeutic tasks.

B.J. Erickson, M.D., Ph.D. (✉)
Department of Radiology, Mayo Clinic, Rochester, MN, USA
e-mail: bje@mayo.edu

R.L. Arenson, M.D.
Department of Radiology and Biomedical Imaging, University of California,
San Francisco, CA, USA
e-mail: ronald.arenson@ucsf.edu

R.A. Greenes, M.D., Ph.D.
Arizona State University, Tempe, AZ, USA

Department of Biomedical Informatics, Mayo Clinic, Rochester, MN, USA
e-mail: greenes@asu.edu

© Springer-Verlag London 2015   659
M.F. Collen, M.J. Ball (eds.), *The History of Medical Informatics in the United States*, Health Informatics, DOI 10.1007/978-1-4471-6732-7_15

Keywords Imaging information systems • Radiology information systems (RIS) • Computer aided diagnosis (CAD) • Computerized tomography (CT) • Digital communications in medicine (DICOM) • Magnetic resonance imaging (MRI) • Picture archival and communications systems (PACS) • Radiology information system (RIS) • Vendor neutral archive (VNA)

The practice of radiology (RAD) and diagnostic imaging includes selection of the best imaging method to determine the cause of symptoms or to assess therapy in a patient; selection of the optimal acquisition technique for the selected imaging modality; the interpretation of the images; and the other management needs including scheduling, billing, staffing, etc. For the first decades, beginning in the 1960s, these functions dealt with images captured on film and video, and were managed manually and with paper-based methods such as card files and film folders. Using computers to acquire, store, and transmit images seems mundane today, but even now this can be a challenge. Furthermore, while the explorations of use of computers in imaging were focused on applications to assist in the interpretation of images, the greatest early successes were in the reporting and management arenas.

15.1 Radiology Information Systems

The Radiology Information System (RIS) manages much of the administrative and textual information that is used in a radiology department, including the referring physician's order for the examination, scheduling of the examination, workflow management and tracking (for the processes of bringing patient and imaging device together, conducting the examination, producing the images, and transporting the images and associated information to the radiologist who will do the interpretation), producing the interpretive report, distributing the report to the referring physician, and capturing charges and billing for the procedure. Ordering and scheduling may also be handled by the electronic health record (EHR) system. Although radiology reports originally were transcribed by transcriptionists, nearly all radiology reports today are created using speech recognition systems (SRSs). In the days before RIS and Picture Archival and Communications Systems (PACS), patients would arrive at the imaging department, sometimes with a hand-written note from the ordering physician indicating what the issue was, and the type of examination the physician desired. The radiologist would review the order and determine the precise testing method and often perform it himself (most radiologists at this time were male). Once the examination was completed, the radiologist would hand-write his impression, to be taken back to the ordering physician. By the mid 1940s, it was becoming more common for the report to be typed, but often it was days after the examination was performed that the transcribed report was available to the ordering physician.

Radiology information systems were first designed in the early 1960s, when radiology was largely performed by capturing x-ray images on transparent film stock, so that they would be most optimally visualized when placed on a board or panel that could be illuminated from behind. Nuclear medicine studies were also film-based, and cine film was used for fluoroscopic examinations. Performing the examination involved preparing work lists for the different areas of a department, preparing folders to hold the films of an examination, collating the images and folders into a master folder for each patient, and tracking the folders as they made their way from the area where the examination was performed, to the area where the interpretation was done by the radiologist. Images were interpreted by hanging the films on a lighted panel. If previous examinations had been performed for the patient, especially of the same body region, it was usually necessary to retrieve the master folder or the subfolder with the relevant examinations of that body region from the film library, bring it to the interpretation area, and hang the prior films on the lighted panel alongside the newer images. Once the interpretation was completed, a film library support person would need to refile the new and older images in the subfolder, place the subfolder back into the patient's master folder, and transport it back to the film library for storage.

The earliest systems for managing the internal work of the Radiology Department, such as examination scheduling, folder management, work list preparation, and workflow tracking were developed at Massachusetts General Hospital (MGH) and Johns Hopkins Hospital (JHH) in the late 1960s [1, 12]. In 1970, JHH initiated a prototype information system to process physicians' written orders, produce work lists for the nurses, and generate daily computer-printed, patient drug profiles for the patients' records. The JHH continued to develop this system, eventually producing a product that would run on an IBM 2760, which included the capability for radiologists to use a touch screen to select terms from a lexicon displayed on the screen to create, edit, and sign off on a report [13]. The reporting application became a commercial product called SIREP by the Siemens Corporation and by 1975 was installed in over 100 radiology departments in the United States and Europe. In 1975, a Minirecord (minimal essential record) system was added, which included encounter forms that were filled out at each patient visit and they also contained an area for medications and procedures [23]. In 1976, a radiology reporting system was implemented using a terminal that permitted the radiologist to select phrases with which to compose descriptions and interpretations of x-ray studies. Its output was a computer-printed report that was available as soon as the radiologist completed his interpretation [31].

Bauman, who had worked on the early systems at JHH with Gitlin, moved to Boston in 1969, where he joined the faculty at MGH while working for the Public Health Service (PHS). A resident at MGH, Arenson had been a systems engineer for IBM during his years as an undergraduate and through medical school and internship, and was working on management systems at that time as well. The two teamed up with several systems developers from the Laboratory of Computer Science at MGH directed by Barnett. Arenson became the principal investigator (PI) of a large grant from the Bureau of Radiological Health (Bauman's employment by the PHS made him ineligible to be the PI). Together, they created a system that included such novel concepts as bar code tracking for film folders and a sophisticated scheduling system. The actual radiology report was added to the system in 1978.

After Arenson completed his residency, he joined the faculty at the Hospital of the University of Pennsylvania (HUP), where he immediately began to replicate the MGH system with a number of enhancements including patient tracking with bar codes and some management reports along the lines of modern dashboards. At that time, Jost at Washington University (WU) in St. Louis was independently developing RIS modules including a number of sophisticated management reports.

Jost and Arenson felt that although they could continue to develop RIS software to be used at their respective institutions, a commercial company would be important to the development of the next generation RIS. This joint effort led to the creation of the Radiology Information Systems Consortium (RISC). The concept was to capture the best of breed from systems that were being developed at MGH, HUP, JHH, and WU. The plan was for experienced users and developers from leading institutions to drive the functionality, priorities, and future enhancements. A vendor would be selected that would be responsible for the actual programming, marketing, sales and support. The vendor would be assured of success and hopefully would also shorten the development time for new functions.

A conference of RISC was held in Philadelphia in 1978, by that time including a total of 12 academic sites plus the U.S. Center for Devices and Radiologic Health (CDRH). A request for proposal (RFP) was developed by the 12 institutions, primarily based on input from MGH, HUP and WU, detailing the functional requirements for the RIS. This was followed by a meeting of interested vendors in Philadelphia; after a review of the responses to the RFP, Digital Equipment Corporation (DEC) was selected. Arenson became the Chairman of the board of RISC, and Bauman became the chair of the development task force. That task force met with DEC developers many times over the next few years, and DECrad was born. DECrad was very successful and rapidly became the dominant RIS. It was the RIS used for demonstrating the value of RIS in several reports [15, 16]. DECrad was sold by DEC to IDX Corporation in 1991 and renamed IDXrad, which continued to be the leading RIS up until it was sold to GE in 2005, when it was renamed Imagecast. Throughout these transitions, RISC remained the driving force for this RIS until GE decided to completely rewrite the application using a different database and an entirely new platform, and it was released in 2004 as version 10.

RISs are now widely deployed in nearly every radiology department in the United States and much of the world. They are increasingly being integrated into the EHR as a module because this allows easier extraction of key information for proper examination execution (e.g. an accurate problem list and medication/allergy list), for efficient Computerized Physician Order Entry (CPOE), and efficient reporting and billing.

Beginning in the 1960s, there was considerable activity aimed at capturing radiology reports. Some of the earliest work occurred at the University of Missouri. The team consisted of Lodwick, Lehr, Dwyer, and Templeton. While they would go on to be better known for their PACS efforts, they did work on the reporting systems as well [30]. In addition to the efforts JHH, MGH, HUP, and WU, other work was being done at the Beth Israel Hospital in Boston, the University of Arkansas, and a few other places. While some efforts were simply to have transcriptionists enter the text into computers, there was also recognition of the value of using controlled vocabularies and structure within a report [5–7, 17, 25, 29]. Despite those early efforts, the convenience of dictation was hard to surpass, and most structured approaches did not get much traction. While most entry of the report text was performed by transcriptionists in the early days of radiology, most departments now use SRSs to directly convert the radiologist speech into text. In some cases, there are transcriptionists that listen to the speech while viewing the output of the SRS to correct errors, but accuracy is now high enough that this is becoming rare. While good, SRS is not perfect, and for some speakers and environments, accuracy can suffer. The result can be nonsense phrases, or worse, phrases that make sense but which are wrong. For example, the dictation might have been "There is no evidence of tumor recurrence." while the SRS might transcribe "There is now evidence of tumor recurrence." Work on algorithms to 'understand' the text and highlight potentially ambiguous words, or phrases that are in conflict with other phrases in the report may help to address these problems. However, for the example above, both sentences make 'sense' and so another approach is to highlight key words (e.g. 'left' and 'right') as well as words that have low scores, and thus are more likely to be incorrect.

Structured reporting (SR) is another approach to improving report accuracy and readability and to make computer mining of reports more feasible. Rather than allowing free text dictation, SR recognizes the type of examination done, and provides a template for the radiologists to fill out. In this way, standardized terms (for example, *RadLex*, the lexicon published by the Radiological Society of North America) can be used which helps reduce ambiguity for humans and computers. Such templates can be expected of all members of a department in order to increase consistency of style. It is also possible to require certain fields to increase compliance with mandates such as the Joint Commission's. An example of this is specific information that must be included in the reports of head CTs performed on patients with suspected acute stroke.

Another potential benefit of SR is templates that promote the use of specific measurements, encouraging quantitative techniques rather than just qualitative assessments. This is becoming more important as better quantitative imaging methods are being developed and validated for certain diseases. SR also appears to improve the completeness of reports by prompting the radiologist to complete each component of the template. One of the most successful applications has been in breast imaging, where a standardized vocabulary for reporting called Breast Imaging Reporting and Data System® (BI-RADS®) developed under the auspices of the American College of Radiology (ACR) has gone through several updates since its introduction in the early 1990s [2]. By its use being required as part of the accreditation process for mammography imaging facilities since the late 1990s, BI-RADS® has enabled many research studies to be conducted that tracked imaging morphology to pathologic findings, imaging performance/quality monitoring, and outcomes.

15.2 Picture Archival and Communications Systems

Radiology information systems contained most of the information to allow radiologists to get their work done. The one important piece they lacked was the images themselves. Initially, most images were on film and would need to be scanned in order to be available in computer form. Even if directly generated by computer, the data files needed to represent images were too large to store, transmit, and display using standard computer technology of the time.

From the time of the first computerized tomography (CT) scanners, scientists were developing ways to render images in a photo-realistic three-dimensional (3D) manner. The first digital images were created in the mid-1970s with the introduction of computerized axial tomography (CAT), as CT was originally called. Since that time, scanners are used to acquire images in other planes, and so the 'axial' part of the name was removed, and today, they are called CT scanners. CT has been considered one of the biggest advances in medical technology since the invention of the x-ray, and earned Cormack and Hounsfield the 1979 Nobel Prize. In the early 1970s they developed the first practical CT scanning system for general health care; and with CT scanning many soft internal tissues could be seen for the first time [3].

In 1975, CT scans used in hospitals cost about 1 million dollars. Typical examinations would consist of 20–50 images, usually 1 cm thick. In the 1980s Kalendar introduced helical or spiral CT, in which the patient is moved through the gantry, while the x-rays are being acquired. This allows more rapid acquisition of CT images. In the early 2000s, multi-detector CT (MDCT) was introduced. Up to that time, there was a single x-ray source, and a single row of detectors. MDCT allows even more rapid acquisition of images because multiple slices are acquired at the same time. Today, a typical CT examination will have 100s to 1,000s of images.

Magnetic resonance imaging (MRI), considered to be a new way of looking inside of living organisms, resulted in Lauterbur sharing with Mansfield the Nobel prize in 2003 for its development. The nuclei of some atoms (particularly hydrogen) act as tiny magnets that tend to align in the presence of a magnetic field; the atoms will emit a radio wave that is proportional to the strength of the magnetic field. Lauterbur created a gradient in the magnetic field so the frequency of the radio could be used to determine the location in a tissue sample. Mansfield developed mathematical techniques for analyzing the data, so the images could be stacked together to form a 3D view [8].

In the 1980s, MRI scanners cost about 2 million dollars. Typical examinations were about 100 images, consisting of two or three image or contrast types (T1-weighted, T2-weighted, and proton-density were common image types). Since the original scanners, important advances include the ability to acquire multiple slices at the same time (3D) or in an interleaved fashion, allowing many more images to be acquired during an examination. Many new image/contrast types have been developed, including fluid-attenuated inversion recovery (FLAIR), suscepti- bility weighted imaging (SWI), magnetic resonance angiography (MRA), fat- and water-saturated sequences, diffusion imaging, perfusion imaging, functional imaging, and many more. Today, typical MRI examinations typically have 100s to 1,000s of images.

Both CT and MRI images were rendered onto film for interpretation in the early days, and transported to reading rooms in that form. Other traditional modalities transitioned to direct digital capture, including plain films, fluoroscopy, nuclear medicine, and ultrasound, but for a while, the exam folders and master folders continued to be the main way of storing and moving the images around the radiology department and hospital. This became increasingly burdensome with the multiplicity of images introduced by the newer modalities such as CT and MRI, and the need for viewing them interactively in order to view the entire dynamic range (gray scale) and contrast (window and level) settings, zoom, view time series and comparisons, do measurements, and as noted above, 3D rendering and feature extraction.

As a result, a separate system called a PACS was developed that had special computing hardware to deal with the images. In particular, the system had special storage to deal with the 'large' size of the images (each radiographic image is typically 10 MB), when the typical hard disk drive at the time could store only 5 MB. Ethernet was invented in 1983 but was not widely available, so special transmission systems were often required (the speed was 10 megabits per second, but the bandwidth was shared among all computers on the network, compared to today's switched networks where each computer often has its own dedicated circuit). Computer displays at the time were usually text terminals, so special graphical displays were required, but again, the images were higher resolution than most graphics terminals could display.

A number of early pioneers created systems that one could call precursors of PACS. Among these were Dwyer, Lodwick, and Kruger, who worked on computer diagnoses on workstations [11, 18, 22]. They faced the challenges of needing to store a sufficient number of images to be clinically relevant. The images could be stored locally, so network performance was not an issue, but local storage devices had small capacity compared to the images. In important issue was the display system. Cathode ray tubes (CRTs) were the dominant display system, using either a raster-scanning system (such as for commercial television) or vector-based graphics (where each 'stroke' of a line had to be drawn individually). One important challenge of using commercial television-class displays was that they had only about 270 unique lines of resolution, far below the resolution of film. Even though display cards could provide higher resolution, the displays also had poor performance over time – the phosphors used decayed, particularly those phosphors that had high brightness, such as were required in most interpretation environments [24]. Despite these limitations, many in the field could see that computer displays were the future.

Other notable steps in the advancement of digital radiology were led by Capp, who was an early investigator of teleradiology in the early 1970s. In 1977, Mistretta created Digital Subtraction Angiography (DSA) that really generated interest in digital imaging. Huang was performing image processing on CT images in 1977, and Kundel worked on image perception in 1979, also with digital images. In the early 1980s Prewitt and Duerinckx were beginning to talk about storing and retrieving digital images and may have been the first to use the term PACS [9]. In 1982,

Arenson at HUP created remote archiving and display for portable chest x-rays in the ICU under a grant from the NIH. With his colleagues, Arenson developed fiber optic transmission to a remote VAX for image processing and storage. The ability to store and transmit images on a network resource seems very mundane today, but it was an important advance for the field.

The first conference on PACS was in Newport Beach, California, in 1982, sponsored by the Society of Photo-optical Imaging Engineers (SPIE). Slightly before this, Dwyer had described what might be the first functional PACS. Because the standard network technology was not able to rapidly transmit the 'large' images, there were two main options that PACS vendors used to address the challenge. These two options were referred to as 'centralized' versus 'distributed' PACS. As the terms imply, a centralized PACS stored all images in a central server, and relied on special high-performance hardware to transmit the images to the display station. In these early days of PACS, there was active debate about the proper architecture for PACS. The LORAL Aerospace PACS installed at some of the military facilities was designed with all images stored on a single high performance server with all workstations connected to it via a dedicated unidirectional fiber optic cable that transmitted the image data to the workstations, plus an Ethernet connection for all other communications. The alternative was a distributed system where images were routed from the imaging device to the appropriate workstation(s) for interpretation, and then routed on to the PACS for storage and retrieval. In cases where the work was predictable, the latter worked well and did not require the dedicated and proprietary data cable. The PACS architecture debate is no longer an issue because standard technology (large central servers and gigabit Ethernet) can store and transmit images to workstations in a timely fashion. LORAL leveraged its expertise in satellite imaging to develop such a system. The system was selected for a large Army hospital contract because of its ability to 'display any image, anywhere in 2 seconds.' The alternative was to build rules about where images are likely to be viewed, and route them prior to the physician request. While this sounds reasonable, in practice, medicine was too unpredictable for this to be successful. Today, the high performance of standard hardware combined with streaming protocols has made centralized systems the standard.

A watershed event for PACS was the Digital Imaging Network/Picture Archiving and Communications System (DIN/PACS) contract, where the Department of Defense released a RFP for a PACS for some of its hospitals. This was an important step in legitimizing PACS as a viable way to practice radiology. The first installation of a PACS that utilized a standard data representation for images known as ACR/NEMA was at Fort Detrick in 1992. (The standard known as American College of Radiology/National Electrical Manufacturers Association or ACR/NEMA is described in greater detail below). Shortly thereafter, a fully filmless installation was successful at Madigan Army Medical Center at Fort Lewis, Washington. The Walter Reed Army Medical Center in Washington, DC, cooperated with Johns Hopkins in conducting a baseline study of the image storage and retrieval equipment for the radiology department. In addition, the National Naval Medical Center at Bethesda had two major interests in utilizing DIN/PACS. The Center in Bethesda was responsible for providing medical care and consults with a number of Navy bases within 100 miles, of which Patuxent Naval Air Station was one of the more important. There were high costs associated with patients traveling between the Naval Air Station and Bethesda Naval Hospital. Having a teleradiology connection and other links available improved the promptness of diagnosis and treatment and reduced the costs of transferring patients to Bethesda.

The first completely filmless hospital in the United States was the Baltimore Veterans Administration hospital, which opened its doors as a filmless facility in 1993. Siegel was selected to be the chair of the department and was instrumental of the design of the department and also played a critical role in implementation, and early studies on the value and best practices for a filmless department [28].

As noted above, PACS implementations used special network technology to transmit images in an acceptable time frame within a hospital. Today, standard network technology is fast enough for PACS. The bigger challenge today is image transmission between hospitals that have merged and which are many miles apart. Such mergers are resulting in the development of workflow systems that are responsible for managing RIS and PACS information across multiple hospitals, and perform routing much like the PACS of the early days. These workflow systems assure that different identifiers for a given patient are properly handled, and assure that prior examinations are available anywhere in the system. They help to assure timely reporting of examinations even when the images are acquired in a location far away from the radiologist.

Another important trend that is changing the original architecture of radiology information systems is the vendor neutral archive (VNA). The key concept of a VNA is that it can store any image and optionally the report, and can respond to a query from any PACS/RIS to provide the images and report. This system relies on the successor of the ACR/NEMA standard known as DICOM, described further below. Some VNAs can also manage the mapping of patient identifiers for different health systems. By centralizing the storage, it is a single location that must be queried when EHRs attempt to display images. By decoupling from the production servers of the PACS, it means that the task of migrating data is not required when a new PACS or RIS is installed.

15.3 Teleradiology

An important category of medicine is the remote provision of medical care. Teleradiology is the interpretation of images obtained at a distant site, and was a particularly interesting capability. One of the earliest production teleradiology systems was developed by Dwyer for Leavenworth prison. Teleradiology and limited wide-area network speeds were strong drivers for the use of irreversible or 'lossy' image compression. Substantial work was put into studying how lossy compression could be used to minimize the impact of relatively slow connections while not degrading diagnostic performance. Many early attempts used mathematical measures (e.g., Peak Signal to Noise Ratio and Root Mean Squared Error) of the information present in an image before and after compression. However, there was disappointingly poor correlation between such measures and diagnostic performance. Ultimately, it was found that observer performance tests needed to be performed for each imaging modality to establish the acceptable compression level, and even then, it was clear that a particular ratio was not appropriate for every image of one type. In some cases, lossy compression was found to actually improve performance, likely because it removes noise [27]. Another surprise was that the use of 3D compression methods did not perform substantially better than 2D methods even for thin-slice CT where there is great similarity in image content from slice to slice [11].

There is now a blending of teleradiology and PACS. While interpretation from home was a large driver for teleradiology in the past, 'nighthawk services' were developed that contracted with radiology groups to interpret examinations during the night. These services (and, increasingly, merged hospitals) have subspecialists interpreting examinations 24 h per day, as a part of a routine shift.

15.4   ACR/NEMA and DICOM

A significant advance in the practice of digital radiology was the development of the ACR/NEMA standard, later renamed Digital Communications in Medicine or DICOM. Challenges in digital imaging and PACS were noted as early as the first SPIE meetings on the topic in the early 1980s. CT and MR scanners were becoming more common, but each vendor and model stored the image data in a proprietary format. One had to view images from a given system on the electronic console that came with that scanner. Researchers that wished to do more than just look at the images had to sign Non-Disclosure Agreements in order to access the digital image data. The desire for multi-function, multi-modality interpretation workstations was also severely hampered by these incompatibilities. It was clear to some leaders in the radiology field that this was hindering progress, and so the American College of Radiology (ACR) worked with the National Electrical Manufacturers Association (NEMA) to develop a standard for image data. The official effort began in 1983, when members of the ACR combined with the NEMA with the expressed purpose of developing a standard for exchanging medical images.

There were many key players from academia involved in the development of the ACR/NEMA standard. Among them were Dwyer, Horii, and Clunie. The role of industry in the standard was critical, and included people from each of the major vendors, including Hindle from Philips and Parisot from GE. The first version of ACR/NEMA was released in 1985, and included not only the information content, but also a hardware mechanism for exchanging images, including a 100-pin connector. This first version was a good start in setting the right direction but was not widely adopted – very few CT or MR scanners ever had the 100-pin connector, for example.

Version 2 was released in 1988, and allowed for transmission over EIA-485, which meant existing computer transmission hardware could be used. Several vendors demonstrated the transmission of images via V2.0 in 1990, with commercial availability of equipment at the 1990 RSNA convention. The first large deployment of V2.0 was at Fort Detrick, Maryland, in 1992. Because few existing image-creating devices existed, the system utilized 'gateways' from DeJarnette Systems to convert the proprietary format images to V2.0 and then transmitted them to the PACS, which had been jointly developed by Siemens and Loral Aerospace Systems.

In 1993, the third version of the ACR/NEMA standard was released under the name DICOM in order to increase the acceptance outside the United States and outside of radiology. It also provided a much more flexibly and object-oriented style information model. The standard described 'tags' for various pieces of information about the image, including required elements like the dimensions of the image, patient name, and examination date. There were also optional fields defined and optional 'private' tags that vendors could use for their own purposes. DICOM continues to be updated (large changes are referred to as 'supplements') as new imaging methods and requirements develop, and is a good example of academic and industry partnership.

Because DICOM is focused on the image component of radiology department activities, items like orders, reports, and billing information are communicated by Health Level 7 (HL7). Compared to the highly specified information model of DICOM (some might say 'rigid'), HL7 is much more flexible in the way that information can be communicated. The problem with such flexibility is that two systems that communicate using HL7 may not be able to work well together. An organization called 'Integrating the Healthcare Enterprise' (IHE) was formed by the Radiological Society of North America (RSNA) and the Healthcare Information Management Systems Society (HIMSS) to define preferred implementations (referred to as 'profiles') for accomplishing specific tasks. As with DICOM, this effort began with a focus on radiology departments, but now has profiles for most of medicine.

One recent focus of effort is on sharing medical information between medical enterprises. IHE profiles describe ways to exchange patient identifiers, and subsequently, medical information, between health care enterprises. One recent effort funded by the National Institute of Biomedical Imaging and Engineering (NIBIB) is focused on using IHE standard mechanisms to provide patients with images in digital form, replacing the widespread use of compact discs for image exchange.

15.5   Three-Dimensional and Computer-Aided Diagnosis

In the 1960s, Warner's medical information system's computer order entry and results reporting (CPOE/RR) application was linked to its HELP decision-support capabilities. When an x-ray order was entered, the computer automatically presented the reason for the order, and retrieved any previous x-ray reports and relevant laboratory data; and a Bayesian analysis was applied to this order to provide the five most probable findings [14]. While this constitutes an important form of decision support for radiology, it is focused on helping the ordering physician.

Computer Aided Diagnosis (CAD) as applied to radiology generally focuses on assisting the radiologist in detecting a lesion (Computer Aided Detection or CADe), determining the most likely diagnoses for a lesion (Computer Aided Differential Diagnosis or CADx), or determining if there is a change in a lesion compared to a prior examination, such as for assessing a cancer therapy (Computer Aided Change Detection or CACD). The adoption of CAD in radiology has been slower than some might have expected. One of the earliest attempts to leverage computation for image interpretation was by Lindberg and Lodwick [19–21].

Current algorithms seem to mostly improve reliability ("Computer Aided Diligence") particularly for less experienced radiologists, or for cases where fatigue might be a factor. One of the earliest successes (and the first CAD algorithm to be reimbursed by CMS) was a CAD system for mammography [7]. This system was widely employed in the 'second look' mode, where a radiologist would first review the images and attempt to identify masses. Then the CAD results would be shown, to help assure masses were not missed. Such algorithms would often show 'false positives' but are generally designed to be more sensitive and let the radiologist decide that possible lesions are not true masses.

CAD algorithms are available for other imaging types. CT colonography (CTC) or virtual colonoscopy involves the laborious task of trying to find polyps in 2D and 3D images made by CT scanners when the colon is insufflated with CO_2 gas. Much like mammography, this is a task that can cause fatigue. Stool can also appear much like polyps, making the task more challenging. The value of CAD for CTC has been debated but now is generally accepted and reimbursed. Detection of small lung metastases and small pulmonary emboli is also a daunting search task where computer algorithms are rather regularly applied.

Another related focus is visualization, which includes a number of approaches such as 3D rendering, rotation, registration of multiple modalities, and changes in images over time or as a result of an intervention. If the surface of a structure of interest can be defined from multiple 2D slices, it is possible to create a 3D rendering of the surface using knowledge of optics. These surface renderings utilize the same ideas and technology as much of the early computer-generated movie industry like PIXAR. One of the popular early 3D rendering systems was Analyze [26], which had tools for reading the proprietary image formats and creating 3D images for the 2D slices, as well as making measurements. Such renderings are now commonplace and expected, particularly for vascular imaging where the shape of vessels is critical.

For some diagnostic and therapeutic tasks, 3D measurements are more important than images. One such example is in surgical planning for liver resections and donations. In such cases where resection of a portion of the liver is contemplated, computer measurement of the volume that would remain with the patient/donor (and contributed to a recipient in case of transplant) must be computed, but reception lines can only occur along anatomic segments. There is a required volume of liver tissue per kilogram of lean body mass to keep a human alive, and only careful 3D measurements allow such treatment options. Another application is in mesial temporal sclerosis, where precise measurement of the hippocampus can enable successful surgery. Precise measurement of a patient's aorta and major branches allows creation of a custom endograft for treatment of aortic aneurysm. In the future, it is likely that more such applications of precise measurement based on 3D imaging.

15.6　Conclusion

Radiology has benefited tremendously from the advent of computers. In tandem with medical informatics generally, radiology has benefited from improved operations management and business execution by using computers. The unique properties of radiology reports, with constrained vocabulary and a characteristics style made some aspects of computerization much more feasible than in many other medical specialties. Radiology also faced unique challenges of having to acquire, transmit, display, and store medical image – images that continue to challenge some of the technologies available to us today.

References

1. Alcox RW, Gitlin JN, Miller JW. Preliminary study of automatic data processing applications to diagnostic radiology at the Johns Hopkins Hospital. The Johns Hopkins University, School of Hygiene and Public Health, Baltimore, MD; 1967.
2. American College of Radiology. Breast imaging reporting and data systems (BI-RADS®). Reston: American College of Radiology; 1992.
3. Baker Jr HL, Campbell JK, Houser OW, Reese DF, Sheedy PF, Holman CB. Computer assisted tomography of the head. An early evaluation. Mayo Clin Proc. 1974;49:17–27.
4. Barnhard H, Long J. Automatic coding and manipulating of radiology diagnostic reports. Proc conf on the use of computers in radiology. 20–23 Oct 1996. University of Missouri; 1968.
5. Bauman R, Pendergrass H, Greenes R, Kalayan B. Further development of an on-line computer system for radiology reporting. Proc conf on computer applications in radiology. DHEW Pub No (FDA) 73-8018. 1972: 409–22.
6. Brolin I. Automatic typing and transmitting of radiological reports. Proc conf on the use of computers in radiology. 20–23 Oct 1996. University of Missouri; 1968.
7. Chan H, Doi K, Lam K, Vyborny CJ, Schmidt RA, Metz CE. Digital characterization of clinical mammographic microcalcifications: applications in computer-aided detection. Proc society photo-optical instrumentation engineers. Med Imaging II. 1988;914-A:591–3.
8. Chang R, Huang S, Moon WK, Lee Y, Chen D. Solid breast masses: neural network analysis of vascular features at three-dimensional power doppler US for benign or malignant classification 1. Radiology. 2007;243:56–62.
9. Duerinckx AJ, Pisa E. Filmless picture archiving and communication in diagnostic radiology. Proc SPIE. 1982;318:9–18. Reprinted in IEEE Computer Society Proc PACS.
10. Dwyer III SJ, Harlow CA, Ausherman D, Lodwick G, et al. Computer diagnosis of radiographic images. Proc Soc Photo-Opt Instrum Eng, Appl Opt Instrum Med. 1972;35:106–30.

11. Erickson BJ, Krupinski E, Andriole KP. A multicenter observer performance study of 3D JPEG2000 compression of thin-slice CT. J Digit Imaging. 2010;23:639–43.
12. Gitlin JN, Margulies S. Application of computer techniques to selected diagnostic radiology operations. Proc Am Pub Health Assn. Detroit, MI; 1968:na.
13. Gitlin JN. Application of automatic data processing techniques to selected diagnostic radiology operations. Rockville: US Department of Health, Education and Welfare; 1974.
14. Johnson D, Ranzenberger J, Pryor TA. Nursing applications of the HELP system. Proc SCAMC. 1984;703–8.
15. Jost RG, Rodewald SS, Hill RL, Evens RG. A computer system to monitor radiology department activity: a management tool to improve patient care. Radiology. 1982;145:347–50.
16. Jost RG, Trachtman J, Hill RL, Smith BA, Evens RG. A computer system for transcribing radiology reports. Radiology. 1980;136:63–6.
17. Kricheff II, Korein J. Computer processing of narrative data: progress and problems. Proc 1966 conf on the use of computers in radiology. 20–23 Oct 1966. University of Missouri; 1968.
18. Lehr J, Lodwick G, Garrotto L, Manson D, Nicholson B. MARS: Missouri Automated Radiology System. Proc Joint Conf Amer Fed Info Proc Societies. ACM. 1972: 999–1003.
19. Lindberg D. Computer failures and successes. South Med Bull. 1969;57:18–21.
20. Lindberg D. Electronic retrieval of clinical data. J Med Educ. 1965;40:753–9.
21. Lindberg DAB. A statewide medical information system. Comput Biomed Res. 1970;3:453–63.
22. Lodwick GS. The history of the use of computers in the interpretation of radiological images. Proc ACM con on history of medical informatics. ACM. 1987: 85–94.
23. McColligan E, Blum B, Brunn C. An automated care medical record system for ambulatory care. In: Kaplan B, Jelovsek RF, editors. Proc SCM/SAMS joint conf on ambulatory med. 1981. p. 72–6.
24. Mizusawa K. The perceptual image formation processes of brightness contrast. Proc society of photo-optical instrumentation engineers. Appl Opt Instrum Med II. 1974;43:59–62.
25. Pendergrass HP, Greenes RA, Barnett GO, Poitras JW, Pappalardo AN, Marble CW. An on-line computer facility for systematized input of radiology reports 1. Radiology. 1969;92:709–13.
26. Robb R, Hanson D, Karwoski R, Larson A, Workman E, Stacy M. Analyze: a comprehensive, operator-interactive software package for multidimensional medical image display and analysis. Comput Med Imaging Graph. 1989;13:433–54.
27. Savcenko V, Erickson BJ, Palisson PM, Persons KR, Manduca A, Hartman TE, et al. Detection of subtle abnormalities on chest radiographs after irreversible compression. Radiology. 1998;206:609–16.
28. Siegel EL, Kolodner RM. Filmless radiology. New York: Springer; 2001.
29. Simon M, Leeming BW, Bleich HL, Reiffen B, Byrd J, Blair D, et al. Computerized radiology reporting using coded language 1. Radiology. 1974;113:343–9.
30. Templeton AW, Lodwick G, Sides S. RADIATE: a radiology and hospital computer oriented communicating system. Proc conf on the use of computers in radiology. 20–23 Oct 1966. University of Missouri; 1968.
31. Wheeler PS, Simborg DW, Gitlin JN. The Johns Hopkins radiology reporting system. Radiology. 1976;119:315–9.

Chapter 16
Public and Personal Health Testing Systems

Morris F. Collen and Harold P. Lehmann

Abstract The explicit relationship between the clinical environment and public health dates from the 1878 Act of Congress, which authorized the U.S. Public Health Service to collect morbidity reports for quarantinable diseases. In the 1970s, hospital infection surveillance programs began to employ computer databases; in the 1980s, state health departments developed computer-based systems to monitor communicable diseases. Subsequent developments of databases and techniques such as data mining improved detection and facilitated alerts; compliance with reporting accelerated once direct connections were instituted between clinical laboratories and public health agencies. Personal health testing systems (HTS) also evolved, with the use of multiple tests in what became known as multiphasic screening. By 1965, Kaiser Permanente was using automated multiphasic health testing (AMHT) systems in two clinics in Northern California to provide systemized personal health checkups, including features described later as clinical decision support. By the early 1970s, AMHT systems had spread into many health care facilities, for a range of uses that included pre-admission screening of hospital patients and online records of outpatient encounters, both nationally and internationally. In the 1980s funding and reimbursement issues led to the termination of most AMHT programs; at Kaiser Permanente, AMHT was integrated into its larger systems. Since 2001, the CDC has funded the development of real time surveillance systems that take daily Health Level 7 feeds directly from clinical information systems as part of syndromic surveillance, a criterion in CDC's meaningful use program.

Keywords Automated multiphasic health testing • Biosurveillance • Public health informatics • Personal health screening • Realtime surveillance systems • Communicable disease monitoring • Infection surveillance • Syndromic surveillance

---

Author was deceased at the time of publication.

M.F. Collen (deceased)

H.P. Lehmann, M.D., Ph.D. (✉)
Division of Health Sciences Informatics, Johns Hopkins School of Medicine,
Baltimore, MD, USA
e-mail: Lehmann@jhmi.edu

© Springer-Verlag London 2015   673
M.F. Collen, M.J. Ball (eds.), *The History of Medical Informatics in the United States*, Health Informatics, DOI 10.1007/978-1-4471-6732-7_16

16.1   Public Health Biosurveillance Systems

The explicit relationship between the clinical environment and public health dates from the 1878 Act of Congress, which authorized the US Public Health Service to collect morbidity reports for quarantinable diseases. The Centers for Disease Control (CDC) in Atlanta established a surveillance system to monitor infectious diseases in the United States. Data collected at the state and local levels were centralized in federal level databases to provide national morbidity reporting and disease-specific surveillance data: Notifiable disease reporting (46 conditions, at that time); laboratory-based surveillance (with links to the Notifiable-disease reporting system); the National Nosocomial Infection Study; the National Electronic Injury Surveillance System; and other disease-specific systems [40].

Since then, the notion of "surveillance" has taken on several meanings: (1) Screen for, locate, and track cases of "notifiable" and other diseases, whether at birth, upon immigration, or intercurrently; (2) Identify outbreaks of disease; and (3) Assess disease burden in the community or even in a hospital or health system.

Prior to the 1800s health screening tests were provided to immigrants as a public health measure by the Marine Hospital Service in order to identify those with a contagious disease such as tuberculosis and syphilis, or with a significant chronic disease, such as diabetes, who might become a healthcare burden to the country. In 1930 mass screening techniques were applied by the US Public Service for the detection of syphilis and tuberculosis [4]. Petrie and associates [32] reported employing mass screening techniques in Atlanta, when between 1945 and 1950 more than one million residents voluntarily took multiple health screening tests; and they introduced the term multiphasic screening as an extension of mass screening.

Breslow [4] and public health associates in San Jose, California, popularized multiphasic screening as an efficient way of providing a group of routine health tests; and Garfield [18] advocated multiphasic testing as an efficient entry mode to patient care, and an effective way to establish databases for multiple diseases.

Thomas [41], a consultant to the international Organization of Economic Cooperation and Development (OECD) in which the United States was a member-country, described the functions of databases in public agencies. He emphasized that their databases were usually very large, and the way their databases were organized had a marked influence on all of their activities. He also advised that since access to public information could mean political power, and since automation often involved great changes in access to information, a balance between the increased efficiency of large database management systems for public administration needed to be balanced with adequate participatory decision making. In the United States centralized procurement for federal agencies was established by the Brooks Act in 1965; however, the control and use of automated data processing were not to be controlled or interfered with in any way. Most of the data in public health databases were composed of appropriate data collected in standardized formats from individual healthcare providers and medical centers, and from city, county, state, and/or national public health agencies. Some of the data in public administration databases were needed to assure accurate personal identification, but most data were used for operative and planning purposes.

In the 1970s hospital infection surveillance programs began to employ computer databases to augment prior manual monitoring methods. In 1980 Hierholzer [23] and Streed at the University of Iowa Hospitals and Clinics initiated and installed an online infection control surveillance database on an IBM 370/3033 system in order to supplant existing manual collation methods as well as to provide a number of summary reports [34]. A team with special training in epidemiology and infection control methods, using criteria established by the CDC, collected, collated, and entered the data. A study comparing the automated methods to the prior manual methods showed the new system saved time for both data collection and report generation. The system provided several new reports, including antibiotic sensitivity reports, surgical infection rate reports, and notification of potential epidemics reports; it also supported related research and education programs [34].

Going beyond the hospital, in 1980 LaVenture and associates [25] at the Wisconsin State Department of Health, initiated a Computer Assisted Disease Surveillance System (CASS) that consisted of a database written in a version of the MUMPS program [2] for individual patient's case records, and provided summary monthly and yearly disease trends. CASS was used to support the needs of their epidemiologists to monitor, prevent, and control communicable diseases. Their objectives were to systematically collect reports of infectious diseases for the population in their specified region; consolidate the data into reports with meaningful summary tables, graphs and charts; interpret the data to detect outbreaks and describe trends of disease or of factors determining disease; and regularly disseminate summary data with interpretation to physicians, hospitals, and to other public health agencies. Wise [44] reported using a Radio Shack TRS-80 Model III microcomputer with floppy disc drives and a set of programs written in Basic language to capture patients' demographic and infection data and to assist with infection control monitoring and reporting at Mt. Sinai Hospital. The database included files that permitted the system to generate appropriate periodic infection surveillance reports, including hospital locations of infected patients, frequencies of the sites of infections of the body, and sensitivities of the infecting organisms to antibiotics.

In 1987 the CDC established a surveillance database in the state of Washington for the reporting of patients infected with *Escherichia coli* serotype O157:H7. This organism was first discovered in 1982, as a human pathogen that caused bloody diarrhea that was sometimes associated with serious complications (hemolytic uremia syndrome) [36]. In 1987 this CDC database reported 93 patients, yielding an annual incidence of 2.1 cases per 100,000 population. Ostroff [31] noted that monitoring the occurrence of such infections improved the detection of outbreaks and provided information leading to better therapy.

In 1988 the Healthcare Cost and Utilization Project (HCUP), a group of healthcare databases was developed through a Federal-State-Industry partnership sponsored by the Agency for Healthcare Research and Quality (AHRQ) [21]. HCUP databases brought together the data collection efforts of state organizations, hospital associations, private data organizations, and the Federal government to create a large national database of patient level healthcare data. Starting in 1988 HCUP data-bases included: (1) the Nationwide Inpatient Sample (NIS) with inpatient data from a sample of more than 1,000 hospitals; (2) the Kids' Inpatient Databases (KID) starting in 1997 with a nationwide sample of pediatric inpatient discharges; (3) the State Inpatient Databases (SID) starting in 1995 with inpatient discharge abstracts from participating states; (4) the State Ambulatory Surgery Databases (SASD) starting in 1997 with data from hospital and freestanding ambulatory surgery encounters, and (5) the State Emergency Department Databases (SEDD) starting in 1999 with data from hospital-affiliated emergency departments for visits not result-ing in hospitalization [21].

Brossette and associates [5], at the University of Alabama at Birmingham, applied data mining techniques based on association rules to attempt to discover early and unsuspected, useful patterns of hospital-based infections and antimicro-bial resistance from the analysis of their hospital's clinical laboratory data. Clinical experts in this field of knowledge developed rule templates for identifying data sets likely to be associated with specified adverse events and a historical database was mined to create specific association rules that fit those templates. During use, when statistical high levels of these rule based datasets occurred within a specified time period, the system would provide an alert signal for the possible occurrence of an adverse event. They reported the results of a version of their Data Mining Surveillance System (DMSS) that analyzed inpatient microbiology culture data col-lected over 15 months in their University Hospital. They found their DMSS was able to provide alerts for a possible increase in numbers of resistant bacterial infec-tions that might have been undetected by traditional epidemiological methods.

The National Center for Biotechnology Information (NCBI) of the NLM devel-oped a pathogen detection pipeline in conjunction with an FDA project which aimed to rapidly identify pathogenic isolates in order to combat outbreaks of foodborne illness and antibiotic resistant hospital infections [29].

Computer applications for the public health essential service of surveillance [33] developed independently of clinical systems [27]. Compliance with reporting accel-erated once direct connections were instituted between clinical laboratories and public health agencies. The 9/11 and the anthrax attacks of 2001 spurred the US government and CDC to fund development of surveillance systems more tied to clinical practice. The focus was on realtime systems that could take daily Health Level 7 feeds (i.e., directly from clinical information systems) of free text patient chief complaints from emergency departments, in a process called syndromic sur-veillance [22]. These systems, established as CDC-funded Public Health Informatics Centers of Excellence, were the Electronic Surveillance System for the Early Notification of Community-based Epidemics, or ESSENCE [26], Real-Time Outbreak and Disease Surveillance, or RODS [42], and Automated Epidemiological Geotemporal Integrated Surveillance, or AEGIS [35]. The success of these systems in multiple localities stimulated the CDC's meaningful use (MU) program to include syndromic surveillance as one of its optional criteria in Stage 1 and a required cri-terion for Stage 2 for eligible professionals, eligible hospitals, and critical access hospitals in order to participate in incentive programs for the Medicare and Medicaid Electronic Health Record (EHR).

In the second edition of *Public Health Informatics and Information Systems,* Magnuson and Fu [28] provide a comprehensive look at public health informatics in areas beyond surveillance.

The early 2000s saw the rise of novel sources of data for surveillance, both Internet search engines [19] and social media [6]. The potential in public health for social media is much broader than surveillance [17]. Hospitals began using these source as signals for patient (customer) "sentiment" and other indicators of quality care [20]. These applications of informatics move beyond patient-based screening, to personal health testing systems, as essential public health services.

16.2 Evolution of Personal Health Testing Systems (HTS)

Before 1900 public health screening was applied to immigrants to identify those with significant disease who might become a burden to the country. In 1930 mass screening techniques were applied by the US Public Service for the detection of syphilis and tuberculosis [4]. Petrie and associates [32] exploited the capabilities of mass screening techniques in Atlanta, where between 1945 and 1950 more than one million residents voluntarily took multiple health screening tests, and applied the term *multiphasic screening* to the extension of mass screening. Breslow and associates in San Jose, California, popularized multiphasic screening as a more efficient way of providing combinations of tests, and advocated follow-up healthcare services in conjunction with screening programs [3]. In 1948 an editorial in the *Journal of the American Medical Association* [24] proposed that in contrast to the periodic health examinations traditionally provided by physicians, and commonly called "health checkups", health screening procedures could be widely applied, were relatively inexpensive, and required relatively little time of physicians.

In 1963 a health risk appraisal (HRA) program was initiated by Robbins, chief of the Cancer Control Branch, Division of Chronic Diseases of the US Public Health Service, and Sadusk at George Washington University School of Medicine. The program related the results of procedures performed in personal health examinations to relative health hazards of an individual, using tables that provided the probability of death on an age and sex basis, based on data that showed 60 % of all deaths in any age group were due to approximately 15 causes. They proposed this approach to appraising probable personal health hazards provided a feasible personal preventive medicine program. Based on the premise that each person had an individual set of health hazards for each age-sex-race group, and supplemented with the person's family and past history findings and the results of a personal health examination, the HRA provided an appraisal of the probable risk of death for a person and advised that person how an individualized preventive medicine plan could decrease the identified health risks [37]. In the 1980s health risk appraisals were used by a variety of healthcare professionals and were reported to be useful for members of health maintenance organizations [16].

16.3   Development of Multiphasic Health Testing Systems (MHTS)

In 1963 Collen and associates [7] at Kaiser Permanente (KP) in Northern California developed and began operating multiphasic health testing (MHT) systems in their San Francisco and Oakland medical centers to provide systemized personal health checkups. In 1965 they added the data processing power of an IBM 1440 computer to develop automated multiphasic health testing (AMHT) systems. The extension of the use of the computer from the clinical laboratory directly into its use for routine periodic health examinations exploited its potential for supporting direct patient care. As online procedures, while the patient was still present, the computer processed the information from: (1) the punched cards for anthropometry and blood chemistry; (2) all data collected from the examinee including a self-reported health questionnaire that was acquired by the examinee sorting a deck of punched cards into separate sets of "Yes" or "No" responses (with comparisons to responses from any prior questionnaires); (3) a group of physiological measurements (blood pressure, spirometry, visual and hearing acuity, height and weight); (4) physicians' interpretations of an electrocardiogram, chest x-ray, and breast x-rays in women over age 50; and (5) urine tests, blood hemoglobin test and a white cell count. The punched cards were read by a card reader into the data communication system; and the data were stored in the central computer in Oakland. An online summary report for the physician contained all test results, any alert flags, and suggested likely diagnoses to consider [7–9, 12].

In the first 3 years, 12,500 examination records were stored on magnetic tape using a fixed field, fixed format design that was economical to program, and also permitted rapid storage and retrieval of any specific data collected for any single examination. The data collected included patient's identification, appointment schedules, registration and referral data, patient's medical histories, physician's physical examinations, diagnoses, follow-up referrals, clinical laboratory tests, x-rays, electrocardiograms, physiological measurements (blood pressure, spirometry, height and weight), specialty procedures (tonometry, visual and hearing acuity), immunization records, and others. As what would be described later as clinical decision support, the system included "alert" signals for test results outside of predetermined normal limits, "advice" rules for secondary sequential testing, "consider" rules for likely diagnoses, comparisons of current history question responses with previous responses, and signals of "new symptoms" when reported by the patient for the first time. The continuing long-term computer patient record (CPR) permitted comparisons of current patient data to prior data for identifying clinically significant changes. Demonstrated reliable and secure, the system provided a large research database for clinical, epidemiological, and health services research [11, 13].

In the 1970s the advent of automated chemical analyzers permitted the development of highly efficient technology systems for combinations of test procedures capable of completing multiple blood chemistry tests from a single blood sample (see Sect. 9.3.1). The surge of interest in *automated multiphasic health testing* in the early 1970s spurred some practitioners who provided personal health checkups to use their automated testing systems to integrate the resultant data into an electronic patient record (EPR).

Altshuler and associates [1] at the St. Joseph's Hospital in Milwaukee, Wisconsin, developed Programmed Accelerated Laboratory Investigation (PALI), using a group of automated chemistry and hematology analyzers to perform at least 18 blood chemistry tests and four hematology tests, with secondary testing when indicated. They used the laboratory information system (CLAS) devised by SPEAR medical systems division of Becton, Dickinson & Company in Waltham, Massachusetts.

Warner and associates [43] at the LDS Hospital in Salt Lake City developed a multiphasic testing program to use as a pre-admission screening procedure for all scheduled patients. Several days prior to admission patients completed a self-administered history and underwent a series of tests and procedures that were entered into a computer-based record. Spirometry and electrocardiography were online tests; blood chemistry was analyzed online in the clinical laboratory; age, sex, height, weight, and blood pressure were taken and entered by nurses; and hematology and urinalysis were entered on remote keyboard terminals. The final screening report, including data from all the tests and a list of any values outside normal limits, was sent to the nursing station and placed on the patient's chart. Data collected during the patient's hospital stay were also entered into the computer-based record.

Cordle [15] at the University of North Carolina described how a clinic made up of a group of general internists in Charlotte implemented an office information system (OIS) for their general practice using precoded encounter forms. An operator keypunched the patient data into cards, which were then read into the computer. The clinic also operated an automated multiphasic health testing system with a self-administered patient history and automated test stations connected directly to the computer to make online reports available at the conclusion of the patient's examination.

In 1965 a subsidiary computer center was established in Kaiser Permanente's Department of Medical Methods Research to develop a prototype medical information system including medical application subsystems for multiphasic testing, clinical laboratory, and pharmacy. These used procedures already operational in the AMHT system for patient identification data, appointment scheduling, daily patient appointment lists, registration, operations control data, statistical reports, and quality control.

16.4 Diffusion of Automated Multiphasic Health Testing Systems (AMHTS)

Shambaugh [38, 39] at the Pacific Health Research Institute in Honolulu, noted that in the late 1960s the US Public Health Service (USPHS), supported by the findings of the KP AMHTS, established four large multiphasic testing centers in Milwaukee, Brooklyn, Baton Rouge, and Providence for the purpose of demonstrating the new technique and developing long term statistics on its medical and cost effectiveness.

In 1969 the US Congress was developing legislation to make *multiphasic health testing* (MHT) an integral part of Medicare, and the USPHS sent out a request for bids for a large, highly automated center to be located on Staten Island, and a new medical industry was born. A prototype online, real time system for multiphasic health testing for the Massachusetts General Hospital was developed by GD Searle and Co.; the firm added Science and Engineering Inc. as a subsidiary and Medidata was formed. In the US, Medidata's customers were hospitals, group practices, and pathologists who saw automated multiphasic health testing centers to be extensions of their automated clinical laboratories.

In the early 1970s AMHT systems had spread into many industrial and private In the 1980s most AMHT programs in the United States were terminated due to: (1) lack of support from Medicare and public health institutions that questioned the cost-effectiveness of annual health evaluations; (2) lack of reimbursement from health care insurers that paid its members only for their care when sick; and (3) opposition from fee-for-service physicians who considered AMHT programs to be financially competitive [30] with health care facilities in the United States. Although the cost effective process of delivering health care as set forth by Garfield [18] had its challenges, some studies supported their effectiveness for early detection [10]. In the 1960s and the 1970s AMHT systems in KP medical centers were actively operational on the principle that periodic health evaluations had an essential role in maintaining personal health; and Garfield [18] proposed that AMHT systems should be the efficient entry to personal total health care.

An economic recession in 1973 led Congress to reduce support for preventive medicine programs. By the 1980s most AMHT programs in the United States had been or were being terminated due to (1) lack of support from Medicare and public health institutions that questioned the cost-effectiveness of annual health evaluations; (2) lack of reimbursement from health care insurers that paid its members only for their care when sick; and (3) opposition from fee-for-service physicians who considered AMHT programs to be financially competitive [30]. University based programs supporting the development of AMHT demonstrations were phased out. The Staten Island Center funding was withdrawn. Grant funding for the Massachusetts General Hospital Center was eliminated. The USPHS demonstration and research centers were phased out entirely. Legislation for Medicare reimbursement was withdrawn. Within Kaiser Permanente, standalone AMHT programs were gradually absorbed by the organization's large centralized medical information system and standalone computer-based clinical subsystems, and capital costs for building space began to soar.

16.5 Summary and Commentary

The extension of the use of the computer from the laboratory directly into routine periodic health examinations exploited its full potential for supporting direct patient care, when the patients' blood and urine tests were collected in an automated multiphasic health testing center, along with a group of other physiological measurements, all stored in a computer, and provided to the physician with a summary report that contained all test results, reference values, alert flags, and likely diagnoses for the physician to consider [12, 14]. Other and broader public health uses of computing grew dramatically after the turn of the century.

Since 2000, we have seen the emergence of the subdiscipline known as infectious disease informatics. As extensively covered in *Infectious Disease Informatics and Biosurveillance* [45], this new field uses surveillance data sources and surveillance analytics (e.g., text mining, spatial and temporal analyses, simulation, etc.) to detect and respond to infectious disease outbreaks and protect the health of the public.

References

1. Altshuler CH. Programmed accelerated laboratory investigation. Hum Pathol. 1973;4:450–1.
2. Barnett GO, Souder D, Beaman P, Hupp J. MUMPS – an evolutionary commentary. Comput Biomed Res. 1981;14:112–8.
3. Breslow L. A health department's role in the cancer program. Calif Med. 1948;68:346–9.
4. Breslow L. An historical review of multiphasic screening. Prev Med. 1973;2:177–96.
5. Brossette SE, Sprague AP, Jones WT, Moser SA. A data mining system for infection control surveillance. Methods Inf Med. 2000;39:303–10.
6. Chew C, Eysenbach G. Pandemics in the age of Twitter: content analysis of tweets during the 2009 H1N1 outbreak. PLoS One. 2010;5:e14118.
7. Collen MF, Rubin L, Davis L. Computers in multiphasic screening. In: Stacy RW, Waxman BD, editors. Computers in biomedical research. New York: Academic; 1965.
8. Collen MF. The multitest laboratory in health care of the future. Hospitals. 1967;41:119.
9. Collen MF. Machine diagnosis from a multiphasic screening program. Proceedings of 5th IBM medical symposium. 1963.
10. Collen MF. Multiphasic screening as a diagnostic method in preventive medicine. Methods Inf Med. 1965;4:71.
11. Collen MF. History of MHTS. In: Collen MF, editor. Multiphasic health testing services. New York: Wiley; 1978. p. 1–45
12. Collen MF. Periodic health examinations using an automated multitest laboratory. JAMA. 1966;195:830–3.

13. Collen MF, Davis LS, Van Brunt EE, Terdiman JF. Functional goals and problems in large-scale patient record management and automated screening. FASEB Fed Proc. 1974;33:2376–9.
14. Collen MF, Rubin L, Neyman J, Dantzig GB, Baer RM, Siegelaub AB. Automated multiphasic screening and diagnosis. Am J Publ Health Nation Health. 1964;54:741–50.
15. Cordle F. The automation of clinic records: an overview with special emphasis on the automation of office records in the primary medical care setting. Med Care. 1972;10(6):470–80.
16. Dion M. Risk assessment and health improvement. In: Squires WD, editor. Patient education and health promotion in medical care. Palo Alto: Mayfield Pub. Co; 1985. p. 201–9.
17. Eysenbach G. Infodemiology and infoveillance tracking online health information and cyber-behavior for public health. Am J Prev Med. 2011;40:S154–8.
18. Garfield SR. The delivery of medical care. Sci Am. 1970;222:15–23.
19. Ginsberg J, Mohebbi MH, Patel RS, Brammer L, Smolinski MS, Brilliant L. Detecting influenza epidemics using search engine query data. Nature. 2009;457:1012–4.
20. Greaves F, Ramirez-Cano D, Millett C, Darzi A, Donaldson L. Harnessing the cloud of patient experience: using social media to detect poor quality healthcare. BMJ Qual Saf. 2013;22:251–5.
21. HCUP. US overview. Healthcare Cost and Utilization Project (HCUP). June 2014.
22. Henning KJ. What is syndromic surveillance? MMWR Morb Mortal Wkly Rep. 2004;53(Suppl):5–11.
23. Hierholzer Jr WJ. The practice of hospital epidemiology. Yale J Biol Med. 1982;55:225–30.
24. JAMA. Editorial: streamlining health examinations. JAMA. 1948;137:244.
25. LaVenture M, Davis JP, Faulkner J, Gorodezky M, Chen L. Wisconsin epidemiology disease surveillance system: user control of database management technology. 1982:156.
26. Lombardo JS. The ESSENCE II disease surveillance test bed for the national capital area. Johns Hopkins Apl Tech Dig. 2003;24:327–34.
27. Lombardo J, Buckeridge D. Disease surveillance: a public health informatics approach. Hoboken: Wiley-Interscience; 2007.
28. Magnuson JA, Fu PC. Public health informatics and information systems. 2nd ed. New York: Springer; 2014.
29. NLM. National Library of Medicine. Programs and services annual report FY2012. nlm.nih.gov/ocpl/anreports/fy2012.pdf. Accessed 2015.
30. Oldfield H. Automated multiphasic health testing: a diagnosis in three parts. J Clin Eng. 1978;3:292–301.
31. Ostroff SM, Hopkins DP, Tauxe RV, Sowers EG, Strockbine NK. Surveillance of *Escherichia coli* O157 isolation and confirmation, United States, 1988. MMWR CDC Surveill Summ. 1991;40:1–6.
32. Petrie LM, Bowdoin CD, McLoughlin CJ. Voluntary multiple health tests. J Am Med Assoc. 1952;148:1022–4.
33. PHFSC. Public health in America. Public Health Functions Steering Committee, Centers for Disease Control and Prevention. 2008.
34. Rasley D, Wenzel RP, Massanari RM, Streed S, Hierholzer Jr WJ. Organization and operation of the hospital-infection-control program of the University of Iowa Hospitals and Clinics. Infection. 1988;16:373–8.
35. Reis BY, Kirby C, Hadden LE, Olson K, McMurry AJ, Daniel JB, et al. AEGIS: a robust and scalable real-time public health surveillance system. JAMIA. 2007;14:581–8.
36. Riley LW, Remis RS, Helgerson SD, McGee HB, Wells JG, Davis BR, et al. Hemorrhagic colitis associated with a rare Escherichia coli serotype. N Engl J Med. 1983;308:681–5.
37. Sadusk JF, Robbins LC. Proposal for health-hazard appraisal in comprehensive health care. JAMA. 1968;203:1108–12.
38. Shambaugh V. MJ Clinics in Asia. Personal communication with M. Collen. 2012.
39. Shambaugh V. The origin of the International Health Evaluation and Promotion Association (IHEPA). Personal communication with M Collen. 2010.

40. Thacker SB, Choi K, Brachman PS. The surveillance of infectious diseases. JAMA. 1983;249:1181–5.
41. Thomas U. OECD informatics studies. Computerized data banks in public administration. 1971.
42. Tsui FC, Espino JU, Dato VM, Gesteland PH, Hutman J, Wagner MM. Technical description of RODS: a real-time public health surveillance system. JAMIA. 2003;10:399–408.
43. Warner HR. Computer-based patient monitoring. In: Stacy RW, Waxman B, editors. Computers in biomedical research, vol. III. New York: Academic; 1972.
44. Wise WS. Microcomputer infection surveillance system. Proc SCAMC. 1984:215–9.
45. Zeng Q, Gainer V, Goryachev S. Using derived concepts from electronic medical records for discovery research in informatics for integrating biology and bedside. Proc AMIA Annu Symp. 2010.

Chapter 17
Decision Support Systems (DSS)

Morris F. Collen and Alexa T. McCray

Abstract In the 1970s, to control costs and comply with Medicare rules, hospitals began to use computer-based systems for utilization review. In the early 1980s, a diagnostic related group (DRG) approach was applied to hospital payments, and increasingly complex data reporting requirements led hospitals to establish quality assurance programs. Medical information, or medical knowledge, databases for clinical decision support (CDS) were developed in the 1980s. The capabilities provided by online real time monitoring, vastly increased data storage, and physician order entry and results reporting (OE/RR) came together in CDS programs in the 2000s; by 2010 most physicians were using systems that provided online practice guidelines as well as clinical reminders and alerts about potential adverse clinical events. These advances build upon techniques from other fields, including artificial intelligence; the emergence of huge clinical databases in the 1990s led to the use of data mining to uncover previously unknown important relationships between clinical data elements, and the use of efficient knowledge discovery algorithms to extract knowledge from data by identifying and describing patterns in a meaningful manner. To support knowledge creation in biomedicine, the National Library of Medicine produces and maintains hundreds of up-to-date scientific databases, including MEDLINE (over 23 million citations with 700,000 posted in 2013 alone), human genome resources, toxicology and environmental databases (searched billions of times a year by millions around the globe).

Keywords Utilization review • Quality assurance • Clinical decision support • Clinical databases • Medical knowledge databases • Data mining • Knowledge discovery • National Library of Medicine

---

Sections of this chapter are reproduced from author Collen's earlier work *Computer Medical Databases*, Springer (2012).

Author Collen was deceased at the time of publication. McCray edited the chapter on his behalf after his death.

M.F. Collen (deceased)

A.T. McCray (✉)
Center for Biomedical Informatics, Harvard Medical School, Boston, MA, USA
e-mail: Alexa_McCray@hms.harvard.edu

© Springer-Verlag London 2015
M.F. Collen, M.J. Ball (eds.), *The History of Medical Informatics in the United States*, Health Informatics, DOI 10.1007/978-1-4471-6732-7_17

685

Some of the earliest computer applications to patient care were to support the decision making processes of health care providers, including administrators, physicians, nurses, technicians, and others. Computer programs were developed to help administrators monitor the utilization of care services and to help assure a high quality of patient care. Soon a great variety of automated online clinical decision support systems (CDSS) and computer-based order entry and results reporting (CPOE/RR) were developed for real time ordering of tests and procedures and to provide alerts, alarms, advice, and help to health care providers when unexpected events or variations from the expected occurred. Large scale clinical knowledge bases allowed sophisticated algorithms to make novel associations and discover new clinically relevant knowledge.

17.1 Administration Decision Support

Utilization review programs have the objectives to help administrators of health care facilities monitor patient care activities to provide an efficient process of care and to utilize appropriate procedures at the lowest cost; and to support the provision of effective care and help achieve desired patient outcomes. Within a hospital, the monitoring of adverse incidents and occurrences, such as a patient falling out of bed, was always an important administrative function.

In 1951 the Joint Commission on Accreditation for Hospitals (JCAH) that was established under the sponsorship of the American College of Surgeons, the American College of Physicians, the American Hospital Association, and the American Medical Association, began to require hospitals to establish routine medical and nursing reviews of patients' records in an expanded goal of monitoring not only the costs but also the quality of care provided. In the 1960s most hospitals did not choose to use their expensive computing resources for this purpose; and some subscribed to a Professional Activity Study (PAS) directed by Slee [111] for the Commission of Professional and Hospital Activities in Ann Arbor, Michigan. As early as 1959, 109 hospitals in 23 states subscribed to PAS [94]. In 1962, 240 hospitals in 32 states participated in Slee's program; participating hospitals ranged in size from 24 to 618 beds; 20 had medical school affiliations [111]. PAS required each hospital's medical record department to complete a case abstract form from the medical record of each discharged patient. PAS edited and entered the data into their computer-stored database and provided monthly and annual compilations of the hospital's routine statistics, as well as an index of their cases by diagnosis, surgical operation, and physician. PAS also provided comparisons among hospitals of length of hospital stay, surgical procedures performed, blood transfusions related to admission value of blood hemoglobin, and many other important data used for reviewing utilization of hospital services and outcomes of patient care.

In 1965 the Health Insurance for the Aged Act, also known as the Medicare Act, was signed into law by President Lyndon Johnson This required all participating hospitals to carry out a utilization review program in order to receive payment for

Medicare patients. Applied to patients in a hospital, utilization review included such questions as: Was the patient's admission to the hospital necessary? Was the treatment of the patient carried out as expeditiously as possible with a minimum of delay? Was the patient discharged as soon as medically ready? [78]. To assess and monitor the utilization of services in their hospitals, administrators needed the ability to compare their current hospital experience to their own hospital's past experience, and compare their performance to that of other hospitals. Using manual review procedures of patients' paper-based records was time consuming and costly, so selecting cases for review involved either random sampling of medical records (such as every tenth chart) or selecting cases that exceeded some predefined average length of hospital stay. By 1966, Slee's Commission on Professional and Hospital Activities had worked for 15 years with information systems and analytic tools, as well as with the evaluation of the quality of medical care. With a pool of data based on 17 million hospitalizations, Slee developed inter-hospital and inter-physician comparisons, such as comprehensive length-of-stay tables, so that for each class of patients the variations in the length-of-stay distributions could be analyzed, such as for average stay, and variance of stay by patient groupings. In the 1970s Slee's Professional Activity Study was augmented to satisfy all the requirements of the Professional Standards Review Organization (PSRO) program [110].

In 1967 Wolfe at the University of Pittsburgh proposed a computer-based screening method for selecting cases for utilization review. Wolfe's method was based on the average length of stay for specific diagnoses determined by the collection of data from five hospitals. The method used 355 variables commonly found in charts, such as patient's age, gender, diagnoses, surgical procedures, and emergency or elective admission. Wolfe [126] also developed a statistical regression approach for estimating the length of stay for a particular condition (for example, operations on the biliary tract), with suggested upper and lower control limits. On entering the major diagnosis for a specific patient and the actual length of stay for the patient, cases of unusual length of stay (if they exceeded the upper control limit or were shorter than the lower control limit) could be selected for further review. The computer application of this approach permitted a more rapid screening review of all of a hospital's patients' records, rather than merely of samples and also provided ready tabulations of length of stay for particular diagnoses.

In the 1970s the increasing costs of hospital care further stimulated the development of hospital utilization review programs to monitor patients' lengths of stay, in an attempt to identify patients who remained in the hospital longer than the generally accepted averages, which implied excessive costs. Administrative personnel, usually nurses, were trained to audit hospital charts for non-standard practices. The retrospective review of patient records began to be replaced by concurrent, online monitoring of computer-based patients' records. By the mid-1970s some mainframe and minicomputer-based hospital information systems were reported to be capable of satisfying PSRO requirements as a byproduct of collecting data for their electronic patient record system. Meldman [88] at Forest Hospital, a 150-bed psychiatric facility in Des Plaines, Illinois, following the recording of admission and patient care data on paper forms, used a PDP11/40 computer to permit a nurse reviewer to interact with a display terminal, and review all data in patients' records to assure that the criteria for good quality patient care were met. The output of the review was a report structured to furnish a detailed patient profile prior to, during, and after psychiatric care.

To ensure that services and payments to Medicare beneficiaries were medically necessary and in accordance with accepted standards of care, in 1972 Congress enacted legislation that directed the Department of Health, Education, and Welfare to establish an Office of Professional Standards Review. An Experimental Medical Care Review Organization was established by Sanazaro et al. [105], then the Director of the National Center for Health Services Research and Development, to develop working models to test the feasibility of conducting systematic and ongoing review of medical care. Trained hospital personnel completed abstracts of the patients' records, from which computer printouts were generated that matched pre-defined criteria for a diagnosis with data abstracted from each patient's hospital discharge. In 1974 the Office of Professional Standards Review Organization issued a PSRO Program Manual. After a review of the increased regulations imposed by Congress requiring regular reviews of health care costs and quality, the American Hospital Association wrote that much of the data required by the PSRO lent itself to automation for ease of handling, review, and reporting [97]. The PSRO require-ments for uniform reporting of data included a hospital discharge data set and other data concerning the number of days certified at admission, and admission review procedures and their outcomes. Soon the American Nurses Association published standards of practice for nursing care.

Forrest [53] summarized studies at Stanford University analyzing data from the Professional Activity Study, and reported that abstracts of patient charts could be used to measure the quality and cost of care in hospitals. However, individual hos-pitals began to install their own systems, since as Ball [10] had concluded, comput-ers in medical care were no longer a choice but a requirement not just to meet the needs for better patient care but also to comply with the government regulations imposed by the PSRO and the National Health Insurance legislation.

As an example of the influence of all these regulations on hospitals, Smith [112] noted that the impetus for the development of the electronic medical record system at Druid City Hospital came primarily from the so called PSRO Amendments to the Social Security Act. Using an IBM System/3 computer for the patient record data-base, the hospital instituted a hospital information system providing an order entry module for the clinical laboratory, pharmacy, and radiology and a module for admis-sion and bed census; all were linked to the business office billing system and were capable of providing a concurrent review of all inpatients.

In 1976 Budkin and associates [35] at the Miami Heart Institute initiated their PSRO computer subsystem. Their 258-bed private hospital had admitted 7,500 patients in 1979; of these 73 % were Medicare patients. Their PSRO computer-based system used a dual-processor Xerox Sigma computer with 128 terminals sta-tioned throughout the hospital. They developed one online and three batch-processed report programs. The online program allowed the patient review coordinator to enter all information generated from reviews of patients' records. Reports were printed each night for each physician, describing each patient's status and alerting the physician to the number of days elapsed since the patient's admission. A monthly report analyzed the number of admissions and the associated lengths of stay and gave comparisons with prior months. A year-end report summarized monthly averages and compared the data for Medicare patients with non-Medicare patients. The researchers noted that although frequent revisions of their subsystem were required by the PSRO agency, overall the system helped to reduce the time that physicians spent in utilization review activities. It also eased the clerical workload required to comply with the PSRO rules and guidelines.

In the 1980s the implementation of the diagnostic related groups (DRG) classification for hospital patients extended the process of utilization review to include length-of-stay criteria. The Utah Professional Review Organization used a centrally managed system of nurse reviewers in Utah's 42 acute care hospitals. As patient records were received, an abstract was completed containing the Uniform Hospital Discharge Data Set together with a record of adverse clinical events that occurred during hospitalization. The abstracts were keypunched into the computer database, from which the organization conducted a variety of studies in utilization and quality of care [76]. In 1982 because the DRG method of payment was considered by some to place so much emphasis on cost containment that it could endanger the quality of care, the PSRO program was replaced by Congress with the Peer Review Organization (PRO). Assigned the major responsibilities for monitoring the implementation of the Medicare Prospective Payment Program that was initiated in 1983, the PRO was to emphasize outcome measures of care rather than process measures [75].

Mullin [92] at the Yale-New Haven Hospital reported a computer-based, concurrent utilization review program that provided standards for length of stay by DRG rather than by diagnosis. Furthermore, for the hospital's individual medical practitioners, Mullin developed profiles that showed the actual versus the expected percentage of a medical practitioner's patients discharged at the 50th, 75th, and 90th length-of-stay percentiles of the comparison norms. Fetter [51] advocated applying the DRG approach to hospital payments as improving utilization review and evaluating hospital performance, since the patients fitting into a DRG required generally similar services.

These complex data reporting requirements resulted in hospitals establishing quality assurance programs that developed criteria for selecting medical records for review and detection of adverse events and of negligent care. These programs functioned as action plans within an institution to establish minimum acceptable standards for patient care, and to monitor the delivery of patient care to assure that these standards were met or surpassed [12]. Quality assurance monitoring required the establishment of uniform criteria for diagnoses and treatment of specific diseases for hospital patients. Previously these review processes had been performed by the manual audit of patients' charts by physicians and nurses. As the costs of medical care increased and computer-based medical information systems became common, quality assurance programs for evaluating and monitoring the quality of care became increasingly important to health care administrators and policy makers.

Time-consuming offline manual audits of paper-based medical records had been the usual basis for quality assurance programs, since the patient care process recorded online in the medical record could be easily compared to predefined standards of care and to published results of evidence-based patient therapy. By the 1970s the capability of computers to support these processes began to be used. Whereas the medical audit of paper-based records had always involved a retrospective review of care, online monitoring of patient care was more effective in detecting any variations from desired practices at the time the care was actually being provided.

Christofferson and Moynihan [37] described process-based methods that evaluated the care provided to individual patients; these methods usually required examining the medical record and comparing the care provided to clinical norms. Outcome oriented methods were typically statistically driven and allowed for the measurement of quality through the comparison of patients' health outcomes with empirically derived norms. Statistical assessments did not evaluate the care rendered to individual patients; rather they combined data for many patients to compare the quality of care across institutions. Outcome methods assumed the availability of computer-based data collection and analysis. Generic screening combined process oriented case review with the outcome oriented statistical method. It relied on the clinical review of the patient record and used a single set of criteria applied uniformly across all diagnostic categories; adverse events that should not occur were defined as those having a high probability of being associated with substandard care. Generic screening had a high potential in automated screening systems; as hospital information systems advanced, the various adverse events monitored as a part of generic screening systems could be integrated into a system that automatically alerted for cases that needed further clinical review. Gabrieli [56] asserted that computers had the potential to mechanize a major portion of the quality assurance work, and the challenge was to codify the medical intelligence necessary to monitor the quality of care provided for a price that was affordable. Gabrieli had developed computer-based patient records and automated analysis techniques for discharge summaries, and had concluded that for audit purposes the discharge summary was well suited as a source document.

In the late 1980s Drazen [47] at A. D. Little reported out that, in addition to managing patients' lengths of stay, some hospital utilization review programs also checked patients' records for unnecessary utilization of resources and omitted services, and provided reminders about services that should be considered. In 1989 the Joint Accreditation Commission for Healthcare Organizations (JACHO), formerly the Joint Commission on Accreditation of Hospitals (JCAH), reported on its progress with developing clinical indicators for obstetrics, anesthesia, and hospital-wide care to pilot test this generic screening approach in 17 hospitals. The commission explained that an indicator was not a direct measure of quality, but rather was a screen or flag that identified or directed attention to specific performance issues within a health care organization that should be the subject of more intensive review [62]. At the end of the 1980s an Institute of Medicine committee recommended that

Congress restructure the PSRO program into Medicare Quality Review Organizations to emphasize more systematic data collection, analysis, and feedback to providers and practitioners, and to be explicitly oriented to quality of care and not to utilization or cost control [75]. By that time computer software programs were available to provide hospital information systems with a comprehensive quality assurance program that generally included support for both review and remedy. These included the review of patients' records for over- or under-utilization of care services; for the appropriateness of the care services provided to patients; for identification and analysis of adverse events or injuries to patients caused by the care process as distinguished from those caused by the disease process; and for provision of incident or occurrence reports (such as a patient falling out of bed). Also included were risk management (such as maintaining the condition of corridor floors to avoid slip-and-fall accidents); infection control (protection from hospital-acquired infections); the monitoring of medical injuries or iatrogenic diseases (conditions resulting from medical interventions, such as a medication overdose); and the institution of appropriate corrective actions in each case.

Although computer-aided systems for utilization review and for quality assurance held great promise, by the end of the 1980s few such systems were in operation. One problem was that few such programs were operational in large, integrated health information systems with computer-based patient records. Another problem was the inability of national agencies to agree on clinically validated criteria for defining the processes and procedures for arriving at diagnoses and for providing treatments for what would be considered appropriate and high quality care. The JACHO concluded that computerization of clinical data collecting activities in hospitals was progressing slowly and that there was as yet no user-friendly national reference database to support hospitals in their efforts to use performance measures to monitor the quality and appropriateness of patient care [96].

In the 2000s evolving clinical decision support programs provided more effective methods to improve the quality of patient care in hospitals, both by decreasing errors through online monitoring and verification of data in real time as they were entered into the computer, and by furnishing information on alternative therapies as orders were entered.

Whenever there was a controversy about the quality of care provided to a patient, the patient's medical record was the primary document used for review, which had to be available at any later review exactly as it existed at the time when the disputed clinical decision was made. For a computer-based medical record, this requirement imposed a high degree of data integrity on the hospital information system, since the patient's medical record stored in the system's databases had to be restored and reconstructed in exactly the same format and content as they appeared to the physician at the time and date in question.

17.2 Clinical Decision Support Systems (CDSS)

Clinical decision support (CDS) is generally expected to be provided to some extent by a medical information system for computer-aided diagnosis and for computer-aided therapy. A diagnosis is a unique combination of a patient's symptoms, signs, and syndromes that distinguish one disease from another; where a symptom is a patient's complaint such as "pain"; a sign is an objective finding of a disease such as a palpable mass or an abnormal laboratory test result; and a syndrome is a specific set of symptoms and signs that occur together and represent a specific diagnosis. A clinical decision support system (CDSS) employs a comprehensive knowledge base. It may also employ an active relevant patient care data base, and applies advanced computer analytics or inference programs to these data bases.

CDSSs were intended for use by physicians who had difficulty in arriving at a diagnosis for a patient who had a complex combination of symptoms and signs, or had a rare disease. When first seeing a patient with a clinical problem, a physician takes the patient's medical history by questioning for important symptoms and completes a physical examination searching for important signs of physical abnormalities. The physician then usually arrives at a first "impression" of the patient's likely diagnosis and then arranges for supplementary diagnostic tests and procedures to confirm the "final" diagnosis. If the physician is still uncertain as to the diagnosis, the patient may be referred to consult with a specialist who is more experienced with such problems, or the physician may search through the available medical literature for help with the differential diagnosis of medical conditions with similar signs and symptoms (syndromes).

As the cost for the storage of large volumes of data greatly decreased, the increased availability of huge clinical databases (data warehouses) stimulated searches for previously unknown medical knowledge associations. It is a basic clinical process when deciding on a patient's medical diagnosis that, if the physician has the required knowledge, and if the patient has a specific group of findings (symptoms, signs, and syndromes), then the patient probably has the suspected diagnosis. Physicians also use symbolic logic, probability, and value theory to arrive at both a diagnosis and the appropriate treatment for each patient [66]. Just as physicians developed clinical decision rules (such as, if the patient has cough, sputum, fever, and chills, then consider the probable diagnosis of pneumonia), so did computer programmers develop algorithms and rules to identify useful associations between data items, such as, if this finding is present, then consider this action. It is difficult to find rules with sufficient sensitivity to identify correctly important true associations, yet have sufficient specificity not to generate false associations.

In the 1950s one of the earliest CDSSs that applied decision rules in direct patient care was the Kaiser Permanente multiphasic health testing program. This program was well publicized when during a federal Congressman's visit, an asymptomatic woman who had asked for a routine health checkup was found to have an abnormally high white blood cell count; and the computer printed an online alert, "consider leukemia." On further testing, this asymptomatic woman was found to have early chronic lymphatic leukemia; she immediately began treatment [122].

In 1966 Barnett and associates at the Laboratory of Computer Science, a unit of the Department of Medicine of the Massachusetts General Hospital and the Harvard Medical School, initiated a pilot project that included a clinical laboratory reporting system and a medications ordering system [13]. Barnett's online, interactive MUMPS-based system could check in real time the medications ordered for a patient against the data in the electronic patient's record for drug interactions with other drugs ordered for the patient, for drug-laboratory test interferences, for known allergic reactions to drugs, or for any other adverse drug events. If this information was not given immediately to the physician at the time of the entry of the order, Barnett considered the CDSS to be less useful, since if there was a significant time delay between writing an order and its entry into the computer system, the responsible physician might have left the patient care unit, and any advised changes in the order by the computer-based order entry system could then be delayed. Barnett recognized that the order entry systems available at that time allowed the physicians to write their orders and notes in the routine fashion, and then employed clerical personnel to enter the information into the computer system. He noted that the inherent weakness in this strategy was that the computer interaction was not with the physician who was generating the order, but with a nurse or clerical staff member who had no decision making power for the specific event [16].

In 1974 Barnett conducted a study of primary care provided to office patients in the Harvard Community Health Plan where the computer-based records in their Computer-Stored Ambulatory Record (COSTAR) were monitored automatically to identify every patient found to have a positive throat culture. If appropriate treatment was not recorded within 4 days of the positive report, the computer generated a printed notice to the responsible physician pointing out the discrepancy from the prescribed standard of care. If the medical record still did not contain a notation of treatment 2 days later, another printed notice was automatically generated. Whereas the traditional method of the notification of a positive culture by a printed laboratory report sent to the health care provider had an incidence of "failure to treat" of about 10 % of the patients with positive cultures, computer-generated feedback practically eliminated this problem. Barnett concluded that an active computer-based care monitoring system offered a unique ability to promote positive changes in medical care practice, and its ability to audit the effectiveness of a quality assurance program. The COSTAR system included a CDSS, and once again Barnett [15] emphasized the requirement for timely feedback of information about a deviation from standard care; the message about the deviation had to be given to the physician within a time period short enough to allow corrective action to be taken to give the appropriate care. Barnett et al.'s [14] approach was to develop a CDSS in which monitoring and feedback were concurrent rather than retrospective; that is, the deviations were detected immediately, rather than later after the event. He emphasized that the attributes of COSTAR permitted it to be used effectively in a program of quality assurance and online clinical decision support, since the data used for quality assurance activities were the same data entered into the system as part of the patient care process. Barnett (1978) concluded that an online CDSS offered a unique technique to promote positive changes in medical care practice.

In 1963 Lindberg and associates [72] at the University of Missouri in Columbia installed an IBM 1410 computer in their medical center, which had 441 hospital beds and admitted 60,000 patients in the year of 1964. Their overall objective was to support the practice and teaching of medicine. A major initial project was the development of a system for reporting all clinical laboratory determinations through the computer [71]. At that time their laboratory data were keypunched into cards, and the test data on approximately 500,000 tests per year were then entered into the computer. Other files of patient material being computer processed included a tumor registry, hospital discharge diagnoses, operations file, and surgical pathology file. The system soon supported the hospital's admission, discharge, and patient census programs, patient billing and accounting, nightly nursing report sheets, dietary department inventory; periodic hospital statistics, and personnel records.

Their system also supported 34 research projects and was used in the teaching of medical students [69]. They used the Standard Nomenclature of Diseases and Operations (SNDO) for the coding of patients' discharge diagnoses and surgical operative procedures [73] and stored these on magnetic tape for all patients admitted to the hospital from 1955 to 1965. Other categories of patient data in the system included a patient master reference file with identification data stored on a random-access disk file. All SNDO-coded diagnoses for autopsy and surgical-pathology specimens and all coded radiology and electrocardiogram interpretations were stored on magnetic tape in fixed-field format. Computer routines were available for recovery of all categories of data stored. All were aimed at medical student and physician inquiries [70].

To query the system, the user keypunched a control card with the code number of each diagnosis about which the user was inquiring. The computer system read the punched cards and searched the magnetic tape records containing all diagnoses. When a record with the specified code was found, the system identified the unit numbers of the patients associated with the diagnosis, and assigned a "flag" in the random access working storage corresponding with each patient who had the diagnosis [34]. In 1965 they replaced the punched card system in their clinical laboratory with IBM 1092/1093 matrix-keyboard terminals to permit entering test results into the computer. The test results were submitted to a "limits" program, which categorized them as reasonable, abnormal, or as unreasonable. The system was programmed to recognize patterns of laboratory test results with other findings recorded in the patient's record, and to advise the physician of patient care actions to consider.

After studying the patterns found in almost 6,000 electrolyte determinations for serum sodium, potassium, chlorides, and carbonate, Lindberg [69] was able not only to identify important combinations of abnormal test values, but also to recognize new patterns and predict the state of kidney function. Their laboratory system, which they had begun to develop in 1963, continued to be a main focus of their hospital information system. By 1968 the team had added an information system for their department of surgery to provide patient identification, admission, and discharge functions; listing of all surgical complications while in the hospital; operating room entries made by the surgeon, anesthesiologist, and circulation nurse; laboratory, surgical-pathology, and autopsy reports; a daily operating room log; and individual patient summary reports.

Lindberg [68] also developed his CONSIDER program, which used the American Medical Association (AMA) publication, *Current MedicalTerminology*, to provide the signs, symptoms, and findings for common diagnoses. If the user submitted a set of signs and symptoms, the computer would then list the diseases the physician should consider. With Kingsland, Lindberg initiated a fact bank of biomedical information for use by practicing physicians and also by scholars and students that contained information from diverse origins, such as textbooks, monographs, and articles.

Collen and colleagues [42, 104] used a symptom frequency approach to differentiate between gastrointestinal diagnoses such as hiatus hernia and duodenal ulcer. In the 1970s Collen [41] provided some clinical decision support rules in a multihealth testing system that included alert and warning signals for patients with clinical laboratory test results outside of predetermined normal limits, and provided advice rules for secondary sequential testing and consider rules for likely diagnoses. All patient data were stored in electronic patient records (EPRs), and also in a research database.

In the early 1970s Warner and associates at the Latter Day Saints (LDS) Hospital in Salt Lake City developed their Health Evaluation through Logical Processing (HELP) program that provided a CDS system with the capability of online monitoring of patient care services, in an effort to detect inappropriate orders by physicians and incorrect administration of medications by nurses. The system at the LDS Hospital had display terminals located at its nursing units that allowed the nurses to select orders from displayed menus, and to review the orders entered and the results reported for their patients. The system also provided discharge and transfer functions. Warner [123] had already published the use of Bayes Rule applied with a very high accuracy to the computer-aided diagnosis of congenital heart disease. In 1972 Warner approached the problem of quality assurance and clinical decision support for ambulatory care patients by using the HELP system. The group provided computer protocols to nurse practitioners who functioned as physician assistants and monitored the patients' care. After patients completed a computer-based self-administered questionnaire, an assistant entered the findings into the system. Based on the patient's history and physical examination data, the interactive protocol system would decide what diagnostic, procedural, and therapeutic decisions should be considered for the patient. These decisions would then be audited by the system according to protocol logic. If any patient data necessary for these decisions were found lacking, the assistant would then be prompted for the collection of those data. Protocols were implemented for upper respiratory infections, urinary tract infections, hypertension, and diabetes. After an initial learning period, data entry error rates of 1 % were reported, significantly less than those of paper protocols, and there were no cases where the assistants failed to collect or enter data prompted by the computer [36].

In the 1980s, Warner's computer-based provider order entry and results reporting program was linked to his HELP decision support program. When an order for an x-ray or laboratory test was entered, the computer automatically retrieved any previous x-ray or laboratory reports; with the physicians' reasons for requesting the order, a Bayesian analysis was applied to provide the radiologist with the five most probable diagnoses [63]. When a medication order was entered, the display suggested an appropriate dosage and dispensing schedule based on data such as the patient's age, weight, other prescribed medications, and laboratory tests results obtained from the electronic patient record; it also suggested alternative medications that should be considered. Warner's group further enhanced its menu-based order entry programs with relevant data added from the complete clinical patient profile in the electronic health record for the dynamic creation of patient adjusted order entry screens that relied on the centralized patient database, a medical knowledge base, and an inference machine that combined these two information sources to create data entry screens fitting the needs of the specific patient. Warner also developed a program that combined a centralized patient care database and a medical knowledge base, and used these two databases to create data entry screens that fit the individual needs of the specific patient. The system also suggested procedures and treatments for the patient's problems [99]. Haug [58] reviewed their extensive experiences in decision support using the HELP system. As their experience increased, Warner's group developed ILIAD, one of the earliest computer-based "intelligent" CDS programs.

In the 1970s McDonald [80] at Indiana University was one of the earliest to develop and use an outpatient information system, known as the Regenstrief Medical Record (RMR). The system included a clinical decision support system to assist in the process of providing clinical reminders, suggestions, recommendations, advice, alerts, or alarms to help ensure that the quality of office care conformed to predefined medical practice guidelines. Patient data were captured automatically by the computer-based laboratory and outpatient pharmacy systems; or were recorded by hand as marks or numbers on computer-printed encounter forms and were then optically scanned. A two-part patient encounter form was generated for each patient's return visit. The physician was able to identify the patient readily, to note the active problems from the last visit, and to see the active treatment profile. The physician recorded numeric clinical data, such as weight and blood pressure, for later optical machine reading into the computer. The problem list was updated by drawing a line through problems that had been resolved and by writing in new problems that had arisen. Progress notes were entered in the space beside the problem list. Space was also provided for writing orders for tests and for return appointments; and within the space for orders, the computer suggested certain tests that might be needed. The patient's current prescriptions were listed at the bottom of the encounter form in a medication profile; the physician refilled or discontinued these drugs by writing "R" or "D/C" next to them and wrote new prescriptions underneath this list. The patient took a carbon copy of this section of the encounter form to the pharmacy as his prescription.

Thus, the encounter form performed many of the recording and retrieving tasks for the physician. Data recorded by physicians on the encounter forms were entered by clerks into the computer. Laboratory information was captured directly from the laboratory system. Pharmacy prescription information was collected from both the hospital and outpatient pharmacy systems. Essential information from hospital stays, such as diagnoses, was transferred from hospital case abstract tapes. The patient summary report was the second report generated for each patient's return visit. This report included laboratory data, historical information, treatment, radiology, EKG, nuclear medicine, and other data in a modified flow sheet format [84]. It also listed the patient's clinic, hospital, and emergency room visits and the results of x-ray and laboratory tests, with test results presented in reverse chronological order. With this time-oriented view of the data, the physician could quickly find the most recent data (for example, blood pressure or blood sugar) and compare them to the previous levels. An asterisk was placed beside each abnormal value for emphasis. The objective of the patient's summary report was to facilitate data retrieval and to perform some data organization tasks for the physician. McDonald [84] reported that the RMR used paper-based reports, rather than displayed reports, as its primary mechanism for transmitting information to the physician since it was cheap, portable, and easier to browse, and paper reports could be annotated with paper and pencil.

By the mid-1970s McDonald's RMR system provided a cumulative summary report that presented the information stored in the computer-based patient record and also printed an encounter summary form to be used for the coming visit. In addition, the RMR system furnished a surveillance report by which the computer transmitted its protocol-generated suggestions as clinical decision support to the physician. Specific clinical situations and their associated advised actions were defined in terms of protocols that the computer could interpret directly. McDonald developed an early computer-based provider order entry/results reporting program that used protocols with specific rules for defined adverse clinical events, including adverse drug events, and provided *alerts* and *advice* with recommended courses of actions necessary to correct the adverse events. The computer screened each patient's medical record for specified events prior to the patient's next clinic visit. If any of the adverse clinical situations were present, they were reported on the surveillance report, along with the recommended actions. The earliest protocols were primarily related to the ordering of some commonly used drugs and were intended to ensure that specified indicated procedures were done at proper intervals. As an example, the program would recommend that a laboratory test be ordered following the prescription of a certain potent drug, or it warned the physician of the possibility of adverse interactions between two prescribed drugs. After conducting a controlled study, McDonald concluded that the computer could change clinician behavior by providing prospective recommendations, and reported that clinicians noticed and responded to more drug-related clinical events with such recommendations than without. The patient's surveillance report was generated for each patient's return visit; this report represented sophisticated data processing involving the selection and interpretation of patient data to assist the physician in clinical decision making.

It also contained statements that served as clinical reminders to physicians regarding diagnostic studies or treatments.

McDonald [80] tested 390 protocols developed on the basis of patient care strategies reported in the medical literature, and reported that physicians responded to 51 % of 327 events when given computer-generated recommendations, and 22 % of 385 events when not given computer suggestions. McDonald found that physicians with a busy practice in an outpatient adult clinic who were given timely computer reminders and recommendations for certain adverse clinical events that were automatically detected, had responded to twice as many events as did a control group of physicians who were not given such computer decision support. Physicians' response rates fell when they left the group who were receiving computer recommendations and joined the control group. McDonald concluded that the difference in response rate was not due to ignorance of the appropriate practice, but rather to the difficulties of contending with the information loads of a busy practice; thus they were errors of omission rather than of commission. In a third study in which 31 practitioners participated, McDonald [83] confirmed a twofold or greater effect on practitioners' behavior, and concluded that the computer reminders had a substantial and reproducible effect on the care providers within their environment.

In the early 1980s the RMR system contained medical records for more than 60,000 patients, with data regarding inpatient, outpatient, and emergency room care [79]. The RMR system shared a DEC VAX 11/780 computer with the clinical laboratory and pharmacy systems, and used a microcomputer-based workstation to display forms, in which the user could enter data using a mouse to select data from menus [79, 85]. The records in the patient care database were of variable length with the data coded or as free-text narrative reports. A dictionary of terms defined the kinds of data that could be stored in the medical record files; and CARE, their own language and retrieval system, permitted non-programmers to perform complex queries of the medical records [79]. Their database files also included their clinical laboratory system data, pharmacy system data, and a patient appointment file. McDonald applied the term *gopher work* to the functions of recording, retrieving, organizing, and reviewing data. In the 1980s the RMR system was operational in the general medical clinic and in the diabetes clinic, and included a hospital and a pharmacy module. By the mid-1980s any patient seen by the General Medicine Service in the emergency room, in the outpatient clinics, or in the hospital wards had been registered with the Regenstrief computer-based medical record system. By 1986 a network of microcomputer-based clinical workstations had been implemented to provide a general medical clinic with a clinical decision support system, using CARE rules, alerts, and advice as a part of online patient care that supplemented their offline reviewing of their electronic patient records [82]. Subsequent studies by McDonald's group showed that computer-generated clinical reminders had a significant effect on improving use of preventive care protocols such as vaccinations [119], and on reducing the number of laboratory tests ordered when prior test results were automatically displayed at the time of such orders [120]. They concluded that the display of clinical reminders could have significant effects on physicians' behavior [81].

In 1988 the RMR system was linked to the local Veterans and University hospitals' laboratory, radiology, and pharmacy systems, and contained more than 24 million observations on 250,000 patients. In 1 year patient information was captured for more than 300,000 outpatient visits and for 20,000 hospital admissions. Thus, Indiana University physicians who rotated their work in those hospitals could use the same RMR programs to find and analyze clinical data for patient care. RMR's query programs permitted users, through the CARE program, to generate clinical care reminders and queries across sets of patients in the RMR medical record database; it also provided a program for statistical analyses of groups of patients.

By the end of the 1990s the RMR system served a large network of hospitals and clinics [87] and had become a leading model in the United States. McDonald's outstanding contribution was to focus on the computer's capabilities for providing real time reminders to physicians about problems reflected in the outpatient care data. In addition, the group scientifically evaluated, by controlled clinical trials, the effects of these computer reminders on the quality of care in an online, practice linked, quality assurance program.

In 1969 the Division of Cardiology at Duke University Medical Center in Durham, North Carolina, began to collect data on their patients hospitalized with coronary artery disease. The information collected included each patient's history, physical examination data, and the results of laboratory and diagnostic tests and of cardiac catheterization. Users entered data from cardiac catheterization by using a coding algorithm that displayed a series of questions; the user entered the responses. A total of ten keystrokes was used to describe the coronary anatomy of a patient. The database was used in their clinical practice to provide automated reports of the testing procedures and results and to provide diagnostic and prognostic profiles of new patients based on their previous experience [100]. These data on cardiac catheterization results and patients' outcomes were aggregated in the Duke Databank for Cardiovascular Disease and used to support clinical research in this field [101].

In 1974 Stead and Hammond at Duke University Medical Center began to use a clinical decision support symptom-oriented protocol used by physicians and paramedical personnel in their Health Services Clinic for managing patients with upper respiratory infections. A list of medical records that contained the diagnostic code for this condition was compiled in the computer, and the manual records for these patients were then audited for data completeness and protocol compliance [4]. By 1980 they used their GEMISCH language CDS program to provide computer-generated reminders to improve physicians' drug prescribing practices in their Community and Family Medicine Clinic. Information that identified each prescription and the prescribing physician was entered into the computer system. Lists of commonly prescribed drugs and their generic equivalents were stored in a computer-based dictionary, with messages detailing the cost savings and therapeutic advantages for each of these generic equivalents or therapeutic alternatives. An individualized feedback profile reported each time a prescriber wrote one of the selected brand name drugs or less desirable therapeutic alternatives. They reported that whereas a control group of physicians prescribed 29 % of drugs generically, the group receiving computer reminders prescribed 62 % generically, a very significant increase in generic drug prescribing [125].

In the 1970s Weed's approach to a problem-oriented medical record (POMR) advocated a standardized process for the collection of the patient's data, by the formulation of a precise list of the patient's medical problems, with a detailed plan for treating each problem. Tufo [121] and associates at the Given Health Care Center of the University of Vermont College of Medicine considered Weed's defined approach to patient care well suited to facilitate the medical audit process in the office, and designated this coupling of the principles of problem-orientation to audit as the problem-oriented system. Based on office practice guidelines, their problem-oriented CDS system was designed to assess, first, whether an agreed upon task had been performed and, second, the accuracy and reliability in performing the task. For example, was an abnormally low blood hematocrit value observed and was an appropriate action taken, or was a goal of blood pressure control to 130/85 mmHg reasonable for this person? Among the controversial issues about the problem-oriented medical record was one Rubin [103]) noted, that although Weed's problem-oriented record was useful to track and audit the specific problems recorded in the Problem List, an abnormality found during the care process (for example, a nurse recording an elevated blood pressure) not identified in the problem list might not be audited.

In the 1980s an Automated Medical Record Audit System (AMRAS) was implemented at the University of Texas Medical School's Ambulatory Clinic, where patients received primary care. Their electronic patient record employed a record audit program that used the latest updated electronic patient record files and applied protocol-driven algorithms as a clinical decision support system to print a report for the physician. Two days before each clinic session, the tape file on each patient scheduled to attend was reviewed. Of its recommendations, 80 % concerned general medicine and preventive care and the remainder for specific clinical specialty problems. In a study of 133 patients with diabetes, physicians followed the automated CDSS suggestions in 50 % of 58 patients, as compared to similar suggested procedures followed in 37 % of 75 diabetic patients in a control group cared for with traditional paper-based records and without the CDSS audits. The average total costs for outpatient plus inpatient care per patient per year was one-half as much for the experimental group who received CDSS audits [118].

In the late 1980s, the Community Health Care Center Plan of New Haven used their outpatient information system electronic patient record to monitor their clinic patient care process. For each patient visit, physicians completed an encounter form to record their findings and treatment. The information system was linked to the pharmacy system for collecting data on dispensed medication prescriptions. Finseth and Brunjes [52] studied the consistency in the recording of blood pressure measurements, the diagnosis of hypertension, and the associated prescribed medications as measures of appropriate quality of care for this condition. They reported that the electronic patient record readily provided the capacity for identification of individual patients who should have their blood pressures regularly checked, those for whom a diagnosis of hypertension was indicated, and those who needed treatment.

They also suggested that the system enabled identification of individual medical practitioners whose performance might need to be modified.

In 1982 Brewster [30] at Little Company of Mary Hospital, a 500-bed facility in Evergreen Park, Illinois, described a hospital information system with a quality assurance program in which continuous concurrent monitoring occurred by having the system check for an appropriate response each time a process was initiated for which criteria had been developed. Automatic reminders were printed to prompt desired responses in the patient care process; inappropriate responses were stopped if the sequence of actions was initiated through the online computer system and did not coincide with previously programmed instructions. The quality assurance program was applied to radiology patient preparation, clinical laboratory specimen requisition and collection, pharmacy medication system, drug-drug interaction and drug-allergy systems, dietary system, and central service order system.

By the end of the 1980s, it was expected that a CDSS with clinical practice guidelines would become an integral part of a computer-based quality assurance program. In 1988 physicians had generally agreed to accept practice guidelines to support effective medical care, in the belief that such rules could preserve quality of care in the face of continued cost-cutting [5].

Research on artificial intelligence (AI), the branch of computer science associated with machines that perform tasks normally thought to require human intelligence, was initiated in the 1950s with a major goal of understanding the processes of intelligent thought [74]. The Dendral Project was one of the first large-scale programs to embody the strategy of using detailed, task-specific knowledge about a problem domain as a source of heuristics; that is, promoting investigations conducive to discovery, seeking generality through automating the acquisition of such knowledge, and attempting to distill from this research lessons of importance to AI research [74]. The heuristics employed were based on specific knowledge of chemistry and knowledge of the atoms and bonds of molecules. The first large implementation of Dendral was done over long-distance telephone lines. When the DEC PDP-6 computer arrived at the Stanford AI Lab, the program was transferred there [32, 33].

Using techniques from the AI field, the MYCIN program was developed by Shortliffe's group at Stanford University School of Medicine in the 1970s [106, 108]. Written in the LISP programming language, MYCIN used medical knowledge acquired from experts in the field of infectious diseases to help assess each patient's needs, and to then give advice and provide explanations for its judgments [44]. MYCIN was composed of three programs. First, a "consultation program" arrived at therapeutic decisions using a built-in knowledge base for micro-biology, as well as the patient's data that had been entered by the physician. After acquiring facts about the infection of interest, such as the specific micro-organism involved, a series of "if-then" production rules based on the stored expert knowledge would provide the appropriate advice. For example, if the causative organism was found to be bacteria "X", then it was advised to prescribe "Y" as the appropriate treatment. If the patient's physician questioned the advice, the program could be interrupted; and it then allowed the entry of questions, such as "Why?" Common questions had pre-programmed answers; and MYCIN then allowed for further questions that produced higher-level explanations. MYCIN allowed physicians who were inexperienced in computing to enter their questions and receive answers in natural language. Second, the "explanation program" allowed MYCIN to justify its recommendations and to answer a physician's questions about its reasoning process. It simultaneously kept a record of what had happened if this information were needed for subsequent reviews. Third, the "knowledge acquisition program" allowed infectious disease experts to update or correct the system's knowledge base. In 1976 MYCIN had more than 400 rules representing the transformation of knowledge from a number of infectious disease experts into decision-making criteria and rules [127].

In 1979, the success of the MYCIN project led the Stanford group to develop ONCOCIN, an oncology protocol management consultant program designed to assist physicians in the treatment of cancer patients. They used OPAL, an icon-based graphical programming language that allowed physician cancer specialists to enter complex cancer treatment protocols that could include groups of drugs for cycles of chemotherapy combined with radiotherapy [93]. A set of programs, ONCOCIN included an "Interviewer" that reviewed data entered from the patient's outpatient visits and passed the data to a second rule-based program, a "Reasoner" that used artificial intelligence techniques to recommend the optimal therapy for the patient based upon its logic of the management protocol and the patient data and allowed the physician to examine and approve or modify the ONCOCIN advice. Any changes were kept available for future review. The "Reasoner" program used parameters and rules (260 rules initially) presented in a natural language stylized format similar to those used in the MYCIN system [107, 109]. The "Interpretation" program helped analyze the data, and an ONYX decision support program recommended cancer chemotherapy for patients whose clinical course was atypical, such as when patients received multiple cycles of modified treatments under different clinical settings over different periods of time [65]. An evaluation of ONCOCIN found a slight divergence from ONCOCIN's advice and the actual clinical treatment given, but both were judged by clinical experts to be acceptable in most cases; recording of relevant data was found to increase when the ONCOCIN system was used [91].

17.3   Computer-Based Provider Order Entry/Results Reporting (CPOE/RR)

Spencer and colleagues [18, 113] proposed that the apex of the pyramid of the patient care process was the physician's order set and that virtually all activities in a hospital were planned to support and implement these patient care orders. Prior to the advent of computer-based medical information systems, the ordering of tests and procedures (such as clinical laboratory tests, x-ray examinations, surgical procedures, and others) by health care providers (physicians, nurses, and other licensed practitioners) had relied on using handwritten, or typed, or pre-printed paper requisitions. Also the reporting of the results of tests and procedures had relied on handwritten, or dictated and typed, or instrument printouts being sent back to the health care providers. To replace these error prone methods, a computer-based medical information system needed a computer-based provider order entry (CPOE) program capable of accepting the direct entry of a request order for a test or procedure to be provided to a patient; and a results reporting (RR) program capable of communicating back the report of the results after the test or procedure was completed. These made up the CPOE/RR that also provided relevant alerts, reminders, or appropriate clinical advice.

Early in the implementation of a medical information system it became important to plan for a CDSS that included a CPOE/RR program. The care provider used the order entry function to enter requisitions for clinical laboratory tests and x-ray procedures, to prescribe medications, order diets, enter preoperative orders for scheduled surgery procedures, send consultation requests, and enter any other orders for the care of a patient; and the CPOE also needed links to the business office system for patient transfer, discharge, accounting and billing functions. The results reporting function communicated the responses to the orders back to the health care providers, supplemented with relevant alerts and advice.

In the 1960s the earliest order entry programs used pre-punched cards containing added punched data that identified the patient and the name of the ordering provider and specified the desired medical orders. The ordering data that had been punched into the cards were then entered by a card reader into the central computer. For results reporting the reports were usually batch-processed, and the results of the tests and procedures were printed centrally. The printouts of results were then dispatched to the nursing stations to be filed in the patients' paper-based charts. Upon the completion of urgent or "stat" clinical laboratory tests, the results of these tests were individually printed out and usually also reported by telephone to the nursing station. When the order entry function transmitted prescriptions ordered by physicians to the pharmacy, then the system periodically generated listings of prescribed medications for patients cared for by each of the nursing stations. Nurses entered into the computer the time, dose, and method of administration for each drug given to each patient.

In the 1960s when a medical information system implemented a clinical support information system (CSIS) that included the clinical laboratory, radiology, pharmacy, and/or the business office subsystems, each subsystem had its own separate communication terminal. As a result, it was time consuming for health care providers when entering new orders or changing old orders for a patient, to have to repeatedly enter the patient's identification data into each of the separate terminals for the laboratory, the pharmacy, radiology, and the business office for a patient's bed transfer, discharge, or billings. Furthermore, many orders were of such a nature that they required associated secondary orders that involved communications to additional departments. For example, an order for an upper gastrointestinal x-ray examination, to be provided to a patient in a bed in the hospital's internal medical service, scheduled to be done at a specific time on a specified day, required the procedure be scheduled in the radiology department. In addition, the nursing and dietetics departments needed to be notified that food and fluids should be withheld from the patient prior to the procedure, that the patient should be transported to arrive in the radiology department at the time of the scheduled procedure, and that appropriate instructions be given as to any special medication and dietary orders for feeding the patient on return to the patient's bed. When such a series of orders was common routine, then they were often simplified by the establishment of standing orders. As Blumberg [28] at the Stanford Research Institute noted, since at that time 20–40 different drugs often accounted for 90 % of the orders written at a single nurse's station, a checklist order form was feasible; and order entry punch cards prepared for the nurses stations were usually used for the order entry of commonly prescribed medications.

By the mid-1960s, some order entry systems used terminals that had multiple-function keyboard buttons, with overlay mats designed for entering different modes for order entry. For example, one overlay was used for ordering laboratory tests, a different overlay for ordering medications from the pharmacy, and so on. In addition, keyboards were used for the entry of non-standard or textual orders [7–9, 11].

In the 1970s with the advent of visual display terminals that used a keyboard or a light-pen for data entry, some physicians began to be able to enter their orders directly into the system; but most continued to write their orders in free text on paper order forms. Nurses edited and encoded the orders; and then the nurses or clerks entered the orders into the computer terminals. It was difficult to standardize orders that were written in free text; and, at that time, the most common method of entering simple orders was by selecting appropriate statements from displayed menus of fixed orders. Complex orders were generated by a series of selections from a branching tree of menu screens, each item of which was defined and coded in a data dictionary.

Physicians' acceptance of order entry in one of the earliest hospital information systems, the Lockheed/Technicon system, increased when they were allowed to construct individualized *personal order sets* to suit their individual practices; they were then able to enter full sets of frequently used routine standing orders with a few strokes of the light pen.

In 1968 an early example of an *order entry* program for patient care was initiated at the Texas Institute for Rehabilitation and Research. As physician's orders were made, the affected departments were notified and made appropriate entries on one of the eight IBM 2260 visual display terminals located throughout the hospital. Computer printouts of scheduled activities were printed each evening, and were placed at each patient's bedside, and each department received a printout of activities expected to be performed during the day for its patients [18]. When the order entry function transmitted to the pharmacy the patients' drug prescriptions ordered by physicians, then the system periodically transmitted listings of prescribed patients' medications to the appropriate nursing stations. Nurses then entered into the computer the time, dose, and method of administration for each drug that had been given to a patient.

The earliest results reporting (RR) systems in the 1960s were usually batch-processed; results reports of all routine non-urgent tests and procedures were usually printed centrally. The paper printouts were then dispatched to the appropriate nursing stations to be filed in the patients' paper-based charts. Upon the completion of a "stat" (urgent) procedure, the results were individually printed out, or reported by telephone to the nursing station. In the 1970s with the advent of visual display terminals, urgent test results became retrievable on demand from the electronic patient record system.

In 1980 Black [22] at the Ohio Department of Mental Health published a detailed guide for planning, implementing, and evaluating an Automated Peer Review System. The great advantage of concurrent review made possible by an online electronic patient record was the ability to provide immediate CPOE feedback for disclosed errors and to permit faster corrective action than was possible by retrospective manual review methods.

In 1982 the 540 bed St. Mary Medical Center in Long Beach, California, used its IBM PCS) system to initiate a CPOE/RR system. This eliminated the need to send paper requisitions to the various clinical support departments and permitted a user to view results from these departments by using a computer terminal located in the nursing unit [89]. Finseth [52] and Brunjes studied the consistency in the recording of blood pressure measurements, the diagnosis of hypertension, and the associated prescribed medications as measures of appropriate quality of care for this condition. They reported that the outpatient information system's patient records readily provided the capacity for identification of individual patients who should have their blood pressures checked, such as those for whom a diagnosis of hypertension was indicated and those who needed treatment. They also suggested that the system enabled identification of individual practitioners whose performance might need to be modified.

Anderson [6] reported that the use of personal order sets by physicians at the Methodist Hospital of Indiana, which had installed the Technicon HIS in 1987, resulted in faster order entry and results reporting, a significant decrease in the error rate for entering orders, decreased nursing paperwork, and greater use of the direct order entry mode by physicians. By the end of the 1980s it was expected that clinical practice guidelines and alerts for adverse events evaluated as clinical decision support would become an integral part of the information system computer-based quality assurance programs and of CPOE/RR systems [5].

In the 1990s Hripcsak and associates [61] at the Columbia-Presbyterian Medical Center in New York developed a generalized clinical event monitor that would trigger a warning about a possible adverse event in clinical care, including possible medication errors, drug allergies, or drug side effects, and then generate a message to the responsible health care provider. Their objective was to generate alerts in real time in order to improve the likelihood of preventing adverse drug events.

By the 2000s most hospital information systems contained online, interactive CPOE modules that facilitated the direct entry of orders by physicians, thereby eliminating clerical intermediaries and any need to send paper requisitions to the various clinical support departments. By using interactive visual-display terminals and clinical workstations located in the nursing units and in the physicians' offices, physicians and nurses were able to view the results of tests and procedures they had ordered that were transmitted from the various clinical support departments; and urgent test results became retrievable on demand from the central computer-stored database of patient records.

In the 2000s clinical workstations began to be used for order entry since they permitted online guidelines for clinical decision support. The results reporting function communicated the results of procedures and tests from the clinical support systems back to the terminals located in the hospital, in the clinic, and in physicians' offices. By 2010 the diffusion of electronic health records and clinical workstations had resulted in most physicians' accepting computer-based CDSS with CPOE/RR programs that provided online practice guidelines, in addition to clinical reminders and alerts, to help define and monitor effective, quality patient care.

17.4   Online Monitoring for Adverse Clinical Events (ACEs)

It is an important requirement for the database management system of a primary medical record, such as an electronic patient record, to have the ability to promptly alert and warn health care providers of a potential adverse clinical event (ACE) that may harm a patient. This is done by designing a system capable of real time continual online monitoring of the healthcare delivery process for specified events capable of affecting the patient's well being and/or the quality of the patient's care. For any clinical procedure, such as measuring a patient's blood sugar or blood pressure and comparing the current test result to the patient's prior test results, programmed rules in the system are able to identify a significant change from prior values and signal an alert notice to the physician of a potential beneficial or harmful effect. This is a common requirement for an electronic patient record system that contains data from the clinical laboratory and/or from the pharmacy [94].

Maronde and associates [77] at the Los Angeles County-University of Southern California Medical Center advocated that, in addition to the entry of prescribed drugs, clinical laboratory tests, and clinical diagnoses into a patient's computer-based record, the database for an online adverse events monitoring system should include an assessment of chemical mutagenesis, including available objective data of chromosomal breaks, deletions, or additions, since they felt that the possible role of drugs in producing mutations had not been given sufficient attention. They advised that monitoring for chemical mutagenesis would entail chromosomal staining and study of chromosome morphology, and assessment of the incidence of discernible autosomal dominant and sex-linked recessive mutations.

With the advent of CPOE/RR programs for electronic patient records, monitoring alerts and warnings began also to provide clinical decision support suggestions and clinical practice guidelines. This was most readily done by implementing a CDSS with a CPOE/RR program to provide monitoring for ACEs together with real time alerts, reminders, and warnings. Results reporting programs for potential adverse clinical events began also to provide clinical decision support with alerts, advice, and clinical practice guidelines. Rind and associates [102] at the Beth Israel Hospital in Boston also described the importance of computer-generated alerts and reminders in monitoring ACEs. They defined a reminder as a communication that was sent to a clinician at the time of seeing a patient and defined an alert as a communication sent as soon as it became evident that an adverse condition had occurred that warranted an alert. A common example was when the pharmacy system employed the results reporting application of the CPOE/RR program to promptly send an alert on the discovery of an adverse drug event; or the clinical laboratory system sent an alert of a possible adverse effect of a drug on a test result.

17.5 Data Mining, Data Analytics, and Knowledge Discovery

In the 1960s Sterling and associates [115] at the University of Cincinnati proposed that a high-speed digital computer could be an ideal instrument with which to review and query a large number of patients' clinical records with the objective of finding within the huge masses of clinical information some important associations between the recorded patient care events. They developed an approach they called "robot data screening." Since the multitude of possible relations among the many variables to be analyzed was much too large for traditional statistical or epidemiological approaches, they studied models for analyzing combinations of two variables, then combinations of three variables, then of four variables; and they soon realized that the numbers of combinations of variables would become impractical even for their current computer when working fulltime. Accordingly, an inspection of the first pair of variables could show those that were not of interest and could be discarded. This process could be repeated and variables that were of interest would be retained and further coupled with other variables of interest, until only associations of interest would remain for the user to study. Sterling reported developing a computer program that applied criteria, or rules, to check each set of combinations of variables, and to eliminate those not to be retained. Depending on the outcome of each check, the machine then repeated the selection process with revised rules, until all uninteresting variables were eliminated. However, even by this elimination process, too many results were still provided for human study. They refined their robot data screening program to more closely simulate an investigator pursuing a number of hypotheses by examining the screened data, and rejecting some variables and accepting others. For a specific field of clinical knowledge, for example cardiology, they developed an algorithm that, when given a set of antecedent conditions, they could expect a certain set of probable consequences to follow; associations located by this screening program could then be scrutinized for the most useful information.

In the 1960s some commercial search and query programs for large databases became available, led by Online Analytic Processing. These systems used relational databases and provided answers to analytic queries that were multi-dimensional

[38, 39]. Database structures were considered to be multidimensional when they contained multiple attributes, such as time periods, locations, product codes, and others, that could be defined in advance and aggregated in hierarchies. Connolly and Begg [43] described a method of visualizing a multi-dimensional database by beginning with a flat two-dimensional table of data; then adding another dimension to form a three-dimensional cube of data called a hypercube; and then adding cubes of data within cubes of data, with each side of each cube being called a dimension, and with the result representing a multi-dimensional database. The combination of all possible aggregations of the base data was expected to contain answers to every query that could be answered from the data.

Blum [27] at Stanford University used the ARAMIS rheumatology database and proposed two different uses for clinical databases: the first use was for retrieving a set of facts on a particular object or set of objects; the second use was for deriving or inferring facts about medical problems. It was for this second use that Blum [25, 26] used a knowledge based approach to develop a computer program called the RX Project, to provide assistance to an investigator when studying medical hypotheses. The RX Project was a method for automating the discovery, study, and incorporation of tentative causal relationships when using large medical databases. Its computer program would examine a time oriented clinical database and use a "Discovery Module" that applied correlations to generate a list of tentative, possible relationships for hypotheses of the form, "A causes B". Then a "Study Module" used a medical knowledge base containing information that had been entered directly into it by clinicians. It also contained automatically incorporated, newly created knowledge and provided a statistical package to help create a study design. The study design followed accepted principles of epidemiological research, and controlled for known confounders of a new hypothesis by using previously identified, causal relationships contained in the knowledge base. The study design was then executed by the online statistical package, and the results were automatically incorporated back into the knowledge base. Blum [23, 24] further refined the RX Project to use causal relationships that had been already incorporated in the RX knowledge base to help determine the validity of additional causal relationships.

Fox [54] at the University of California in Los Angeles described their database-management system, A Clinical Information System (ACIS). Their system was developed for patient record applications, registries, and clinical research. It used linguistic methods for encoding and retrieving information in natural language. ACIS processed both hierarchical and inverted data files, and provided facilities to manipulate any of the variables in the retrieved data. Its databases could be examined using single English words or phrases; the inverted files could be manipulated using the Boolean commands, AND, OR, NOT. Systematized Nomenclature of Medicine (SNOMED) codes could be used to translate and explore items of interest.

By 1980 rapid advances had occurred in automated information retrieval systems for science and technology [45]. At that time, more than 1,000 databases were available for computerized searching, and more than two million searches were made in these databases. By the 1990s the availability of large, inexpensive data storage devices meant that it was possible to store very large datasets. However, since traditional methods for querying databases to search for desired information were still slow and expensive, a need developed for a new generation of techniques to more efficiently search through voluminous collections of data. The concept of robot data screening was then expanded to automated data mining.

Data mining was a concept introduced in the 1990s for finding data correlations or patterns in very large databases (today sometimes called "big data") or in collections of multiple large databases called data warehouses. Algorithms for data mining were developed initially for management applications, such as for planning stock keeping units for large grocery retailers where huge numbers of food items would move through scanners each day. Algorithms used rules to guide decisions and actions for a final solution, or for an intermediate action, or for the next observation to make. Algorithms could be deterministic or probabilistic in nature.

Most early data mining algorithms were based on Bayes' essay [17] on probability theory published in 1763, in which he proposed that the probability of the occurrence of an event could be expressed as the ratio between the current actual rate of occurrence of the specific event of interest and the total rate of all possible events of interest occurring within a specified time interval. Ledley and Lusted [66] explicated the application of Bayes' formula for estimating the probability of a diagnosis when given a set of symptoms or for estimating the likelihood of an adverse drug event when a patient had received a specific drug. Data mining required highly efficient and scalable algorithms with which to process ('mine') the ever-increasing sizes of clinical databases. These large databases typically held millions of data items, as opposed to the thousands of data items usually studied by classical statistical data analysis techniques. This necessitated the creation of extremely fast algorithms that usually incorporated simple pruning strategies for deciding when whole sections of the analysis data could be skipped as not likely to contain data that would produce new useful results. A consequence of this approach was that it was possible (given sufficient computing resources) to find all patterns in the data for which the support exceeded a specified support threshold level. There were many techniques used for data mining, including record linkage, outlier detection, Bayesian approaches, decision tree classification, nearest neighbor methods, rule induction, and data visualization. However, since traditional statistical methods were generally not well suited to evaluating the probability of 'true' and 'false' relationships identified in huge volumes of clinical data, methods began to be developed to try to better establish the sensitivity (for detecting 'true' positive associations) and the specificity (for detecting 'false' positive or 'true' negative) of the identified associations.

Data mining was defined by Prather and associates [98] at Duke University as the search for relationships and global patterns that were hidden among vast amounts of data. Prather and colleagues applied data-mining techniques to the database of their computerized patient record system. They initiated a data mining project using their Duke Perinatal Database for a knowledge discovery project to identify factors that could contribute to improving the quality and cost effectiveness of perinatal care. Multiple queries made in Structured Query Language (SQL) were run on their perinatal database to create a 2-year data set sample containing 3,902 births. As each variable was added to the data set, it was cleansed of erroneous values by identifying any problems, correcting errors, and eliminating duplicate values. Some alphanumeric fields were converted to numerical variables in order to permit statistical analysis. Factor analysis was conducted on the extracted dataset and several variables were identified which could help categorize patients and lead to a better understanding between clinical observations and patient outcomes.

Connolly and Begg [43] defined data mining as the process of extracting valid, previously unknown information from large databases to support decision making, and described four data mining techniques: (1) predictive modeling that involved building a training data set with historical known characteristics, and then developing rules that are applied to a new data set to determine their accuracy and physical performance; (2) database segmentation to develop clusters of records of similar characteristics; (3) link analysis to discover associations between individual records; and (4) deviation detection to identify outliers that express deviations from some previously defined expectation or norm.

Hand [57] described data mining as a new discipline at the interface of statistics, database technology, pattern recognition, and machine learning that is concerned with the secondary analysis of large databases in order to find previously unsuspected relationships that could be of interest. Hand further described data mining as the analysis of large observational datasets to find relationships between data elements, and to summarize the data in novel ways that were understandable and provided useful information. In a medical context, data mining was often used for the discovery of new relationships between clinical events; and for the surveillance or monitoring of adverse events. Often the data had been collected for some primary purpose other than for data mining analysis. Unlike hypothesis-driven data analyses in which data are analyzed to prove or disprove a specific hypothesis (for example, the hypothesis that there was an increased incidence in gastrointestinal bleeding among users of non-steroidal anti-inflammatory drugs), data mining made no (or few) prior assumptions about the data to be analyzed. It therefore has the potential to discover previously unknown relationships or patterns among the data. It would not assess causality in relationships between variables, but would only identify associations in which certain sets of values occurred with greater frequency than would be expected if they were independent. To prove causality in an association, further studies (for example, a randomized controlled clinical trial) would be necessary to confirm or refute that hypothesis. The relationships and summaries derived with data mining have been also referred to as 'models' or 'patterns'. Examples of such patterns could include linear equations, rules, clusters, graphs, tree structures, and recurrent patterns in a time series.

Hand also noted that since data mining was a relatively new field, it had developed some new terminology. An important difference between data mining and statistics was the emphasis of the former on algorithms; and the association of data mining with the analysis of large datasets was a key differentiating factor between data mining and classical exploratory data analysis as traditionally pursued by statisticians. The presence of large datasets could give rise to new problems, such as how to analyze the data in a reasonable amount of time, how to decide whether a discovered relationship was purely a chance finding or not, how to select representative samples of the data, or how to generalize the models found for sample datasets to the whole dataset. Seeking relationships within a dataset involved determining the nature and the structure of the representation (model) to be used; then deciding how to quantify and compare how well different representations (models) fitted the data; choosing an algorithmic process to optimize the 'score function'; and deciding what principles of data management were required to implement this process efficiently. Data mining approaches involve (1) model building, i.e., describing the overall shape of the data, and included regression models and Bayesian networks; and (2) pattern discovery, i.e., describing data as a local structure embedded in a mass of data, such as when detecting signals of adverse drug events, and then having experts in the field of knowledge decide what data was interesting.

Knowledge discovery was defined by Frawley and associates [55] at GTE Laboratories in Waltham, Massachusetts, as the non-trivial extraction of previously unknown and potentially useful information and patterns from large databases. They defined a pattern as a statement that described with some degree of certainty the relationships among a subset of the data. They defined knowledge as a pattern that was interesting to the user; and when the output of a computer program that monitored a database produced a new pattern, such output could be considered to be discovered knowledge. For such discovered knowledge they advised that the user needed to consider: (1) its certainty, since that depended upon the integrity and size of the data sample; (2) its accuracy, since seldom was a piece of discovered knowledge true across all of the data; (3) its interest to the user, especially when the discovered knowledge was novel, useful, and non-trivial to compute; and (4) its efficiency, in that the running time on a computer should be acceptable. They further advised that efficient discovery algorithms needed to be designed to extract knowledge from data by identifying interesting patterns representing a collection of data that shared some common interest, and describing the patterns in a meaningful manner.

Berman and associates [20] at Yale University School of Medicine also addressed the difficulty in maintaining and updating knowledge bases over the long-term. They explored the utility of interfacing their knowledge database with information stored in external databases in order to augment their system's information retrieval capabilities. To support their expert system for the clinical management of a disease, for example, asthma, they developed a knowledge database that integrated biomedical information relevant to asthma, and used their knowledge base to answer clinical questions and to guide relevant external database queries. When a clinician initiated a request for the name of a suspected occupational compound causing asthma, the system first looked for this substance in their internal knowledge base of agents known to cause asthma. If a match was not found, their system then automatically accessed databases at the National Library of Medicine (NLM), such as TOXLINE, to find a match for a possible causative agent. If a match was found, the system then looked in its knowledge database to see if any related substances could be found there. If at any point in the process a match was found then the results were presented to the user. The user was then offered the option of directing further queries to the NLM databases.

Agrawal and associates [1–3] at IBM's Almaden Research Center developed what they called the Quest Data Mining System. They took the approach that depending on the overall objective of the data analysis and the requirements of the data owner, the data mining tasks could be divided into: (1) exploratory data analysis, that typically used techniques that were interactive and visual, and might employ graphical display methods; (2) descriptive modeling, that described all the data by overall probability distributions, cluster analysis, and by models describing the relationship between variables; (3) predictive modeling, that permitted the value of one variable to be predicted from the known values of other variables; and (4) discovering patterns and association rules of combinations of items that occurred frequently. Agrawal further identified a variety of relationships that could be identified by data mining, including: associations, which were relationships in which two or more data elements (or events) were found to frequently occur together in the database. The data elements (or events) were usually referred to individually as items and collectively as item-sets; and the number of times an item or item-set occurred in a defined population was known as its support. Data mining methods found all frequent item-sets; that is, all associations among items whose support exceeded a minimum threshold value that exceeded what would be expected by chance alone. Rules were similar to associations, except that once identified, each frequent itemset was partitioned into antecedents and consequents; and the likelihood that the consequents occurred, given that the antecedents had occurred, was calculated, and this value was known as the confidence of the rule. Given a dataset, classical data mining methods were able to find all rules whose support and confidence exceeded specified threshold values. Yet discovering rules with high confidence did not necessarily imply causality. Sequential patterns were relationships for which the order of occurrence of events was an important factor in determining a relationship. A frequent sequential pattern was a group of item-sets that frequently occurred in a specific order. Clusters were data elements or events that were grouped according to logical relationships; for example, a cluster of influenza cases might be found during certain seasons of the year.

Bohren and associates [29] at the University of North Carolina at Charleston used a general classification system called INC2.5 that was capable of uncovering patterns of relationships among clinical records in a database. They described their system as an algorithm working in an incremental manner by incorporating new data, one patient at a time. The system was based on concept formation, a machine-learning method for identifying a diagnosis from patients' descriptions. Patients with common symptoms were grouped together and were represented by a description formed by a patient-symptom cluster that summarized their medical condition. INC2.5 used a similarity-based, patient evaluation function that optimized patient outcomes with respect to previously seen patients with the most similar group of symptoms, and it would provide for the physician a list of information possibly relevant to the diagnosis in question. They tested INC2.5 on datasets for patients with breast cancer, general trauma, and low back pain. Testing involved an initial learning phase, followed by adjusting the certainty threshold to increase confidence in its performance for accurate predictions. Finally, an attempt was made to reduce computer running time and reduce costs by determining the optimal variable threshold level and the minimal number of variables consistent with an acceptable accuracy of prediction. They concluded that the algorithm had the ability to automatically provide quality information concerning both the predictability of an outcome variable and the relevance of the patient's variables with respect to the outcome; and that its performance could be altered by adjusting the certainty threshold, adjusting the variable threshold, and by eliminating irrelevant variables.

Fayyad and associates [50] considered data mining as a method to analyze a set of given data or information in order to identify new patterns. They published a comprehensive review of the evolution of "Knowledge Discovery in Databases" (KDD), a term they noted to be first used in 1989. They defined KDD as the use of data mining primarily for the goal of identifying valid, novel, potentially useful, and ultimately understandable patterns in data; and they distinguished between verifying the user's hypothesis and automatically discovering new patterns. They described the process as involving the following steps: (1) define the user's goal; (2) select the data set on which KDD is to be performed; (3) clean and preprocess the data to remove 'noise', handle missing data, and account for time-sequence information changes; (4) reduce the effective number of variables under consideration; (5) select the data mining method (summarization, classification, regression, or others); (6) select the data mining algorithms, and which models and parameters are appropriate; (7) conduct data mining and search for patterns of interest; (8) interpret the mined patterns; and (9) act on the discovered knowledge and check for potential conflicts with previously known knowledge. The process could involve significant iterations and might require loops between any of these steps. They emphasized that KDD for the data mining of clinical databases needed natural language processing since some important patient care data, such as reports of procedures, were usually stored in their original textual format.

Fayyad et al. [50] described two primary goals of data mining: first, description, that focused on finding interpretable patterns describing the data, goals achievable by using a variety of data mining methods; and, second, prediction, that involved using some variables from the database to predict unknown or future values of other variables of interest. Most data mining methods were based on techniques from machine learning, pattern recognition, and statistics; and these included (1) classification methods for mapping a data item into a predefined group, (2) clustering a set of similar data, (3) regression of a data item into a real-valued prediction variable, (4) summarization by finding a compact description of a subset of data, and (5) probabilistic models such as those frequently used for clinical decision support modeling. These methods were used to develop best fitting algorithms and were viewed as consisting of three primary types: model representation, that used knowledge (stored data) to describe a desired discoverable patterns; search algorithms, designed to find the data in the database that best satisfied the desired patterns or models; and model evaluation, that used statements as to how well the particular discovered pattern met the goals of the search process.

Evans and associates [48, 49] at Creighton University used data mining methods for the automatic detection of hereditary syndromes. They reported that they could apply algorithms to family history data and create highly accurate, clinically oriented, hereditary disease pattern recognizers.

Wilcox and Hripcsak [124] at Columbia University also considered data mining to be a form of knowledge discovery. Their objective was to automatically build queries for interpreting data from natural language processing of narrative text, since valuable clinical information could reside in clinical progress notes, in radiology and other procedure reports, in discharge summaries, and in other documents. They developed a system to generate rules for the output of a natural language processor called Medical Language Extraction and Encoding System (MedLEE) that automatically generated coded findings from any narrative report entered into it. Berndt and associates [21] at the University of South Florida described their system for comprehensive tracking for community health (CATCH), and evaluating trends in health care issues. Nigrin [95] and associates at Boston's Children Hospital developed the Data Extractor (DXtractor) system that allowed clinicians to enter a query for a defined population or patient group, explore and retrieve desired individual patient data, find previously seen patients with similarities to the current patient, and generate a list of patients with common attributes. Based on their work with DXtractor, Nigrin described in some detail the development of a new data mining tool called Goldminer that allowed non-programming clinicians, researchers, and administrators to more effectively mine both clinical and administrative data in a large database. From primary patient record databases, they developed a separate clinical research database to run Goldminer. The data were maintained in an Oracle-8 database kept updated by routinely running Structured Query Language (SQL) scripts that copied new or modified data from their patient record databases. A web-based Java applet, Goldminer performed a population survey and guided the user through a variety of parameter specifications to retrieve a particular group of patients. Then, using logical Boolean set operations (AND, OR, and NOT), as well as temporal set operators to combine data sets, it provided the ability to generate complex overall queries, despite relatively simple individual data requests.

Johnson [64] described an extension to SQL that enabled the data analyst to designate groups of rows, and then manipulate and aggregate these groups in various ways to solve a number of analytic problems, such as performing aggregations on large amounts of data as when doing clinical data mining. Tenabe and associates [117] at the National Cancer Institute described an Internet-based hypertext program, called MedMiner, which filtered and organized large amounts of textual and structured information extracted from very large databases, such as NLM's PubMed. Benoit [19], at the University of Kentucky, described an information retrieval framework, based on mathematical principles, designed to organize and permit end-user manipulation of a retrieved set of data. By adjusting the weights and types of relationships between query and set members, it was possible to expose unanticipated, novel relationships between the query-and-document pair. Holmes and associates [60] at the University of Pennsylvania applied a learning classifier system, called EpiCS, to a large surveillance database to create predictive models described as robust that could classify novel data with a 99 % accuracy. Brossette and associates [31] at the University of Alabama at Birmingham developed their Data Mining Surveillance System for infection control for the automatic early detection of any increased rate of hospital infections, and of any increased frequency in resistant bacterial infections. By applying data mining algorithms to their hospital clinical laboratory data, they could automatically detect adverse patterns and events that would not have been detected by existing monitoring methods.

Lee and associates [67] at Rensselaer Polytechnic Institute in Troy, New York, applied several data mining techniques to heart disease databases to identify high-risk patients, define the most important variables in heart disease, and build a multivariate relationship model that corresponded to the current medical knowledge and could show the relationship between any two variables. They found that for the classification of patients with heart disease, neural networks yielded a higher percentage of correct classifications (89 %) than did discriminant analysis (79 %). Downs and Wallace [46] and associates at the University of North Carolina at Chapel Hill applied data mining algorithms to a large set of data from their Child Health Improvement Program and studied associations between chronic cardiopulmonary disease and a variety of behavioral health risks including exposure to tobacco smoke and to poverty. They concluded that, even though their data were relatively sparse and inconsistently collected, and some of their findings were spurious or had been previously described, data mining still had the potential to discover completely novel associations.

Srinivasan and Rindflesch [114] expanded the concept of data mining to text mining, by using the National Library of Medicine's MESH headings and subheadings to extract related information from MEDLINE, with the goal of searching related concept pairs to discover new knowledge. For example, the method could specify a pair of MESH subheadings, such as 'drug therapy' and 'therapeutic use', to approximate the treatment relationship between drugs and diseases; and then combine the pair with another conceptual pair to form a summary view for the study of the interrelationships between the concepts. Szarfman et al. [116] reported that since 1998 the Food and Drug Administration had been exploring automated Bayesian data mining methods using the Multi-Item Gamma Poisson Shrinker program to compute scores for combinations of drugs and events that were significantly more frequent than their usual pair-wise associations. In a review of software packages for data mining, including SAS Enterprise Miner, SPSS Clementine, GhostMiner, Quadstone, and an Excel add-on XLMiner, Haughton et al. [59] concluded that SAS Enterprise Miner was the most complete, while the SAS and SPSS statistical packages had the broadest range of features.

17.6 National Library of Medicine (NLM)

Through its many public resources and services, the National Library of Medicine supports scientific discovery, clinical research, health care delivery, public health, and education, for professionals and for the general public. One of the 27 Institutes and Centers at the National Institutes of Health (NIH) in Bethesda, Maryland, NLM celebrated its 175th anniversary in 2011. A compendium of NLM's milestones throughout its history, as well as annual reports dating back as early as the 1940s, are available on the NLM web site at http://apps.nlm.nih.gov/175/milestones.cfm and http://www.nlm.nih.gov/pubs/reports.html. An early history of the NLM was written by Miles [90], and a recent history of NLM by Collen [40].

NLM creates and maintains a large number of scientific databases, including MEDLINE, the online bibliographic database that grew out of the MEDLARS system which originated in 1964. MEDLINE contains more than 23 million citations to journal articles in the life sciences covering publications from 1946 to the present. Thousands of citations are added each day, with a reported 700,000 citations posted in 2013 alone. The PubMed search interface provides free access to MEDLINE as well as links to PubMed Central, NLM's full text archive of publicly available articles.

NLM produces several hundred electronic information resources on a wide range of topics that are searched billions of times each year by millions of people around the globe. Notable resources include a broad range of human genome resources, including GenBank, Entrez Gene, GEO, and dbGaP; a large number of toxicology and environmental databases, including TOXNET, an integrated database system of hazardous chemicals, toxic releases and environmental health; and resources designed primarily for the general public, including the flagship MedlinePlus and ClinicalTrials.gov, a database of information about clinical trials being conducted around the world.

NLM also supports and conducts research, development, and training in biomedical informatics and health information technology.

17.7 Summary and Commentary

The computer-aided systems for utilization review and quality assurance of the 1970s were superseded in the 1980s by more robust medical information, or medical knowledge, databases. These databases provided information about specific medical problems and were primarily designed to help clinicians make appropriate decisions in the diagnosis and treatment of their patients. Rapid advances in computer storage capabilities as well as greater processing capabilities during this era meant that medical knowledge bases could be commonly used to support clinical decision making. At the same time, it became clear that computer-based medical information systems needed programs that allowed direct order entry for tests and procedures together with the return of the results of those tests and procedures as well as alerts and warnings for actual or potential adverse clinical events. This was followed by the further incorporation of clinical decision support, advice and clinical practice guidelines in medical information systems.

In the 1990s the process of data mining applied to very large clinical databases became possible as computer storage became cheaper and computational processing became faster. Using techniques from statistics and information science, data mining has the potential to discover new information and uncover previously unknown important relationships and associations between clinical data elements.

A major problem encountered in any field, and this is certainly true for biomedicine, is keeping knowledge bases up-to-date. In the domain of biomedicine only the National Library of Medicine has the resources to satisfy this essential requirement. Through its many public resources and services, NLM has consistently played and continues to play a vital role in supporting scientific discovery, clinical research, and health care delivery.

References

1. Agrawal R, Srikant R. Fast algorithms for mining association rules. Proc 20th Int Conf Very Large Data Bases (VLDB). 1994;1215:487–99.
2. Agrawal R, Imielinski T, Swami A. Database mining: a performance perspective. IEEE Trans Knowl Data Eng. 1993;5:914–25.
3. Agrawal R, Mehta M, Shafer JC, Srikant R, Arning A, Bollinger T. The Quest data mining system. Proc Int Conf Data Min Knowl Disc. 1996;96:244–9.
4. Ahlers P, Sullivan RJ, Hammond WE. The cost of auditing outpatient records. South Med J. 1976;69:1328–32.
5. AMA News. Medicine by the book. Am Med Assoc News. 1989;32:1.
6. Anderson JG, Jay SJ, Perry J, Anderson MM. Diffusion of computer applications among physicians. In: Salamon R, Protti D, Moehr J, editors. Proceedings of international symposium medicine information and education. Victoria: University of Victoria; 1989. p. 339–42.
7. Ball MJ. An overview of total medical information systems. Methods Inf Med. 1971;10:73–82.
8. Ball MJ, Hammon GL. Maybe a network of mini-computers can fill your data systems needs. Hosp Financ Manage. 1975;29:48.
9. Ball MJ, Jacobs SE, Colavecchio FR, Potters JR. HIS: a status report. Hospitals JAHA. 1972;46:48–52.
10. Ball MJ. Computers: prescription for hospital ills. Datamation. 1975;21:50–1.
11. Ball MJ. Fifteen hospital information systems available. In: Ball MJ, editor. How to select a computerized hospital information system. New York: S. Karger; 1973. p. 10–27.
12. Ball MJ, Hannah KJ, Browne JD. Using computers in nursing. Reston: Reston Pub. Co; 1984.
13. Barnett GO. Computers in patient care. N Engl J Med. 1968;279:1321–7.
14. Barnett GO, Winickoff R, Dorsey JL, Morgan MM, Lurie RS. Quality assurance through automated monitoring and concurrent feedback using a computer-based medical information system. Med Care. 1978;16:962–70.
15. Barnett GO. Quality assurance through computer surveillance and feedback. Am J Public Health. 1977;67:230–1.

16. Barnett GO. The modular hospital information system. In: Stacy RW, Waxman BD, editors. Computers in biomedical research. New York: Academic; 1974. p. 243–85.
17. Bayes T. An essay toward solving a problem in the doctrine of chances. Philos Trans R Soc Lond. 1763;53:370–418.
18. Beggs S, Vallbona C, Spencer WA, Jacobs FM, Baker RL. Evaluation of a system for on-line computer scheduling of patient care activities. Comput Biomed Res. 1971;4:634–54.
19. Benoit G, Andrews JE. Data discretization for novel resource discovery in large medical data sets. Proc AMIA. 2000; 61–5.
20. Berman L, Cullen M, Miller PL. Automated integration of external databases: a knowledge-based approach to enhancing rule-based expert systems. Comput Biomed Res. 1993;26:230–41.
21. Berndt DJ, Hevner AR, Studnicki J. CATCH/IT: a data warehouse to support comprehensive assessment for tracking community health. Proc AMIA. 1998; 250–4.
22. Black GC, Saveanu TI. A search for mental health output measures. Proc SCAMC. 1980;3:1859–71.
23. Blum BI. A data model for patient management. Proc MEDINFO. 1983;83:748–51.
24. Blum RL. Automated induction of casual relationships from a time-oriented clinical database. Proc AMIA. 1982; 307–11.
25. Blum RL. Discovery and representation of casual relationships from a large time-oriented clinical database: the RX project. In: Lindberg DA, Reichertz P, editors. Lecture notes in medical informatics. New York: Springer; 1982. p. 38–57.
26. Blum RL. Automating the study of clinical hypotheses on a time-oriented clinical database: the Rx project. Proc MEDINFO. 1980; 456–60.
27. Blum RL, Wiederhold G. Inferring knowledge from clinical data banks: utilizing techniques from artificial intelligence. Proc SCAMC. 1978; 303–7.
28. Blumberg MS. Requirements for a computer system to process physician orders in hospital. Digest of the 1961 Intern Conf Med Electronics. 1961; 32.
29. Bohren BF, Hadzikadic M, Hanley EN. Extracting knowledge from large medical databases: an automated approach. Comput Biomed Res. 1995;28:191–210.
30. Brewster C. Concurrent quality assurance using a medical information system. Top Health Rec Manage. 1982;3:38–47.
31. Brossette SE, Sprague AP, Jones WT, Moser SA. A data mining system for infection control surveillance. Methods Inf Med. 2000;39:303–10.
32. Buchanan BG, Shortliffe EH. Rule based expert systems: the MYCIN experiments of the Stanford Heuristic programming project. Reading: Addison-Wesley; 1984.
33. Buchanan BG, Feigenbaum EA. DENDRAL and Meta-DENDRAL: their applications dimension. Artif Intell. 1978;11:5–24.
34. Buck Jr CR, Reese GR, Lindberg DA. A general technique for computer processing of coded patient diagnoses. Mo Med. 1966;63:276–9. passim.
35. Budkin A, Jacobs WA, Smith CD, Daily JD, Button JH, Berman RL. An automated PSRO-utilization review system. J Med Syst. 1982;6:139–47.
36. Cannon SR, Gardner RM. Experience with a computerized interactive protocol system using HELP. Comput Biomed Res. 1980;13:399–409.
37. Christofferson J, Moynihan CT. Can systems measure quality? Comput Healthc. 1988 (April); 24–7.
38. Codd EF. A relational model of data for large shared data banks. Commun ACM. 1970;13:377–87.
39. Codd EF, Codd SB, Salley CT. Providing OLAP (on-line analytical processing) to user-analysts: an IT mandate. San Jose: Codd Inc.; 1993.
40. Collen MF. Specialized medical databases. In: Collen MF, editor. Computer medical databases. London: Springer; 2012. p. 53–69.
41. Collen MF. Patient data acquisition. Med Instrum. 1977;12:222–5.
42. Collen MF, Rubin L, Neyman J, Dantzig GB, Baer RM, Siegelaub AB. Automated multiphasic screening and diagnosis. Am J Public Health Nations Health. 1964;54:741–50.

43. Connolly TM, Begg CE. Database management systems: a practical approach to design. New York: Addison-Wesley; 1999.
44. Davis RM. Evolution of computers and computing. Science. 1977;195:1096–102.
45. Doszkocs TE. CITE NLM: natural-language searching in an online catalog. Inf Technol Libr. 1983;2:365–80.
46. Downs SM, Wallace MY. Mining association rules from a pediatric primary care decision support system. Proc AMIA. 2000; 200–4.
47. Drazen EL. Utilization review in medical care: opportunities for computer support. In: Towards new hospital information systems. Amsterdam: North Holland; 1988. p. 14–7.
48. Evans S, Lemon SJ, Deters CA, Fusaro RM, Lynch HT. Automated detection of hereditary syndromes using data mining. Comput Biomed Res. 1997;30:337–48.
49. Evans S, Lemon SJ, Deters C, Fusaro RM, Durham C, Snyder C et al. Using data mining to characterize DNA mutations by patient clinical features. Proc AMIA. 1997; 253–7.
50. Fayyad U, Piatetsky-Shapiro G, Smyth P. From data mining to knowledge discovery in databases. AI Mag. 1996;17:37–54.
51. Fetter RB. Information systems requirements for case mix management by DRG. In: Towards new hospital information systems. Amsterdam: North Holland. 1988; 161–7.
52. Finseth K, Brunjes S. Quality of care and an automated medical record: blood pressure and hypertension. In: Hinman EJ, editor. Advanced medical systems: the 3rd century. Miami: Symposia Specialists; 1977. p. 161–7.
53. Forrest WH. Assessment of quality review in health care systems: the hospital. In: Hinman EJ, editor. Miami. Advanced medical systems: an assessment of the contributions. Miami: Symposia Specialists; 1979. p. 21–9.
54. Fox MA. Linguistic implications of context dependency in ACIS. Proc MEDINFO. 1980; 1285–9.
55. Frawley WJ, Piatetsky-Shapiro G, Matheus CJ. Knowledge discovery in databases: an overview. AI Mag. 1992;13:57.
56. Gabrieli ER. Computer-assisted assessment of patient care in the hospital. J Med Syst. 1988;12:135–46.
57. Hand DJ. Data mining: statistics and more? Am Stat. 1998;52:112–8.
58. Haug PJ, Gardner RM, Tate KE, Evans RS, East TD, Kuperman G, et al. Decision support in medicine: examples from the HELP system. Comput Biomed Res. 1994;27:396–418.
59. Haughton D, Deichmann J, Eshghi A, Sayek S, Teebagy N, Topi H. A review of software packages for data mining. Am Stat. 2003;57:290–309.
60. Holmes JH, Durbin DR, Winston FK. Discovery of predictive models in an injury surveillance database: an application of data mining in clinical research. Proc AMIA. 2000; 359–63.
61. Hripcsak G, Clayton PD, Jenders RA. Design of a clinical event monitor. Comput Biomed Res. 1996;29:194–221.
62. JACHO. Agenda for change: characteristics of clinical indicators. QRB. 1989;15:330–9.
63. Johnson D, Ranzenberger J, Pryor TA. Nursing applications of the HELP system. Proc SCAMC. 1984; 703–8.
64. Johnson SB, Chatziantoniou D. Extended SQL for manipulating clinical warehouse data. Proc AMIA. 1999; 819–23.
65. Kahn MG, Fagan LM, Shortliffe EH. Context-specific interpretation of patient records for a therapy advice system. Proc MEDINFO. 1986;86:26–30.
66. Ledley RS, Lusted LB. The use of electronic computers in medical data processing: aids in diagnosis, current information retrieval, and medical record keeping. IRE Trans Med Electron. 1960;ME–7:31–47.
67. Lee S-L. Data mining techniques applied to medical information. Inform Health Soc Care. 2000;25:81–102.
68. Lindberg D. The computer and medical care. Springfield: CC Thomas; 1968.
69. Lindberg D. Electronic retrieval of clinical data. J Med Educ. 1965;40:753–9.

70. Lindberg D. Operation of a hospital computer system. J Am Vet Med Assoc. 1965;147:1541–4.
71. Lindberg D. A computer in medicine. Mo Med. 1964;61:282–4.
72. Lindberg D, Van Pelnan HJ, Couch RD. Patterns in clinical chemistry. Low serum sodium and chloride in hospitalized patients. Am J Clin Pathol. 1965;44:315–21.
73. Lindberg D, Reese GR, Buck C. Computer generated hospital diagnosis file. Mo Med. 1964;61:581–2. passim.
74. Lindsay RK, Buchanan BG, Feigenbaum EA, Lederberg J. DENDRAL: a case study of the first expert system for scientific hypothesis formation. Artif Intell. 1993;61:209–61.
75. Lohr KN, Schroeder S. Special report: a strategy for quality assurance in medicare. New Engl J Med. 1990;322:707–12.
76. MacFarlane J, Britt M. The computer as a support tool in a multi-hospital medical peer review system. Proc SCAMC. 1981; 647–9.
77. Maronde RF, Rho J, Rucker TD. Monitoring for drug reactions including mutations, in outpatients. In: Computer aid to drug therapy and to drug monitoring. Proceedings of IFIP working conference. New York: North Holland; 1978. p. 63–8.
78. McClenahan JE. Medicare: utilization review under Medicare. Hospitals. 1965;39:55.
79. McDonald C, Blevins L, Glazener T, Haas J, Lemmon L, Meeks-Johnson J. Data base management, feedback control, and the Regenstrief medical record. J Med Syst. 1983;7:111–25.
80. McDonald CJ. Protocol-based computer reminders, the quality of care and the nonperfectability of man. N Engl J Med. 1976;295:1351–5.
81. McDonald CJ, Tierney WM. Computer-stored medical records: their future role in medical practice. JAMA. 1988;259:3433–40.
82. McDonald CJ, Tierney WM. The medical gopher: a microcomputer system to help find, organize and decide about patient data. West J Med. 1986;145:823–9.
83. McDonald CJ, Wilson GA, McCabe GP. Physician response to computer reminders. JAMA. 1980;244:1579–81.
84. McDonald CJ, Murray R, Jeris D, Bhargava B, Seeger J, Blevins L. A computer-based record and clinical monitoring system for ambulatory care. Am J Public Health. 1977;67:240–5.
85. McDonald CJ, Hui SL, Smith DM, Tierney WM, Cohen SJ, Weinberger M, et al. Reminders to physicians from an introspective computer medical record. Ann Intern Med. 1984;100:130–8.
86. McDonald CJ, Wilson G, Blevins L, Seeger J, Chamness D, Smith D et al. The Regenstrief medical record system. Proc SCAMC. 1977; 168–9.
87. McDonald CJ, Overhage JM, Tierney WM, Dexter PR, Martin DK, Suico JG, et al. The Regenstrief medical record system: a quarter century experience. Int J Med Inf. 1999;54:225–53.
88. Meldman MJ. Clinical computing in psychiatry: an integrated patient data base approach. Comput Med. 1975;4:1–2.
89. Mikuleky MP, Ledford C. Model for implementation of order system in department of nursing. Proc AAMSI. 1982; 436–40.
90. Miles WD. A history of the National Library of Medicine: the nation's treasury of medical knowledge. Washington, DC: National Library of Medicine; 1982.
91. Miller RA, Schaffner KF, Meisel A. Ethical and legal issues related to the use of computer programs in clinical medicine. Ann Intern Med. 1985;102:529–36.
92. Mullin RL. Utilization review based on practitioner profiles. J Med Syst. 1983;7:409–12.
93. Musen MA, Fagan LM, Shortliffe EH. Graphical specification of procedural knowledge for an expert system. Proc IEEE computer society workshop on visual languages. 1986; 167–78.
94. Myers RS, Slee VN. Medical statistics tell the story at a glance. Mod Hosp. 1959;93:72.
95. Nigrin DJ, Kohane IS. Scaling a data retrieval and mining application to the enterprise-wide level. Proc AMIA. 1999; 901–5.
96. O'Leary D. The joint commission's agenda for change. J Med Assoc Ga. 1987;76:503–7.

97. Phillips DF. Regulations and data systems: questions of demands versus needs. Hospitals. 1977;51:85.
98. Prather JC, Lobach DF, Goodwin LK, Hales JW, Hage ML, Hammond WE. Medical data mining: knowledge discovery in a clinical data warehouse. Proc AMIA. 1997; 101–5.
99. Prokosch HU, Pryor TA. Intelligent data acquisition in order entry programs. Proc SCAMC. 1988; 454–8.
100. Pryor DB, Stead WW, Hammond WE, Califf RM, Rosati RA. Features of TMR for a successful clinical and research database. Proc SCAMC. 1982; 79–83.
101. Pryor DB, Califf RM, Harrell FE, Hlatky MA, Lee KL, Mark DB, et al. Clinical data bases: accomplishments and unrealized potential. Med Care. 1985;23:623–47.
102. Rind DM, Davis R, Safran C. Designing studies of computer-based alerts and reminders. MD Comput. 1995;12:122.
103. Rubin AD, Risley JF. The PROPHET system: an experiment in providing a computer resource to scientists. Proc MEDINFO. 1977; 77–81.
104. Rubin L, Collen M, Goldman GE. Frequency decision theoretical approach to automated medical diagnosis. Proceedings of the 5th Berkeley Symp on mathematical statistics and probability. San Francisco: University of California Press; 1967.
105. Sanazaro PJ, Goldstein RL, Roberts JS, Maglott DB, McAllister JW. Research and development in quality assurance: the experimental medical care review organization program. N Engl J Med. 1972;287:1125.
106. Shortliffe EH. Update on ONCOCIN: a chemotherapy advisor for clinical oncology. Inf Health Soc Care. 1986;11:19–21.
107. Shortliffe EH, Scott AC, Bischoff MB, Campbell AB, Van Melle W, Jacobs CD. An expert system for oncology protocol management. In: Rule based expert systems: the MYCIN experiments of the Stanford heuristic programming project. Proc Internal Joint Conf on Artificial Intelligence. 1984; 653–65.
108. Shortliffe EH. A rule-based approach to the generation of advice and explanations in clinical medicine. In: Schneider W, Sagvall-Hein AL, editors. Computational linguistics in medicine. Amsterdam: North-Holland; 1977. p. 101–8.
109. Shortliffe EH, Scott AC, Bischoff MB. ONCOCIN: an expert system for oncology protocol management. In: Proceedings of 7th international joint conference on artificial intelligence. 1981; 876–81.
110. Slee VN. PSRO and the hospital's quality control. Ann Intern Med. 1974;81:97–106.
111. Slee VN. Automation in the management of hospital records. Circ Res. 1962;11:637–45.
112. Smith LH. Computerized medical record systems. Proc of a forum: medical record systems, an examination of case studies 1977. Chicago: AHA; 1–11.
113. Spencer WA, Baker RL, Moffet CL. Hospital computer systems: a review of usage and future requirements after a decade of overpromise and underachievement. Adv Biomed Eng. 1972;2:61–138.
114. Srinivasan P, Rindflesch T. Exploring text mining from MEDLINE. Proc AMIA. 2002; 722–6.
115. Sterling T, Pollack S, Gleser M, Haberman S. Robot data screening: a solution to multivariate type problems in the biological and social sciences. Commun ACM. 1966;9:529–32.
116. Szarfman A, Machado SG, O'neill RT. Use of screening algorithms and computer systems to efficiently signal higher-than-expected combinations of drugs and events in the US FDA's spontaneous reports database. Drug Saf. 2002;25:381–92.
117. Tanabe L, Scherf U, Smith LH, Lee JK, Hunter L, Weinstein JN. MedMiner: an internet text-mining tool for biomedical information, with application to gene expression profiling. Biotechniques. 1999;27:1210–4.
118. Thomas JC, Moore A, Qualls PE. The effect on cost of medical care for patients treated with an automated clinical audit system. J Med Syst. 1983;7:307–13.
119. Tierney WM, Hui SL, McDonald CJ. Delayed feedback of physician performance versus immediate reminders to perform preventive care: effects on physician compliance. Med Care. 1986;24:659–66.

120. Tierney WM, McDonald CJ, Martin DK, Hui SL. Computerized display of past test results: effect on outpatient testing. Ann Intern Med. 1987;107:569–74.
121. Tufo HM, Bouchard RE, Rubin AS, Twitchell JC, VanBuren HC, Weed LB, et al. Problem-oriented approach to practice: I. Economic impact. JAMA. 1977;238:414–7.
122. US Congress. Detection and prevention of chronic disease utilizing multiphasic health screening techniques. Hearings before the subcommittee on health of the elderly of the special committee on aging. Washington, DC: US Congress, 1966.
123. Warner HR. A mathematical approach to medical diagnoses: applications to congenital heart disease. JAMA. 1961;177:177–83.
124. Wilcox A, Hripcsak G. Knowledge discovery and data mining to assist natural language understanding. Proc AMIA. 1998; 835–9.
125. Wilkinson WE, Gehlbach SH, Hammond WE, Clapp NE. Using computer-generated feedback to improve physician prescribing. Proc SCAMC. 1982; 76–8.
126. Wolfe H. A computerized screening device for selecting cases for utilization review. Med Care. 1967;5:44–51.
127. Wraith SM, Aikins JS, Buchanan BG, Clancey WJ, Davis R, Fagan LM, et al. Computerized consultation system for selection of antimicrobial therapy. Am J Health Sys Pharm. 1976;33:1304–8.

Part IV
Epilogue

Chapter 18
Medical Informatics: Past and Future

Morris F. Collen and Robert A. Greenes

Abstract Led in its earliest decades by a few pioneers and supported by a small number of professional organizations and universities, medical informatics was funded primarily by federal grants and contracts until 1980, when industry began to enter the marketplace. Despite technology advances, diffusion across health care was slow, and computers were used predominately for business functions. In the 1980s specialized subsystems were developed for the clinical laboratory, radiology, and pharmacy, but by 1989 only a few medical information systems were operational, most of them in academic health centers that had received federal funding. In the 1990s, distributed information systems allowed physicians to enter orders and retrieve test results using clinical workstations; and hospital networks integrated data from all the distributed clinical specialty databases in an electronic patient record. By the end of 1990s, systems were up and running in the Department of Defense and Veterans Administration. In the 2000s, more clinicians in the United States were using electronic health records, due in part to steps taken to adjust the computer to its professional users. Diffusion was further advanced in 2010, when direct federal funding was extended to health care providers using systems that met "Meaningful Use" requirements in caring for Medicare and Medicaid patients. Advances expected in the next decade include precision medicine and patient genotyping; telehealth care; cloud computing; support for elder care with multiple chronic diseases and polypharmacy; advanced clinical decision support; patient data security; big data analytics, improved population health, public health, and disaster management; and interoperability and integration of care across venues.

Keywords Medical informatics • Clinical support systems • Electronic health record • Technology diffusion • Physician adoption • Historical development • Technological innovations • Federal role

Author was deceased at the time of publication.

M.F. Collen (deceased)

R.A. Greenes, M.D., Ph.D. (✉)
Arizona State University, Tempe, AZ, USA

Department of Biomedical Informatics, Mayo Clinic, Rochester, MN, USA
e-mail: greenes@asu.edu

© Springer-Verlag London 2015
M.F. Collen, M.J. Ball (eds.), *The History of Medical Informatics in the United States*, Health Informatics, DOI 10.1007/978-1-4471-6732-7_18

18.1 The First Six Decades: Review and Commentary

18.1.1 Evolution of Electronic Health Records, Clinical Support Systems, and the Field of Medical Informatics

Health care has been much slower to adopt the computer than it was to adopt two other important technologies – the telephone and the automobile. In 1876 Bell patented the telephone as a device for electronic speech transmission. While Hollerith was working on punched cards for the 1880 census, at that time Bell was beginning to market the telephone. According to Starr [31], in the late 1870s physicians were among the first to use telephone exchanges to connect their offices with local pharmacies, and to communicate with patients who were requesting house calls.

The great automobile race was held in 1895 from Paris to Bordeaux and back. In 1908 Ford put out his first Model T automobile. In the early 1900s, the *Journal of the American Medical Association* reported that automobiles were already generally accepted by the medical profession as its usual mode of travel; and that they enabled doctors to considerably decrease the time required for making house calls; and in addition that they made it easier for patients to visit physicians in their offices [17]. A Chicago dentist is reported to have purchased in 1927 the first Model A Ford on the market [18].

Starr [31] credited the telephone and the automobile with the greatest early improvements in the productivity of the medical practitioner. Clearly the automobile and the telephone quickly and dramatically affected the way the medical profession provided patient care. The automobile was much more efficient than the horse in transporting the busy physician to his home, office and hospital. The telephone was more efficient than was the postal mail in getting urgent messages to and from the physician.

Billings could not have foreseen the long-term consequences from his advice to engineer Hollerith to use punched cards to machine process the 1890 United States census data. The resulting invention of electronic data processing was probably the most important innovation of the twentieth century. In 1946 the first electronic digital computer built in the United States was called the ENIAC (Electronic Numerical Integrator and Calculator). In 1951 the UNIVAC, the first commercial computer with thermionic vacuum tubes became available. It was replaced in 1959 by the International Business Machines (IBM) 7090 computer that used transistors. In the 1940s computer programming began with von Neumann's invention of the stored computer program. These early innovations were quickly followed by many generations of specialized computer programming languages, together with advances in computer hardware, networking, data storage, and other devices, and in the software and hardware engineering disciplines to support them.

While computing quickly revolutionized many industries and fields, its advance in health care was much slower. Physicians have always used the physical and chemical sciences to gather information from patients regarding abnormalities in anatomical structure and in physiological function. Examples of medical physics that have used the sciences of mechanics and hydraulics are the mercury sphygmomanometer, aerodynamics for the spirometer, acoustics for the stethoscope, heat for the thermometer, and optics for the microscope and ophthalmoscope. Biochemistry was the basis for clinical laboratory analyses of a patient's blood and urine. Roentgenography exploited the absorption of x-rays by body tissues to study variations in anatomical structures. Nuclear medicine used radioisotopes to identify variations in physiology. Medical electronic analog devices recorded electrical signals from the heart (electrocardiography), from the brain (electroencephalography), and from the muscles (electromyography). Medical electronic digital devices measured pulse rates and body temperature. Enhanced digital imaging using three-dimensional reconstruction in computerized tomography (CT), magnetic resonance imaging (MRI), ultrasound imaging, and other modalities, is based on measurements of x-ray absorption of tissues, changes in tissue hydrogen molecule nuclear spin and orientation when deflected by a magnetic field, or other physical properties.

The 1950s through the 1980s were remarkable for medicine in the United States, not only because of the rapid diffusion of technological innovations, but because of the important changes in legislation and in the financing of health care. The country's economy continued to be strong as the Dow Jones industrial average climbed from 500 in the 1950s and, except for a recession in the 1970s, to the 2,000s in the 1980s. Health became a major potential political issue when, in 1953, Hobby became the first Secretary of Health, Education, and Welfare (HEW). In the 1950s, about one-half of the U.S. population was covered by some sort of voluntary health insurance. President Johnson signed the Medicare Act in 1965; as a result, Medicare and Medicaid extended health care to the elderly and the indigent. By the end of the 1980s, most people had some type of health insurance. Under this type of arrangement, third-party payers and health insurers helped to finance medical technology. In the 1950s, national expenditures for health care were about 3 % of the national gross product, or about $100 per-person per-year. In the 1960s, these expenditures were about 5 %, or $150; by 1987 health care expenditures had risen to 11 %, or almost $2,000 per-person per-year. Within this environment, the evolution and the diffusion of computers into medicine were sporadic.

Based on the continuing technological advances, and stimulated by increasing needs for managing the processes of health care, a new domain of knowledge and professional expertise has taken shape over the past six decades, known as medical informatics [14, 28]. In a sense this field was enabled by six trends:

- increased volumes and types of data that were independent of either the physician's or the patient's judgments
- the more solid basis resulting from this for the claim to objective decisions
- increased physicians' dependence on technology
- increasing variety of physician specialists needed to conduct and interpret the results of particular procedures such as radiographs, electrocardiograms, and other technology-based interventions
- a growing emphasis on need to monitor the quality of patient care
- recognition by health professionals of the need for formal organizations and collective care by cooperating groups and corporate re-orientation.

The first six decades of medical informatics were ones of high expectations and frequent disappointments. Medical informatics evolved as health care professionals learned to exploit the computer to help meet the immense and complex information needs of patient care. Led in its earliest decades by a few pioneers and supported by a relatively small number of professional organizations and universities, this new field was funded primarily by federal grants and contracts. Pressured by increasingly complex and expensive patient care, medical informatics gradually diffused throughout the United States and the world. Blum et al. [5] categorized the 1950s as "phase zero," when most computer biomedical applications began to process text and some images and signals. Blum also called the 1960s "phase one," when computers began to provide some direct applications to patient care; and he considered the 1970s "phase two," when medical informatics began to mature with more applications for clinical information systems and clinical decision support.

The personal computer moved rapidly into doctors' offices in the 1980s, but even by the end of the decade, it was not yet a day-to-day tool of physicians. It did not significantly affect patient care services or alter visibly the quality or the costs of medical care. Given the recognized need at that time to finance increasingly expensive medical care, one would hope that the potential of the computer to increase the performance of health care professionals and to increase the quality of medical care, yet to decrease the costs of care, would stimulate a more rapid diffusion of medical informatics for patient care. However, this rapid diffusion did not occur until the beginning of the next century.

Despite the slow initial diffusion of medical informatics for its first four decades, noteworthy accomplishments in each decade were the relatively rapid advances of computer hardware, software, data communications, and their applications to medicine; greatly increased computer memory, data storage, and data processing speed; and significantly decreased costs. The field evolved from expensive slow mainframe computers in the 1960s, to minicomputers with integrated circuits in the 1970s, to microcomputers and personal computers communicating by using local area networks in the 1980s, to networked clinical workstations using the Internet and the World Wide Web for global communications in the 1990s, and on to mobile smartphones and electronic tablets, smart sensors and wearables and ubiquitous computing and social networking in the 2000s. The development of the electronic health record (EHR) was a gradual process, evolving in capability from the 1960s to the present, with the diffusion of EHR systems in hospitals and medical offices accelerating in the 2000s, with expanding cloud data services, translational informatics, and telehealth in the 2010s.

In the 1950s, the earliest application of computers in the United States for health care purposes was pioneered by Ledley [19] when he conducted research applications for dentistry while at the National Bureau of Standards. In the 1950s, large mainframe, time-sharing computers were used for the earliest computer applications in medicine, when most data were entered into the computer by punched cards, and the printed output was produced in batches. During the 1950s, the medical community began to learn to use computers, and shared visions of their remarkable potential for medicine; however, only a few biomedical pioneer investigators actually had access to a computer.

In the 1960s, IBM introduced its 360-series of computers that used integrated circuits on silicon chips; and that became the basis of modern commercial computing. A major competitor appeared in 1962 with the invention of the first minicomputer, a general-purpose Laboratory Instrumentation Computer (LINC) that evolved into the Digital Equipment Computer (DEC) PDP series; these soon became the most widely used computers for medical applications. Using a DEC PDP-7 minicomputer initially (subsequently upgraded to later models), the Massachusetts General Hospital Utility Multi-Programming System (MUMPS) [13] was reported in 1969, and became commercially available shortly thereafter; it became the most commonly used programming language for medical computing applications in the United States – and is still widely used over 45 years later.

In the 1960s, lower-cost minicomputers were introduced and used for many medical applications, especially where data could be collected directly from automated and semi-automated instruments, and then undergo some limited data processing. The 1970s saw the advent of even cheaper and faster minicomputers and microcomputers, following the fabrication of the central processing unit (CPU) on a microprocessor chip by a group at Intel in 1969. In 1976 the Apple II computer appeared on the market. The first computer to feature a graphical user interface (GUI) was developed at the Xerox Palo Alto Research Center (PARC); and the GUI became the basis for the Macintosh computer that was released by Apple in 1984. The 1980s produced a rapid diffusion of personal computers (PCs) and the incorporation of microprocessors in a variety of medical applications, along with the expansion of computer networks both locally and nationally. Any computer-based system that had evolved for a clinical support information system (CSIS) usually became a subsystem of a larger medical information system (MIS). In the 1990s computer applications in many clinical support services were operational; some progress was becoming apparent in the use of computers for patient care and for electronic medical records (EMRs) in hospitals and medical offices; and the Internet made commonplace international communications using computers.

In the 1960s, the US Congress authorized several streams of research support for biomedical computer applications. The National Institutes of Health (NIH) was the greatest contributor through its Division of Research Resources, with several Institutes providing additional support for specialized applications; and the National Library of Medicine (NLM) supporting training programs in medical informatics beginning in the late 1970s. The Chronic Disease Division of the U.S. Public Health Service supported computer applications for health testing services and preventive medicine. The National Center for Health Services Research supported many demonstration and evaluation projects. The Regional Medical Program supported some computer projects with direct applications to patient care. In the Department of Defense (DoD), the Defense Advanced Research Projects Agency (DARPA) supported research, including the development of DoD's multihospital information systems for the medical facilities of its three armed services. The Veterans Administration (VA) supported the development of its own large multihospital information system.

The Public Health Hospitals and the Indian Health Service independently developed their own multihospital information systems. The National Aeronautics and Space Administration (NASA) developed remote health care projects for its staff in space missions. NASA was notable in another way: in the 1960s its remarkable achievement of putting a man on the moon led many to believe that computer technology could solve any problem.

In 1968 a survey conducted for the National Center for Health Services Research and Development reported that in the United States about half of the 1,200 hospitals with more than 200 beds used computers for some business functions, but only about 15 % of these had some operational medical or medical research computing applications [15]. The majority of hospitals subscribed to out-of-hospital, shared computing services [2] until the mid-1970s, when lower-cost, smaller special-purpose minicomputers were introduced with the capabilities of being located in different clinical departments, all linked to one or more central hospital, large main-frame computers [3]. At that time, a survey of computer applications in approximately 100 hospitals in the United States reported that only about one-third had clinical laboratory or other patient care applications [30].

By the end of the 1970s, a survey conducted by Maturi and DuBois [22] for the National Center for Health Services Research and Development assessed the state of commercially available laboratory, radiology, and pharmacy information systems. They reported that the major vendors of clinical laboratory systems at that time were Becton Dickenson, Technicon, Medlab, and Community Health Computing. The major vendors of radiology systems were Siemens and General Electric; and the major vendors of pharmacy systems were Becton Dickenson, International Business Machines, and Shared Medical Systems [22]. A second survey, conducted by Young and associates [34] at the University of Southern California, identified minicomputer-based information systems in medium-sized hospitals with 100–300 beds. They found that less than one-fourth of the hospitals had clinical laboratory applications that included the preparation of laboratory work sheets and schedules; very few had applications with two-way data transmission and laboratory test results reporting. They concluded that, as of that date, the smaller systems with minicomputers fell short of the more sophisticated systems in larger hospitals with mainframe computers.

In the 1960s and 1970s, the most satisfied users of computers in health care were business and administrative personnel. It was a time of somber realization that developing a comprehensive, efficiently functioning hospital information system (HIS) was a more complex project than putting a man on the moon, since the HIS was extremely complicated technology and was very costly to develop and to maintain. Furthermore, the somewhat crude systems, elementary user interfaces, and limited technology at the time had provided few immediate benefits and had frustrated many medical practitioners. Yet it was in the 1970s, perhaps in part because of the frustrations and unmet needs, and recognition of the potential importance of this area of endeavor, that medical informatics was identified as a new specialty to represent the broad field of computers, communications, information science, and biomedical technology as applied to medical practice, medical research, and medical education.

In 1980 a survey by Ball and Jacobs of vendors of hospital information systems (HISs) found that 18 vendors provided some nursing, pharmacy, laboratory, and radiology functions [1]. By 1987 about 20 % of hospitals in the United States had computer links between their hospital information systems and affiliated physicians' offices. Some already had workstation terminals that enabled data to be exchanged, copied, and modified; and some permitted direct access to laboratory and radiology reports from an office information system [25]. Linkages of a hospital information system to their staff physicians' offices were encouraged by the facilitation of the transfer of test results to the physicians [23]. In 1987 a Medical Software Buyer's Guide listed more than 900 products that included software for laboratory, pharmacy, and radiology systems [27]. In 1989 Dorenfest reported that the number of hospitals using some sort of computerization outside of finance had risen dramatically as computers moved into patient registration, pharmacy, nursing, and laboratory [10].

In the 1980s, IBM introduced its personal computer (PC) which readily operated on data in text mode; together with its many clones, it was in that decade the most successful personal computer on the market. Also in the 1980s, an important innovation for medical information systems (MISs) was the development of the local area network (LAN), which permitted the linking of mainframe, mini- and microcomputers of different vendors, located in different departments of hospitals and clinics.

The 1980s brought some maturation to the field of medical informatics with the acceptance of more realistic scenarios for the applications of computers to direct patient care in hospitals and clinics. Some of the greatest advances in that decade for medical informatics were in the clinical support information systems (CSISs), specialized subsystems developed for the clinical laboratory, radiology, and pharmacy. However, even at the end of the 1980s when most physicians already had a personal computer, the computer's use for direct patient care in hospitals and clinics was disappointingly limited; and it was evident that, for clinical applications, medical informatics was still an evolving field. Physicians found that the available computer terminals were still too difficult to use for handling common forms of patient data, for entering narrative information into the computer, and for retrieving meaningful textual statements from the computer. Health care practitioners wanted terminals that could accept continuous speech and cursive handwriting. As a consequence, in the 1980s most practicing physicians still wrote their notes in paper-based patients' charts similar to those they had used in the 1950s. Although they saw great changes in the generation and transmission of laboratory and radiology results, most physicians still reviewed the results of these procedures recorded in traditional paper-based patient charts. In the 1980s, nurses were generally accepting their hospital's information systems that used display terminals equipped with keyboard data entry. By the end of the 1980s, hospital administrators could use the computer to monitor the patient-care process as it was happening, rather than reviewing paper-based medical charts retrospectively. Computer-based utilization review and quality assurance programs began to impose rules to control hospital admissions and discharges, and to advise in patient care plans. The implementation of diagnostic related groups

(DRGs) by Medicare in the 1980s stimulated the implementation of computer-based claims reimbursement.

Since faulty clinical judgments often resulted from inaccurate or incomplete data, the initiation of computer-based provider order entry (CPOE) and results reporting (RR) with programmed alerts and advice, were expected to improve the quality of patient care by providing reminders and suggesting treatment alternatives. However, CPOE, especially the use of predefined order sets for specific indications, had the potential of having physicians place too much reliance on consensus-developed protocols, which might not exactly fit an individual patient's needs. For complex medical problems, physicians still wanted to rely on their clinical judgment based on experience derived from their having treated many similar patients.

Throughout the 1970s and 1980s, most of the medical information systems (MISs) with both inpatient and ambulatory care applications were developed in academic centers, primarily with federal funding. These included the systems at the Johns Hopkins Medical Center in Baltimore and at the Latter Day Saints (LDS) Hospital in Salt Lake City where many of the LDS Hospital's clinical modules soon became available from a commercial vendor. The successful systems at the Massachusetts General Hospital and the University of Missouri-Columbia grew out of initial clinical laboratory modules. The University of Missouri-Columbia system had a unique statewide communications network, and the Johns Hopkins Medical Center made substantive contributions to MIS development by devising a local area network (LAN) that linked different computers from different vendors. A MIS that was entirely developed commercially and was available in the 1970s and 1980s was the Lockheed/Technicon/TDS system. In the 1970s and 1980s, effective outpatient information systems (OISs) were Harvard's COSTAR, the Regenstrief Medical Record (RMR), and Duke's The Medical Record (TMR) systems. Each was partially supported by federal funds; all eventually became available from commercial vendors. The enormous difficulty in developing a comprehensive integrated EMR system was demonstrated by the remarkable fact that even by 1989 few EMR systems were operational in this country. An early comprehensive MIS with an integrated EMR with all of the basic associated CSISs was completed at the end of the 1990s by DoD with its Composite Health Care System (CHCS). The VA soon followed with its Decentralized Hospital Computer Program (DHCP).

In the 1990s, health care professionals were beginning to hope that acceptable EMR systems and national data standards would be adopted to facilitate data transfer between different medical facilities visited by a patient, and that computer terminals would also allow data entry by handwriting and voice. It should be noted that the terms "EMR" and "EHR" (electronic health record) are now used somewhat interchangeably, but the intent when the term EHR was introduced the late 2000s was that it was to connote a more comprehensive record system that includes data from multiple sources pertaining to the health and health care of a patient.

In the 1990s, most hospitals had or were linked to a variety of CSISs such as the clinical laboratory and radiology. In the 1990s distributed information systems allowed physicians to enter orders and retrieve test results using clinical workstations connected to client-server minicomputers in local area networks that linked the entire hospital. Patient data from all of the distributed clinical specialty databases were integrated in an EHR. The advent of clinical workstations linked by local area networks to the clinical support services made a CPOE system more acceptable for clinicians to use [9, 12]. Health care professionals were beginning to hope that acceptable EHRs and national data standards would be adopted to facilitate data transfer between different medical facilities visited by a patient; and that computer terminals would also allow data entry by handwriting and voice.

In the 2000s, increasing numbers of clinicians in the United States were using EHRs in their daily practice, but still not most of them. Clinical workstations helped the physicians manage office practices and provide patients' records with text, graphics, voice, and high resolution images. In some systems they were helped with difficult clinical decisions by linking to NLM's MEDLINE and PubMed, and to knowledge and factual databases; retrieving online guidelines to alternative diagnostic and therapeutic procedures, and receiving built-in decision support in the form of order sets, documentation templates, "infobuttons", and alerts (regarding adverse clinical events, drug-drug interactions, allergies), and reminders (tests or immunizations due).

As discussed further in Sect. 18.1.2, in the late 2000s Congress passed the American Recovery and Reinvestment Act (ARRA) that provided, among many other things, financial support for EHR systems, and for their diffusion in hospitals and in physicians' offices. With funding and incentives from several Federal agencies, notably the extraordinary financial support of the Combined Medicare-Medicaid System (CMS), EHR systems diffused rapidly over the next several years into most physicians' offices, medical clinics, and hospitals in the United States; and the use of traditional paper-based patients' charts and handwritten pharmacy prescriptions rapidly decreased. An important aspect of the legislation was that the financial support be tied to demonstration of "Meaningful Use," the requirements for which were designed to be more comprehensive in periodic stages over several years, in fostering increasing interoperability and interchange of clinical data, patient access, use of decision support, quality reporting, public health reporting, and other capabilities. The EHRs now included text, graphics, voice, and high-resolution images; users received help with built-in clinical decision support, more routinely available although by no means pervasive (see Chap. 16). In the 2010s, some physicians began to find the computer to be indispensable although perhaps not as friendly as the telephone.

It was hoped that a universal patient identifier would be adopted with appropriate safeguards that could protect patient data confidentiality; and that interoperability between different vendors of EHRs would become easier. However, to date this goal has been met by significant resistance from privacy advocates, and is not likely to happen in the near future.

In the 2010s, low-cost smartphones and tablets capable of transmitting text, voice, audio, and video became pervasive. Patients were beginning to use their smart phones and their personal mobile records to conduct mobile health with their health care providers and to access health care organization records through dedicated patient portals. There was also some use of personal health records (PHRs) by patients – dedicated systems controlled by patients for their personal health and health care recordkeeping and management – but to date this has lacked a strong financial model and has not been widely adopted.

18.1.2 Financial and Other Drivers for Progress

The experiences of these six decades confirmed that altering human behavior is very difficult; and for physicians to change their patient care practices and accommodate the use of computers was certainly no exception. The majority of clinicians did not readily adjust to giving up dictating to secretaries or writing in their paper-based medical charts, until they became accustomed to keyboard data entry and/or to mouse-type data selectors with visual display terminals, or until they could dictate directly into the EHRs. It became evident that the key to the successful diffusion of computers in medicine was to adjust the computer to its professional users, and not vice versa. Physicians have often been blamed for the lag in the diffusion of computer applications to patient care. However, history has shown that when new technology seemed likely to improve the efficiency or the quality of patient care, physicians were not reluctant to embrace such innovations, as evidenced by the immediate and wide diffusion of CT and MRI scanning, held back only by regulations requiring cost-benefit justifications for such expensive technologies. It was predictable that when necessary enhancements became available, physicians would eventually embrace computer workstation terminals and electronic health records.

Although federal government agencies funded much of the early research and development in medical informatics, the government provided, other than for the DoD's Composite Health Care System, little direction or coordination of these activities until the late 2000s. This resulted in a general "bottom-up" approach to the development of medical informatics and health IT solutions in this country. Even such federal agencies as the Veterans Administration, the Public Health Service, and the Indian Health Service independently developed their own MISs. This was in contrast to some other countries, notably Japan, where a top-down approach was taken for their MIS development. In the United States, other than the National Library of Medicine's program to develop a Unified Medical Language System (UMLS), there was little evidence of a nationwide coordinated effort in MIS development until the late 2000s and beyond. At that point, the federal government, with an eye to reining in continually rising costs of health care and providing a more accountable, high value health system, generously supported the diffusion of EHRs. Whereas in the 1960s and 1970s, federal government agencies had provided most of the funding for health research and development, including early health information technology (IT), in the 1980s industry began to financially support an increasing share of research and development in health IT in the United States; and in the 1990s industry became the largest supporter of the development of health IT.

By the 1980s, the increasing expenditures for health care became a great national concern, and efforts to control the costs of care became a matter of high priority. In 1983 the Health Care Financing Administration (HCFA) instituted for hospital patients a scheme of fixed Medicare payments for 468 diagnosis-related groups (DRGs) based on International Classification of Diseases (ICD) codes. In each hospital in the United States that accepted Medicare patients, this led to a rapid and often a major change in its hospital computer system, to allow collecting the necessary data to satisfy Medicare billing requirements. Since Medicare accounted for about 40 % of all hospital beds in use in the United States, it became evident that a federal agency could be a powerful force in the diffusion of health IT in this country. By the end of the 1980s, HCFA began to consider requiring physicians to similarly provide in their claims for payments the codes for the diagnoses of Medicare office patients; and HCFA began to explore the electronic processing and payments of claims. As the concerns in the 1980s about the rising costs of medical care grew, there was a concomitant increased competition among medical care organizations to build more efficient and cost-effective integrated delivery networks, a trend toward industrialization of medical care and the formation of medical conglomerates developed; this in turn provided the stimulus for multi-facility health information systems; and the health care industry had become one of the largest industries in the United States. In 1988, *The Fifth Annual Market Directory of Computers in Health Care* listed 750 vendors of medical computer systems, their applications and supplies [8]. In 1989 a compendium in the journal *MD Computing* listed almost 400 manufacturers or vendors selling more than 1,000 different medical computing products; most were designed for personal computers, and only about one-third were for clinical purposes [16].

The daunting complexity of a large hospital and the enormous number of technical requirements for a comprehensive EHR system are clearly evidenced by the relatively slow major achievements in EHR systems during these past six decades. Probably the greatest increments of change in the function, design, development, and diffusion of EHRs in the United States occurred when the federal government funded these changes, as when (1) in 1983 the changes in government reimbursement policies for the payment of claims for the care of Medicare patients required hospitals to use diagnosis-related groupings (DRGs) when billing for reimbursement for medical services provided to eligible patients; and (2) in 2009 when the US Congress passed the American Recovery and Reinvestment Act (ARRA), Title XIII of which was the Health Information Technology for Economic and Clinical Health (HITECH) Act. The HITECH Act included and resulted in the establishment in 2010 of the Office of the National Coordinator for Health Information Technology (ONC) to directly fund health care providers to implement in their offices electronic health record (EHR) systems that satisfied Meaningful Use of certified information technology used to provide care to the Center for Medicare and Medicaid (CMS) patients. Regrettably, Congress did not require at this date, as it had in 1983, standardized data coding and interoperability of patients' records so that a patient could choose to be seen by different physicians in different EHR systems and yet have all their data integrated wherever they received their care.

18.1.3 Perspectives on Health Information Technology Advances to Date

Considering health IT relative to other technology activities in our society, it is helpful to step back and reflect on what one might consider as truly *great* technology achievements over the past century or so. Among many achievements, we can cite the following as truly remarkable technology events: (1) In the 1900s sending a telegram by cross-country wires; or going to a telephone attached to a wall and turning its crank to generate a call signal on the telephone party line and then completing a personal telephone call. (2) In the early 1920s using a crystal set, and bare copper wire wrapped around a cylindrical box so that by sliding a wire leader from an outside aerial along the coiled copper wire, an amateur radio operator could thus vary the wavelengths of incoming radio signals; and with ear phones hear transmitted voices and music from all over the country. (3) Then came the wireless transmission of images; and television was first used to announce the results of a presidential election. (4) The Russians shot Sputnik into space; and President Eisenhower reacted by initiating Defense Department's DARPA that created ARPANET, that evolved into the Internet, that grew to include electronic mail and the World Wide Web. (5) When NASA put a man on the moon, this was generally thought to be man's greatest technology achievement. (6) In the 1990s electronic mail (email) was becoming generally available and began to compete with postal mail; and later the use of smartphones included the ability to similarly exchange voice and text messages.

Thus as we look back at the progress in this difficult and complex field, it has been allowed to evolve, as with many technology advances, in somewhat uncoordinated fashion, with growing efforts to align these efforts as the needs and challenges of our health care system continue to increase. In considering the next decade, we describe some advances that provide both further challenges and growing opportunities to create a robust health information technology framework for the future, and an informatics discipline, methodologies, skills, and cadre of experienced professionals to bring it about.

18.2 Some Projections for the Next Decade

It can be reasonably projected that in the next decade important advances will occur in: (1) increasing use of patient genotyping, (2) telehealth care as well as connected care, also known as m-health for mobile applications, (3) greatly enhanced cloud computing services and integrated care; (4) care of the elderly and monitoring of adverse drug events (ADEs); (5) clinical decision support systems (CDSS); (6) improved patient data security; (7) big data analytics, improved population health, public health, and disaster management; and finally, (8) interoperability and integration of care across venues.

18.2.1 Precision Medicine

Precision (or personalized or individualized) medicine refers to the increasing specificity of patient characterization now possible, through genomic, proteomic, and other "omic" analytic methodologies. For several decades, clinical support systems, such as the clinical laboratory, the imaging department, and the pharmacy have become increasingly essential aspects of an EHR system. Just considering the clinical laboratory, during the past several decades, physicians have become increasingly dependent upon ir and its computer-based subsystem. In 1991 several hundred different tests were already available; and in 2012 the numbers and the demand for laboratory tests had greatly increased due to the increase in numbers of patients, especially the elderly patients with diabetes, heart disease, and Alzheimer's disease. New omics analyses are rapidly becoming available and affordable. From the outset, it has been increasingly necessary to employ computers to develop enhanced automated laboratory systems to meet these demands; and the quantitative nature of most laboratory tests make them ideal for automation [6]. In the next decade it can be projected that patients admitted to large medical centers will routinely receive genotyping of their genome, and other omics analyses, in addition to the usual phenomic data obtained by recording the many other tests and procedures routinely performed along with the history taking and physical examination of a patient.

With the increasing use of both genomic and phenomic medical data in personal patient care, HIPAA can be expected to issue appropriate further restrictions to protect each patient's electronic health record (EHR), specify protection for transfer of a patient's data between legal health care providers; and yet allow medical research to benefit from the use of all types and sources of patient data. The increasing use of advanced computer analytics, using warehouses with huge clusters of servers providing cloud computing, will benefit CDS for complex medical diagnosis and treatment problems by using both phenomic and genomic patient data.

Hopefully in the next decade with further advances in pharmacogenomics, the study of how genetic variations in individual patients can influence medication therapy will further improve the safety and effectiveness of prescribed drugs. See Sect. 18.2.4.

18.2.2 Telehealth and Connected Care (m-Health)

Telehealth, or connected care, also called mobile health care (*m-health*), refers to any communications used by health care providers to care for distant patients. Telehealth can range from telecommunications between one patient and one health care provider, to advanced high-quality online voice and video interactions with a patient's EHR. Patients with mobile devices can monitor and report on their own vital signs and manage treatment and thus decrease the need for some visits to the doctor's office. In the 2010s outpatient information systems (OISs) and hospital information systems (HISs) already had the capability of accepting patient care orders generated wherever a patient was located, by a health care practitioner using the order entry module (OE) of the CPOE program of the medical center; and the results reporting (RR) module could display test results using mobile terminals such as smartphones or electronic laptops.

In the next decade telehealth care for patients located outside of a major medical center that holds the patients' EHRs will be greatly expanded due to the increasing numbers of elderly patients with diabetes, heart disease, kidney disease, arthritis, Alzheimer's disease and other chronic disorders. M-health will be commonly and more efficiently provided in patients' homes, with the health care providers, using smartphones, electronic laptops or tablets equipped with mobile broadband access, to directly transfer the patient's data to-and-from the health care provider and the patient's record stored in the clinic or hospital EHR database. A major driver for this trend is the rapid growth in variety and capabilities in recent years of a wide range of personal biosensors for temperature, weight, blood pressure, p02, heart rate, glucose level, respiratory parameters, etc., and environmental sensors for such things as motion/activity, air quality, and ambient temperature, as well as sensors embedded in home appliances and in the automobile. We will see increasing numbers and varieties of wearable and implanted sensors and devices, including those embedded in smartphones, along with increasingly capable mobile apps and internet-enabled things. Interfaces will increasingly support voice recognition, text-to-speech; and even some touchless gesture controls for applications where keypads and touch screens are used on smartphones, as well as 3D sensing such as now done in some gaming consoles. Of course the expected cautions must be raised in such scenarios; such use can sometimes be dangerous, such as when a person is driving an automobile while texting or engaging in other multifunction tasks.

Together with cloud computing to manage this wealth of data, and tools to analyze it, and to provide summaries/dashboards, reminders, and notifications of both patient and provider, as necessary, we can expect a major expansion in this realm of development. This will be augmented further by policies and reimbursement strategies that emphasize wellness, early detection of disease, and more active care coordination, e.g., post-discharge, as well as incentives for reimbursement of providers for telehealth services and easing of some of the geographic and professional restrictions currently limiting the licensing of providers to perform such services.

It can be reasonably projected for the next decade, therefore, that remote biosensors, hand-held portable devices, and cloud computing will become not only routine tools and resources for the consumer/patient, but also for health care providers, to enable them to communicate with each other and with their patients, to review their patients' data any time at any site, to transmit advice to patients, to transmit orders to pharmacies and to laboratories, and to obtain web-based clinical decision support.

Virtual consultation and remote diagnosis offer incredible potential to shape surgery practices of the future, and to increase access to clinical specialist services from within the primary care system. Telehealth technology could significantly reduce the burden on the provision of secondary health care, and could result in a major transformation of primary care, as for example, with the creation of remote diagnosis and observation rooms, allowing patients to be diagnosed via video links and subsequently treated remotely by specialists. Such mobile telehealth methods could also reach many nurses, support staff, and doctors, thereby broadening access to conveniently accessible care. Telehealth also has the potential to create high-definition conferencing suites by enabling clinical experts to discuss together care options, irrespective of their geographical location, leaving more time for the delivery of other vital services. Telehealth is continually evolving and can be adapted to many different situations. Robotic surgery is already well developed and used for distance surgery. Renal care and optometry have already been identified as areas where telehealth can be used effectively. Patients with kidney failure using dialysis machines in their own homes can be monitored remotely by their renal specialists. Eye examinations by optometrists can be carried out via a video link. The opportunities for education and training, including virtual skill-based training, are also exciting.

18.2.3 Cloud Computing Services and Big Data

Cloud computing is a term applied to internet-based and web-enabled access to groups of computer servers, and is often represented symbolically in network diagrams as a cloud. The term cloud storage is generally applied to a group of servers or distributed data resources functioning as one integrated data warehouse that can be shared by multiple clients; and the concept of a "cloud" in this context is simply represented as storing online the client's data using a network of storage devices (servers) instead of storing it on the client's own hard drive.

In the next decade cloud computing services will greatly expand not only their storage but also their computing capabilities; and they will allow linked desktop computers to be replaced by smaller mobile devices such as smartphones and electronic tablets. Whereas, prior to the Web, a hospital computer network was often served by a large mainframe computer that shared stored data files, after the establishment of the Internet and the Web, the term computer server was applied to a computer system that provided services to clients; and the client-server model employed a communicating network that used the Web and the Internet Protocol (IP) to link a group of distributed data resources that functioned as one integrated data warehouse that could be shared by multiple clients. By using the Web, cloud computing enables a client's computer applications to run off-site on the provider's cloud storage equipment and to link back to the client, thereby reducing the client's infrastructure costs; it also enables the client to quickly scale the system up or down to meet changing needs, and to pay only for the amount of services needed for a given time. Global wireless communication has evolved to the point that using huge collections of cloud-based storage servers can create translational networks that link data warehouses in collaborating medical centers in the nation, and can support mobile e-health care for many individual patients. However, for patients' medical data, any shared storage by servers increased the risk of potential invasions of patients' data security and data privacy.

The increasing use of advanced computer analytics is also being seen and will expand. A prominent example has been the Watson program developed by IBM to harness large databases, text resources, and knowledge bases to create advanced CDS for complex medical diagnosis and treatment problems using both phenomic (based on the traditional phenotype characterization data in EHRs – history, physical, lab, imaging, etc.) and genomic patient data.

The subdiscipline of translational research informatics emerged in the 2000s to address the transfer of large volumes of patients' data between different data warehouses and clouds, and to support the querying of diverse information resources located in multiple institutions. The National Center for Biomedical Computing (NCBC) grants program of NIH funded development of a number of technologies to address locating, querying, composing, combining, and mining biomedical resources.

In the next decade the Internet likely will be a maze of thousands of servers and clients; and *cloud storage* services will be provided by multiple vendors, including Amazon, Apple, Google, IBM, Microsoft and other commercial vendors, each allowing the transfer of files between computers, smartphones, and electronic tablets. Barret [4] reported that Dropbox developed by Houston, was already storing on remote servers about 20 billion documents for 4 million client-users with their 500,000 computers. When a user downloaded the Dropbox software to the user's computer, it created a folder for placing documents that the user wanted to access remotely, e.g., from the Web, and to synchronize with other instances on different computers. Despite these capabilities, with various high visibility data breaches in the early 2010s, the cloud storage of electronic medical records continues to raise concern about the need for added security and privacy.

Virtualization is a term sometimes used to describe the moving of data from a fixed storage site into a cloud. The journal *Economist* [33] considered computing clouds to be essentially digital-service factories that were global utilities accessible from all corners of the planet; and described a "cloud of clouds" as having three levels of service: (1) one level called "software as a service" (SaaS) included Web-based applications; (2) another level called "platform as a service" (PaaS) allowed developers to write applications for Web and mobile devices; and (3) a level called "infrastructure as a service" (IaaS) allowed basic computing services that companies, like Amazon, used as its computer center. Lev-Ram [20] reported that Intel was developing cloud services that could work seamlessly on any device, and software developers could build applications using a standard set of tools. Intel's Cloud Builders program provided step-by-step guidance to companies that wanted to move data and services to the cloud; and Intel brought together a group of about 70 companies to develop cloud computing software and hardware standards.

18.2.4   Elderly Care and Adverse Drug Events

During the past six decades, the increasing use of prescribed drugs in patient care has resulted in an alarming increase in the number of adverse drug events (ADEs) especially in patients older than 60 years. One of the most important contributions computers have made to the quality and safety of medical care has been in pharmacotherapy and in ADE monitoring.

Whereas prior to the 1960s, hospitals stocked full lines of medications at patient care units in cabinets managed by nurses, the advent in the 1970s of automated medication dispensing from unit-dose machines led to automated, ward-based medication cabinets in the 1980s. Prior to the introduction of hospital unit-dose systems, drugs were sometimes obtained out of general supplies in nursing stations; their administration to patients could take place in different hospital locations and was often recorded in different paper-based records. The earliest PHARM systems were used for improving drug administration, but it was soon realized that the most important application of the increasing computing power, associated with the greatly expanding data-storage capacities, needed to be applied to the development of automated PHARM systems for monitoring and detecting ADEs in order to improve the quality and safety of patient care.

Beginning in the 1960s, it was realized that developing computer-based drug monitoring systems for studying, detecting and preventing ADEs could be especially useful for hospitalized patients who usually have accessible a full record of information on all events occurring for each patient; and this information is especially important for patients over the age of 60 years who usually take multiple prescription drugs, referred to as polypharmacy, and for whom ADEs are more common. In the 2010s, even though it was estimated that less than 1 % of the three billion prescriptions written in the United States per year were entered by a computer, the electronic entry of prescriptions, a key component of e-prescribing, CPOE, and the EHR, was expected to accelerate the process [29]. It can be projected that in the next decade the advances in pharmacogenomics, the study of how genetic variations in individual patients can better influence medication therapy, and further improve the safety and effectiveness of prescribed drugs (see also Chap. 13). It can also be projected that the Food and Drug Administration (FDA) will need to increase its national automated ADE monitoring system to include every EHR system in this country.

Because of the increase in chronic diseases, patients need to increasingly be managed across multiple venues of care, from home to workplace, to provider office, to specialist offices or imaging centers, to hospital, or extended care facilities; access to medication data, as well as to an integrated problem list, allergies, and labs across venues will be needed more than ever. To coordinate care across such venues, a higher degree of interoperability and exchange of information will be needed. This is partially addressed in our discussion of telehealth and connected care in Sect. 18.2.2. We will come back to this point in Sect. 18.2.8.

18.2.5   Clinical Decision Support

Physicians have always sought the best advice for the diagnosis and treatment of their patients' medical problems, either by consulting with more experienced specialists or by searching in medical publications for the best outcomes of patients reported to have had been treated for similar problems. With the advent of computers and medical information systems, the earliest informaticians explored the use of computers to help clinicians provide better quality of care to their patients. Programs for clinical decision support (CDS) have been continually developed and enhanced to try to provide better computer aided diagnosis (CAD) for patients with rare and/ or complex medical conditions; and more effective computer-aided therapy (CAT) for patients with complicated associated medical problems. CPOE and RR are already essential components of EHR systems. The aforementioned advances in precision medicine, increase in numbers and complexity of elderly patients with multiple chronic diseases, the growth of polypharmacy, and the increasing recognition of need for coordination of care across multiple venues are adding dramatically to the need for CDS tools.

It can be projected that meeting this need will come from several areas:

- *Improved methods for generating knowledge.* These include advances in text mining from the literature, data mining and predictive modeling from the increasingly large and varied clinical databases, and improved capture of clinical trial data in standardized form and expansion in requirements for registering and making such data available.
- *Knowledge representation.* Formal methods will mature for organizing knowledge through ontologies, and knowledge processing formalisms such as rule systems, especially evolution of the semantic web and associated technologies. A major aspect of this will be the formalization of the metadata, e.g., relating to source and provenance of the knowledge, the domain of application, the setting and context, in increasingly fine-grained and yet standardized form, that will allow the knowledge to be searched and retrieved for highly specific use.
- *Standardization.* Interoperability of data and knowledge are essential at many levels, and this will continue to be a major focus of effort as work to harmonize the many competing standards and approaches continues. This includes data models, vocabularies and terminologies, ontologies, reasoning formalisms, transport protocols, grouping methods (such as for order sets or documentation templates), workflow and guideline formalisms, quality measures, and decision support as a service.
- *Knowledge management.* Efforts to formalize knowledge in its many forms and associated metadata are leading to increasingly robust approaches to managing a knowledge base, update it, and access for specific needs. It is unclear where the authoritative knowledge will reside, but possibilities include national level repositories hosted by agencies such as the NLM, those supported by professional specialty or disease-focused organizations, large health care organizations or payers, or by knowledge vendors. There may be opportunities for internation-

ally hosted knowledge resources, such as by the World Health Organization. It can be expected that over the next decade, the gap will be filled by selective repositories for specific needs, such as national resources defining data elements and rules for quality measurement to support Meaningful Use, drug interaction data as available through various knowledge vendors, and guidelines for particular clinical problems, by panels for evidence-based recommendation either through government agencies or professional or disease-focused organizations.

- *Decision support as a service.* Increasingly we can expect CDS and workflow process recommendations to be available from a clinical application in or independent of an EHR system through invocation of an external service, either provided by commercial or public or health care enterprise sources. Such services are available in experimental form, currently, such as the OpenCDS resource [26] for evaluation of clinical rules; and various commercial offerings of infobutton manager-enabled retrieval of context-specific published reference content.

- *New knowledge capabilities.* CDS has had limited penetration over the last several decades, due to lack of ability to share knowledge because of proprietary data models and systems, lack of adoption of standards-based approaches for sharing despite several possible standards, poorly devised CDS that has frustrated users by inappropriate alerts, interruptions of workflow, or poor user interface, and other issues. The primary forms of knowledge have been rules for alerts and reminders, order sets for various clinical indications, documentation templates for organizing the capture of key information or the production of focused outputs, and infobuttons, to deliver context-specific information. Each of these methods has considerable room for improvement over the next decade. In addition, we can expect advances in cognitive models for presentation, visualization, and manipulation of complex data; increased use of natural language processing (NLP) to extract data from clinical narrative content for use in CDS; use of big data analytics directly to compare a particular patient being evaluated to similar patients, e.g., in terms of expected response to a particular therapy or comparison of alternative therapies; advanced knowledge tools such as IBM's Watson and others that can obtain data from multiple sources and reason with them to answer specific queries; and other approaches that will likely emerge.

18.2.6 Patient Data Security and Privacy

Enacted on August 21, 1996, the Health Insurance Portability and Accountability Act of 1996 (HIPAA), Public Law 104–191, requires the Secretary of Health and Human Services (HHS) to publicize standards for the electronic exchange, privacy, and security of health information. As enacted, it required the Secretary to issue privacy regulations governing individually identifiable health information, if Congress did not enact privacy legislation within 3 years of the passage of HIPAA. Because Congress did not do so, HHS developed a proposed rule and released it for public comment on November 3, 1999. The Department received over 52,000 public comments. The final regulation, the Privacy Rule, was published December 28, 2000. In March 2002, the Department proposed and released for public comment modifications to the Privacy Rule. The Department received over 11,000 comments. The final modifications were published in final form on August 14, 2002. A text combining the final regulation and the modifications can be found at 45 CFR Part 160 and Part 164, Subparts A and E.

Against this backdrop, it is nevertheless hoped that in the next decade a national patient identifier will be adopted to facilitate the transfer of a patient's data, and yet protect the security and confidentiality of the patient's data. With the evolution of the automated generation of the summaries of computer-based patient records, and electronic claims reporting as a byproduct of patient care transactions, and data from a patient's records of different services received from a variety of separate health care providers in different medical facilities, the need developed for the patient's data to be linked by a common patient identification number. In the past, each health care provider assigned to each patient a medical record number that was unique for that provider's patient database.

It would be ideal to give every person a unique health record identification (ID) number for nationwide use that would *not* be the same as the Social Security number; since if pragmatists and economists were to prevail in using the Social Security numbers for patients' health records, it would still be a problem to fully protect the confidentiality of each patient's medical information.

Matching algorithms based on patient demographic characteristics can be highly accurate, but still have errors. Also, they are cumbersome to use when one is trying to create a large-scale database, say for genomic-phenomic correlation, for population health, or for other research purposes, especially where data on individual patients' health status needs to be analyzed over time. For such purposes, either an actual unique ID or generation of a consistent pseudo-ID is needed to achieve linkage of data from multiple sources and episodes of care.

Researchers recognized early that it was necessary to place restrictions on the research use of medical databases to protect the identity of the patients and to preserve the confidentiality of the data without interfering unduly with the enhancement of analytic power inherent in computer technology [24]. Lindberg [21] wrote that in the 1970s the increased number of collaborative studies using networked medical computer systems created a definite problem for protecting patient confidentiality. In the 1980s the increasing mobility of patients across state lines, and the emergence of multistate health care providers resulted in a need for uniform regulations in all states governing the use and disclosure of health care information. In recognition of this problem, the Uniform Healthcare Information Act was drafted in 1985 and was recommended for enactment in all states [7]. By the end of the 1980s, the usual forms of data protection included frequent changes of assigned codes or passwords to medical information system users that authorized access to patient data from certain terminals; yet the highest risk to system security at that time continued to be from unauthorized access by telephone terminals into computer networks.

The databases themselves can be encrypted to a high degree. Cryptography can transform messages into forms that render them unintelligible to unauthorized persons. When one considers that every cryptography security program ever invented has been broken, including the German and the Japanese wartime cryptography programs, it is realistic to accept that this problem will never be solved and must be continually challenged.

Data security also involves the protection of data from unauthorized alteration, and from accidental or intentional disclosure to unauthorized persons. Data security is dependent on adequate system security to protect the system from unauthorized access. *System security* includes protection from risks such as illegal access to computer rooms or to computer databases, illicit use of data communications by hackers, or illegal modification of programs. This is clearly a national/international issue of growing concern as a number of episodes in the early 2010s have shown. It can be expected that this will continue to be an area of active advance by system developers and security experts, but as experience has shown, this is typically like an arms race, with advances by systems developers countered by advances by hackers, and then by the systems developers, etc.

The goal of having a unique identifier to facilitate record linkage for individual care and the construction of large population databases – for population health, biosurveillance, quality and outcomes measurement, and research – is fraught with politics, fueled by the recognition that even the most "secure" systems can be hacked. Thus one must be sanguine about the expectations for progress in this area. The best hope is to ensure that health data systems continually have the maximum levels of security available, and that policy and regulations define sufficiently suitable and enforceable rules for role-based authorization and access to data to establish sufficient public confidence.

18.2.7 *Communications in Catastrophic Disasters*

In 2010 Stroud observed that during a wide-reaching catastrophic public health emergency or disaster, the existing surge capacity plans may not be sufficient to enable health care providers to continue to adhere to normal treatment procedures and to follow usual standards of care [32]. Global climate changes are expected to produce periodic disasters that will require maintaining essential communications under extreme adverse conditions of crisis. This is a particular concern for emergencies that may severely strain resources across a large geographic area, such as a pandemic influenza or, as seen in 2014, a large-scale Ebola virus outbreak (largely confined to western Africa), or the detonation of a nuclear device. Under these circumstances, it may be impossible to provide care according to the standards of care used in non-disaster situations, and, under the most extreme circumstances, it may not even be possible to provide basic life.

Wireless networks are evolving that do not depend on a fixed communications infrastructure; and can allow for ubiquitous connectivity regardless of the environment and the situation. In disaster events where power shortages can interrupt standard line and mobile phone communications, the development of specially programmed mobile phones or other wireless communication devices within range of one another can each act as both transmitter and receiver in an ad-hoc network, and pass information from device to device to form a web of connections. The networks need to be so designed and constructed that even when one or more devices fails, a message can still get through, such as by sending the message along several paths and thereby increasing the likelihood that the message will be received [11].

We also need to have comprehensive cloud-based repositories and redundancy that permit access to data despite disruptions in local resources. This touches on sections above on cloud computing, big data, and security and privacy.

18.2.8   Health Information Systems Architecture

Our current health information systems are still saddled with legacy assumptions and architectures that make it difficult to respond to some of the priorities of the current and future decades – such as coordination of care across multiple venues, telecare/connected care harnessing patient-controlled and patient-generated data, a focus on wellness, prevention of disease, and early and aggressive management of disease outside of the hospital, and the harnessing of big data for population health, research, and other social benefits. The current systems are silos and largely proprietary. The initiative known as the Health Information Exchange (IHE) helps with the transfer of care summary documents and messages, and provides connections "around the edges". But we are still far away from having an integrated longitudinal health and health care record for individuals, and from a fully integrated system of care delivery.

Impetus for change may well come from reimbursement practices for health care services such as pay-for-value rather than fee-for-service and payment for telecare-based consultation; it may come from the increasing embrace of personal health records by consumers driven by advances in personal sensors, wearables, and apps; or from increased confidence in privacy and security fostering more aggregation and sharing of data where appropriate.

On the technical side, there is advancement in opening up access to EHRs through standard application program interfaces (APIs) delivered through web-based service-oriented architectures (SOAs), common data models and terminology servers to translate EHR-specific data elements into standard data representations, master patient index identity services, role-based authorization and access services, CDS services, and other capabilities. This begins to enable the evolution of three-tiered architectures in which applications (both mobile and desktop) can be built as a top layer, interacting only with the middle-tier services, that in turn interact with the lower tier data sources such as EHR system. This enables apps to be independent of underlying systems, interoperable, and able to access data from a variety of data sources. Thus these new apps can begin to address some of the priorities for health and health care that traditional legacy-based systems with their silos and proprietary boundaries cannot.

The extent to which this occurs will depend on standards development and acceptance, health care organizations and purchasers demanding service oriented architecture-based interfaces for important services, vendors finding business value or need to comply with such demands, and evolution of an ecosystem where businesses based on this model can thrive.

18.3 Conclusion: Looking Back, Looking Forward

We can say that the progress over the past six decades, although slow and difficult, has finally established the value and in fact necessity of health information systems. The discipline of medical informatics, now more ubiquitously referred to as clinical or health informatics, has evolved to be part of a broader field known as biomedical informatics, which also embraces bioinformatics, focused on the "omics" field and its translation to practice, imaging informatics, focusing on tissue and organ system data and knowledge, typically embedded in imaging and sensor technologies, and population/public health informatics dealing with large-scale and aggregate health data.

As this book is published in the mid-2010s, it is also positioned at what may be regarded as an inflection point. At this point we are seeing increased recognition of the role of health care in the larger health of the individual and the population and the need to integrate and interact with other components of the health system, changing priorities, and greatly expanded technological capabilities. These factors are all converging to open up the potential of the field to what can be expected to be exponential growth in the next decade and beyond.

With admiration for all the pioneers of the field over the past six decades, who have laid the groundwork for an essential part of our lives, this work has reached the stage where it is now a major part of the economy, provides career paths for a rapidly growing workforce, and represents a major opportunity to continue to innovate and create systems and methods for better health and for the advances in knowledge to support it.

References

1. Ball MJ, Jacobs SE. Hospital information systems as we enter the decade of the 80's. Proc Annu Symp Comput Appl Med Care. 1980;1:646.
2. Ball MJ, Hammon GL. Maybe a network of mini-computers can fill your data systems needs. Hosp Financ Manag. 1975;29:48.
3. Ball MJ. Computers-prescription for hospital ills. Datamation. 1975;21:50–1.
4. Barret V. Best small companies. Forbes. 2011;188:82–92.
5. Blum BI, Lenhard Jr RE, McColligan EE. An integrated data model for patient care. IEEE Trans Biomed Eng. 1985;32:277–88.

6. Bronzino JD. In: Bronzino JD, editor. Computers and patient care. Saint Louis: C.V. Mosby; 1977. p. 57–102.
7. Burnett KK, Battle H, Cant GD. Uniform Health-Care Information Act. Chicago: National Conference of Commissioners on Uniform State Laws; 1985.
8. Cardiff Publishing. Fifth annual market directory of computers in healthcare. Englewood: Cardiff Pub. Co; 1988.
9. Collen MF. A history of medical informatics in the United States, 1950 to 1990. Indianapolis: American Medical Informatics Association; 1995.
10. Dorenfest SI. The decade of the 1980's: large expenditures produce limited progress in hospital automation. US Healthc. 1989;6:20–2.
11. Effros M, Goldsmith A, Medard M. Wireless networks. Sci Am. 2010;302:73–7.
12. Friedman C, Hripcsak G, Johnson SB, Cimino JJ, Clayton PD. A generalized relational schema for an integrated clinical patient database. Proc SCAMC. 1990; 335–339.
13. Greenes RA, Pappalardo AN, Marble CW, Barnett GO. Design and implementation of a clinical data management system. Comput Biomed Res. 1969;2:469–85.
14. Greenes RA, Shortliffe EH. Medical informatics. An emerging academic discipline and institutional priority. JAMA. 1990;263:1114–20.
15. Herner & Co. The use of computers in hospitals: Report III-Survey analysis; Report IV-Descriptions of computer applications. Bethesda: National Center for Health Services Research; 1968.
16. Hoffman T. The 6th annual medical hardware and software buyers guide. MD Comput. 1989;6:334–77.
17. King LS. The automobile makes an impact. JAMA. 1984;251:2352–5.
18. Lacey R. Ford, the men and the machine. Boston: Little, Brown; 1986.
19. Ledley RS. A personal view of sowing the seeds. In: Blum BI, Duncan KA, editors. History of medical informatics. New York: ACM Press; 1990. p. 84–110.
20. Lev-Ram M. Intel's sunny vision for the cloud. Fortune. 2011;164:95–100.
21. Lindberg D. Special aspects of medical computer records with respect to data privacy. In: Williams B, editor. Proc 2nd Illinois Conf Med Inform Syst, University of Illinois Urbana. Pittsburgh: Instrument Society of America; 1975. pp. 35–38.
22. Maturi VF, DuBois RM. Recent trends in computerized medical information systems for hospital departments. Proc SCAMC. 1980;3:1541–9.
23. McDonald CJ, Tierney WM. Computer-stored medical records: their future role in medical practice. JAMA. 1988;259:3433–40.
24. Miller RF. Computers and privacy: what price analytic power? Proc Annu Conf ACM. New York: ACM. 1971; 706–716.
25. Newald J. Hospitals look to computerization of physician office linkage. Hospitals. 1987;61:92–4.
26. Open CDS. Open clinical decision support tools and resources. http://www.opencds.org/, 10 Jan 2015.
27. Polacsek RA. The fourth annual medical software buyer's guide. MD Comput. 1987;4:23.
28. Reiser SJ, Anbar M. The machine at the bedside: strategies for using technology in patient care. New York: Cambridge University Press; 1984.
29. Schiff GD, Rucker TD. Computerized prescribing: building the electronic infrastructure for better medication usage. JAMA. 1998;279:1024–9.
30. Spencer WA. An opinion survey of computer applications in 149 hospitals in the USA, Europe and Japan. Inform Health Soc Care. 1976;1:215–34.
31. Starr P. The social transformation of American medicine. New York: Basic Books; 1982.
32. Stroud C, Altevogt BM, Lori Nadig L, Hougan M. Forum on medical and public health preparedness for catastrophic events; Institute of Medicine. Washington, DC: National Academies Press; 2010.
33. The Economist. Tanks in the cloud. De Economist. 2011;402:49–50.
34. Young EM, Brian EW, Hardy DR, Kaplan A, Childerston JK. Evaluation of automated hospital data management systems (AHDMS). Proc SCAMC. 1980;1:651–7.

Proceedings of Major Professional Meetings

Proc AAMSI Conf 1982. Proceedings of the First Annual Conference, American Association for Medical Systems & Informatics, Bethesda, MD: AAMSI, 1982.

Proc AAMSI Conf 1983. Proceedings of the Second Annual Conference, American Association for Medical Systems & Informatics, Bethesda, MD: AAMSI, 1983.

Proc AAMSI 1983. Proceedings of the AAMSI Congress on Medical Informatics, AAMSI Cong 83 Lindberg DAB, Van Brunt EE, Jenkins MA (eds). Bethesda, MD: AAMSI, 1983.

Proc AAMSI 1984. Proceedings of the Congress on Medical Informatics, AAMSI Congress 84. Lindberg DAB, Colleen MF (eds). Bethesda, MD: AAMSI, 1984.

Proc AAMSI 1985. Proceedings of the Congress on Medical Informatics, AAMSI Congress 85. Levy AH, Williams BT (eds). Washington, DC: AAMSI, 1985.

Proc AAMSI 1986. Proceedings of the Congress on Medical Informatics, AAMSI Congress 86. Levy AH, Williams BT (eds). Washington, DC: AAMSI, 1986.

Proc AAMSI 1987. Proceedings of the Congress on Medical Informatics, AAMSI Congress 87. Levy AH, Williams BT (eds). Washington, DC: AAMSI, 1987.

Proc AAMSI 1988. Proceedings of the Congress on Medical Informatics, AAMSI Congress 88. Hammond WE (ed). Washington, DC: AAMSI, 1988.

Proc AAMSI 1989. Proceedings of the Congress on Medical Informatics, AAMSI Congress 89. Hammond WE (ed). Washington, DC: AAMSI, 1989.

Proc AMIA 1982. Proceedings of the First AMIA Congress on Medical Informatics, AMIA Congress 82. Lindberg DAB, Collen MF, Van Brunt EE (eds) New York: Masson, 1982.

Proc AMIA 1994. Proceedings of the Eighteenth Annual Symposium on Computer Applications in Medical Care. Ozbolt JG (ed). JAMIA Symposium Supplement. Philadelphia: Hanley & Belfast, Inc., 1994.

Proc AMIA 1995. Proceedings of the Nineteenth Annual Symposium on Computer Applications in Medical Care. Gardener RM (ed). JAMIA Symposium Supplement. Philadelphia: Hanley & Belfast, Inc., 1995.

Proc AMIA 1996. Proceedings of the 1996 AMIA Annual Fall Symposium. Cimino JJ (ed). JAMIA Symposium Supplement. Philadelphia: Hanley & Belfast, Inc., 1996.

Proc AMIA 1997. Proceedings of the 1997 AMIA Fall Symposium. Masys DR (ed). JAMIA Symposium Supplement. Philadelphia: Hanley & Belfast, Inc., 1997.

Proc AMIA 1998. Proceedings of the 1998 AMIA Fall Symposium. Chute CG (ed). JAMIA Symposium Supplement. Philadelphia: Hanley & Belfast, Inc., 1998.

Proc AMIA 1999. Proceedings of the 1999 AMIA Fall Symposium. Lorenzi NM (ed). JAMIA Symposium Supplement. Philadelphia: Hanley & Belfast, Inc., 1999.

© Springer-Verlag London 2015

M.F. Collen, M.J. Ball (eds.), *The History of Medical Informatics in the United States*, Health Informatics, DOI 10.1007/978-1-4471-6732-7

Proc AMIA 2000. Proceedings of the 2000 AMIA Fall Symposium. Overhage JM (ed). JAMIA Symposium Supplement. Philadelphia: Hanley & Belfast, Inc., 2000.

Proc AMIA 2001. Proceedings of the 2001 AMIA Symposium. Bakken S (ed). JAMIA Symposium Supplement. Philadelphia: Hanley & Belfast, Inc., 2001.

Proc AMIA 2002. Proceedings of the 2002 AMIA Fall Symposium. Kahane IS (ed). JAMIA Symposium Supplement. Philadelphia: Hanley & Belfast, Inc., 2002.

The following proceedings are available at http://knowledge.amia.org/all-proceedings

Proc AMIA Annu Symp 2003. Proceedings of the 2003 AMIA Fall Symposium. Musen M (ed).

Proc AMIA Annu Symp 2004. Proceedings of the 2004 AMIA Fall Symposium. AMIA did not have a symposium that year because it hosted MEDINFO 2004.

Proc AMIA Annu Symp 2005. Proceedings of the 2005 AMIA Fall Symposium. Friedman C (ed).

Proc AMIA Annu Symp 2006. Proceedings of the 2006 AMIA Fall Symposium. Bates D (ed).

Proc AMIA Annu Symp 2007. Proceedings of the 2007 AMIA Fall Symposium. Teich J (ed).

Proc AMIA Annu Symp 2008. Proceedings of the 2008 AMIA Fall Symposium. Suermondt J (ed).

Proc AMIA Annu Symp 2009. Proceedings of the 2009 AMIA Fall Symposium. Ohno-Machado L (ed).

Proc AMIA Annu Symp 2010. Proceedings of the 2010 AMIA Fall Symposium. Kuperman G (ed).

Proc AMIA TBI 2009. Proceedings of the AMIA Summit on Translational Bioinformatics (TBI), Lussier Y (ed).

Proc AMIA TBI 2010. Proceedings of the AMIA Summit on Translational Bioinformatics (TBI), Tarczy-Hornoch P (ed).

Proc AMIA TBI 2011. Proceedings of the AMIA Summit on Translational Bioinformatics (TBI), Sarkar IN (ed.)

Proc AMIA TBI 2012. Proceedings of the AMIA Summit on Translational Bioinformatics (TBI), Shah N (ed).

Proc AMIA TBI 2013. Proceedings of the AMIA Summit on Translational Bioinformatics (TBI), Tenenbaum J (ed).

Proc AMIA TBI 2014. Proceedings of the AMIA Summit on Translational Bioinformatics (TBI), Denny J (ed.)

Proc AMIA CRI 2010. Proceedings of the AMIA Summit on Clinical Research Informatics (CRI), Embi P (ed).

Proc AMIA CRI 2011. Proceedings of the AMIA Summit on Clinical Research Informatics (CRI), Payne P (ed).

Proc AMIA CRI 2012. Proceedings of the AMIA Summit on Clinical Research Informatics (CRI), Kahn M (ed).

Proc AMIA CRI 2013. Proceedings of the AMIA Summit on Clinical Research Informatics (CRI), Bernstam E (ed).

Proc AMIA CRI 2014. Proceedings of the AMIA Summit on Clinical Research Informatics (CRI), Richesson R (ed).

Proc MEDINFO 1974. Proceedings of the First World Conference on Medical Informatics, MEDINFO 74, Stockholm. Anderson J, Forsythe JM (eds). Amsterdam: North-Holland, 1974.

Proc MEDINFO 1977. Proceedings of the Second World Conference on Medical Informatics, MEDINFO 77, Toronto. Shires DB, Wolf H (eds). Amsterdam: North-Holland, 1977.

Proc MEDINFO 1980. Proceedings of the Third World Conference on Medical Informatics, MEDINFO 80, Tokyo. Lindberg DAB, Kaihara S (eds). Amsterdam: North-Holland, 1980.

Proc MEDINFO 1983. Proceedings of the Fourth World Conference on Medical Informatics, MEDINFO 83, Amsterdam. Van Bemmel JH, Ball MJ, Wigertz O (eds). Amsterdam: North Holland, 1983.

Proc MEDINFO 1986. Proceedings of the Fifth World Conference on Medical Informatics, MEDINFO 86, Washington. Salamon R, Blum BI, Jorgenson M (eds). Amsterdam: North-Holland Pub Co., 1986.

Proc MEDINFO 1989. Proceedings of the Sixth World Conference on Medical Informatics, MEDINFO 89, Beijing. Barber B, Cao D, Qin D, Wagner G (eds). Amsterdam: North-Holland, 1989.

Proc MEDINFO 1992. Proceedings of the Seventh World Congress on Medical Informatics, MEDINFO 92, Geneva. Lun KC, Degoulet P, Piemme TE, Rienhoff O (eds). Amsterdam: North-Holland, 1992.

Proc MEDINFO 1995. Proceedings of the Eighth World Congress on Medical Informatics, MEDINFO 95, Vancouver, BC. Greenes RA, Peterson HE, Protti DJ (eds). Amsterdam: North-Holland, 1995.

Proc MEDINFO 1998. Proceedings of the Ninth World Congress on Medical Informatics, MEDINFO 98, Seoul, Korea. Cesnik B, McCray, AT, Scherrer JR (eds). Amsterdam: IOS Press, 1998.

Proc MEDINFO 2001. Proceedings of the Tenth World Congress on Medical Informatics, MEDINFO 2001, London, England. Patel VL, Rogers R, Haux H (eds). Amsterdam: IOS Press, 2001.

Proc MEDINFO 2004. Proceedings of the Eleventh World Congress on Medical Informatics, MEDINFO 2004, San Francisco, California, USA. Fieschi M, Coiera E, Li Y-C J (eds). Amsterdam: IOS Press, 2004.

Proc MEDINFO 2007. Proceedings of the Twelfth World Congress on Medical Informatics, MEDINFO 2007, Brisbane, Australia. Kuhn KA, Warren JR, Leong T-Y (eds). Amsterdam: IOS Press, 2007.

Proc MEDINFO 2010. Proceedings of the Thirteenth World Congress on Medical Informatics, MEDINFO 2010, Capetown, South Africa. Safran C, Reti S, Marin HF (eds). Amsterdam: IOS Press, 2010.

Proc MEDINFO 2013. Proceedings of the Fourteenth World Congress on Medical Informatics, MEDINFO 2013, Copenhagen, Denmark. Lehman CU, Ammenwerth E, Nøhr C (eds). Amsterdam: IOS Press, 2013.

Proc SAMS 1973. Proceedings of the Society for Advanced Medical Systems. Colleen MF (ed). San Francisco: ORSA, 1973.

Proc SCAMC 1977. Proceedings of the First Annual Symposium on Computer Applications in Medical Care. Orthner FH, Hayman H (eds). New York: IEEE 1977.

Proc SCAMC 1978. Proceedings of the Second Annual Symposium on Computer Applications in Medical Care. Dunn RA, Orthner FH (eds). Silver Springs, MD: IEEE Computer Society Press, 1978.

Proc SCAMC 1979. Proceedings of the Third Annual Symposium on Computer Applications in Medical Care. Dunn RA (ed). New York: IEEE, 1979.

Proc SCAMC 1980. Proceedings of the Fourth Annual Symposium on Computer Applications in Medical Care. O'Neill JT (ed). New York: IEEE, 1980.

Proc SCAMC 1981. Proceedings of the Fifth Annual Symposium on Computer Applications in Medical Care. Hefferman HG (ed). New York: IEEE, 1981.

Proc SCAMC 1982. Proceedings of the Sixth Annual Symposium on Computer Applications in Medical Care. Blum BI (ed). New York: IEEE, 1982.

Proc SCAMC 1983. Proceedings of the Seventh Annual Symposium on Computer Applications in Medical Care. Dayhoff RE (ed). New York: IEEE, 1983.

Proc SCAMC 1984. Proceedings of the Eighth Annual Symposium on Computer Applications in Medical Care. Cohen GS (ed). New York: IEEE, 1984.

Proc SCAMC 1985. Proceedings of the Ninth Annual Symposium on Computer Applications in Medical Care. Ackerman MJ (ed). New York: IEEE, 1985.

Proc SCAMC 1986. Proceedings of the Tenth Annual Symposium on Computer Applications in Medical Care. Orthner HF (ed). New York: IEEE, 1986.

Proc SCAMC 1987. Proceedings of the Eleventh Annual Symposium on Computer Applications in Medical Care. Stead WW (ed). New York: IEEE, 1987.

Proc SCAMC 1988. Proceedings of the Twelfth Annual Symposium on Computer Applications in Medical Care. Greenes RA (ed). New York: IEEE, 1988.

Proc SCAMC 1989. Proceedings of the Thirteenth Annual Symposium on Computer Applications in Medical Care. Kingsland L (ed). New York: IEEE, 1989.

Proc SCAMC 1990. Proceedings of the Fourteenth Annual Symposium on Computer Applications in Medical Care. Miller RA (ed). Los Alamitos, CA: IEEE, 1990.

Proc SCAMC 1991. Proceedings of the Fifteenth Annual Symposium on Computer Applications in Medical Care. Clayton PD (ed). New York: McGraw-Hill, Inc., 1991.

Proc SCAMC 1992. Proceedings of the Sixteenth Annual Symposium on Computer Applications in Medical Care. Frisse ME (ed). New York: McGraw-Hill, Inc., 1992.

Proc SCAMC 1993. Proceedings of the Seventeenth Annual Symposium on Computer Applications in Medical Care. Safran C (ed). New York: McGraw-Hill., 1993.

Index

© Springer-Verlag London 2015　　　　　　　　　　　　　　　　　753
M.F. Collen, M.J. Ball (eds.), *The History of Medical Informatics*
in the United States, Health Informatics, DOI 10.1007/978-1-4471-6732-7

Printed in the United States
By Bookmasters